T0345097

Mental Health Practice

for the

Occupational Therapy Assistant

Mental Health Practice
for the
Occupational Therapy Assistant

Christine A. Manville, EdD, OTR/L
Associate Professor and Residency Coordinator
Belmont University
Nashville, Tennessee

Jeremy L. Keough, MSOT, OTR/L
Staff Occupational Therapist
Blount Memorial Hospital
Maryville, Tennessee

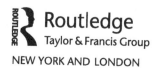

Routledge
Taylor & Francis Group

NEW YORK AND LONDON

Mental Health Practice for the Occupational Therapy Assistant includes ancillary materials specifically available for faculty use. Included are Test Bank Questions, Student Study Guides, and PowerPoint slides. Please visit www.routledge.com/9781617112508 to obtain access.

First published 2016 by SLACK Incorporated

Published 2024 by Routledge
605 Third Avenue, New York, NY 10158

and by Routledge
4 Park Square, Milton Park, Abingdon, Oxon OX14 4RN

Routledge is an imprint of the Taylor & Francis Group, an informa business

Library of Congress Cataloging-in-Publication Data

Mental health practice for the occupational therapy assistant / [edited by] Christine A. Manville, Jeremy L. Keough.
      p. ; cm.
  Includes bibliographical references and index.
  ISBN 978-1-61711-250-8 (alk. paper)
  I. Manville, Christine A., 1957- , editor. II. Keough, Jeremy L., editor.
  [DNLM: 1. Mental Health Services. 2. Occupational Therapy--psychology. 3. Allied Health Personnel. 4. Mental Disorders--therapy. 5. Occupational Therapy--methods. 6. Professional-Patient Relations. WM 450.5.O2]
  RM735.3
  615.8'515--dc23
                        2015034408

ISBN: 9781617112508 (hbk)
ISBN: 9781003525073 (ebk)

DOI: 10.4324/9781003525073

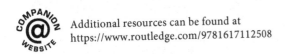

Additional resources can be found at
https://www.routledge.com/9781617112508

DEDICATION

To Linda Anderson from the University of Wisconsin Madison for her instruction regarding the practice area of mental health and her inspiration to work with individuals who have been diagnosed with mental illness; and to my clients and colleagues who continue to teach me about mental illness and recovery.

Christine A. Manville, EdD, OTR/L

To Belmont University for their support as a student and continued professional support and to all those who assisted in the creation of this textbook.

Jeremy L. Keough, MSOT, OTR/L

CONTENTS

Mental Health Practice for the Occupational Therapy Assistant includes ancillary materials specifically for faculty use. Included are Test Bank Questions, Student Study Guides, and PowerPoint slides. Please visit www.routledge.com/9781617112508 to obtain access.

ACKNOWLEDGMENTS

I would like to thank Christine Manville for her tireless effort, mentorship, and leadership that has enabled this excellent book to become a reality and create a positive impact on mental health practice in occupational therapy.

Jeremy L. Keough, MSOT, OTR/L

ABOUT THE AUTHORS

Christine A. Manville, EdD, OTR/L, is an Associate Professor of Occupational Therapy and the OTD Residency Coordinator at Belmont University in Nashville, Tennessee. Her research interests include adults, adolescents, and children diagnosed with mental illness; teenagers at risk for failure in the public school system; teaching and learning in secondary and postsecondary education; and professional development. Dr. Manville earned her undergraduate degree in occupational therapy from the University of Wisconsin, Madison, and her doctoral degree in educational leadership from Johnson and Wales University in Providence, Rhode Island. Her professional experience includes 34 years working in the practice area of mental health. Dr. Manville held the position of pioneer Program Director for the Occupational Therapy Assistant Program at the Community College of Rhode Island from 1997 to 2006 and has been employed at Belmont University since 2007.

Jeremy L. Keough, MSOT, OTR/L, is currently a staff occupational therapist for Blount Memorial Hospital in Maryville, Tennessee. Jeremy earned his undergraduate degree in occupational therapy from Eastern Kentucky University in Richmond, Kentucky and a post-professional master's degree from Belmont University in Nashville, Tennessee. His professional experiences include long-term care, inpatient rehabilitation, outpatient rehabilitation, work hardening, acute care, and occupational therapy assistant education. Jeremy served as the Occupational Therapy Assistant Program Director at Roane State Community College in Oak Ridge, Tennessee and instructed students in mental health coursework and in a nontraditional level-II fieldwork setting. Currently, Jeremy's interests include neurorehabilitation approaches, occupation-based practice, and promoting occupational therapy.

CONTRIBUTING AUTHORS

Lori T. Andersen, EdD, OTR/L, FAOTA (Chapter 1)
Retired Associate Professor
Department of Occupational Therapy & Community Health
Florida Gulf Coast University
Fort Myers, Florida

Susan S. Bazyk, PhD, OTR/L, FAOTA (Chapter 3)
Professor, Occupational Therapy
School of Health Sciences
Cleveland State University
Project Director
Every Moment Counts: Promoting Mental Health
Cleveland, Ohio

Lea C. Brandt, OTD, MA, OTR/L (Appendix C)
Co-director, MU Center for Health Ethics
MHPC OTA Program Director
Associate Professor
University of Missouri
Columbia, Missouri

Tina Champagne, OTD, OTR/L (Chapter 4, 5)
Champagne Conferences & Consultation
Cutchins Programs for Children and Families
Northampton, Massachusetts

Lee Ann Fallett, MA, CRC, OTR/L (Chapter 6)
Board of Directors
Keystone House, Inc.
Norwalk, Connecticut

Cathy H. Ficzere, PharmD, BCPS (Appendix B)
Associate Professor of Pharmacy Practice
Belmont University College of Pharmacy
Nashville, Tennessee

Yvette Hachtel, JD, MEd, OTR/L (Appendix C)
Professor, School of Occupational Therapy
Belmont University
Nashville, Tennessee

J. Michael McGuire, PharmD, BCPP (Appendix B)
Assistant Professor of Pharmacy Practice
Belmont University College of Pharmacy
Nashville, Tennessee

Janice Ryan, OTD, OTR/L (Chapter 10, 11)
Certified Human Systems Dynamics Professional
Human Systems Occupational Therapy
Chattanooga, Tennessee

Renee R. Taylor, PhD (Chapter 12)
Professor
Director, Model of Human Occupation Clearinghouse
Department of Occupational Therapy
University of Illinois at Chicago
Chicago, Illinois

Su Ren Wong, BOccThy, OTR/L (Chapter 12)
Department of Occupational Therapy
University of Illinois at Chicago
Chicago, Illinois

Preface

Mental Health Practice for the Occupational Therapy Assistant illustrates an integrated approach to learning for the occupational therapy assistant. It addresses the development of knowledge, skills, and competencies needed by the entry-level occupational therapy assistant to effectively address the psychosocial, emotional, behavioral, and mental health needs of clients. The information and treatment applications presented can be applied within multiple practice settings and environments. Specific aspects that are highlighted in this book include incorporation of the *Occupational Therapy Practice Framework, 3rd edition* (OTPF), the use of organization and structure to enhance learning, and provision of instructor/student resources to reinforce the learning experience.

This text expands upon the basic foundation of occupational therapy mental health practice. The OTPF is infused throughout the text to fully present and describe provision of occupational therapy mental health services. It is also used as a guide to define the scope of practice of the occupational therapy assistant in the area of mental health. The impact of mental illness on the client's ability to participate in significant occupations throughout the lifespan is examined using a developmental lens. The text addresses the provision of occupational therapy services in a wide variety of settings. Students learn how to identify the occupational environment and, under the supervision of the occupational therapist, evaluate a client's participation in occupation. They also learn how to collaborate with the occupational therapist to create and implement treatment plans that include one-on-one intervention and the use of therapeutic groups. Information on the design of therapeutic groups, development of leadership skills, and the implementation of group process is also incorporated in this text.

The structure and presentation of information are designed to enhance learning for the occupational therapy assistant student. Bloom's taxonomy was used to guide the organization of information throughout the text. *The Diagnostic and Statistical Manual V* (DSM) and *International Classification of Functioning* (ICF) are described as systems that create a common language between occupational therapy practitioners and other health care providers.

Instructor and student resources provide an enhanced learning opportunity for students. Test questions, PowerPoint slides, student study guides, and learning activities are included to supplement the text. The book includes appendices on the topics of pharmacology and ethical and legal issues, website resources, and epilogues of case studies. These appendices are included to augment and reinforce the understanding of occupational therapy services and the efficacy of treatment.

In conclusion, occupational therapy services for the treatment of psychosocial, emotional, behavioral, and mental health needs of clients are evolving and emerging. We have created a textbook that will aid students to develop the knowledge, skills, and confidence required by the entry-level occupational therapy assistant to effectively provide mental health services in a variety of settings. Focus is placed on client-based services, population- and community-based services, and traditional occupational therapy services as appropriate for the occupational therapy assistant.

Christine A. Manville, EdD, OTR/L and Jeremy L. Keough, MSOT, OTR/L

Unique Features of This Text

- Specific thought was applied to incorporate the principles of Bloom's taxonomy throughout this text to aid the learning process
- Teacher resources include PowerPoint slides, student study sheets, test questions, and application questions for each chapter
- Mental health practice is viewed through a developmental lens to ensure that occupational performance throughout the lifespan is addressed
- Current practice trends in community-based occupational therapy are described
- The text incorporates the *Occupational Therapy Practice Framework, 3rd edition* to enhance student learning.
- Written specifically for the occupational therapy assistant
- Provides information students will need to know to work effectively with clients on a one-on-one basis, as well as in groups
- Includes the most current information on mental health occupational therapy assistant practice

Scope of Practice in Mental Health Occupational Therapy

Lori T. Andersen, EdD, OTR/L, FAOTA and Jeremy L. Keough, MSOT, OTR/L

KEY TERMS

- Affordable Care Act
- Arts and Crafts Movement
- Asylums
- Biopsychosocial
- CMHP/QMHP
- Community Mental Health Act

- Deinstitutionalization
- Early Occupations
- Founding Members
- Habit Training
- Institutionalization
- Medical Model

- Moral Treatment
- President's New Freedom Commission
- Psychobiology Model
- Recovery Model
- Transinstitutionalization

CHAPTER LEARNING OBJECTIVES

After completion of this chapter, students should be able to:

1. Recognize the significance of the history of occupational therapy on the current role of occupational therapy practitioners in mental health practice.

2. Discuss cultural, legislative, and financial influences that affect mental health care in the United States.

3. Explain the shift toward community-based practice in mental health care.

4. Classify models of practice currently used in mental health occupational therapy services.

5. Examine how the Recovery Model incorporates key aspects of the philosophy of occupational therapy.

Manville, C.A., & Keough, J. L.
Mental Health Practice for the Occupational Therapy Assistant (pp 1-24).
© 2016 Taylor & Francis Group.

CHAPTER OUTLINE

INTRODUCTION

National Society for the Promotion of Occupational Therapy (NSPOT) Founding Vision, 1917:

The particular objects for which this corporation is formed are as follows: The advancement of occupation as a therapeutic measure; for the study of the effect of occupation upon the human being; and for the scientific dispensation of this knowledge.

American Occupational Therapy Association (AOTA) Centennial Vision, 2017

By the year 2017, we envision that occupational therapy is a powerful, widely recognized, science-driven, and evidence-based profession with a globally connected and diverse workforce meeting society's occupational needs.

The formal origin of the profession of occupational therapy dates back to its founders and the initial proponents of the profession. In the very early part of the 20th century, a number of people were using occupation as a therapeutic measure to treat mental and physical impairments. Each of these individuals brought to the table a set of different experiences, skills, values, and beliefs that shaped and influenced the development of the field. They included, among others, social reformers who were involved in significant events in history, including the mental hygiene movement, arts and crafts movement, progressive era reform, women's rights movement, settlement movement, and educational reform (Quiroga, 1995).

The founding members of the profession shared the belief that meaningful work and occupation facilitate the restoration of health. Their common interest in the healing power of occupation resulted in the development of a new profession that they named *occupational therapy*. These individuals corresponded with one another to share their ideas and establish a scientific basis for the use of occupation as a healing agent. In particular, George E. Barton and William Rush Dunton, Jr. focused on the task of organizing a meeting at which to discuss the creation of a formal association to promote the therapeutic use of occupation (Quiroga, 1995). Due to the slow speed of correspondence at that time in history, however, it took more than two years to arrange that first meeting.

The inaugural meeting of the NSPOT met March 15, 1917, in Clifton Springs, New York. Eleanor Clark Slagle, George E. Barton, William Rush Dunton, Jr., Thomas B. Kidner, Susan Cox Johnson, and Isabel G. Newton attended this meeting. Although Herbert J. Hall and Susan E. Tracy could not attend, they are also considered early proponents of the profession. The NSPOT would later become known as the AOTA in 1921.

Although this chapter primarily focuses on the history of occupational therapy in mental health practice, it would be irresponsible to neglect the broader context of the history of the profession as a whole. Occupational therapy has its roots in psychiatry; however, the profession developed within a wider context of society and medicine. Numerous sociocultural, political, economic, and technological factors have shaped the profession since its creation and continue to influence development of the field of occupational therapy today.

Figure 1-1 displays the complex interaction of numerous influences as they interact to form what is termed *mental health occupational therapy*. Singularly, a thread may not appear significant; however, each provides a contribution to the substance of mental health occupational therapy services. Some threads have been left blank to represent unidentified influences that have yet to be determined.

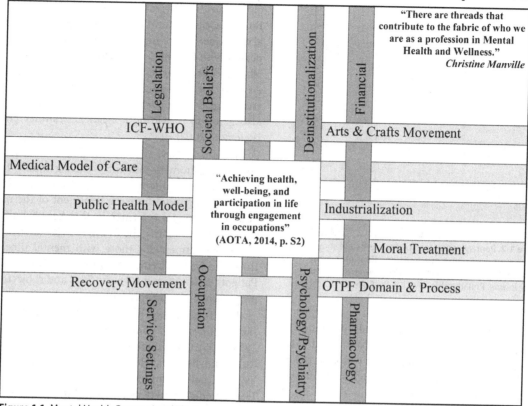

Figure 1-1. Mental Health Occupational Therapy.

These threads/themes are covered in greater detail in subsequent chapters. Discussion of these influences is intended to help the reader understand the profession's past, present, and future direction. As Robert Bing, past president of the AOTA, wrote:

> ... history can tell us that the seeming hardship, the self-doubts of efficacy, the searching for our roots are actually precursors for establishing a new strategic vision and plan that could put us in the forefront of progress. (Bing, 1983, p. 376)

PART 1: EARLY DEVELOPMENT OF OCCUPATIONAL THERAPY

Credo

That occupation is as necessary to life as food and drink.

That every human being should have both physical and mental occupation.

...That sick minds, sick bodies, sick souls, may be healed through occupation.

William Rush Dunton, 1919

Mental Health Care Before the 1900s

Although the profession of occupational therapy was formally incorporated in 1917, the interest in the use of occupation as a therapeutic measure started many centuries before that time. The concept that meaningful work and occupation help to maintain and restore health was first promoted in early history by Galen. Galen was a prominent Roman physician who wrote that "employment is nature's best physician and is essential to human happiness" (Dunton, 1947, p. 1; Haas, 1944, p. 3). Although the use of occupation in early Greek and Roman cultures was recognized as effective in the treatment of mental and physical illness, it was a cure most often reserved for the wealthy (Haas, 1944, p. 6).

In medieval times, mental illness was thought to be caused by disturbances within the humors or body fluids (blood, phlegm, yellow bile, and black bile) and related to a person's religious faith and beliefs. Society thought that

	M.	F.	T.		M.	F.	T.
Ill health of various kinds	100	90	190	Nostalgia	—	1	1
Intemperance	66	5	71	Want of employment	18	1	19
Loss of property, failures, &c.	43	18	61	Mortified pride	2	1	3
Dread of poverty	2	—	2	Celibacy	1	—	1
Disappointed affections	10	9	19	Anxiety for wealth	1	—	1
Intense study	11	1	12	Use of opium	1	4	5
Domestic difficulties	11	26	37	Use of tobacco	3	—	3
Fright	6	10	16	Puerperal state	—	39	39
Grief, loss of friends, &c.	19	37	56	Lactation too long continued	—	3	3
Intense application to business	9	—	9	Uncontrolled passion	2	3	5
Religious excitement	26	24	50	Tight lacing	—	1	1
Political excitement	3	—	3	Injuries of the head	9	3	12
Metaphysical speculations	1	—	1	Masturbation	10	—	10
Want of exercise	3	1	4	Mental anxiety	27	30	57
Engagement in a duel	1	—	1	Exposure to cold	2	—	2
Disappointed expectations	4	4	8	Exposure to direct rays of the sun	11	1	12
				Exposure to intense heat	—	1	1
				Stock speculations	2	—	2
				Unascertained	259	200	459
					663	513	1176

Figure 1-2. Pennsylvania Hospital for the Insane showing the supposed cause of admission. (Reprinted from Kirkbride, T. S. (1847). *Report of the Pennsylvania Hospital for the Insane.* Philadelphia, PA: TK & PG Collins.)

people with mental illness were possessed by demons and were being punished for sins they had committed (Pinel, 1806 trans., p. xxi). Treatment focused on restoring the balance of the humors and body fluids through such interventions as bloodletting and purging.

Individuals suffering from mental illness were perceived to be irrational and a danger to themselves and society. For their own protection and the protection of others, they were confined to poorhouses, madhouses, and prisons. There, they were often subjected to beatings and torture. The image of an unkempt, wild-looking person restrained in shackles and lying on a filthy bed of straw is representative of how society dealt with individuals with mental illness in medieval times.

By the end of the 18th century, society's view of mental illness was changing. Although humoral pathology, or an imbalance of body fluids, was still perceived as a cause of mental illness, people afflicted with mental illness were now thought to be human beings capable of rational thought and not individuals under the influence of demons. Consequently, a belief in rehabilitation of the mentally ill, as promoted by Galen, was rekindled. People with mental illness were admitted to *asylums* for their treatment. Figure 1-2 illustrates the supposed cause for admission to the Pennsylvania Hospital for the Insane in 1847 and preceding years. In the table, "M" represents males, "F" represents females, and "T" represents total.

Moral Treatment

Moral treatment was considered a psychological treatment in contrast to the physical treatment of balancing body humors (Peloquin, 1994). Dr. Philippe Pinel, the superintendent at Bicêtre Asylum in Paris in the late 18th century, was an early supporter of moral treatment. He wrote *Treatise on Insanity*, which discussed historical views

of the causes and treatments of mental illness. In his work, Pinel described Moral Treatment as providing an individual with laborious or interesting occupation and treating that person with kindness and firmness (Pinel, 1806 trans., pp. 38, 48). Pinel incorporated this philosophy into the Bicêtre Asylum by removing the restraints from patients and encouraging their participation in activities. Attention was also given to providing a cleaner, healthier environment (Paterson, 2002).

William, Henry, and Samuel Tuke were also early proponents of moral treatment. When a family friend died in an asylum, William Tuke, a Quaker living in England, advocated for more humane treatment of the mentally ill. Tuke was a social reformer in the Age of Enlightenment who wanted to rectify the living conditions in asylums and improve treatment for those with mental illness. At that time, the typical living conditions in asylums were filthy. Patients were chained with shackles and subjected to whippings, immersion in cold baths, and other types of brutality.

The Tuke family held the firm belief that those with mental illness have some control over their behavior (Tuke, 1813, p. 35). Consequently, in the late 18th century, William Tuke and his son, Henry, founded the York Retreat, an asylum that championed Moral Treatment. Here, traditional medical practices were combined with more humane treatment. The ideals of the Quaker religion greatly influenced the philosophy of York Retreat. The residents were called "friends," just as those in the Quaker religion were known as "friends." The retreat, located on a country estate, was designed to provide a comfortable, peaceful, and healthy environment that encouraged spiritual reflection (Charland, 2007). It was believed that boredom and idleness compromised recovery by allowing the minds of patients to focus on unhealthy, negative thoughts. Therefore, patients were encouraged to participate in meaningful occupations such as exercise, homemaking tasks, arts and crafts, and other leisure activities to occupy their minds with healthy thoughts. Spotlight 1-1 illustrates an account of the York Retreat in 1813 as written by Samuel Tuke.

In 1844, the *American Journal of Insanity*, Volume 1, also published a report on asylums in England. This report might very well have been describing the York Retreat. In particular, the report stated:

Occupation and exercise in the open air is deemed very useful for the insane: they should be employed as much as possible. Spacious yards and pleasure grounds should be provided, and music and dancing and various games may be resorted to with benefit to many cases. In the better conducted Asylums, books are procured and placed at the disposal of patients; the exercise of trades and other in-door employments encouraged—employments is in some cases rewarded; and out-of-door occupation is provided by means of large gardens

---

SPOTLIGHT 1-1. RECALLING YORK RETREAT IN 1813

"In regard to melancholies, conversation on the subject of their despondency, is found to be highly injudicious. The very opposite method is pursued. Every means is taken to seduce the mind from its favourite but unhappy musings, by bodily exercise, walks, conversations, reading, and other innocent recreations. The good effect of exercise, and of variety of object, has been very striking in several instances at this Institution." (Tuke, 1813, p. 96)

"The female patients in the Retreat, are employed, as much as possible, in sewing, knitting, or domestic affairs; and several of the convalescents assist the attendants. Of all the modes by which the patients may be induced to restrain themselves, regular employment is perhaps the most generally efficacious; and those kinds of employment are doubtless to be preferred, both on a moral and physical account, which are accompanied by considerable bodily action; that are most agreeable to the patient, and which are most opposite to the illusions of his disease." (Tuke, 1813, p. 99)

---

or farms, in which patients regularly labor in the proper seasons. (Metropolitan Commissioners in Lunacy, 1844, p. 174)

It must be noted that the staff-to-patient ratio at York Retreat was very high, allowing for more individualized care and attention. Perhaps this may have accounted for the success of the York Retreat in helping people recover from mental illness. Through systematic clinical observation, it was noted that patients who were treated with more humane care and kindness did better and had higher discharge rates compared with patients experiencing traditional medical treatment (Charland, 2007). The York Retreat became a model for treatment of the mentally ill, and soon people from the United States visited the retreat to see the phenomena first hand (Quiroga, 1995, p. 21).

The United States also had several notable individuals in the late 18th century who sought to reform systems and provide more humane treatment for the mentally ill. One of the most famous was Dr. Benjamin Rush of Philadelphia. Considered the "Father of Psychiatry," he was also the superintendent of the Pennsylvania Hospital. Medical knowledge in the United States at the time was similar to Europe. Perceptions had shifted from considering those with mental illness as subhuman, possessed by demons, and incapable of rational thought to the view that mental illness was a disease of the mind to be cured by treatments that focused on body fluid equilibrium.

In his book, *Medical Inquiries and Observations Upon the Diseases of the Mind*, Dr. Rush described the current treatments of that time, including bloodletting, purging the body, withholding food, cold baths, strait waistcoats (straitjackets), and tranquilizing chairs (a type of restraining chair). These treatments were thought to have an effect on body fluids and circulation of blood within the body. Dr. Rush was also proud of the fact that his patients were no longer in chains or punished by whipping. Instead, treatments focused on providing patients with a pleasant environment, fresh air and light, kind yet firm treatment,

and activities such as music and book readings to occupy the mind (Rush, 1812, pp. 174-176, 243). In addition, Dr. Rush recommended using work activities as a treatment for those with mental illness (Dunton, 1947, p. 2).

Another example of the use of moral treatment in the United States was at the early New York State Lunatic Asylum in Utica, New York. Dr. Amariah Brigham, an alienist (early terminology for a psychiatrist), was the first superintendent at New York State Lunatic Asylum when it opened in 1843. This asylum was the first state-run facility in New York. As an advocate of Moral Treatment, Brigham (1847) promoted the following changes:

> …removal of the insane from home and former associations, with respect and kind treatment upon all circumstances, and in most cases manual labor, attendance on religious worship on Sunday, the establishment of regular habits of self-control, diversion of the mind from morbid trains of thought. (p. 1)

In 1844, Dr. Brigham founded and became editor of the *American Journal of Insanity*, which was the precursor to the *American Journal of Psychiatry*. The first issue described the asylum at Utica:

> The State Lunatic Asylum at Utica, when the arrangements authorized by the wise and benevolent foresight of the last Legislature, and which are now in progress, are completed,—will be among the best constructed Institutions for the insane in the world,—capable of accommodating five hundred patients, and enabling them to be divided into twelve distinct classes, or families, for each sex, exclusive of a large chapel, shops, schoolrooms, and hospitals. Attached to the Asylum, is an excellent farm, of above one hundred and forty acres, affording pasturage and hay for the cows and horses that will be necessary, and good land for raising all the vegetables required by the household. The patients, in good weather, perform much

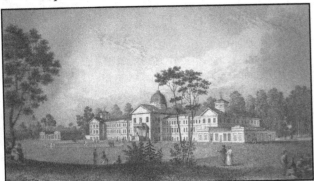

Figure 1-3. Pennsylvania Hospital for the Insane. (Reprinted from Kirkbride, T. S. (1847). *Report of the Pennsylvania Hospital for the Insane.* Philadelphia, PA: TK & PG Collins.)

labor on the farm, and in the garden, by which they are gratified and improved. Some also work in the joiners' shop, some make and repair mattresses, and several work at making and mending shoes. The women make clothing, bedding, and do the ironing, and assist in various household duties. They also manufacture many useful and fancy articles for sale. (Brigham, 1844, pp. 5-6)

Many of these activities mentioned helped to provide for the needs of the institution. These activities promoted the benefit of gainful or profitable employment, as well as labor that helped sustain the institution (Haas, 1944, p. 10).

Another example of humane care could be seen at the early Pennsylvania Hospital for the Insane. Thomas Story Kirkbride became superintendent of Pennsylvania Hospital in 1840. Figure 1-3 illustrates the Pennsylvania Hospital in 1847 when Thomas Kirkbride was employed there. In the 1847 yearly report of the Pennsylvania Hospital, Thomas Kirkbride not only emphasized the number of admissions, but also the number of patients who had recovered as a significant outcome of Moral treatment. As a strong advocate of Moral treatment, he also worked to reform the system. Dr. Kirkbride addressed the duties of teachers or companions, who were perhaps the first occupational therapists (Dunton, 1947, p. 3).

> They will advise the patient in the selection of books, encourage them to engage in the different kinds of employment, suggest means of amusement and occupation, and by their conversation and example do all in their power to promote their happiness, and general harmony, and aid in carrying out the wishes of the physicians. (Kirkbride, 1878, p. 24)

Kirkbride developed the Kirkbride Plan, which promoted the building of asylums on spacious estates and grounds far away from noisy cities. The common design used for facilities was a tall central building with long wings on either side. The floor plans of resident housing allowed for plenty of natural light and fresh air to provide a comfortable, pleasant environment. It was believed that this type of environment helped one to recover from mental illness. Several psychiatric hospitals in the United States were built using this plan and are known as *Kirkbride Hospitals* (Geller & Morrissey, 2004). Many Kirkbride Hospitals are still operating today.

Whereas people of means were being admitted to hospitals with better living conditions and treatment, people with limited income and more severe symptoms of insanity found themselves imprisoned or put into almshouses (poorhouses). As time went on, in an effort to provide them with more humane treatment and improved living conditions, they were placed into asylums. Although well-intentioned, this resulted in overcrowding and a subsequent lack of personal attention, as attendants were not able to work with the volume of patients and involve them in various occupations (Peloquin, 1994). Consequently, the previous level of success that the asylums had reached in helping to facilitate recovery from mental illness declined.

The use of moral treatment and therapeutic occupation continued until the midpoint of the century, circa 1850, and then declined in the United States (Haas, 1944, p. 11). This was partly due to decreased success in facilitating recovery, as well as changes in the economic, political, and social conditions in the country with the approach of the Civil War (Bing, 1981). President Franklin Pierce vetoed the Indigent Insane Bill of 1854, which would have provided grants of land for asylums that would utilize the moral treatment approach (Sharfstein, 2000). This required Dorothea Dix and others to advocate at the state level to meet the needs of those with mental illness.

Socially and culturally, beliefs about the cause of mental illness changed again in the mid-1800s. Medicine now believed that mental illness was caused by brain lesions. Unfortunately, because the use of moral treatment had been linked with the restoration of the balance in body humors, it was concluded that the concept of moral treatment alone would be ineffective. As such moral treatment took a minor role as there was thought to be no cure for mental illness (Peloquin, 1994).

Influences on the Development of Early Occupational Therapy

The latter part of the 19th century was again a time of great social and political change. In part, it was a result of the perceived ills associated with the Industrial Revolution and age of machines and manufacturing. The Industrial Revolution was viewed as both a blessing and a curse, as it improved and decreased the quality of life for many. This period of history included tremendous social, economic, political, and technological change. A number of social and political movements were initiated in reaction to those changes. One of the social reform movements resulted in the development of settlement houses, a concept that originated in England and soon spread to the United States. Settlement houses were usually run by wealthy young men and women with an interest in social and political reform. In the United States, these facilities helped immigrants to adjust to their new country, advocated for the development of child labor laws, and improved care for the mentally ill. The most famous settlement house in the United States was Hull House in Chicago run by Jane Addams (Quiroga, 1995, p. 37). Figure 1-4 illustrates what Hull House looked like in 1925.

One movement that began in reaction to the ills of industrialization and mass production was the ***Arts and Crafts Movement***. Proponents of the Arts and Crafts Movement believed industrialization would be the downfall of civilization, with a decline in standards and moral values associated with an increased emphasis on materialism. Although mass production made it possible for more people to afford products, especially those in the lower class, items created through mass production were considered to be of poor quality. A major promoter of the movement was William Morris, a British social reformer who advocated that society place increased value on hard work and quality products over materialism (Schemm, 1994). Morris embraced a socialist view critical of societal problems caused by the Industrial Revolution such as poor working conditions.

In the United States, people embraced the Arts and Crafts Movement, but not because of the socialist viewpoint (Schemm, 1994). Americans held onto the value of handicrafts as being of higher quality and contributing to an improved quality of life for the individuals who create them through their participation in satisfying work. The process of mass production was believed unsatisfying, as the person was merely an extension of the machine and could not celebrate or be personally satisfied with completion of a product (Levine, 1987). The Arts and Crafts Movement espoused the view that handicrafts integrated the mind and the body through a labor of love that was satisfying (Schemm, 1994). Mary Reilly furthered this concept in her well-known quote from her 1961 Eleanor Clarke Slagle lecture, "That man, through the use of his hands as they are energized by mind and will, can influence the state of his own health" (Reilly, 1962). Many applied the tenets of the Arts and Crafts Movement to therapeutic programs in asylums, hospitals, and settlement houses (Schemm, 1994).

Arts and crafts societies formed in a number of cities in the United States, including Boston. The Boston Society of Arts and Crafts was formally incorporated on June 28, 1897. Twenty-four people signed the incorporation documents, including architect George Edward Barton. The mission was to "develop and encourage higher standards in the handicrafts" (Society of Arts and Crafts, 2013). As mentioned earlier, Barton would later become one of the founders of the National Society for the Promotion of Occupational Therapy. The Chicago Arts and Crafts

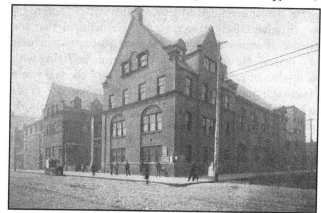

Figure 1-4. Hull House in 1925. (Reprinted from Hull House. (1925). Hull House Year Book 1925, Author: Frederick Hildmen Printing Co.)

Society was incorporated at Hull House in Chicago on October 22, 1897.

In the early 20th century, a paradigm shift occurred once again as medicine started to focus on a scientific foundation that incorporated new technologies such as x-rays. Illness was perceived as stemming from a physiological process (Levine, 1987) rather than environmental problems. A person was viewed as a conglomeration of body parts, and illness seen as a problem with the interaction among or within those parts. Dr. Herbert J. Hall, Dr. Adolph Meyer, and Dr. William Rush Dunton, Jr. were among those who did not agree with the shifting paradigm and held to a holistic view of care. This holistic view of man included a mind–body union called ***psychobiology***, a term coined by Dr. Meyer. These three physicians became promoters of the use of occupation as a therapeutic measure.

Dr. Hall advocated for the work cure, a return of handicapped workers to productive living that was self-supporting, rather than a life of bed rest, idleness, and dependence. He pointed to past successes of client participation in occupations such as simple work, housekeeping, laundry, kitchen, manufacture of items, and farming, which also provided economic rewards and incentives to an institution. Dr. Hall started a handicraft program for those afflicted with mild nervousness in 1904 (Quiroga, 1995, p. 96). His workshop was set up in Marblehead, Massachusetts, and was based on the philosophy of the Arts and Crafts Movement. He believed that participation in crafts was more appealing to patients than the occupations or employment offered by asylums in the past. Harvard's Proctor Fund awarded Dr. Hall a $1,000 grant to study the effectiveness of his work cure (Quiroga, 1995, p. 96). In Hall's workshop, patients learned how to create artistic products such as pottery, weaving, and woodcarvings that could be sold as a means of partial self-support (Hall & Buck, 1915). Hall hired Arthur Baggs to run Marblehead Pottery as part of the therapy program. Today, Marblehead Pottery pieces are sought as prized functional art products (Marblehead Pottery, 2013).

Dr. Meyer articulated the theoretical basis concerning the curative effects of occupation. He believed that the essence of man was not based on the parts or structures of a person. He stated, "...a live organism pulsating with its rhythm of rest and activity ... constitute the real world of actual living" (Meyer, 1922/1977). Therefore, one needs to have a healthy rhythm and balance of time use in work, play, rest, and sleep. According to Dr. Meyer, mental problems were "problems of living" and disorganized habits, not structural or humoral problems (Meyer, 1922/1977). Dr. Meyer's wife, Mary Potter Brooks Meyer, successfully used occupation to facilitate recovery of patients at Worcester State Hospital in Massachusetts (Levine, 1987). Meanwhile, Dr. Meyer observed his patients' contentment and engagement when participating in crafts and other activities. He supported the use of occupation in his clinic, stating:

> A real pleasure in achievement, a real pleasure in the use and activity of one's hands and muscles, and a happy appreciation of time began to be used as incentives in the management of our patients, instead of abstract exhortation to cheer up and to behave according to abstract or repressive rules. (Meyer, 1922/1977, p. 640)

Dr. Meyer developed a professional relationship with Julia Lathrop, a social worker and civic activist affiliated with Hull House. Lathrop had taken an interest in mental health reform after reading a book written by Clifford Beers, *A Mind That Found Itself* (Quiroga, 1995, pp. 41-42). Beers had been treated at a number of asylums while suffering from periods of depression. His autobiographical account exposed the harsh treatment of the individuals confined to asylums. Beers helped initiate the mental hygiene movement and started the National Committee for Mental Hygiene (Peloquin, 2000, p. 11). A member of this committee, L. Vernon Briggs, documented his political activities to enact hospital reform in his book *Occupation as a Substitute for Restraint in the Treatment of the Mentally Ill: A History of the Passage of Two Bills Through the Massachusetts Legislature*. One bill introduced by Briggs in 1911 sought to prohibit the use of restraints in hospitals for the insane except under certain conditions. Another bill was intended to provide for instruction in occupational therapy for nurses and attendants working in hospitals for the insane (Briggs, 1923, pp. 67-70).

In 1908, after reading the book written by Clifford Beers, philanthropist Henry Phipps provided an endowment to start a psychiatric clinic at Johns Hopkins Hospital. Dr. Adolph Meyer was hired to develop the clinic in 1913. Meyer "borrowed" Eleanor Clarke Slagle, taking her from Chicago to Baltimore to work with him (Baum, 2002; Peloquin, 1991a). Treatment at the Phipps Clinic focused on "**habit training**," helping patients to independently follow daily routines and use time appropriately (Meyer, 1922/1977; Peloquin, 1991b). An early model of practice,

the habit training model developed by Slagle sought to help patients organize and balance the daily activities of work, play, rest, and sleep by following a prescribed daily routine (Reed, 1993, p. 36).

Dr. William Rush Dunton, Jr. was a physician who worked at Sheppard-Pratt Hospital. He advocated for restoring the use of both moral treatment and arts and crafts in asylums for the treatment of mentally ill individuals. Dunton believed that a person with mental illness had difficulty with focusing attention. He hypothesized that those with depression tended to have a narrow focus on depressive thoughts; those in an excited stage were unable to organize the many thoughts rapidly entering the mind; those with dementia could not form clearly organized ideas. He believed that the use of occupation helped to facilitate recovery by substituting healthy thoughts and helping the person to refocus his or her attention (Dunton, 1921, pp. 27-28).

Early Training Programs

In the early 1900s many mental hospitals started to employ craft teachers to work with patients (Dunton, 1921, pp. 15-20). Also during this time, a number of programs were started throughout the country in order to train hospital attendants, nurses, and others on the use of occupations to treat individuals with mental illness.

Dr. Meyer and Julia Lathrop of Hull House, home of the Chicago Arts and Crafts Society, applied the Arts and Crafts Movement philosophy to the treatment of people with mental illness (Levine, 1987). In 1908, Lathrop started a course at the Chicago School of Civics and Philanthropy to teach the use of crafts to hospital attendants working with the mentally ill. She was assisted by Rabbi Hirsch and artisans from the Chicago Arts and Craft Society (Dunton, 1921, pp. 15-16; Dunton, 1947, pp. 4-5). Eleanor Clarke Slagle was one of the first to take the course and eventually became the head of this school from 1915 to 1920. The school was renamed the Henry B. Faville School (Dunton, 1947, p. 4). In 1914, prior to her taking charge of the Henry B. Faville School, Slagle designed a 3-week course in occupation, which was offered at the Henry Phipps Psychiatric Clinic (Henry Phipps Psychiatric Service, 2013).

Dunton (1921, p. 15) credits Susan E. Tracy with providing the very first course on the use of occupation for those with mental illness in 1906. Tracy worked at Adams Nervine Hospital in the Boston area and used occupation in her work with individuals who were diagnosed with mild mental health issues. Tracy saw the healing nature of participation in various occupations. She noted that patients who were occupied were happier and less irritable, contributing to a positive change in mental attitude to life (Fuller, 1910, p. 3). Tracy promoted the therapeutic use of self, including expressing empathy, support, and enthusiasm when working with patients. She believed that occupational therapy should be a subspecialty of nursing, and

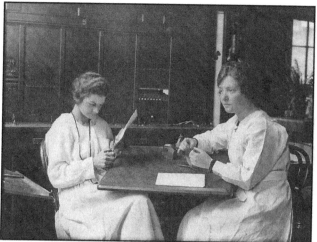

Figure 1-5. Reconstruction aides in training.

she developed and directed training programs for nurses in New York, Chicago, and Boston (Quiroga, 1995, p. 76).

In 1910, Tracy wrote a widely used textbook called *Studies in Invalid Occupations* for use in her training courses. The book focused, in part, on teaching the instructor of occupation courses (Dunton, 1921, p. 15). Tracy's book described how to use various craft activities for different types of patients in different settings. Some of the book chapters offered instruction on how to use various crafts with children or grandmothers, those confined to hospital rooms, and those who might be in restricted positions for healing (Tracy, 1910). Tracy emphasized that it is not enough for someone to know how to accomplish the various crafts. Rather, it is imperative that the person working with invalids have knowledge of the individual needs and conditions of the patient (p. 18). Her book is considered the first occupational therapy textbook.

Many other courses were starting around the country. Reba G. Cameron, also a nurse, started an occupational training program for nurses in 1911 at Taunton State Hospital in Massachusetts. Dr. William Rush Dunton, Jr. initiated a training program in 1911 at Sheppard Asylum (now the Sheppard-Pratt Hospital) in Towson, Maryland. Milwaukee-Downer College started a "somewhat informal" training course in the use of occupations for invalids in 1913. Elizabeth Upham Davis was the major force behind the development of the Milwaukee-Downer program of study (Dunton, 1947, p. 5). In 1914, Miss Evelyn Collins, whose background included training in the manual and industrial arts combined with some experience working with the mentally ill, provided courses in invalid occupations at Teacher's College, Columbia University (Dunton, 1921, p. 18).

Ideology and Education for the New Profession

In its infancy, the new profession worked to define itself. The varied beliefs and opinions of the early founders and proponents were at times in concert and at other times in conflict. Influencing and overlaying these beliefs and opinions were the political, social, economic, and technological issues of the times. Moral treatment promoted humanistic care. A central tenet of moral treatment was that those afflicted with mental illness were not possessed by the devil or demons or at fault for their illness. Rather, they were human beings capable of rational thought if treated well. The use of occupation and moral treatment in the asylums was based on the healing effect of diverting one's mind from illness and replacing abnormal thoughts with positive thoughts. Occupation, employment, and work were perceived as beneficial psychologically, physically, and economically.

There were conflicting ideas, though, on the value of the product versus the process for patients participating in occupations. Proponents of the Arts and Crafts Movement and its ideology believed that participation in the craft helped to cure. They also perceived that a well-crafted end product was of utmost importance and curative in and of itself (Levine, 1987). These proponents, sometimes classified as *diversionists*, believed that the education of attendants on how to use occupations in a therapeutic manner should focus only on training to become skilled in various crafts. Others believed that the process of the craft or activity was the most important aspect rather than the product. They believed that patients were not always capable of producing high-quality art objects. Careful selection of the occupation was required to match the abilities of the patient, and the project should match the interest, values, needs, and rehabilitation goals of the patient (Dunton, 1947, p. 10; Fuller, 1910, p. 2; Schemm, 1994). As such, many advocated for the inclusion of medical information, as well as craft instruction, in the education of attendants and nurses using crafts with patients (Tracy, 1910, p. 18).

World War I

On April 6, 1917, shortly after NSPOT was established, the United States was drawn into World War I. This political event provided a great impetus for the development of occupational therapy. The founders of NSPOT were instrumental in convincing the Medical Department of the Army to hire reconstruction aides in occupational therapy (Dunton, 1918). Reconstruction aides included occupational therapy aides and physical therapy aides. Both professions were still in their infancy, so there was a lack of formal educational programs (Hartwick, 1992). The army required occupational therapy aides to have skills in crafts, teaching, and hospital experience, and physical therapy aides were expected to have experience in numerous physical agent modalities. Figures 1-5 and 1-6 illustrate reconstruction aides in training dated May 13, 1918.

Because World War I created the need for educated reconstruction aides, a number of schools or war emergency courses opened to meet this need. The St. Louis School

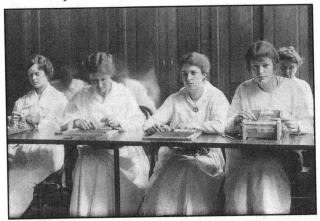

Figure 1-6. Reconstruction aides in training.

for Reconstruction Aides opened in 1918 and remains one of the few original programs that is still in operation. The name of the school was changed, however, to the St. Louis School of Occupational Therapy. It is now known as the Program in Occupational Therapy at Washington University. Similarly, the Boston School of Occupational Therapy was established for the same purpose. It continues today under the name of Tufts University – Boston School of Occupational Therapy.

Although most reconstruction aides were stationed in the United States, a number went to France to work in base hospitals with the American Expeditionary Forces. Those trained in occupational therapy worked with soldiers who were *shell-shocked*—a term used to describe a condition of functional war neurosis, anxiety, and/or hysteria that results from dealing with the stresses of frontline battle. The psychological consequences, physical ailments, and poorly defined illnesses associated with war were the subject of Herbert Hall's book, *Wartime Nerves* (Hall, 1918). Hall's book advocated for occupational therapy treatment to heal the "spirit." Reconstruction aides employed crafts to help these men forget the stresses of war and return them to the frontlines as quickly as possible (Low, 1992). Their efforts were successful in returning soldiers to active duty (Low, 1992; Peloquin, 1991b).

Although the role of occupational therapy in mental health was becoming well developed in the early 20th century, World War I added the impetus for the growth of the profession. The use of crafts and vocational activities for the restoration of physical abilities of injured soldiers helped establish occupational therapy's role for the treatment of physical limitations. Three types of therapeutic occupations or occupational therapy were identified. These *early occupations* included (1) those that provide a diversion from pain and troubles of life; (2) those that restore mental and physical function; and (3) vocational education to return one to gainful employment (Dunton, 1919 pp. 43-44). The article "Bedside Occupational Therapy," a publication for disabled soldiers, described a fourth occupation

as one that "…gives a start in a kind of avocation, 'side-line,' or hobby" (Vaughn, 1919, p. 14). Spotlight 1-2 distinguishes the different types of occupations used by early occupational therapy approaches.

Although World War I gave impetus to the growth of occupational therapy in the areas of psychosocial practice, physical rehabilitation, and vocational rehabilitation, the end of the war and the onset of the Great Depression saw a decreased need for occupational therapists. The Arts and Crafts Movement was also waning. The movement's ideals and the philosophy that helped give rise to the profession, the public reaction to the ills of industrialization, and use of occupation to develop self-esteem and work ethic were concepts lost on a new generation (Levine, 1987). Many in the medical community perceived occupational therapy as providing merely diversional craft activities for patients and lacked a scientific base (Levine, 1987).

Social, Financial, and Legislative Influences Leading to Deinstitutionalization

Societal beliefs, financial implications, and legislation influenced the development and provision of mental health care in the United States. Deinstitutionalization is an example of how societal beliefs led to the passing of legislation that opposed lifelong institutionalization of individuals with mental illness. An example of legislation with financial implications is the bill that funded the creation of community mental health centers as a way to provide affordable treatment for those individuals who were discharged from institutions into the community as a result of deinstitutionalization. Such examples illustrate how the context of time and the chronological relationship of events have influenced the present and future status of mental health services and treatment for individuals with mental illness.

Figure 1-7 provides an illustration of how social/cultural, legislative/governmental, and economic/financial factors influence the provision of mental health services.

Following World War II, significant changes occurred in how mental health was perceived, both socially and culturally. These changes may have been influenced by the many soldiers who returned home with physical and psychological impairments. Significantly, concepts of curability replaced concepts of incurability for those affected by mental illness (Sharfstein, 2000). Additionally, the discovery of pharmacological treatment approaches hastened the social acceptance of the concept of curability. Subsequently, society identified the need to change the care process for individuals with mental illness.

Prior to the mid-20th century, the majority of individuals with mental health impairments were placed into institutions. Some community-based treatment settings existed; however, these were not commonly available alternatives. Examples included Hull House run by Jane Addams, Consolation House with George E. Barton, or the arts and crafts workshop supported by Herbert J. Hall described previously in this chapter. Asylums for the insane, in the Kirkbride tradition, were designed to be "retreats" or places where a patient could escape the pressure of daily life. The pleasant environment and treatment, and participation in occupations and manual labor, were designed to cure and return the person to his or her previous home and community (Geller & Morrisey, 2004). At that time, institutionalization was viewed as humane care. Institutionalization was also perceived as an acceptable method of protecting society from individuals with mental illness. Significantly, society as a whole deemed it necessary to accept responsibility for the care and needs of individuals who were institutionalized. Societal beliefs that fostered institutionalization included the belief that people with mental illness could not make choices for themselves and were totally incapacitated by their disorder. Those perceptions changed by the middle of the 20th century.

In the first half of the 20th century, most asylums were renamed *hospitals*. These hospitals became "... a dumping ground for all manner of people who could not care for themselves. The once-grand asylums deteriorated into snake pits and hellholes..." (Geller, 2004). It seemed as if history was repeating itself with the horror stories of squalid conditions and inhumane care. The early successes of moral treatment in asylums could not be achieved with the increasing number of patients. The therapeutic use of self and personal kindness previously found to be helpful in the recovery of many individuals with mental illness were unattainable with the limited staffing of hospitals. In 1903, 150,000 patients were institutionalized. By 1954, that number had risen to 556,000 (Geller, 2000). Patients with mental illness occupied one out of every two hospital beds (Geller, 2000; Scull, 2011a).

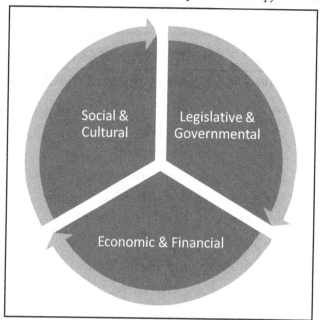

Figure 1-7. Contextual influences.

Around the mid-20th century, society as a whole gained a greater understanding for the need to maintain the respect and dignity of institutionalized persons (Barton, 2000; Klerman, 1977). News articles shared the plight of institutionalization in journalistic exposés written to educate the public on this topic (Sharfstein, 2000). Problems of institutionalization included dependency in the hospital environment, lack of meaningful relationships, loss of privacy, impaired personal identity, and absence of fulfillment (Krieg, 2001). Hayes and Baxley (1998) identified that institutional behaviors resulted in the inability to make choices or decisions and maintain habits or routines. Klerman (1977) identified that institutionalization isolated staff and clients, dehumanized people, took away individual responsibility, and created a sense of rebellion toward authoritarian rule. Problems with institutionalization were often compounded by a lack of hygiene, overcrowding, poor living conditions, and reported cases of ill treatment at some facilities (Priebe & Fakhoury, 2007). Risk for abuse of power and corruption were possible at times. The beginning of the deinstitutionalization movement was created.

Deinstitutionalization refers to the provision of care to meet an individual's needs within the community rather than in an institution. Table 1-1 highlights positive and negative factors associated with deinstitutionalization. Although not all-inclusive, they include economic, social, and technological variables, as well as the values of self-respect and dignity, and the belief that persons with mental health impairments should be able to seek their treatment in the least restrictive environment (Krieg, 2001; Novella, 2010; Priebe & Fakhoury, 2007; Sawyer, 2011).

TABLE 1-1

POSITIVE AND NEGATIVE FACTORS OF DEINSTITUTIONALIZATION

POSITIVE FACTORS AND VARIABLES ASSOCIATED WITH DEINSTITUTIONALIZATION

+ Greater opportunity for dignity and self-respect

+ Greater freedom over self

+ Greater individual responsibility

+ Evolution of medical (i.e., neuroleptic medicines) and technological treatment (i.e., x-rays)

+ The opportunity for improved quality of life

+ Patients no longer imprinted with behaviors learned in the context of institutionalized care

+ The ability to achieve social integration

+ Less intrusive care; care in the community

+ Decreased stigma from society

+ Decreased costs for mental health care (hospitalization)

NEGATIVE FACTORS AND VARIABLES ASSOCIATED WITH DEINSTITUTIONALIZATION

- A significant number of mentally ill individuals are jobless

- Substandard housing; lack of availability of appropriate housing

- Greater risk for living in poverty

- May lack familial structure and social integration supports

- Greater risk for reinstitutionalization and transinstitutionalization

- Lack of funding for community-based services to treat mental illness

- Significant variation in the quality of care between towns, cities, and states

- Greater risk for poor life decisions affecting overall health and quality of life

- Greater risk for homelessness

- Greater risk for involvement in ethical and social problems such as crime and violence

- Greater risk for participation in fringe expressions of self that bound on the edge of socially accepted and appropriate behavior.

Compiled from Krieg, R. G. (2011). An interdisciplinary look at the deinstitutionalization of the mentally ill. *The Social Science Journal, 38*, 367-380.; Novella, E. J. (2010). Mental health care in the aftermath of deinstitutionalization: A retrospective and prospective view. *Health Care Analysis, 18*, 222-238.; Priebe, S. & Fakhoury, W. (2007). Deinstitutionalization and reinstitutionalization: Major changes in the provision of mental healthcare. *Psychiatry, 6*(8), 313-316.; Sawyer, A. (2011). Translating mental health policy into practice: Ongoing challenges and frustrations. *Health Sociology Review, 20*(2), 114-119.

The values of freedom, respect, and dignity were addressed with deinstitutionalization; however, the responsibility for care of individuals with mental illness changed as well. The government or state institution was no longer viewed as the locus of responsibility for individuals with mental health impairments (Krieg, 2001). Instead, the locus of responsibility was transferred to the individual and his or her family and influenced by the supporting mental health care system.

Many people believed deinstitutionalization to be inadequate to meet the needs of people with mental health impairments, perhaps even more so for those with severe and persistent mental illness. This perception continues today, partly due to negative stereotypes, as well as a lack of sufficient state funds to provide adequate mental health services. Negative stereotypes include the beliefs that people with mental illness are dangerous, not able to care for themselves, and not able to make decisions or choices. These stereotypes form the basis of the argument to maintain institutionalization. In addition, these stereotypes show where the mental health care system has failed

CHECKPOINT 1-1. LIST OF THE EARLY LEGISLATION INFLUENCING MENTAL HEALTH CARE IN THE UNITED STATES	
Year	*Legislation*
1854	Indigent Insane Bill
1955	Mental Health Study Act
1956	Health Amendments of 1956
1946	National Mental Health Act (created the National Institute of Mental Health)
1948	Vocational Rehabilitation Act
1959	Training of Professional Personnel Act

to support individuals in meeting their needs, usually due to a lack of funding.

Following deinstitutionalization, another trend emerged, termed re*institutionalization* or *transinstitutionalization* of clients. **Transinstitutionalization** refers to the process of leaving one institutional environment only to return to another. Johnny and Suzie show two examples of transinstitutionalization. Johnny is a 19-year-old male who was recently discharged from a state institution to live in a group home in the city. Johnny had great difficulty obtaining a job due to his lack of work experience. When he did find employment on an evening shift as a dishwasher, he was unable to maintain it due to his inability to focus and maintain a consistent work pace in such a hectic environment as the restaurant kitchen. Johnny started hanging out with "friends" during the day who encouraged him to steal beer and liquor for them from the local store. Eventually, Johnny was caught by the police, resulting in his incarceration for his crimes. Thus, Johnny went from one institution (the state hospital) to live in another (jail).

Suzie, on the other hand, is a 63-year-old female recently discharged from the psychiatric unit at the general hospital. Suzie was treated for an acute episode of depression and discharged home. However, Suzie was unable to successfully complete her daily tasks of living, as home supports had not been established during her short length of stay in the hospital. In addition, Suzie's depression had masked an early onset of dementia that ever so slightly was encroaching on her independence. Several weeks later, Suzie returned to the hospital and was subsequently discharged to an assisted-living facility.

The transfer of clients to the community has resulted in the relocation of health services, changes in the philosophy of care, and variation in the types of mental health services offered (Sawyer, 2011). State institutions are relinquishing their responsibility for the care of individuals with persistent mental illness to multiple and diverse private and community-based systems of support. This includes community mental health centers, crisis intervention units, private hospitals, and nonprofit group programs. Deinstitutionalization may have started with a change in sociocultural beliefs in the United States; however, it could not have been successful without consideration of legislative action and economic support.

Early shifts in the economy of mental health care in the United States affected how mental health services were provided. These shifts include indirect costs. One aspect of indirect costs is associated with the efforts of deinstitutionalization. Indirect costs include aspects other than financial expenses and affect the consumer or client, community, families, taxpayers, and state and local government. Examples of indirect costs associated with deinstitutionalization include a higher risk for suicide, increased medical care needs, increased need for utilization of family resources, increased need for supportive housing, and higher levels of incarceration in prisons (Priebe & Fakhoury, 2007). Lifestyle choices made by clients living in the community (i.e., drug and alcohol use, diet, cigarette smoking) may lead to higher medical and legal costs. Smaldone and Cullen-Drill (2010) determined that people with mental illness die about 25 years earlier than those without mental illness. With deinstitutionalization, clients obtained greater individual responsibility and control over their own lives; however, they lost a certain level of structure, security, and established level of health care.

Indirect costs also include the support of community-based programs and services. For example, a nonprofit, community-based program may provide general services to the homeless. Other programs are created for a specific purpose, such as a food pantry or group home. Community-based programs and groups often utilize volunteers, churches, church groups, and other community-based agencies.

Legislation has significantly affected mental health care in the United States. Legislation can be helpful to create initiatives toward a specific goal, such as parity in metal health care, as well as provide funding for programs and initiatives. State legislation also affects mental health care and varies from state to state. Examples at the state level include practice acts that define and describe occupational therapy services. Another example is state and federal definitions of a qualified mental health practitioner. Checkpoint 1-1 identifies significant legislative efforts that have occurred in the first half of the 20th century in the United States.

Barton (2000) identified that, before the 1950s, the government was primarily interested in promoting research, developing manpower resources, and supporting training. The National Mental Health Act of 1946 enabled the creation of the National Institute of Mental Health. It also created grants for new programs in the community to serve the mentally ill (Accordino, Porter, & Morse, 2001). The United States government was attempting to validate practices at the time. In the 1950s and 1960s, the passage of a number of laws by Congress paved the way for the shift of care from institutions to the community. One example of legislation includes the Mental Health Study Act of 1955. This act called for a study of the problems associated with mental illness. The Health Amendments of 1956 also facilitated development of community mental health centers through implementation of pilot projects, evaluation studies, and research studies (Geller, 2000). Other examples include the Captioned Films Act of 1958 and the Training of Professional Personnel Act of 1959. Such legislation continued up until the mid-1960s.

PART 2: INFLUENCES ON CURRENT MENTAL HEALTH OCCUPATIONAL THERAPY

Shifting Paradigms and the Medical Model

In the early 20th century, occupational therapy "tied" itself to medicine. This was in part because of the socio-economic and political situations at the time. Women preferred to work with patients and sought legitimacy for the fledgling profession by working under the supervision of male physicians. These same physicians were in a position to promote the profession, sponsor program development, and implement research to demonstrate the effectiveness of occupational therapy, ultimately developing a scientific base (Quiroga, 1995, p. 73). During World War I, reconstruction aides worked under the supervision of physicians (orthopedists), who established a hierarchical system in which the physician determined appropriate treatment (Gutman, 1995; Quiroga, 1995, p. 157). Naturally, reconstruction aides would be influenced more by these physicians than by the competing service of vocational re-educators who devalued occupational therapy reconstruction aides at the time (Gutman, 1995). Eleanor Clarke Slagle implored occupational therapists to secure "prescriptions" for occupational therapy from physicians so that the profession could grow and be recognized as a health care profession (Quiroga, 1995, p. 235).

Around the 1930s, the status of medicine began to rise as physicians became more science driven. There was an emphasis on research and, in particular, measuring the effectiveness of intervention. Stemming from the close association between orthopedists and occupational therapists in World War I, the role of occupational therapy in working with patients with physical disabilities grew. In this practice area, the emphasis was on choosing, grading, and adapting activities for improving motor function, strength, and range of motion. Medicine's view of mankind was becoming more mechanistic (the human body is like a machine) and reductionistic (a human being is the sum of body parts); this viewpoint became known as the *medical model.* During this time, there was significant growth of occupational therapy in the area of physical rehabilitation in conjunction with the medical model. This growth continued during the 1930s and expanded even more with the start of World War II.

Occupational therapy strengthened ties with medicine in 1935, when the profession worked with physicians to establish educational standards. The AOTA asked the American Medical Association to evaluate their existing occupational therapy education programs, as the American Medical Association had prior experience in standards setting for medical education. In addition, they had the power to establish occupational therapy as a legitimate medical profession (Dunton, 1947, p. 7; Hopkins, 1988, p. 24). This was the start of occupational therapy working within a strong medical model.

When working within the medical model, health care disciplines often incorporate the use of the *biopsychosocial model.* The biopsychosocial model focuses on the biological components of disease and disability. At the same time it incorporates social and psychological dimensions of health and illness (Substance Abuse and Mental Health Services Administration [SAMHSA], 2011). For clarity, there are at least three different viewpoints of the biopsychosocial model expressed within the literature. The first, as described earlier, is the biopsychosocial model as it is incorporated into medicine. Another reference to the biopsychosocial model, proposed by Anne Mosey, is found in the occupational therapy literature. This version of the model later became known as the *Person-Environment-Occupational Model.* Finally, the biopsychosocial model is again described in the *International Classification of Functioning, Disability, & Health.* This definition will be covered in greater depth in Chapter 2. By the mid-1950s, the biopsychosocial model began to give greater emphasis to the biological nature of disability. This shift in focus led to an increased use of psychiatric medications to cure mental illness.

In the mid-20th century, there was a "renewed interest in the biochemical aspects of mental illness" (Barton, 1957, pp. 193-195). Drugs were used to treat the symptoms and behaviors associated with severe mental illness, such as psychosis and anxiety, and allowed for more client participation in activities, including occupational therapy.

However, the medications also had side effects that needed to be monitored, such as drowsiness and changes in motor function (Barton, 1957, pp. 194-195). Appendix B in this text discusses current medications used to treat individuals with mental illness, along with their potential side effects.

Some individuals point to the use of medications as a significant element in facilitating deinstitutionalization. Although the use of drugs was perceived as a revolutionary advance in psychiatric care, it was not seen as a means to "cure" mental illness; rather, drugs were viewed as a way to exert social control on behavior (Moncrief, 1999). The biological or biochemical view of psychiatry and psychopharmacology began to take the place of psychoanalysis at an accelerated pace in the 1970s, with the introduction of new, effective medications such as Prozac (fluoxetine), Valium (diazepam), and Zoloft (sertraline) to control moods (Scull, 2011b).

Psychiatric occupational therapy was still a valued service during World War II. In 1942, a study by the Surgeon General's Office found that 40% of medical discharges were due to psychiatric conditions. Dr. Walter Barton, a major in the army, was in charge of psychiatric occupational therapy. Purposeful activity was successfully used as an intervention at that time. A strong advocate for occupational therapy, Barton recommended that occupational therapy departments establish programs for physical fitness, sports activities, singing, dancing, gardening, arts and crafts, and other activities. He believed in the philosophical tenets of occupational therapy that were espoused by Adolph Meyer and William Rush Dunton, Jr. and considered the soldiers' psychiatric problems to be situational rather than deep, emotional conflicts. Major Walter Barton appointed Winifred Kahmann as chief of Occupational Therapy Services and Wilma West and H. Elizabeth Messick as her special assistants. They worked with the AOTA to develop courses to train occupational therapists (Ellsworth, 1983).

Outside of the army, occupational therapy struggled with the changing paradigm in the treatment of mental health patients. Prior to the 1940s and 1950s, occupational therapy provided mental health services in institutions that were primarily based on principles of moral treatment and the psychobiological approach of Adolph Meyer, and which incorporated the influences of the early Arts and Crafts Movement. Occupational therapy used activity analysis in its treatment approaches, and discharge from the institution was not a focal point in treatment planning (Gutman, 2011). However, the view of mental illness and treatment philosophies began to change as Sigmund Freud's psychodynamic theories gained popularity (Quiroga, 1995, pp. 62-63). As a result, by the 1940s and 1950s, occupational therapists working in mental health settings increasingly utilized occupational therapy interventions based on the psychodynamic theories of Sigmund Freud.

Freud considered the etiology of mental illness to be within the person, especially the unconscious mind. His theory proposed that man had a conscious mind and an unconscious mind, with many psychological problems stemming from repressed or hidden thoughts. As his work developed, he characterized the human psyche as having an id (unconscious, childlike part acting on the pleasure principle seeking immediate gratification and pleasure), an ego (based in reality and helping the person to act in socially appropriate ways), and a superego (the internalization of values and morals to guide judgment). Freud also identified defense mechanisms that he claimed are used by a person when tasks or life became difficult. Checkpoint 1-2 describes these defense mechanisms.

According to Freud, a balance between the id, ego, and superego, combined with the ability to use defense mechanisms, was needed for mental health. Psychoanalysis was used to help people see the hidden aspects and root of their psychological problems.

The psychodynamic theory considered the origin of mental illness as within the person; therefore, treatment focused on fixing the person by bringing unconscious thoughts into the conscious mind through dialogue and analysis. This view was in contrast to that of William Rush Dunton Jr., whose therapy emphasized the contexts of the person and participation in occupations that diverted the mind from unpleasant thoughts.

Closer ties with the medical model and specialization in treatment came at a cost of decreased association with other health care professions, such as vocational rehabilitation (Gutman, 1995). The medical model also challenged the profession to identify the theoretical base used as the foundation for its therapeutic approaches at the time. The medical model and reductionistic viewpoint of man became evident as early as the 1920s, when psychiatric occupational therapists incorporated the psychodynamic perspective into their therapy (Friedland, 1988). The general objective was to "...provide opportunities for the expression or sublimation of emotional needs and drives" (West, 1959, p. 1). Occupational therapists employed therapeutic use of self, use of groups and group techniques, and craft activities to achieve that end (West, 1959, p. 24). In some occupational therapy clinics, however, the use of activities was declining in favor of discussion groups that focused on helping patients gain insight into problems (Kielhofner & Barris, 1984).

Around the mid-20th century, psychology and occupational therapy flourished with the development of other therapeutic models and approaches. Table 1-2 includes some of the models and approaches developed by occupational therapy, as well as models established by psychology and adapted for use by occupational therapy. Table 1-2 is not an all-inclusive list. These models and approaches will

---

CHECKPOINT 1-2. DESCRIPTIONS OF DEFENSE MECHANISMS

Conversion: The unconscious transformation of mental conflict into physical symptoms with no organic cause.

Denial: Escaping unpleasant thoughts, events, facts, feelings, wishes, or needs by simply ignoring their existence.

Displacement: The transference of emotions associated with a particular person, object, or situation to a less threatening person, object, or situation.

Identification: Consciously or unconsciously attributing to oneself the characteristics of another person or group who is admired.

Intellectualization: The process in which events are analyzed based on remote, cold facts and without emotion, rather than incorporating feeling into the processing.

Projection: The unconscious rejection of emotionally unacceptable or unwanted thoughts, behaviors, and feelings by projecting or attributing them to someone else.

Rationalization: Subconscious justifications or excuses given to make unreasonable or illogical ideas, behaviors, or feelings seem logical and acceptable.

Reaction formation: Unconsciously dealing with unacceptable feelings and behaviors by developing and demonstrating the opposite behavior or emotion.

Regression: Reverting to an earlier, more primitive, and childlike pattern of behavior that may or may not have been previously exhibited.

Repression: Painful, frightening, or threatening emotions, memories, impulses, or drives are subconsciously pushed, or "stuffed," into the unconscious.

Sublimation: Unconscious redirection of undesirable, immature, or destructive impulses into socially acceptable activities.

Suppression: Conscious denial of painful, frightening, or threatening emotions, memories, impulses, or drives.

---

be seen in other chapters of this text and will be described in greater detail when applicable.

Contemporary Financial and Legislative Influences Affecting Mental Health Care

Recent shifts in legislation and the economy of mental health care in the United States have affected how services are provided. One shift in the economy of mental health care is associated with the change in financial responsibility for the care of individuals with mental illness. Prior to deinstitutionalization, the state paid for the costs associated with state-run mental institutions. Deinstitutionalization created a shift whereby financial responsibility and control of services changed from the state and community level to that of the federal government. To carry out this responsibility, the federal government utilized grant money and eventually instituted the fee-for-service program of Medicare. Additionally, Social Security disability, Veterans Administration (VA) disability income, and supplemental Social Security income all contribute to support community living for persons with mental illness. States continue to provide financial support to these individuals through Medicaid, along with the assistance from the federal government. Mechanic (2012) identifies that Medicaid covers one-fourth of all mental health expenditures in the United States. As more uninsured persons with mental illness gain access to health care through an expansion of Medicaid by the Affordable Care Act, Medicaid may assume an even larger share of mental health expenditures in the United States

The most recent shift occurring in the economy of mental health care in the United States took place with the move to fee-for-service reimbursement models. Medicare and Medicaid were created in 1965. They began the shift to a for-profit model by identifying what treatment services were eligible for reimbursement (Kleinman, 1992). Medicare set definitions for services, as well as set standards of care (Barton, 2000). One consequence of the introduction of Medicare was that a greater number of clients with mental illness were seen in skilled nursing facilities, acute care, and general hospital psychiatric settings.

Today, private insurance may also offer mental health benefits within their covered services, and typically utilize the fee-for-service model. This model influenced the creation of managed health care, which attempts to lower or maintain costs by prioritizing the services and needs of clients. At times, managed care can contribute to limitations in services due to utilization reviews, prior authorization, controlled health networks and providers, and restrictions imposed by managed behavioral health care

TABLE 1-2	
MODELS OF PRACTICE UTILIZED IN MENTAL HEALTH OCCUPATIONAL THERAPY SERVICES*	
MODEL	**PROPONENT**
Sensory Integration	Lorna Jean King
	A. Jean Ayres
Cognitive Disabilities	Claudia Allen
Model of Human Occupation	Gary Kielhofner
Psychodynamic	G. S. Fidler/J. W. Fidler
Developmental	Lorna Jean King/Lela Llorens
Group Development and Adaptation	Anne C. Mosey
Behavioral and Role Acquisition	Mary A. Reilly
Biopsychosocial/Person-Environment-Occupation Model	Anne C. Mosey/Mary Law
Occupational Science	Florence Clark/Ruth Zemke
Psychobiological Approach	Originally developed by psychology and adapted for use within occupational therapy.
Psychoanalytic Approach	
Gestalt Therapy	
Milieu Therapy	
Behavioral Therapy	
Family Therapy	
Psychiatric Rehabilitation Model	
Recovery Model	Developed from a civil rights movement.

*This is not an all-inclusive list of approaches utilized by mental health occupational therapy services. The context, stakeholders, client, and therapist will help determine the best approach to apply.

Compiled from Brown, C., & Stoffel, V. C. (Eds.) (2011). *Occupational therapy in mental health: A vision for participation.* Philadelphia: PA: F. A. Davis Company; Early, M. B. (2000). *Mental health concepts and techniques for the occupational therapy assistant* (3rd ed.). New York, NY: Lippincott Williams & Wilkins.

organizations (Buchmueller, Cooper, Jacobson, & Zuvekas, 2007). Managed care also attempts to enhance stakeholder value and consolidation in the behavioral health industry (Sharfstein, 2000). The economics of mental health care are often influenced and mirrored by legislative efforts.

Contemporary legislation has also affected the delivery of mental health care in the United States. Contemporary legislation was selected to include legislation from the last quarter of the 20th century to the present time. Table 1-3 identifies a timeline of contemporary legislative influences that have affected mental health care in the United States.

The 1975 Education for all Handicapped Children's Act, amended in 1986, would later set the foundation for the creation of the 1997 Individuals with Disabilities Act. The 1975 legislation included children from 3 to 21 years of age, whereas the 1986 amendment allowed coverage of children

from birth (U.S. Department of Education, 2007). The purpose of this legislation was to support states and localities in their efforts to protect the rights and meet the needs of children. Its mission was to improve access to education for children with disabilities. As of 2007, it has affected nearly 6 million children and youth through the provision of special education and services to meet their needs (U.S. Department of Education, 2007). It has enabled children with disabilities to be educated in schools, improved graduation rates, and increased the number of children with disabilities advancing to college education. Currently this program covers children from birth to the transition from high school to adult living.

In the 1980s, the Mental Health Systems Act of 1980 was passed, which later became the Omnibus Reconciliation Act of 1981. This legislation established block grants to

TABLE 1-3

CONTEMPORARY LEGISLATION INFLUENCING MENTAL HEALTH CARE IN THE UNITED STATES

YEAR	LEGISLATION
1965	Community Mental Health Centers Act*
1975	Education for All Handicapped Children's Act
1981	Omnibus Reconciliation Act of 1981 (previously the Mental Health Systems Act of 1980)
1986	Amendments to the Education for All Handicapped Children's Act
1990	Americans with Disabilities Act (ADA)*
1996	Mental Health Parity Act
1997	Individuals with Disabilities Act (IDEA)*
2008	Mental Health Parity and Addictions Equality Act*
2008	Medicare Improvements for Patients and Providers Act*
2009	Affordable Care Act*
2012	The Occupational Therapy Mental Health Act

*Will be discussed in greater detail in Chapter 6 of this textbook.

states to improve accessibility and availability of community supports for deinstitutionalized persons (Mechanic, 2012). It also ended the federal government's commitment to the community mental health centers (Werner & Tyler, 1993). New areas of revenue were added with increased coverage by Medicare and Medicaid (Accordino, Porter, & Morse, 2001). Additionally, the Mental Health Parity Act of 1996 was passed, which was intended to lessen the disparity between mental health coverage and health care plans. Many exceptions were included, though, limiting the impact of this law. The act did not mandate mental health coverage. It did require lifetime limits to be the same for both mental health coverage and medical coverage, but only if the insurance plan covered both aspects of care (Buchmueller, Cooper, Jacobson, & Zuvekas, 2007). Later, this act would lead to the passing of the 2008 Mental Health Parity and Addiction Equality Act. The 2008 act sought similar copays and deductibles for mental health coverage and medical coverage (Forman, 2012). Once again, however, this law did not mandate that benefits for mental health coverage be offered.

The 1990s offered a greater possibility for social integration of persons with mental illness. The Americans with Disabilities Act (ADA) of 1990 attempted to eliminate discrimination toward individuals with disabilities. The ADA does not require equal provisions for individuals with physical and mental disabilities. It does, however, prohibit the exclusion from employment based on a disability, whether a physical or mental disability. The ADA identifies the differences between reasonable accommodations, essential job functions, and "undue hardship" in determining if a person with a disability is able to fulfill an employment opportunity. In part, this law attempted to address inclusion in the community for individuals with disabilities.

More recently, the *Affordable Care Act* of 2009 and the Medicare Improvement for Patients and Providers Act of 2008 were passed. The Affordable Care Act offers the possibility of insurance benefits through an expansion of Medicaid. Mechanic (2012) identified that this benefit could help 3.7 million people without insurance at this time. Additionally, insurance could not deny claims based on pre-existing conditions, and people could stay on their parents' insurance plan up to the extended age of 26. Health care plans were also required to cover an essential set of services to include mental health and substance abuse by 2014. The Medicare Improvement for Patients and Providers Act also provides significant changes to coverage. At the time the law passed, copays for mental health coverage by Medicare were set at 50%. This law lowers the copay to 20% by the year 2014 to be consistent with other Medicare health benefits. This drop is significant, as 22% of persons with severe mental illness receive Medicare benefits (Smaldone & Cullen-Drill, 2010).

The profession of occupational therapy is very active in advocating for mental health coverage and practice. The Occupational Therapy Mental Health Act (HR 3762) was proposed; however, Congress failed to bring the motion for a vote in 2012, causing it to fail. This act offered the chance to increase the number of mental health providers in occupational therapy. Its passage would have resulted in recognition of occupational therapists as mental health and behavioral health professionals by the National Health Service Corps, and allowed for loan repayment and scholarships. More importantly, this act would have assisted occupational therapy to be recognized as a *Qualified Mental Health Profession* **(QMHP)** by states and a *Core Mental Health Professional* **(CMHP)** at the federal level (AOTA, 2006). Currently, QMHP and CMHP include psychologists, psychiatrists, clinical social workers, licensed marriage and family therapists, and psychiatric nurse practitioners.

Recovery Model and the Scope of Practice of the Occupational Therapy Assistant

…through participation in everyday activities that are needed and desired, persons with mental illness and/or substance use disorders will achieve a state of health, well-being, and recovery. (Stoffel, 2010, p. 3)

The AOTA has identified mental health as a vital practice area for the profession of occupational therapy in the next century. Mental health is defined as "a state of successful performance of mental function, resulting in productive activities, fulfilling relationships with other people, and the ability to adapt to change and to cope with adversity" (United States Department of Health and Human Services [USDHHS], 1999). AOTA (2010) recognizes that occupational therapy promotes mental health through the presence of four characteristics found in a positive state of functioning. These characteristics include the following:

1. Positive affect or emotional state
2. Positive psychological and social function
3. Productive activities
4. Resilience in the face of adversity and ability to cope with life stressors

This definition of mental health applies to children and youth up through the aged. It not only covers those with mild-to-severe persistent mental illness, but also individuals in the well population. Mental health is essential to each person's overall health and productivity and as it affects their ability to participate in the family, community, and society (Bonder, 2010; USDHHS, 1999).

Occupational therapy applies various therapeutic approaches to meet the specific needs of clients. Most recently, as therapeutic approaches have evolved, occupational therapy has incorporated approaches within a *recovery model* and a public health model of care. Brown and Stoffel (2011) define recovery as:

A journey of healing and transformation enabling a person with a mental health problem to live a meaningful life in a community or his or her choice while striving to achieve his or her full potential. (p. 787)

Recovery includes two aspects: recovery from mental illness and recovery within mental illness (Gibson, D'Amico, Jaffe, & Arbesman, 2011). Recovery from mental illness refers to improved functioning and decreased symptom levels over time. Recovery within mental illness refers to the attainment of a meaningful life. Occupational therapy has a role in helping an individual in recovery to access and participate in meaningful activities. Meaningful activities can include (but are not limited to) areas such as job and career, education, volunteering, and advocacy efforts (AOTA, 2006).

The recovery model is a civil rights movement that emphasizes a person-centered and empowering approach to health care. The recovery movement was started by consumers and is led by those in recovery. It was started in response to a mental health care system that supported social inequities and discrimination and hampered community inclusion and recovery (SAMHSA, 2011). The participants in the movement are attempting to return control and responsibility of care to the recipient of services, rather than the therapist, institution, government, or third-party payers. The person receiving care needs to be an active participant and drive the recovery process. Therapists cannot do recovery for the client alone; it must start with the person receiving services. Treatment is not recovery, but rather leads to positive advances toward recovery goals. Champagne and Gray (2011) identified 10 fundamental components of recovery. The 10 fundamental components of recovery include the following:

1. Self-directed
2. Individualized and person-centered
3. Empowering
4. Holistic
5. Nonlinear
6. Strengths based
7. Peer supported
8. Respect
9. Consumer responsibility (catalyst of the recovery process)
10. Hope

Occupational therapy fits well within the recovery model. Occupational therapy practitioners have a unique set of skills, knowledge, and abilities that can be used to help persons improve their functioning in everyday life roles. Occupational therapy promotes the development of habits, roles, and actions that have meaning in a person's life (Costa, Molinsky, Kent, & Sauerwald, 2011). Emphasis on the elements of holism, function, participation, and partnership support the development of skills, engagement in activities of interest, and attainment of recovery goals.

Occupational therapy promotes and provides interventions for mental health and participates in the prevention of mental illness. The occupational therapy assistant, under supervision of the occupational therapist, accomplishes this through the use of occupations and activities, preparatory methods and tasks, education and training, advocacy and self-advocacy, and group interventions (AOTA, 2014). The occupational therapy assistant's role also depends on several factors. Factors that influence the role of the occupational therapy assistant include the following:

- Each clinician's level of ability. Examples include experience and service competency.

- Work setting demands. Examples include state laws, reimbursement, and supervision requirements.

- Complexity and stability of the client population. Examples include chronic versus acute, mild to severe, age over the lifespan.

A clinician's skills, knowledge, and ability will vary depending on whether he or she is a new graduate, a seasoned professional, or a new practitioner to mental health practice. As new graduates, occupational therapy assistants are expected to be able to provide entry-level services.

After demonstrating competency, and under the supervision of an occupational therapist, they may serve in the role of clinician, advocate, and group facilitator. Roles that an occupational therapy assistant may fulfill with additional training and experience include clinical administrator, consultant, case manager, and community support worker. It should be noted, however, that they may not use their credentials as an occupational therapy practitioner in those roles unless they are receiving supervision from an occupational therapist. Additionally, state and federal regulations, third-party payers, and employers may have further educational requirements.

Occupational therapy assistants may provide services in a variety of institutional and community-based systems. They may be found in public schools, hospital psychiatric units, mental health institutes, community mental health centers, and correctional/forensic facilities, among others. Occupational therapy assistants may also provide services in after-school programs, worksites, senior centers, homeless shelters, assisted living centers, mental health clinics, drug treatment programs, home-based case management, group homes, transitional/supported employment programs, assertive community treatment, and rehabilitative clubhouses such as Fountain House. Work demands vary between settings, as well as from state to state. Again, state laws, reimbursement prerequisites, and supervision requirements will all influence the role of the occupational therapy assistant.

Regardless of setting, occupational therapy assistants need to have an understanding of the system in which care is provided, including the different professionals who work in mental health settings (Bonder, 2010). This will facilitate communication and collaboration with other disciplines and members of the team. Mental health professionals may include psychiatrists, psychologists, social workers, general practitioners, community psychiatric nurses, certified school teachers, drug abuse counselors, rehabilitation coordinators, vocational rehabilitation, and other allied health professionals.

The level of the complexity and stability of the client population will present different challenges. Clients in an acute phase of their disorder will require different services than a person living in the community who is participating in his or her recovery plan. Additionally, approaches designed for children will be different than those for adults or persons in the late lifespan. Occupational therapy assistants must obtain a clear understanding of each client's needs in order to provide effective services, as the setting, age, and type of client will influence the role of the occupational therapy assistant. Additionally, the term *client* can refer to individuals, groups of individuals, organizations, and populations requiring variations in approach (AOTA, 2010).

SUMMARY

Mental health care in the United States continues to change to meet the needs of consumers and stakeholders. Checkpoint 1-3 highlights some of the historical influences affecting occupational therapy services that were covered in this chapter. Again, this is not an all-inclusive list. More recent influences on mental health care include the Affordable Care Act and the President's New Freedom Commission on Mental Health.

The ***President's New Freedom Commission on Mental Health*** offers one of the most significant influences on mental health care. President George W. Bush created the New Freedom Commission in 2002 to better understand the problems in the current mental health service delivery system that prevent people from getting the excellent health care they need. These problems include the stigma that surrounds mental illness, unfair treatment and financial limitations in private health insurance, and a fragmented mental health delivery system. The commission identified six goals that include the following:

1. Americans must understand that mental health is essential to overall health.

2. Mental health care is consumer and family driven.

3. Disparities in mental health services are eliminated.

4. Early mental health screening, assessment, and referral to services are common practice.

5. Excellent mental health care is delivered to all, and research is accelerated.

6. Technology is used to access mental health care and information.

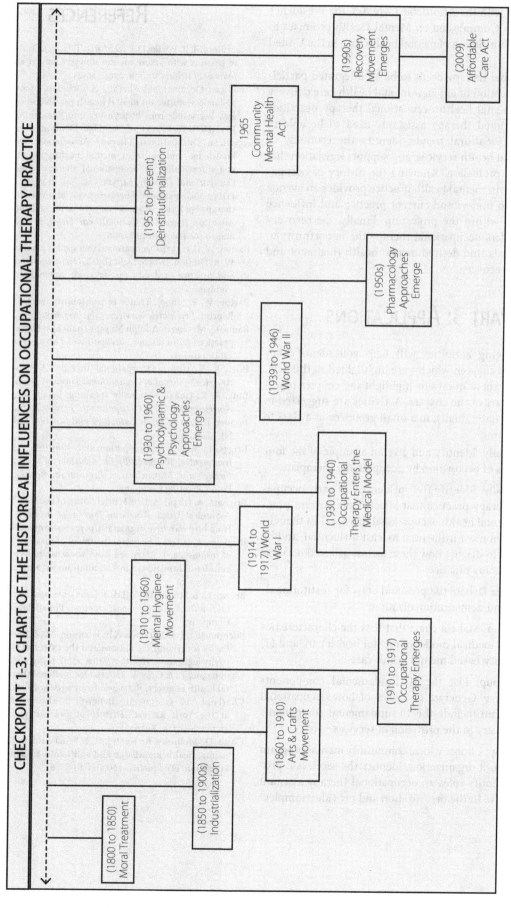

CHECKPOINT 1-3. CHART OF THE HISTORICAL INFLUENCES ON OCCUPATIONAL THERAPY PRACTICE

(1800 to 1850) Moral Treatment

(1850 to 1900s) Industrialization

(1860 to 1910) Arts & Crafts Movement

(1910 to 1917) Occupational Therapy Emerges

(1910 to 1960) Mental Hygiene Movement

(1914 to 1917) World War I

(1930 to 1940) Occupational Therapy Enters the Medical Model

(1930 to 1960) Psychodynamic & Psychology Approaches Emerge

(1939 to 1946) World War II

(1950s) Pharmacology Approaches Emerge

(1955 to Present) Deinstitutionalization

1965 Community Mental Health Act

(1990s) Recovery Movement Emerges

(2009) Affordable Care Act

Combined with the Affordable Care Act, the President's New Freedom Commission on Mental Health promises to lead to a transformation of mental health care in the United States.

Occupational therapy needs to be an integrated participant in the creation of any new mental health care delivery system. As mental health occupational therapy practitioners, occupational therapy assistants need to be able to recognize sociocultural trends, identify the economy of care for mental health services, and support legislation that promotes the profession. Knowing the history of occupational therapy in mental health practice provides an avenue from which to understand current practice and influence future trends within the profession. Finally, the recovery movement offers occupational therapy the opportunity to help individuals find desired mental health treatment and their path to recovery.

PART 3: APPLICATIONS

The following activities will help you identify key aspects of this chapter, which were highlighted in this text. In particular, these questions highlight the chapter objectives at the start of the chapter. Activities are suggested to be completed individually, in a small group, or as a class to enhance learning.

1. Individually: Identify and give an example of the four early uses of occupation by occupational therapists.

2. Individually: Identify five influences on early occupational therapy practice that affected the current practice of mental health occupational therapy. List them in order from most influential to least influential, and be prepared to discuss how these factors affected occupational therapy practice.

3. As a class: Debate the pros and cons for institutionalization and deinstitutionalization.

4. As a group: Make a chart that lists the characteristics of (1) the medical model of mental health care and (2) community-based mental health care.

5. As a group: List the 10 fundamental components of recovery. Generate examples of how occupational therapy can include the 10 fundamental components in a recovery in the provision of services.

6. As a group: Choose a local community mental program or nonprofit organization. Identify the services it provides. Identify roles an occupational therapy assistant could serve in the organization and provide examples.

REFERENCES

Accordino, M. P., Porter, D. F., & Morse, T. (2001). Deinstitutionalization of persons with severe mental illness: Context and consequences. *Journal of Rehabilitation, 67*(2), 16-21.

American Occupational Therapy Association. (2006). Report of the ad hoc committee on mental health practice in occupational therapy. Retrieved from http://uspra.info/Education/Conference2011/HANDOUTS/Report_of_Ad_Hoc_Committee_on_MH.pdf

American Occupational Therapy Association. (2010). Specialized knowledge and skills in mental health promotion, prevention, and intervention in occupational therapy. *American Journal of Occupational Therapy, 64*, 313-323.

American Occupational Therapy Association. (2014). Occupational therapy practice framework: Domain and process (3rd ed.). *American Journal of Occupational Therapy, 68*(Suppl. 1), S1-S48. doi: 10.5014/ajot2014.682006.

Barton, W. E. (1957). Occupational therapy for psychiatric disorders. In W. R. Dunton, Jr. & S. Licht (Eds.), *Occupational therapy: Principles and practice* (3rd ed., pp. 177-196). Springfield, IL: Charles C. Thomas.

Barton, W. E. (2000). Trends in community mental health programs: Reprint. *Psychiatric Services, 51*(5), 611-615.

Baum, C. M. (2002). Adolph Meyer's challenge: Focus on occupation in practice and in science. *Occupational Therapy Journal of Research, 22*(4), 130-131.

Bing, R. K. (1981). Occupational therapy: A paraphrastic journey. *American Journal of Occupational Therapy, 35*(8), 499-518.

Bing, R. K. (1983). Nationally speaking: Beliefs at a new beginning. *American Journal of Occupational Therapy, 37*(6), 375-379.

Bonder, B. (2010). *Psychopathology and function* (4th ed.). Thorofare, NJ: Slack, Inc.

Briggs, L. V. (1923). *Occupation as a substitute for restraint in the treatment of the mentally ill: A history of the passage of two bills through the Massachusetts Legislature.* Boston, MA: Wright & Potter Printing Company.

Brigham, A. (1844). Article I: Brief notice of the New York State Lunatic Asylum at Utica. *American Journal of Insanity, 1*, 5-6. Retrieved from http://archive.org/details/psyamericanjourn01ameruoft.

Brigham, A. (1847). The moral treatment of insanity. *American Journal of Insanity, 4*, 1. Retrieved from www.disabilitymuseum.org/dhm/edu/detail.html?id=1246&annotations=13&paragraphs=1%2C44-47%2C57-58.

Brown, C. & Stoffel, V. C. (Eds.). (2011). *Occupational therapy in mental health: A vision for participation.* Philadelphia, PA: F. A. Davis Company.

Buchmueller, T. C., Cooper, P. F., Jacobson, M., & Zuvekas, S. H. (2007). Parity for whom? Exceptions and the extent of state mental health parity legislation. *Health Affairs, 26*(4), w483-w487.

Champagne, T., & Gray, K. (2011). Occupational therapy's role in mental health recovery. Retrieved from www.aota.org.

Charland, L. C. (2007). Benevolent theory: Moral treatment at the York Retreat. *History of Psychiatry, 18*(1), 61-80. doi: 10.1177/0957154X07070320.

Costa, D., Molinsky, R., Kent, J. P., & Sauerwald, C. (2011). Integrating mental health knowledge and skills into academic and fieldwork education. *OT Practice, 16*(19), CE1-CE8.

Dunton, W. R. (1918). *Report of the president: Proceedings of the Second Annual Meeting of the National Society for the Promotion of Occupational Therapy* (pp. 15-16). Towson, MD: Sheppard and Enoch Pratt Hospital.

Dunton, W. R. (1919). *Reconstruction therapy*. Philadelphia, PA: W. B. Saunders.

Dunton, W. R. (1921). *Occupation therapy: A manual for nurses*. Philadelphia, PA: W. B. Saunders.

Dunton, W. R. (1947). History and development of occupational therapy. In H. S. Willard & C. S. Spackman (Eds.), *Principles of occupational therapy* (pp. 1-9). Philadelphia, PA: J. B. Lippincott Company.

Early, M. B. (2000). *Mental health concepts and techniques for the occupational therapy assistant* (3rd ed.). New York, NY: Lippincott Williams & Wilkins.

Ellsworth, P. D. (1983). Army psychiatric occupational therapy: From the past and into the future. *Occupational Therapy in Mental Health, 3*(2), 1-6.

Forman, A. (2012). Health costs: Mental care is covered. *Wall Street Journal*. Retrieved from www.wsj.com/articles/ SB10000872396390444620104578006141320966754.

Friedland, J. (1988). Diversional activity: Does it deserve a bad name? *American Journal of Occupational Therapy, 42*(9), 603-608.

Fuller, D. H. (1910). The need of instruction for nurses in occupations for the sick. In S. E. Tracy (Ed.), *Studies in invalid occupations* (pp. 1-15). Boston: Whitcomb & Barrow.

Geller, J. L. (2000). The last half-century of psychiatric services as reflected in Psychiatric Services. *Psychiatric Services, 51*(1), 41-67. doi: 10.1176/ps.51.1.41.

Geller, J. L. & Morrissey, J. P. (2004). Asylum within and without asylums. *Psychiatric Services, 55*(10), 1128-1130. doi: 10.1176/appi.ps.55.10.1128.

Gibson, R. W., D'Amico, M., Jaffe, L., & Arbesman, M. (2011). Occupational therapy interventions for recovery in the areas of community integration and narrative life roles for adults with serious mental illness: A scientific review. *American Journal of Occupational Therapy, 65*(3), 247-256.

Gutman, S. A. (1995). Influence of the US military and occupational therapy reconstruction aides in World War I on the development of occupational therapy. *American Journal of Occupational Therapy, 49*(3), 256-262.

Gutman, S. A. (2011). From the desk of the editor: Special issue: Effectiveness of occupational therapy services in mental health practice. *American Journal of Occupational Therapy, 65*(3), 235–237.

Haas, L. (1944). *Practical occupational therapy for the mentally and nervously ill*. Milwaukee, WI: The Bruce Publishing Company.

Hall, H. J. (1918). *Wartime nerves*. Boston, MA: Houghton Mifflin Company.

Hall, H. J., & Buck, M. M. C. (1915). *The work of our hands: A study of occupations for invalids*. New York, NY: Moffat, Yard, & Company.

Hartwick, A. M. R. (1992). *The Army Medical Specialist Corps, 45*[th] *anniversary*. Washington, DC: Center of Military History, United States Army.

Hays, C., & Baxley, S. (1998). The roles of the state, psychiatric hospital and the occupational therapy practitioner, *Mental Health Interest Section Quarterly, 21*(1), 3-4.

Henry Phipps Psychiatric Service. (2013). Our history. Retrieved from www.hopkinsmedicine.org/psychiatry/about/history.html.

Hopkins, H. L. (1988). An historical perspective on occupational therapy. In H. L. Hopkins & H. D. Smith (Eds.), *Willard and Spackman's occupational therapy* (7th ed., pp. 16-37). Philadelphia, PA: J. B. Lippincott Company.

Hull House. (1925). Hull House Year Book 1925, Author: Frederick Hildmen Printing Co.

Kielhofner, G., & Barris, R. (1984). Mental health occupational therapy: Trends in literature and practice. *Occupational Therapy in Mental Health, 4*(4), 35-50.

Kirkbride, T. S. (1847). *Report of the Pennsylvania Hospital for the Insane*. Philadelphia, PA: TK & PG Collins.

Kirkbride, T. S. (1878). *Code of rules and regulations for the government of those employed in the care of patients of the Pennsylvania Hospital for the Insane at Philadelphia* (3rd ed.). Philadelphia, PA: Collins. Retrieved from http://archive.org/details/39002086342947.med.yale.edu.

Kleinman, B. L. (1992). The challenge of providing occupational therapy in mental health. *American Journal of Occupational Therapy, 46*(6), 555-557.

Klerman, G. L. (1977). Better but not well: Social and ethical issues on the deinstitutionalization of the mentally ill. *Schizophrenia Bulletin, 3*(4), 617-631.

Krieg, R. G. (2001). An interdisciplinary look at the deinstitutionalization of the mentally ill. *The Social Science Journal, 38*, 367-380.

Levine, R. E. (1987). Looking back: The influence of the Arts-and-Crafts movement on the professional status of occupational therapy. *American Journal of Occupational Therapy, 41*(4), 248-254.

Low, J. F. (1992). The reconstruction aides. *American Journal of Occupational Therapy, 46*(1), 38-43.

Marblehead Pottery. (2013). Marblehead pottery history. Retrieved from http://marbleheadpottery.net/marblehead_pottery_site/HISTORY.html.

Mechanic, D. (2012). Seizing opportunities under the Affordable Care Act for transforming the mental and behavioral health system. *Health Affairs, 31*(2), 376-382.

Metropolitan Commissioners in Lunacy. (1844). Article VI: Insanity and asylums for the insane in England and Wales. *American Journal of Insanity, 1*, 155-185.

Meyer, A. (1922/1977). The philosophy of occupation therapy. *American Journal of Occupational Therapy, 31*(10), 639–642.

Moncrief, J. (1999). An investigation into the precedents of modern drug therapy in psychiatry. *History of Psychiatry, 10*(40), 475-490. doi: 10.1177/0957154X9901004004.

Novella, E. J. (2010). Mental health care in the aftermath of deinstitutionalization: A retrospective and prospective view. *Health Care Analysis, 18*, 222-238.

Paterson, C. F. (2002). A short history of occupational therapy in psychiatry. In J. Creek (Ed.), *Occupational therapy and mental health* (3rd ed., pp. 3-14). London, England: Churchill Livingstone.

Peloquin, S. M. (1991a). Looking back: Occupational therapy service: Individual and collective understandings of the founders, part 1. *American Journal of Occupational Therapy, 45*(4), 352-360.

Peloquin, S. M. (1991b). Looking back: Occupational therapy service: Individual and collective understandings of the founders, part 2. *American Journal of Occupational Therapy, 45*(8), 733-744.

Peloquin, S. M. (1994). Looking back: Moral treatment: How a caring practice lost its rationale. *American Journal of Occupational Therapy, 48*(2), 167–173.

Peloquin, S. M. (2000). The philosophy of occupational therapy. In A. J. Punwar & S. M. Peloquin (Eds.) *Occupational therapy: Principles and practices* (3rd ed., pp. 7-20). Baltimore, MD: Lippincott Williams & Wilkins.

Pinel, P. H. (1806). *A treatise on insanity* (D. D. Davis, MD, Trans.). Sheffield, England: W. Todd. Retrieved from http://archive.org/details/treatiseoninsanioopine.

Priebe, S., & Fakhoury, W. (2007). Deinstitutionalization and reinstitutionalization: Major changes in the provision of mental healthcare. *Psychiatry, 6*(8), 313-316.

Quiroga, V. A. M. (1995). *Occupational therapy: The first 30 years: 1900 to 1930*. Bethesda, MD: American Occupational Therapy Association.

Reed, K. L. (1993). The beginnings of occupational therapy. In H. L. Hopkins & H. D. Smith (Eds.), *Willard and Spackman's occupational therapy* (8th ed., pp. 26-43). Philadelphia, PA: J. B. Lippincott Company.

Reilly, M. (1962). Occupational therapy can be one of the great ideas of 20th century medicine. *American Journal of Occupational Therapy, 16,* 1-9.

Rush, B. (1812). *Medical inquiries and observations, upon the diseases of the mind.* Philadelphia, PA: Kimber & Richardson. Retrieved from http://archive.org/details/medicalinquiries1812rush.

Sawyer, A. (2011). Translating mental health policy into practice: Ongoing challenges and frustrations. *Health Sociology Review, 20*(2), 114-119.

Schemm, R. L. (1994). Looking back: Bridging conflicting ideologies: The origins of American and British occupational therapy. *American Journal of Occupational Therapy, 48*(11), 1082–1088.

Scull, A. (2011a). The mental health sector and social sciences in post-World War II USA: Part 1: Total war and its aftermath. *History of Psychiatry, 22*(1), 3-19. doi: 10.1177/0957154X10388366.

Scull, A. (2011b). The mental health sector and social sciences in post-World War II USA: Part 2: The impact of Federal research funding and drugs revolution. *History of Psychiatry, 22*(3), 268-284. doi: 10.1177/0957154X10391131.

Sharfstein, S. S. (2000). Whatever happened to community mental health?. *Psychiatric Services, 51*(5), 616-620.

Smaldone, A., & Cullen-Drill, M. (2010). Mental health parity legislation: Understanding the pros and cons. *Journal of Psychosocial Nursing, 48*(9), 26-34.

Society of Arts and Crafts. (2013). The Society of Arts and Crafts: Background and history. Retrieved from www.societyofcrafts.org/about/about.asp.

Stoffel, V. C. (2010), Recovery, In C. Brown & V. Stoffel (Eds.), *Occupational therapy in mental health: A vision for participation.* (pp. 3-15). Philadelphia, PA: FA Davis.

Substance Abuse and Mental Health Service Administration. (2011). Recovery to practice: Frequently asked questions. Retrieved from https://www.providerexpress.com/content/dam/ope-provexpr/us/pdfs/clinResourcesMain/rrToolkit/samhsaRecoveryFAQ.pdf

Tracy, S. E. (1910). *Studies in invalid occupation: A manual for nurses and attendants.* Boston, MA: Whitcomb & Barrows.

Tuke, S. (1813). *Description of the retreat, an institution near York for insane persons.* Philadelphia, PA: Isaac Peirce. Retrieved from http://collections.nlm.nih.gov/muradora/objectView.action?pid=nlm:nlmuid-2575045R-bk.

U.S. Department of Education. (2007). Special education and rehabilitation services. Archived: A 25 yr history of the IDEA. Retrieved from www2.ed.gov/policy/speced/leg/idea/history.html.

U.S. Department of Health and Human Services. (1999). *Mental health: A report of the Surgeon General* (Executive Summary). Rockville, MD: U.S. Department of Health and Human Services, Substance Abuse and Mental Health Services Administration, Center for Mental Health Services, & National Institute of Mental Health.

Vaughn, S. J. (1919). Bedside occupational therapy. *Carry On: A Magazine on the Reconstruction of Disabled Soldiers and Sailors, 1*(6), 13-15.

Werner, J. L., & Tyler, J. M. (1993). Community-based interventions: A return to community mental health centers' origins. *Journal of Counseling and Development, 71,* 689-692.

West, W. L. (Ed.) (1959). *Changing concepts and practices in psychiatric occupational therapy.* New York, NY: American Occupational Therapy Association.

2

Standards of Practice in Mental Health Occupational Therapy

Jeremy L. Keough, MSOT, OTR/L and Christine A. Manville, EdD, OTR/L

KEY TERMS

• Activity Limitations	• Core Knowledge and Skills	• Occupational Therapy Process
• Biopsychosocial Model	• *Diagnostic and Statistical Manual*	• Participation Restrictions
• Bloom's Taxonomy	• *International Classification of Functioning*	• People-First Language
• Body Functions		• Service Competency
• Body Structures	• Occupation	• Specialized Knowledge and Skills
• Client-Centered	• *Occupational Therapy Practice Framework*	• Supervision
• Client Factors		

CHAPTER LEARNING OBJECTIVES

After completion of this chapter, students should be able to:

1. Define the term *foundational knowledge*. Distinguish the foundational knowledge that occupational therapy practitioners have in common with core mental health practitioners.

2. List the components of the *International Classification of Functioning, Disability, and Health* (ICF).

3. Describe how the *Diagnostic and Statistical Manual* (DSM; 5th ed.) is used by individuals who work with individuals diagnosed with metal illness.

4. Compare and contrast the roles of the occupational therapy assistant and occupational therapist in the provision of mental health services.

5. Discuss the influence of state and mental health service organizations on the provision of mental health occupational therapy services.

6. Distinguish advanced practices of occupational therapy assistants from entry-level skills in providing mental health services.

Manville, C.A., & Keough, J. L.
Mental Health Practice for the Occupational Therapy Assistant (pp 25-52).
© 2016 Taylor & Francis Group.

CHAPTER OUTLINE

INTRODUCTION

[T]he vision of mental health as not merely the absence of mental illness, but the presence of something positive. (Keyes, 2007)

Absence of mental illness does not imply the presence of mental health, and the absence of mental health does not imply the presence of mental illness. (Keyes, 2007, p. 100)

Achieving health, well-being, and participation in life through engagement in occupations. (American Occupational Therapy Association [AOTA], 2014)

Occupational therapy assistants provide wellness and mental health services to clients using the knowledge and skills each practitioner attains in his or her education and training. Occupational therapy, founded in psychiatry, shares foundational knowledge and skills in mental health treatment with other core mental health professionals. Foundational knowledge refers to information needed to practice in mental health settings. This knowledge is gained through completion of general undergraduate coursework, as well as course-specific occupational therapy assistant education. The AOTA document "Specialized Knowledge and Skills in Mental Health Promotion, Prevention, and Intervention in Occupational Therapy Practice" identifies some of these common knowledge and skills (2010a). In addition, the *International Classification of Functioning, Disability and Health* (ICF) and *Diagnostic and Statistical Manual* (DSM-5) also describe common knowledge and skills occupational therapy assistants share with other mental health professionals.

This chapter focuses on the ***specialized knowledge and skills*** required of the occupational therapy assistant who works in the practice area of mental health. Contextual influences on mental health service delivery are introduced. Finally, government and state agencies, as well as national and community organizations, that provide mental health services to clients are identified.

PART 1: FOUNDATIONAL KNOWLEDGE IN MENTAL HEALTH SERVICE DELIVERY

International Classification of Functioning, Disability, and Health

The ***ICF*** was created by the World Health Organization (WHO) to provide a common language to describe health and health-related states in an individual. The aim was to design a document that could aid scientific research, improve communication, and enable improved comparison of information gathered from groups in different locations. The ICF is considered a ***biopsychosocial model*** (see Chapter 1). The ICF incorporates both the medical model of care delivery and a social model of disability. Health care in the United States will increasingly incorporate the organizational structure of the WHO. Occupational therapy practitioners will need to be familiar with the ICF to be able to provide adequate services.

In the ICF, the WHO describes the context of health as including activity and participation. The ICF defines activity as "the execution of a task or action by an individual" and participation as "involvement in a life situation"

CHECKPOINT 2-1. IDENTIFYING THE CORRESPONDING LEVELS OF FUNCTION AND DYSFUNCTION		
Levels of Functioning	Levels of Dysfunction	Description
Body function and body structures	Impairments	Significant variation or deficit with a body function or body structure
Individual or whole person	Activity limitations	Troubles a person may have performing activities
Societal	Participation restrictions	Complications a person may experience performing life situations
Adapted from World Health Organization. (2001). *International Classification of Functioning, Disability, and Health (ICF)*. Geneva, Switzerland: Author.		

(WHO, 2001, p. 234). Although the concepts of *activity* and *participation* are used in the ICF to help identify potential problems, they also are utilized to explore other variables that may affect a person's ability to function. The ICF has moved away from "the consequence of a disease to the focus on the components of health that enable functioning" (WHO, 2001). As a result, the ICF utilizes a more client-centered approach. Within the ICF, levels of function have been created, as well as their corresponding levels of dysfunction. Levels of function and dysfunction assist in the identification of intact systems that enable participation in life. Levels of function may be at the body function or body structure level, individual or whole-person level, and societal level. The corresponding levels of dysfunction are labeled **impairments**, **activity limitations**, and **participation restrictions** (Checkpoint 2-1). "Understanding" identifies three levels of functioning with their corresponding level of dysfunction within the ICF.

Occupational therapy services often address all three levels of dysfunction. At times, this can be accomplished in one therapy session. More frequently, the occupational therapy practitioner must prioritize focus on one level of dysfunction and look for carryover in the other areas of functioning. For example, whereas the provision of mental health occupational therapy services may be clear-cut when working with individuals who are hospitalized for acute symptoms, providing services for individuals who live in the community and are experiencing activity limitations and participation restrictions can be more challenging to the entry-level practitioner.

Diagnostic and Statistical Manual

The DSM is published by the American Psychiatric Association. It is a handbook that establishes the standard by which doctors in the United States, as well as other parts of the world, classify, diagnose, and treat mental disorders. A mental disorder is a medical condition that disrupts a person's thinking, feeling, mood, and ability to relate to others, thereby affecting the individual's ability to function in everyday life. There have been five revisions to the DSM since it was first published in 1952.

The DSM provides a common language that permits a wide range of health and mental health professionals, including occupational therapy assistants, to communicate with one another when sharing information about clients. In addition to diagnostic classifications and criteria, the text includes an introduction that discusses how to use the DSM and a section that provides self-assessment tools. This section also includes a discussion on diagnostic categories that require more research.

The DSM-5 is the manual's first major revision in nearly 20 years. The chapters are organized to demonstrate how disorders are related to one another, and each mental disorder is framed by age, gender, and developmental characteristics. The text itself has three major components: diagnostic classification, diagnostic criteria, and descriptive text. All three factors should be considered by physicians and clinicians before a diagnosis of mental illness is made. Although the role of an occupational therapy assistant does not include the task of diagnosing a mental illness, general knowledge of the symptoms associated with mental health disorders is important in order to understand the potential impact these factors have on an individual's ability to participate in meaningful activities and occupations and participate fully within the community.

The *diagnostic classification* refers to the list of the mental disorders that are included in the DSM system. The process of making a diagnosis consists of selecting those disorders from the DSM that best characterize the symptoms currently being exhibited by the individual undergoing evaluation. Accompanying each diagnostic label is a diagnostic code, which is derived from the *International Classification of Diseases, Ninth Edition, Clinical Modification*. These diagnostic codes are used by institutions and agencies for billing purposes and for collecting research data.

Each disorder included in the DSM has a corresponding set of *diagnostic criteria*. These criteria specify the symptoms that must be present and the duration that must have been experienced by the individual who is being evaluated. Other considerations include the symptoms, disorders, and conditions that must not be present in order to qualify for a particular diagnosis. These criteria help to increase

CHECKPOINT 2-2. UNDERSTANDING HOW DIAGNOSTIC CRITERIA ARE USED IN THE DSM 5

Generalized Anxiety Disorder (Code)

A. Excessive anxiety or worry that happens more days than not for a minimum of 6 months.

B. The individual cannot control the anxiety

C. The anxiety and worry are associated with at least three of the following symptoms:

- Restlessness
- Fatigue
- Difficulty with concentration
- Demonstrated irritability
- Tense muscles
- Difficulty with sleep

D. The symptoms cause substantial distress or impairment in everyday life.

E. The disturbance is not due to substance use or a different medical condition.

F. The disturbance is not better explained by another mental illness.

Adapted from American Psychiatric Association. (2013). *Diagnostic and statistical manual of mental disorders* (5th ed.). Washington, D.C.: Author.

CHECKPOINT 2-3. APPLYING PEOPLE-FIRST LANGUAGE

Say	*Instead of*
Individuals diagnosed with mental illness	The mentally ill
She has been diagnosed with autism spectrum disorder.	She's autistic.
He has a mental health condition.	He is mentally disturbed.
She receives Special Education Services.	She's in special ed.
He has a brain injury.	He is brain damaged.

diagnostic reliability. It is important, however, to remember that diagnostic criteria are meant to be used as guidelines and not as a means to describe or stereotype individuals. Checkpoint 2-2 offers an example of the diagnostic criteria associated with a diagnosis of generalized anxiety disorder.

To avoid defining a person by his or her illness, occupational therapy practitioners should always use **people-first language**. People-first language puts the person before the disability and describes the type of mental illness that the person has, not who a person is. In other words, an individual is *diagnosed* with schizophrenia; he is not a "schizophrenic." When people define others by their illness or use blanket statements like "the mentally ill," they promote the use of stereotypes. Stereotypes are assumptions made about individuals that are based on the presumed qualities of the group to which they belong. An example of a stereotype that incorporates a blanket statement is the sentence "The mentally ill are all dangerous." Stereotypes can lead to inaccurate assessments of an individual's skills and ability to participate fully within a community. They are associated

with stigma, prejudice, and discrimination, all of which lead to the reluctance of individuals who are experiencing symptoms of mental illness to seek treatment. Checkpoint 2-3 offers examples of people-first language.

In the DSM, *descriptive text* accompanies each mental disorder. The text of the DSM systematically describes each disorder using the following headings:

- Diagnostic Features
- Associated Features
- Supporting Diagnosis
- Subtypes and/or Specifiers
- Prevalence
- Development and Course
- Risk and Prognostic Factors
- Diagnostic Measures
- Functional Consequences
- Culture-Related Diagnostic Issues

- Gender-Related Diagnostic Issues
- Differential Diagnosis
- Recording Procedures

Currently, more than 200 mental disorders are listed in the DSM-5. These disorders may be caused by a combination of factors, including but not limited to biochemical imbalances, environmental stressors, and biologic stressors. Because the understanding of mental health and the causes of mental disorders are constantly expanding, the diagnostic criteria in the DSM must be updated periodically. In each revision, mental health conditions that are no longer considered accurate are removed or altered, and newly defined conditions are added. Historically, agreement among health care professionals regarding such revisions has been difficult to achieve. Some of the recent and controversial changes to the DSM-5 include combining the subcategories of autism into one single category labeled *autism spectrum disorder* and the creation of a new category called *disruptive mood dysregulation* disorder to describe intense outbursts and irritability beyond what is considered normal in young children (Grohol, 2011). The following are categories of disorders from the DSM-5 that include the diagnoses more commonly seen by occupational therapy practitioners in the individuals whom they treat:

- Neurodevelopmental disorders
- Schizophrenia spectrum and other psychotic disorders
- Bipolar and related disorders
- Depressive disorders
- Anxiety disorders
- Trauma and stressor-related disorders
- Neurocognitive disorders
- Personality disorders

These diagnoses will be described in more detail in subsequent chapters, along with treatment interventions utilized by the occupational therapy assistant to address symptoms associated with each of them.

Core Mental Health Professional Knowledge and Skills

The education of the occupational therapy assistant prepares the student with core knowledge and skills similar to that of other mental health professionals. Shared core mental health knowledge and skills are taught in general education courses that include topics such as general psychology,

human development, abnormal psychology, and group dynamics. Core mental health professional knowledge and skills for occupational therapy practitioners are identified in the document "Specialized Knowledge and Skills in Mental Health Promotion, Prevention, and Intervention in Occupational Therapy Practice" (AOTA, 2010a). Table 2-1 illustrates a brief statement for each of the various core mental health professional knowledge and skills that apply to the occupational therapy assistant. More detailed descriptions of these knowledge and skills can be found in the document mentioned earlier.

Core mental health professional knowledge and skills are divided into three domains that include evaluation and intervention, professional role and service outcome, and mental health systems. Additionally, knowledge and skills of each domain are further described into categories that include knowledge, performance skills, and reasoning skills. Occupational therapy assistants utilize each domain as they provide mental health occupational therapy services. The domain of evaluation and intervention describes how occupational therapy assistants work in collaboration with the occupational therapist during non–profession-specific evaluations and provision of services. The domain of professional role and service outcome reflects that occupational therapy assistants are part of a team of stakeholders that is interested in the mental health of their clients as well as achieving effective and efficient outcomes. Finally, the domain of mental health systems recognizes how multiple diverse systems affect mental health service delivery.

Occupational therapy assistant practitioners possess the knowledge and skills to provide services covered in each domain with supervision from and in collaboration with the occupational therapist. It is important to note that although occupational therapy assistant practitioners are competent at entry-level practice for some tasks, they are not expected to master knowledge and skills in all treatment techniques used by occupational therapy practitioners in mental health. It is assumed that some skills will be developed through experience after entry-level practice has been attained. *Service competency* describes a clinician's attainment of skills or abilities that may be utilized or expected at a particular setting. Throughout this text, students will be cued when service competency may be necessary for advanced-level practice. Entry-level practice expectations for the occupational therapy assistant are identified for each skill and knowledge. Entry-level practice expectations include the following:

- *Competent at entry level:* The occupational therapy assistant is capable of independent performance for this knowledge or skill at entry level.

TABLE 2-1

Core Mental Health Professional Knowledge and Skills for the Occupational Therapy Assistant Applied to Occupational Therapy Services

Knowledge of: Occupational therapy assistant practitioners demonstrate specific knowledge in the following three domains of the core mental health professional knowledge and skills. The first column under each domain identifies the level of knowledge entry-level occupational therapy assistant practitioners have with other core mental health professionals. The second column under each domain identifies the common knowledge entry-level occupational therapy assistant practitioners share with other core mental health professionals. The numbers correspond with each common knowledge item identified in "Specialized Knowledge and Skills in Mental Health Promotion, Prevention, and Intervention in Occupational Therapy Practice" (AOTA, 2010a).

EVALUATION AND INTERVENTION

Competent at entry level practice to demonstrate and apply knowledge	
	(1) Factors affecting psychiatric conditions
	(2) Traditional and concurrent viewpoints on mental health care
	(3) The current DSM-5 and its uses
	(4) Common symptoms with mental illness
	(5) Actions and side effects of medicine management
	(6) Interdisciplinary, evidence-based practice and service delivery models

PROFESSIONAL ROLE AND SERVICE OUTCOME

Competent at entry level practice to demonstrate and apply knowledge	
	(19) Mental health care roles in service delivery
	(20) Role differentiation and collaboration between mental health professionals
	(21) Measuring client outcomes in mental health services
	(22) Approaches and standards used to identify needs and produce recommendations

MENTAL HEALTH SYSTEM

Competent at entry-level practice to demonstrate and apply knowledge	(28) Political, organizational, and legal influences on mental health care
Competent at entry level practice to analyze and integrate knowledge	(29) Reimbursement and funding structures for mental health care
Competent at entry level practice to demonstrate and apply knowledge	(30) Variety of mental health service settings
	(31) Stakeholders of mental health care
	(32) Organizations and their standards that influence mental health care

(continued)

TABLE 2-1 (CONTINUED)

MENTAL HEALTH PROFESSIONAL KNOWLEDGE AND SKILLS FOR THE OCCUPATIONAL THERAPY ASSISTANT APPLIED TO OCCUPATIONAL THERAPY SERVICES

Performance Skills: Occupational therapy assistant practitioners demonstrate specific performance skills in the following three domains of the core mental health professional knowledge and skills. The first column under each domain identifies the level of performance skill entry-level occupational therapy assistant practitioners have with other core mental health professionals. The second column under each domain identifies the performance skill entry-level occupational therapy assistant practitioners share with other core mental health professionals. The numbers correspond with each performance skill item identified in "Specialized Knowledge and Skills in Mental Health Promotion, Prevention, and Intervention in Occupational Therapy Practice" (AOTA, 2010a).

EVALUATION AND INTERVENTION		PROFESSIONAL ROLE AND SERVICE OUTCOME		MENTAL HEALTH SYSTEMS	
Assist at entry level	(7) Evaluate mental health status	**Competent at entry level**	(23) Write mental health care documentation and behavioral objectives	**Assist at entry level**	(33) Retrieve pertinent information and confirm service delivery and documentation complies with current standards
	(8) Form rapport and foster behavioral change				
	(9) Select, direct, and enable crisis resolution one-on-one and in groups				
	(10) Execute functional assessments	**Assist at entry level**	(24) Display fundamental skills with program development and consultation services	**Competent at entry level**	(34) Foster consumer, family-driven, and community-focused delivery systems
	(11) Recognize medical necessity for service provision				
	(12) Create and implement intervention approaches one on one and in groups				

(continued)

TABLE 2-1 (CONTINUED)

MENTAL HEALTH PROFESSIONAL KNOWLEDGE AND SKILLS FOR THE OCCUPATIONAL THERAPY ASSISTANT APPLIED TO OCCUPATIONAL THERAPY SERVICES

Reasoning Skills: Occupational therapy assistant practitioners demonstrate specific reasoning skills in the following three domains of the core mental health professional knowledge and skills. The first column under each domain identifies the level of reasoning skill entry-level occupational therapy assistant practitioners have with other core mental health professionals. The second column under each domain identifies the reasoning skill entry-level occupational therapy assistant practitioners share with other core mental health professionals. The numbers correspond with each reasoning skill item identified in "Specialized Knowledge and Skills in Mental Health Promotion, Prevention, and Intervention in Occupational Therapy Practice" (AOTA, 2010a).

EVALUATION AND INTERVENTION		PROFESSIONAL ROLE AND SERVICE OUTCOME		MENTAL HEALTH SYSTEM	
Assist at entry level	(13) Assess human development and behaviors over the lifespan	**Assist at entry level**	(25) Combine and assess viewpoints of stakeholders to maximize client outcomes	**Assist at entry level**	(35) Appraise factors affecting health, wellness, and participation
Competent at entry level	(14) Incorporate client-centered and recovery oriented approaches		(26) Combine and integrate factors into consultation and program planning		(36) Assess the interactions of systems and their effect on mental health
	(15) Understand how personal values, beliefs, and attitudes affect recovery potential		(27) Appraise obstacles to programs and mental health services	**Competent at entry level**	(37) Incorporate consumer, survivor, and ex-patient movement as applicable to services and systems of care
Assist at entry level	16) Assess culture, diversity, societal, and values on individuals				
	(17) Appraise present medical and mental health methods and interventions				
	(18) Create theories and models to guide the provision of mental health care				

Adapted from American Occupational Therapy Association. (2010b). Specialized knowledge and skills in mental health promotion, prevention, and intervention in occupational therapy practice. *American Journal of Occupational Therapy, 64*(6), 313-323.

- *Assist at entry level:* The occupational therapy assistant requires assistance at entry level for this knowledge or skill. Some knowledge and skills will always require assistance from the occupational therapist. Other knowledge and skills may be mastered after entry-level practice has been attained by developing service competency. Service competency for some knowledge and skills may be developed through cross-training, collaboration with the occupational therapist, on-the-job training, and continuing education.

- *Competent at entry-level practice to analyze and integrate knowledge to make judgments about occupational therapy provision:* This aspect of entry-level practice reflects Level 4 of the cognitive domain Analyzing. This level of ability is characterized by being able to break concepts and material into parts and determine how each is related to the others. This action reflects clinical reasoning used by the occupational therapy assistant in the provision of occupational therapy services.

- *Competent at entry-level practice to demonstrate and apply it to occupational therapy practice:* This aspect of entry-level practice reflects Level 3 of the cognitive domain, *applying*. This level of ability is characterized by carrying out procedures and implementing learned materials in new and concrete circumstances. This action reflects part of the clinical reasoning of the occupational therapy assistant, as well as the application of occupational therapy services.

The ICF, the DSM, and the document "Knowledge and Skills of Core Mental Health Professionals" all provide valuable information an occupational therapy assistant practitioner needs to effectively provide services, and in particular, mental health care services. At the entry level, occupational therapy assistant practitioners must also display profession-specific skills in the areas of mental health promotion, prevention, and intervention. These skills will be described in the second half of this chapter.

PART 2: STANDARDS OF PRACTICE FOR MENTAL HEALTH CARE SERVICES

Specialized Knowledge and Skills in Mental Health Services

The AOTA document "Specialized Knowledge and Skills in Mental Health Promotion, Prevention, and Intervention in Occupational Therapy Practice" describes profession-specific knowledge and skills required of occupational therapy assistant practitioners in mental health practice (AOTA, 2010a). Specific knowledge and skills are divided into four domains to include foundations, evaluation and intervention, professional role and service outcome, and mental health systems. Each domain is the same except for the addition of the domain foundations. This domain refers to knowledge that allows for mental health service promotion, prevention, and intervention delivery.

The knowledge and skills of each domain are further delineated into categories that include knowledge, performance skills, and reasoning skills. Entry-level practice expectations for the occupational therapy assistant are identified for each skill and knowledge level. Descriptions for practice expectations for the occupational therapy assistant are the same as described earlier in this chapter. They include the following:

- Competent at entry level
- Assist at entry level
- Competent at entry-level practice to analyze and integrate knowledge to make judgments about occupational therapy provision
- Competent at entry-level practice to demonstrate and apply it to occupational therapy practice

Table 2-2 illustrates the specialized knowledge and skills of occupational therapy assistants in mental health services. A more detailed description of each knowledge and skill can be seen by referencing the AOTA source document (AOTA, 2010b).

Core mental health professional knowledge and skills and specialized profession knowledge and skills of the occupational therapy assistant are generally reflected in educational standards for occupational therapy assistant programs. The AOTA identifies entry-level practice competency through the Accreditation Council for Occupational Therapy Education (ACOTE) (AOTA, 2006). ACOTE created the "Accreditation Standards for an Educational Program for the Occupational Therapy Assistant." These standards are used by occupational therapy assistant education programs to design curriculum that will prepare students for entry-level practice.

ACOTE identifies many general entry-level competencies in their standards that apply to mental health and other areas of occupational therapy practice. Examples of these general competencies related to core and specialized knowledge and skills of mental health care include the following:

- B.1.5: Demonstrate knowledge and understanding of human development throughout the lifespan

- B.1.6: Demonstrate knowledge and understanding of the concepts of human behavior to include behavioral and social sciences

- B.1.7: Demonstrate knowledge and appreciation of the role of sociocultural, socioeconomic, and diversity factors in society

TABLE 2-2

SPECIALIZED KNOWLEDGE AND SKILLS APPLIED TO MENTAL HEALTH PROMOTION, PREVENTION, AND INTERVENTION

Knowledge Of: Occupational therapy assistant practitioners demonstrate specific knowledge in the following four domains of specialized knowledge and skills applied to mental health promotion, prevention, and intervention. The first column under each domain identifies the level of knowledge and skills applied to mental health promotion, prevention, and intervention. The first column under each domain identifies the level of knowledge entry-level occupational therapy assistant practitioners have with mental health expertise specific to occupational therapy practice. The second column under each domain identifies the specific specialized knowledge of entry-level occupational therapy assistant practitioners. The numbers correspond with each specialized knowledge item identified in "Specialized Knowledge and Skills in Mental Health Promotion, Prevention, and Intervention in Occupational Therapy Practice" (AOTA, 2010a).

FOUNDATIONS	EVALUATION AND INTERVENTION	PROFESSIONAL ROLES AND SERVICE OUTCOMES	MENTAL HEALTH SYSTEMS
Competent at Entry Level to Demonstrate Knowledge and Apply to Occupational Therapy Practice	**Competent at entry level to demonstrate knowledge and apply to occupational therapy practice**	**Competent at Entry level to analyze and integrate knowledge to make judgments about occupational therapy service provision**	**Competent at entry level to demonstrate knowledge and apply to occupational therapy practice**
(38) Nonpsychiatric conditions and occupational therapy practice	(43) The role of occupational therapy in evaluation and intervention of well-impaired populations	(84) Scope and standards of practice related to mental health occupational therapy	(107) Settings and environments where mental health occupational therapy services are provided
	Competent at Entry level to analyze and integrate knowledge to make judgments about occupational therapy service provision	**Competent at entry level to demonstrate knowledge and apply to occupational therapy practice**	(108) Supporting systems of available resources
	(44) Influences of mental health on individual occupations	(85) Intervention, education, and consultation occupational therapy roles in mental health services	
	(45) Influence of mental health systems and medications on performance skills	(86) Occupational Therapy and other mental health providers scope of practice	
	(46) How values, beliefs, spirituality, self-efficacy, and lived experience affect meaning and occupation	**Competent at entry level to analyze and integrate knowledge to make judgments about occupational therapy service provision**	
		(87) Financial resources for occupational therapy services in mental health systems	

(continued)

TABLE 2-2 (CONTINUED)

SPECIALIZED KNOWLEDGE AND SKILLS APPLIED TO MENTAL HEALTH PROMOTION, PREVENTION, AND INTERVENTION

FOUNDATIONS	EVALUATION AND INTERVENTION	PROFESSIONAL ROLES AND SERVICE OUTCOMES	MENTAL HEALTH SYSTEMS
	(47) Evaluation of occupational engagement and component parts	**Competent at entry level to demonstrate knowledge and apply to occupational therapy practice**	(88) Methods to assess occupation-based outcomes and client satisfaction with mental health occupational therapy services
	(48) Environmental assistance and adaptation to support participation in different contexts		
	(49) Cognitive skills training and adaptive strategies		
	(50) Sensory processing and modulation skill development and adaptive strategies		
	(51) Contextual adaptation and methods to affect mental health systems, impairments, and disabilities		
	(52) Learning styles and instructional delivery to meet the mental health care needs of clients		

(continued)

TABLE 2-2 (CONTINUED)

SPECIALIZED KNOWLEDGE AND SKILLS APPLIED TO MENTAL HEALTH PROMOTION, PREVENTION, AND INTERVENTION

Performance Skills: Occupational therapy assistant practitioners demonstrate specific performance skills in the following four domains of specialized knowledge and skills applied to mental health promotion, prevention, and intervention. The first column under each domain identifies the level of performance skill entry-level occupational therapy assistant practitioners have with mental health expertise specific to occupational therapy practice. The second column under each domain identifies the specific specialized performance skills of entry-level occupational therapy assistant practitioners. The numbers correspond with each specialized performance skill item identified in "Specialized Knowledge and Skills in Mental Health Promotion, Prevention, and Intervention in Occupational Therapy Practice" (AOTA, 2010a).

FOUNDATIONS		EVALUATION AND INTERVENTION		PROFESSIONAL ROLES AND SERVICE OUTCOMES		MENTAL HEALTH SYSTEMS	
Competent at entry level to demonstrate knowledge and apply to occupational therapy practice	(39) Assess the relationship of health, well-being, and participation in occupations over the lifespan	Able to assist at entry level	(53) Create an occupational profile	Competent at entry level	(89) Select strategies that encourage professional relationships with stakeholders	Competent at entry level	(109) Utilize interventions to comprehend the obstacles to occupational performance
	(40) Assess activities, occupations, environments, and contexts that have an influence on the client		(54) Integrate awareness of co-commitment factors that influence occupational performance		(90) Describe how occupational therapy services complement and assist other services		(110) Assist clients to gain access to support systems
			(55) Evaluate occupational performance and occupational engagement	Able to assist at entry level	(91) Provide a needs assessment of how occupational therapy services may be utilized in a system	Able to assist at entry level	(111) Make changes and accommodations for systems to enhance services
			(56) Evaluate performance skills		(92) Collaborate with stakeholders to evaluate mental health and services	Competent at entry level	(112) Acquire and discern information about systems

(continued)

TABLE 2-2 (CONTINUED)

SPECIALIZED KNOWLEDGE AND SKILLS APPLIED TO MENTAL HEALTH PROMOTION, PREVENTION, AND INTERVENTION

FOUNDATIONS	EVALUATION AND INTERVENTION	PROFESSIONAL ROLES AND SERVICE OUTCOMES	MENTAL HEALTH SYSTEMS
	(57) Evaluate client performance patterns	(93) Utilize standardized assessments, procedures, and tools	**Able to assist at entry level** (113) Describe the role of occupational therapist as it applies to different stakeholders
	(58) Evaluate client factors	(94) Create procedures for quality improvement	(114) Recommend leadership roles and opportunities in mental health systems
	(59) Evaluate the environment and contextual factors	(95) Utilize evidence-based practice to create and apply needs assessments	(115) Make use of organizational data to help systems provide services
	(60) Identify medical necessity for occupational therapy mental health services	(96) Incorporate consultative services in systems	(116) Acquire and discriminate information about reimbursements systems for occupational therapy services
	Competent at entry level (61) Work together with clients to identify desired outcomes	(97) Improve occupational therapy services through process and administrative changes	
	Able to assist at entry level (62) Work together with clients to identify and aid clients to complete life tasks and roles		

(continued)

Table 2-2 (continued)

Specialized Knowledge and Skills Applied to Mental Health Promotion, Prevention, and Intervention

Foundations	Evaluation and Intervention		Professional Roles and Service Outcomes		Mental Health Systems	
		(63) Integrate various approaches to optimize occupational performance				
	Competent at entry level	(64) Facilitate competency development for clients				
		(65) Create interventions through the use of activities				
	Able to assist at entry level	(66) Create and apply group and individual interventions				
		(67) Educate clients on the use of their sensory system				

(continued)

TABLE 2-2 (CONTINUED)

SPECIALIZED KNOWLEDGE AND SKILLS APPLIED TO MENTAL HEALTH PROMOTION, PREVENTION, AND INTERVENTION

FOUNDATIONS	EVALUATION AND INTERVENTION	PROFESSIONAL ROLES AND SERVICE OUTCOMES	MENTAL HEALTH SYSTEMS
	(68) Educate clients on their strengths and obstacles		
	(69) Create adaptations to environments and contexts		
	(70) Choose and share evidence-based practice with stakeholders		
	(71) Choose optimal instructional delivery methods to meet individual client needs		

(continued)

TABLE 2-2 (CONTINUED)

SPECIALIZED KNOWLEDGE AND SKILLS APPLIED TO MENTAL HEALTH PROMOTION, PREVENTION, AND INTERVENTION

Reasoning Skills: Occupational therapy assistant practitioners demonstrate specific reasoning skills in the following four domains of specialized knowledge and skills applied to mental health promotion, prevention, and intervention. The first column under each domain identifies the level of reasoning skill entry-level occupational therapy assistant practitioners have with mental health expertise specific to occupational therapy practice. The second column under each domain identifies the specific specialized reasoning skills of entry-level occupational therapy assistant practitioners. The numbers correspond with each specialized reasoning skill item identified in "Specialized Knowledge and Skills in Mental Health Promotion, Prevention, and Intervention in Occupational Therapy Practice" (AOTA, 2010a).

FOUNDATIONS		EVALUATION AND INTERVENTION		PROFESSIONAL ROLES AND SERVICE OUTCOMES		MENTAL HEALTH SYSTEMS	
Able to assist at entry level	(41) Assess and choose occupational therapy theories, frames of reference, and intervention models to provide mental health care services	**Able to assist at entry level**	(72) Put together different information to apply appropriately to the occupational therapy process	**Able to assist at entry level**	(98) Evaluation key outcomes for clients receiving occupational therapy services	**Competent at entry level**	(117) Distinguish between consumer-driven, community-focused care and staff-controlled, institutional-driven goals
	(42) Evaluate and identify how to influence the interaction of the person, environment, and activity among well, at risk, and impaired clients to affect occupational participation	**Competent at entry level**	(73) Identify when appropriate to refer clients for other services	**Competent at entry level**	(99) Reason how recovery affects occupational engagement		(118) Distinguish between "recovery," "resilience," and "strength based" from deficit-based care
		Able to assist at entry level	(74) Assess how contextual factors positively or negatively support a client	**Able to assist at entry level**	(100) Assess and identify appropriate outcome assessment method and tools to meet client and stakeholder needs	**Able to assist at entry level**	(119) Differentiate and produce consumer–family-driven mental health care for clients and stakeholders

(continued)

Table 2-2 (continued)

Specialized Knowledge and Skills Applied to Mental Health Promotion, Prevention, and Intervention

Foundations	Evaluation and Intervention	Professional Roles and Service Outcomes	Mental Health Systems
	75) Identify the result of mental health treatment on occupational performance	101) Select treatment services that are appropriate for the recipient of the services and services provider	120) Assess the relationship with the client and stakeholders on mental health and occupational participation
	76) Recognize and assess obstacles to occupational participation from the influence of past lived experiences	102) Recognize and appraise conditions that influence change for clients	121) Distinguish how systemic changes in mental health delivery affect occupational participation on the client
	77) Put together information to produce appropriate interventions in multiple contexts	103) Recognize and appraise conditions that deter or encourage occupational therapy services	
	78) Prepare for obstacles to participation to maximize engagement in occupations	104) Validate rationale for changes in occupational therapy services for clients	
	79) Combine occupational therapy services and available supports to maximize participation in occupations	105) Relate occupational therapy outcome measures to outcome measures used by stakeholders of mental health services	

(continued)

Table 2-2 (continued)

Specialized Knowledge and Skills Applied to Mental Health Promotion, Prevention, and Intervention

FOUNDATIONS	EVALUATION AND INTERVENTION		PROFESSIONAL ROLES AND SERVICE OUTCOMES	MENTAL HEALTH SYSTEMS
	(80) Plan the most appropriate occupational therapy services for a client		(106) Combine the OTPF language with language used by stakeholders of mental health services.	
	(81) Assess how factors influence a client in the community and identify methods to decrease obstacles			
	(82) Describe the occupational therapy process to stakeholders and the client in a clear explicable manner			
	(83) Describe how occupational participation is important in relation to recovery	**Competent at entry level**		

Adapted from American Occupational Therapy Association. (2010b). Specialized knowledge and skills in mental health promotion, prevention, and intervention in occupational therapy practice. *American Journal of Occupational Therapy, 64*(6), 313-323.

- B.5.6: Provide therapeutic use of self...as part of the therapeutic process
- B.5.8: Modify environments and adapt processes

These general competencies reflect that occupational therapy practitioners are educationally prepared for entry-level practice in mental health care.

Occupational Therapy Practice Framework

A discussion of the current practice of occupational therapy in mental health would be incomplete without knowing how to apply the *Occupational Therapy Practice Framework: Domain and Process, 3rd ed.* (OTPF; AOTA, 2014). Although specialized knowledge and skills in mental health practice are specific to occupational therapy mental health services, the OTPF describes the general domains and process of occupational therapy. The OTPF expresses the occupation-based, client-centered, and evidenced-based nature of occupational therapy.

Some students may already be very familiar with the OTPF, whereas other students may be just learning how the OTPF applies to the practice of occupational therapy. As such, this review of the OTPF will provide a refresher for some students while allowing other students to further develop their understanding of how to apply the OTPF. Like the most recent revisions of the DSM to the current DSM-5, the OTPF was created to complement the WHO's view on health. This is described in a document called the *ICF*. As this text illustrates terminology used in the OTPF, knowledge of the OTPF will strengthen the learning experience.

The OTPF was revised in 2013 and published in 2014 as the third edition. The AOTA updates major documents on a 5-year review cycle. A summary of the major changes from the second edition to the third edition of the OTPF are listed here. They include the following:

- Group interventions were added to the interventions list.
- Spirituality received a new definition.
- Clients were defined to include persons, groups, and populations.
- Therapeutic use of self is integrated into the processes as a standard component of intervention.
- Activity demands was removed as a domain and made part of the process of activity analysis.
- A new overarching goal for the outcome of occupational therapy was created. This statement is "Achieving health, well-being, and participation in life through engagement in occupations" (AOTA, 2014, p. S2).
- Areas of occupations are now referred to as *occupations*.

There are five domains in the OTPF. These include occupation, client factors, performance skills, performance patterns, and context/environment. Aspects in each domain interact to affect a person's participation and engagement in occupations. For example, client factors and performance skills that everyone experiences in participation in everyday occupations include thought, emotion, behavior, personality, cognition, sensation, communication, motivation, and pain (Bonder, 1993). Performance patterns of habits, roles, routines, and rituals are also examples of influences that affect a person's participation in everyday occupations. The domains in occupational therapy are identified in Table 2-3.

No OTPF domain is necessarily more important than any other, and each domain can have positive and negative aspects to function. Although the OTPF and ICF are different documents, they have corresponding components. The ICF has two domains with two parts each, compared with the OTPF, which has six domains. Checkpoint 2-4 illustrates the ICF model compared with the OTPF.

The OTPF describes and defines occupational therapy practice with a focus on performance of occupations. Occupations are defined as everyday activities that have meaning and purpose to a person. Although occupational therapy may address those components that affect function, the overall concern is on the individual's ability to participate in daily occupations of interest.

Occupations can include a host of activities that can be grouped under activities of daily living, rest/sleep, education, work, play, leisure, and social participation. The OTPF provides a framework that illustrates occupational therapy practice as it is applied to different populations and within different settings. The OTPF, like the ICF, takes a holistic view of the person and is client centered. It focuses on "[a]chieving health, well-being, and participation in [life] through engagement in occupations" (AOTA, 2014, p. S4). Both the OTPF and ICF models identify participation in activities and the interaction of the environment as important factors to mental health.

However, there are important differences between the OTPF and ICF. The OTPF, being specific to the profession, expands on certain areas to better define and describe the services that may be provided by occupational therapy. The coding system utilized by the ICF for body structures and body functions is not widely utilized in the OTPF. Cohn and Lew (2010) also identify that occupational therapy makes recommendations to structure, modify, and adapt the environment and context to affect performance.

The OTPF emphasizes client-centered care and therapeutic use of self across the occupational therapy process. Therapeutic use of self will be described in Chapter 12 of this book. The OTPF defines **client-centered** care as an "approach to service that incorporates respect for and partnership with clients as active participants in the therapy process" (AOTA, 2014, p. S41). This emphasis corresponds well with the Recovery Model. The Recovery Model is very

TABLE 2-3

DOMAINS OF THE *OCCUPATIONAL THERAPY PRACTICE FRAMEWORK,* 3RD EDITION

OTPF DOMAINS	EXAMPLES	DEFINITION
Occupations	Activities of Daily Living Instrumental Activities of Daily Living Rest and Sleep Education Work Play Leisure Social Participation	Various kinds of life activities in which people engage
Client Factors	Values Beliefs Spirituality Body Functions Body Structures	Factors within a person that affect the ability to participate or perform in occupations
Performance Skills	Motor and Praxis Skills Sensory Perceptual Skills Emotion Regulation Skills Cognitive Skills Communication Skills Social Skills	The abilities an individual demonstrates during actions that have a functional purpose and allow persons to participate in occupations. Performance skills consist of multiple capacities.
Performance Patterns	Habits Routines Roles Rituals	Patterns of behavior that are habitual and repetitive
Context and Environment	Cultural Personal Physical Social Temporal Virtual	Inter-related factors within and surrounding a person that can affect engagement in occupations

Adapted from American Occupational Therapy Association. (2014). Occupational therapy practice framework: Domain and process (3rd ed.). *American Journal of Occupational Therapy, 68*(Suppl. 1), S1-S48.

client-centered whereby the client is controlling and directing his or her own care needs.

Client-centered therapy is important in occupational therapy in order to achieve what is important to the client. It combines actively listening to the person with sensitive reflection on what was heard in order to gain insight on the client and his or her life story. It also includes forming a collaborative relationship for the purpose of treatment planning and service provision, and acknowledges the client as a member of the community. In other words, therapy is client centered when it is grounded in the client's daily life and experiences. Client-centered therapy is more than just a certain number of therapy sessions, clinical pathways, or generic preset goals. It focuses on the needs of the client,

CHECKPOINT 2-4. COMPARING THE INTERNATIONAL CLASSIFICATION OF FUNCTIONING MODEL WITH THE OCCUPATIONAL THERAPY PRACTICE FRAMEWORK		
International Classification of Functioning		*Occupational Therapy Practice Framework Domains*
Part 1	Body Functions and Body Structures	Client Factors
Part 1 (cont.)	Activity and Participation	Performance Patterns and Performance Skills
		Occupations
Part 2	Environment and Personal Factors	Context and Environment
Adapted from American Occupational Therapy Association. (2014). Occupational therapy practice framework: Domain and process (3rd ed.). *American Journal of Occupational Therapy, 68*(Suppl. 1), S1-S48.; World Health Organization. (2001). *International Classification of Functioning, Disability, and Health (ICF)*. Geneva, Switzerland: Author.		

from the client's perspective, and therapy goals that originate from the client.

As mentioned earlier in this chapter, the use of people-first language is important as a way to direct focus on the client and not the stigma attached to the label of a diagnosis. In the medical model, a person diagnosed with a mental health disorder is viewed as an individual with a host of impairments, and health is achieved by elimination of those symptoms. Deficit-based treatment protocols or practices are often applied to persons based on diagnostic labels. However, in occupational therapy treatment, the client has moved being from a passive recipient of care to an active participant who determines his or her own health care needs. It is no longer appropriate or acceptable to describe a person by the disease.

Occupational Therapy Assistant and the Occupational Therapy Process

Understanding the occupational therapy process is an integral part of student development and learning to provide entry-level occupational therapy services. The occupational therapy process is a process that occurs between the occupational therapist, occupational therapy assistant, and client within the domains of occupational therapy. The occupational therapy process is defined as a "[w]ay in which occupational therapy practitioners operationalize their expertise to provide services to clients" (AOTA, 2014, p. S44). The occupational therapy process includes the following:

- Evaluation Process
  - Occupational Profile
- Analysis of Occupational Performance
  - Intervention Process
  - Intervention Plan
  - Intervention Implementation
  - Intervention Review

- Targeting Outcomes
  - Select Outcomes and Measures
  - Use Outcomes to Measure Progress and Adjust Goals and Interventions
  - Assess Outcome Results

Although depicted in a sequential format, the occupational therapy process occurs in a continuous, adaptable method to meet the needs of the client. Occupational therapy practitioners incorporate aspects of clinical reasoning, activity analysis, therapeutic use of self, and understanding of environments and contexts throughout the occupational therapy process. Additionally, the occupational therapy practitioner takes into account the influence of activity and/or occupational demands and the occupational therapy approach used during the occupational therapy process. The end goal is to "achieve health, well-being, and participation in life through engagement in occupation" (AOTA, 2014, p. S4).

Mental health is an important consideration in the evaluation and treatment of clients (Costa, Molinsky, Kent, & Sauerwald, 2011). The evaluation process includes the creation of an occupational profile and analysis of occupational performance. The occupational profile reflects aspects of a client's history, interests, values, activities of daily living capacity, instrumental activities of daily living responsibilities, and individual needs (AOTA, 2014). The occupational therapy assistant may participate in the creation of an occupational profile and analysis of occupational performance in collaboration with the occupational therapist after demonstrating service competency and practicing within state, federal, and professional guidelines.

"Guidelines for Supervision, Roles, and Responsibilities During the Delivery of Occupational Therapy Services" identifies general roles and responsibilities of the occupational therapy assistant throughout the occupational therapy process, which includes evaluation (AOTA, 2009). This document identifies that occupational therapy assistants can assist and participate in the evaluation phase of

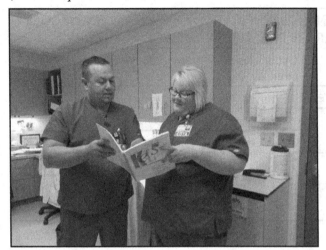

Figure 2-1. Occupational therapist and occupational therapy assistant collaborating.

the occupational therapy process. The occupational therapy assistant may participate in evaluation by the following:

- Participating in screening procedures
- Implementing delegated standardized assessments
- Assisting the occupational therapist in the development of the occupational profile
- Observing a client's performance during engagement in occupation
- Educating stakeholders on the scope of occupational therapy services and process for initiating occupational therapy
- Creating verbal or written reports of client capabilities and observations
- Identifying possible treatment approaches
- Assisting the development of client-centered practices and therapeutic use of self
- Providing the occupational therapist assistance in the creation of short-term goals
- Partnering with the occupational therapist in the evaluation process

The provision of intervention follows the evaluation. Intervention includes the creation of an intervention plan, implementation of the plan, and a review of the intervention or services provided. This phase includes the occupational therapist, occupational therapy assistant, and especially the client to create meaningful change. Examples of intervention approaches may include health promotion, remediation/restoration, maintenance, modification, and disability prevention. In particular, a demonstration of service competency may be needed before the occupational therapy assistant is able to perform certain tasks during the intervention process.

"Guidelines for Supervision, Roles, and Responsibilities During the Delivery of Occupational Therapy Services" identifies general roles and responsibilities of the occupational therapy assistant throughout the occupational therapy process, which includes intervention (AOTA, 2009).

In the intervention phase, the occupational therapy assistant collaborates with the occupational therapist and client to develop the intervention plan. Examples of how the occupational therapy assistant may participate in intervention include the following:

- Providing input to the plan, based on knowledge of the occupational therapy goals
- Selecting, implementing, and modifying interventions to meet client needs in collaboration with the client and the occupational therapist
- Creating verbal or written reports of client capabilities and observations
- Documenting occupational therapy services upon established expectations and standards
- Assisting the development of client-centered practices and therapeutic use of self
- Partnering with the occupational therapist to make recommendations to the intervention plan
- Coordinating the development and implementation of occupational therapy services
- Incorporating evidence-based practice approaches and services with attainment of service competency
- Utilizing knowledge of resources available to support the client and occupational therapy services

Figure 2-1 illustrates the occupational therapy assistant and occupational therapist collaborating to create an intervention plan to meet the needs of a person receiving occupational therapy services.

Another responsibility of the occupational therapy assistant in the occupational therapy process is to assist the occupational therapist to target outcomes (AOTA, 2009). Targeting outcomes includes the selection of measures that are used to evaluate progress and adjust goals and interventions. It also includes assessing outcome results. Outcomes in occupational therapy may focus on occupational performance, adaptation, health/wellness, participation, prevention, quality of life, role competency, self-advocacy, and occupational justice. The broad outcome of occupational therapy intervention is "[a]chieving health, well-being, and participation in life through engagement in occupation" (AOTA, 2014). The occupational therapy assistant may participate in targeting outcomes by doing the following:

- Providing information and documentation related to outcome achievement in collaboration with the occupational therapist

TABLE 2-4		
THE OCCUPATIONAL THERAPY PROCESS		
OCCUPATIONAL THERAPY PROCESS	**COMPONENTS OF THE OCCUPATIONAL THERAPY PROCESS**	**EXAMPLES OF ACTIONS**
EVALUATION	• Occupational profile • Analysis of occupational performance	• Screens • Standardized evaluations • Nonstandardized evaluations • Interviews • Occupational profile • Client observation
INTERVENTION	• Intervention plan • Intervention implementation • Intervention review	• Occupations and activities • Preparatory methods and tasks • Education and training • Advocacy • Group interventions • Activity and occupational demands
OUTCOMES "Achieving health, well-being, and participation in life through engagement in occupations"	• Select outcomes and measures • Use outcomes to measure progress and adjust goals and interventions • Assess outcome results	• Occupational performance • Health and wellness • Quality of life • Prevention • Participation • Role competence

Compiled from American Occupational Therapy Association. (2014). Occupational therapy practice framework: Domain and process (3rd ed.). *American Journal of Occupational Therapy, 68*(Suppl. 1), S1-S48

- Facilitating the transition or discontinuation of services with the client, other professionals, resources, and organizations
- Contributing to the safety and effectiveness of occupational therapy services
- Assisting the development of client-centered practices and therapeutic use of self
- Implementing delegated standardized assessments
- Reporting a client's performance during engagement in occupation
- Making recommendations in partnership with the occupational therapist concerning interventions and progress toward goals
- Making recommendations in partnership with the occupational therapist concerning the future of occupational therapy services

Table 2-4 illustrates the occupational therapy process and examples of actions that can occur throughout.

Occupational therapy assistants work under the supervision of and in collaboration with occupational therapists. It is the responsibility of the occupational therapy assistant to seek out and demonstrate service competency pertaining to delegated tasks. Service competency reflects a level of mastery over tasks that will be performed accurately and sufficiently. It is also the responsibility of the occupational therapist to delegate adequate responsibilities and provide the appropriate level of supervision for occupational therapy services provided. Both work under a plan of care and with clients to attain established goals. Ideally, the occupational therapist and occupational therapy assistant collaborate to meet each other's needs and the needs of the client, setting, and other stakeholders. Checkpoint 2-5 directs the reader to review the current occupational therapy practice act in his or her state and explore the role of the occupational therapy assistant in the occupational therapy process.

Overall, the occupational therapist has responsibility for the evaluation, intervention, and outcome measurement phases of the occupational therapy process. Occupational therapy assistants utilize their knowledge and skills to deliver services, administer standardized assessments, and aid in the plan of care development. These actions assist in meeting a client's individualized recovery goals.

Contextual Influences on Mental Health Care and Service Delivery

The OTPF domain and process describes the role of the occupational therapy assistant; however, contextual influences in mental health care service delivery also influence the role of the occupational therapy assistant. Multiple stakeholders affect the provision of mental health care in the United States through reimbursement, services covered, and access to services. These stakeholders include the following:

- Community-based volunteer, profit, and nonprofit organizations
- Government groups and initiatives
- State mental health agencies and departments

It is important to be familiar with each stakeholder and the influences each group or system has on mental health care service delivery.

Community-based organizations are often developed by stakeholders when they identify a new need within the community or when a previously identified need has not yet been adequately addressed. Organizations may also develop community-based groups to meet an identified need. Community-based groups can be specific in nature or cover a wide scope of services and needs. Grant funding, national initiatives, and directives aid in the development of community-based organizations by providing resources.

Community-based volunteer, profit, and nonprofit organizations include a variety of groups. Examples of organizations include the National Alliance on Mental Illness (NAMI), Center for School Mental Health – -University of Maryland (CSMH), International Mental Health Research Organization (IRHRO), and the National Council for Behavioral Health (NCBH). Examples of for-profit organizations can include third-party organizations that provide health coverage. Additional organizations can include certification groups such as The Joint Commission: Accreditation, Health Care, Certification (JCAHO), Commission on Accreditation of Rehabilitation Facilities (CARF), ACOTE, and National Board for the Certification of Occupational Therapy (NBCOT). Table 2-5 lists some of these important community-based organizations. Each organization's mission statement is also included. Mission statements are brief summaries of the aim and values of each organization.

Government agencies and departments vary in their scope and purpose. Examples of government agencies include the Center for Medicare and Medicaid Services (CMS), Substance Abuse and Mental Health Service Administration (SAMHSA), and the National Institute of Mental Health (NIMH), which are all part of the U.S. Department of Health and Human Services. Additional agencies include the Rehabilitation Services Administration (RSA) and the Office of Special Education and Rehabilitative Services (OSERS). These two agencies are part of the U.S. Department of Education. All of these agencies influence the provision of mental health care services through research, funding, development of guidelines, identification of services covered, and advocacy. Further information on these agencies can be found in the appendix, as well as the reference list at the end of this chapter. Table 2-6 identifies each organization and their mission statements.

Additional governmental influences on mental health include the Health Insurance Portability and Accountability Act of 1996 and the President's New Freedom Commission Report. Although not government agencies, these directives do influence the provision of mental health care service delivery. The President's New Freedom Commission Report was mentioned in Chapter 1.

A variety of state agencies also influence the provision of mental health care and service delivery through advocacy, provision of services, and determining which services to be provided within the state. These agencies include the state Medicaid agency, vocational rehabilitation, Department of Mental Health, Department of Substance Abuse, occupational therapy licensure board, and state mental health authorities. State agencies will be different for each state.

One significant state agency is the occupational therapy licensure board, which creates the rules for the practice of occupational therapy. State rules provide a guideline for what occupational therapy practitioners can and cannot

TABLE 2-5

NATIONAL AND COMMUNITY-BASED ORGANIZATIONS INFLUENCING MENTAL HEALTH CARE

ORGANIZATION	MISSION OF EACH ORGANIZATION
CSMH: Center for School Mental Health	"To strengthen policies and programs in school mental health to improve learning and promote success for America's youth."
NAMI: National Alliance on Mental Illness	NAMI is a grassroots organization consisting of individuals with mental illness, family members, and friends with the mission: "To advocate for effective prevention, diagnosis, treatment, support, research, and recovery that improves the quality of life of persons of all ages who are affected by mental illnesses."
IRHRO: International Mental Health Research Organization	"To alleviate human suffering from mental illness by funding scientific research into causes, prevention, and new treatments."
NCBH: National Council for Behavioral Health	"Advance our members' ability to deliver integrated health care through advocating and consulting, coordinating the Mental Health First Aid program, operating the SAMHSA-HRSA Center for integrated Health Solutions, and offering the National Council for Behavioral Health Conference."
The Joint Commission	"To continuously improve health care for the public, in collaboration with other stakeholders, by evaluating health care organizations and inspiring them to excel in providing safe and effective care of the highest quality and value."
CARF: Commission on Accreditation of Rehabilitation Facilities	"To promote the quality, value, and optimal outcome of services through a consultative accreditation process and continuous improvement services center on enhancing the lives of persons served."
Health Insurance Provider	Organizational missions vary depending on each health insurance provider.

Compiled from Commission for Accreditation of Rehabilitation Facilities International. (2012). CARF's mission, vision, core values and purposes. Retrieved from www.carf.org/about/mission.; International Mental Health Research Organization. (2013). International Mental Health Research Organization. Retrieved from www.imhro.org/about.; Joint Commission. (2013). About the Joint Commission. Retrieved from http://jointcommission.org.; National Alliance on Mental Illness. (2013). National Alliance on Mental Illness. Retrieved from www.nami.org/About-NAMI.; National Council for Behavioral Health. (2013). National Council for Behavioral Health. Retrieved from www.thenationalcouncil.org.; University of Maryland. (2013). Center for School Mental Health. Retrieved from http://csm.umaryland.edu/aboutus/index.html.

do in specific states. Each state that licenses occupational therapy practitioners will have different rules governing the practice of occupational therapy. Each state determines the rules of occupational therapy applicable to the constituents of the state. State practice acts may be more rigorous, but not less stringent, than AOTA standards of practice. Rules that apply to occupational therapy assistant practitioners in the state of Tennessee, for example, are seen in Rule 1150-02-10 on pages 22-23 of the document. Examples of rules pertaining to occupational therapy assistants include the following:

(3) (b) The [Occupational Therapist] shall be responsible for the evaluation of the patient and the development of the patient/client treatment plan. The Occupational Therapy assistant may

contribute information from observations and standardized test procedures to the evaluation and the treatment plans.

(3) (c) The Occupational Therapy Assistant can implement and coordinate intervention plan under the supervision of the licensed Occupational Therapist.

(3) (d) The Occupational Therapy Assistant can provide direct services that follow a documented routine and accepted procedure under the supervision of the Occupational Therapist (Tennessee Department of Health, 2010; p. 22-23).

The rules for the state of Tennessee correspond with the AOTA document, "Guidelines for Supervision, Roles,

TABLE 2-6	
GOVERNMENT AGENCIES INFLUENCING MENTAL HEALTH CARE	
GOVERNMENT AGENCY	**MISSION OF EACH ORGANIZATION**
SAMHSA: Substance Abuse and Mental Health Service Administration	"To reduce the impact of substance abuse and mental illness on America's communities."
CMS: Centers for Medicare and Medicaid Services	"As an effective steward of public funds, CMS is committed to strengthening and modernizing the nation's health care system to provide access to high quality care and improved health at lower costs."
NIMH: National Institute of Mental Health	"To understand mind, brain, and behavior and thereby to reduce the burden of mental illness through research."
RSA: Rehabilitation Services Administration, US Dept. of Education	Provides grant program funds to vocational rehabilitation programs to provide counseling, medical and psychological services, job training, and other individualized services.
OSERS: Office of Special Education and Rehabilitative Services, US Dept. of Education	"To provide leadership to achieve full integration and participation in society of people with disabilities by ensuring equal opportunity and access to, and excellence in, education, employment, and community living."
Compiled from United States Department of Health and Human Services, Centers for Medicare & Medicaid Services. (2013). History. Retrieved from www.cms.gov.; United States Department of Education, Office of Special Education and Rehabilitation. (2013). www2ed. gov.; OSERS. Retrieved from www2ed.gov.; United States Department of Education, Rehabilitation Services Administration. (2013). RSA. Retrieved from United States Department of Health and Human Services, National Institutes of Mental Health. (2013). About NIMH. Retrieved from www.nimh.nih.gov.; United States Department of Health and Human Services, Substance Abuse and Mental Health Services Administration. (2013). SAMHSA. Retrieved from http://beta.samhsa.gov.	

and Responsibilities During the Delivery of Occupational Therapy Services" (AOTA, 2009). It is the responsibility of both the occupational therapist and occupational therapy assistant to understand their state's practice act where occupational therapy services are provided.

SUMMARY

This chapter highlights the standards of practice for occupational therapy assistants as they provide mental health services. Occupational therapy assistants provide services that incorporate core knowledge and skills, related to mental health as well as profession-specific knowledge and skills. These specialized skills are mirrored in the accreditation standards for occupational therapy assistant education programs and the domains of occupational therapy. They are also utilized in the application of the occupational therapy process.

The occupational therapy assistant must demonstrate competency throughout the occupational therapy process. Occupational therapy assistant practitioners are competent at entry level with many aspects of service; however, the number of skills they may use increases with work experience under the appropriate level of supervision by an occupational therapist. Occupational therapy assistant

practitioners can apply many more knowledge and skills throughout the occupational therapy process with the assistance of the occupational therapist. Service competency and supervision are utilized by the occupational therapist and occupational therapy assistant throughout the occupational therapy process to provide quality, evidenced-based services.

Environment and context also influence the provision of mental health care services. Occupational therapy practitioners are trained to look for and consider the effect of environment and context across the lifespan. Contextual influences affecting occupational therapy mental health care service delivery include community-based volunteer, profit, and nonprofit organizations, government groups and initiatives, and state mental health agencies and departments. Chapter 2 covers the occupational therapy standards of practice and influences of occupational therapy mental health care service delivery.

PART 3: APPLICATIONS

The following activities will help you apply knowledge of the terminology used in the OTPF, ICF, and DSM, which will also be used throughout this text. Activities can be completed individually or in small groups to enhance learning.

Individually

1. Identify and list all core mental health professional knowledge and skills for the occupational therapy assistant that are classified as "Competent at entry level." Refer to Table 2-2.

2. Identify and list all occupational therapy assistant profession-specific knowledge and skills applied to mental health promotion, prevention, and intervention that are classified as "Competent at entry level." Refer to Table 2-3.

3. Explain how the following terms are different. Give an example of how the occupational therapy assistant would respond in a therapy session to each level of service expectation.

   a. "Competent at entry level"

   b. "Assist at entry level"

   c. "Competent at entry-level practice to analyze and integrate knowledge to make judgments about occupational therapy provision"

   d. "Competent at entry-level practice to demonstrate and apply it to occupational therapy practice"

In Small Groups

4. Contrast how the DSM-5 and the ICF classification can be incorporated into occupational therapy mental health service provision.

5. Examine the occupational therapy process. Contrast different parts of the occupational therapy process by providing two examples of what an occupational therapy assistant might do for each part.

6. Examine the occupational therapy assistant and occupational therapist role in providing mental health services. Give three examples of how the occupational therapy assistant can collaborate with the occupational therapist throughout the occupational therapy process.

Occupational Therapy Process

- Evaluation Process
  - Occupational Profile
  - Analysis of Occupational Performance
- Intervention Process
  - Intervention Plan
  - Intervention Implementation
  - Intervention Review

- Targeting Outcomes
  - Select Outcomes and Measures
  - Use Outcomes to Measure Progress and Adjust Goals and Interventions
  - Assess Outcome Results

7. Select one of the organizations/systems in Tables 2-5 and 2-6. Gather further information on the organization/system to present to the class and instructor. Identify:

   a. What specific services are offered?

   b. What is the impact of the organization on mental health services in the local community as well as nationally?

   c. What is the history of the organization?

   d. How can occupational therapy services be provided within this organization?

REFERENCES

American Occupational Therapy Association. (2006). Accreditation Standards for an Educational Program for the Occupational therapy Assistant. Retrieved from www.aota.org.

American Occupational Therapy Association. (2009). Guidelines for supervision, roles, and responsibilities during the delivery of occupational therapy services. *American Journal of Occupational Therapy, 63*(6), 797-803.

American Occupational Therapy Association. (2010a). Specialized knowledge and skills in mental health promotion, prevention, and intervention in occupational therapy practice. *American Journal of Occupational Therapy, 64*(6), 313-323.

American Occupational Therapy Association. (2010b). Occupational therapy code of ethics and ethics standards. *American Journal of Occupational Therapy, 64* (Suppl.), S17-S26.

American Occupational Therapy Association. (2014). Occupational therapy practice framework: Domain and Process (3rd ed.). *American Journal of Occupational Therapy, 68*(Suppl. 1), S1-S48.

American Psychiatric Association. (2013). *Diagnostic and statistical manual of mental disorders* (5th ed.). Washington, D.C.: Author.

Bonder, B. (1993). Issues in assessment of psychosocial components of function. *American Journal of Occupational Therapy, 47*, 211-216.

Commission on Accreditation of Rehabilitation Facilities International. (2012). CARF's Mission, Vision, Core Values and Purposes. Retrieved from www.carf.org/about/mission/.

Cohn, E. & Lew, C. (2010). Occupational therapy's perspective on the use of environments and contexts to support health and participation in occupations. *American Journal of Occupational Therapy, 64*(6), 557-569.

Costa, D., Molinsky, R., Kent, J.P., & Sauerwald, C. (2011). Integrating mental health knowledge and skills into academic and fieldwork education. *OT Practice, 16*(19), CE-CE8.

Grohol, J. (2011). Some of the Empty Arguments Against the DSM-5. *Psych Central.* Retrieved from http://psychcentral.com/blog/archives/2011/12/31/some-of-the-empty-arguments-against-the-dsm-5/.

Holmquist, B. B. (2004). Incorporating the occupational therapy practice framework into a mental health practice setting. *Mental Health Special Interest Section Quarterly, 27*(2), 1-4.

International Mental Health Research Organization. (2013). International Mental Health Research Organization. Retrieved from www.imhro.org/about.

Joint Commission. (2013). About the Joint Commission. Retrieved from http://jointcommission.org.

Keyes, C. L. (2007). Promoting and protecting mental health as flourishing: A complementary strategy for improving national mental health. *American Psychologist, 62,* 95-108.

National Alliance on Mental Illness. (2013). National Alliance on Mental Illness. Retrieved from www.nami.orgAbout-NAMI

National Council for Behavioral Health. (2013). National Council for Behavioral Health. Retrieved from www.thenationalcouncil.org.

Tennessee Department of Health. (2010). Chapter 1150-02: General Rules Governing the Practice of Occupational Therapy. Retrieved from www.tn.gov/sos/rules/1150/1150-02.20100119.pdf.

University of Maryland. (2013). Center for School Mental Health. Retrieved from http://csmh.umaryland.edu/aboutus/index.html.

U.S. Department of Education, Rehabilitation Services Administration (2013). RSA. Retrieved from http://www2.ed.gov/about/offices/list/osers/rsa/index.html.

U.S. Department of Education, Office of Special Education and Rehabilitative Services. (2013). OSERS. Retrieved from http://www2.ed.gov/about/offices/list/osers/index.html.

U.S. Department of Health and Human Services, Centers for Medicare & Medicaid Services. (2013). History. Retrieved from www.cms.gov/Research-Statistics-Data-and-Systems/Computer-Data-and-Systems/Privacy/index.html?redirect=/privacy.

U.S. Department of Health and Human Services, National Institutes of Mental Health. (2013). About NIMH. Retrieved from www.nimh.nih.gov/about/index.shtml.

U.S. Department of Health and Human Services, Substance Abuse and Mental Health Services Administration. (2013). SAMHSA. Retrieved from www.samhsa.gov/about-us.

World Health Organization. (2001). *International classification of functioning, disability and health (ICF)*. Geneva, Switzerland: Author.

3

A Public Health Approach to Children's Mental Health in Occupational Therapy

Susan S. Bazyk, PhD, OTR/L, FAOTA

KEY TERMS

- Intensive Individualized
- Mental Health
- Mental Health Literacy
- Mental Illness
- Multi-Tiered System of Support

- Participation and Structured Recreation and Leisure Activities
- Positive Behavioral Interventions and Supports (PBIS)
- Prevention

- Promotion
- Sensory Processing
- Social and Emotional Learning (SEL)
- Targeted Services
- Universal Services

CHAPTER LEARNING OBJECTIVES

After completion of this chapter, students should be able to:

1. Identify the difference between mental health and mental ill health.

2. Recognize the four characteristics associated with positive mental health.

3. State how the continuum of care is applied by the Multi-Tiered System of Supports (MTSS).

4. Describe how the occupational therapy process can be applied at each level of the MTSS.

5. Explain major approaches used in mental health promotion, prevention, and intervention.

6. Apply the occupational therapy process to tiers of the MTSS and to the major approaches used in mental health promotion, prevention, and intervention.

Manville, C.A., & Keough, J. L.
Mental Health Practice for the Occupational Therapy Assistant (pp 53-74).
© 2016 Taylor & Francis Group.

CHAPTER OUTLINE

INTRODUCTION

Raising children … is vastly more than fixing what is wrong with them. It is about identifying and nurturing their strongest qualities, what they own and are best at, and helping them find niches in which they can best live out these strengths. (Seligman & Csikszentmihalyi, 2000, p. 6)

Occupational therapy was founded on a commitment to mind–body unity, resulting in a rich history of promoting mental health in all areas of practice (Bing, 1981). "The psychosocial perspective in occupational therapy is not an add-on or special technique. It is rather an integrated, everyday way of thinking about what the client needs and wants to do" (Jackson & Arbesman, 2005, p. 5). Unfortunately, the term *mental health* is often confused with *mental illness* and the interventions used to ameliorate mental health challenges. How occupational therapy practitioners think about "mental health," however, has a significant impact on how occupational therapy services are perceived, articulated to others, and implemented (Bazyk, 2011). This chapter provides a foundation for "framing" mental health broadly by applying a public health approach to children's mental health. In addition to addressing the needs of youth with identified mental illness, there is a critical need to promote positive mental health in all children and youth. Examples include building positive qualities and personal strengths in addition to remediating problems. A description of occupational therapy's role in mental health promotion, prevention, and intensive interventions with children and youth is presented. Practical strategies for implementation in a variety of settings are also provided. Occupational therapy practitioners have specialized knowledge and skills in addressing the social participation and mental health needs of children and youth. Occupational therapy is well positioned to positively contribute to all three levels of intervention.

PART 1: THE MENTAL HEALTH CONTINUUM

Mental Health

It is critical for occupational therapy practitioners to be clear about what mental health means. Keyes (2007) has advocated for the adoption of a mental health continuum with mental health viewed as a state of functioning separate from mental illness. He asserts that mental health is not merely the absence of mental illness, but the presence of something positive. In the same way that a diagnosis of major depressive disorder is based on symptoms of negative emotions and malfunctioning, a diagnosis of mental health consists of symptoms of positive emotions and positive psychological and social functioning. The continuum of mental health as described by Keyes (2007) can be viewed as ranging from mental illness and/or "languishing in life" at one end to "moderately mentally healthy" and "complete mental health and flourishing" at the other end (p. 100). Checkpoint 3-1 illustrates the continuum of mental health as described by Keyes. Higher degrees of impairment and disability have been noted in individuals without complete mental health and flourishing, even those without a diagnosed mental illness (Keyes, 2007). In contrast, positive mental health is associated with greater physical health and everyday functioning. These research findings support the need for occupational therapy practitioners to emphasize mental health promotion in addition to ongoing efforts to prevent and treat mental illness.

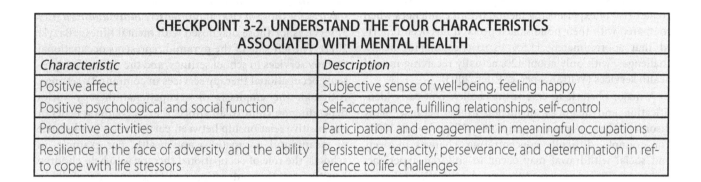

CHECKPOINT 3-1. REMEMBER: THE CONTINUUM OF MENTAL HEALTH
• Mental Illness ("Languishing in Life") • Moderate Mental Health • Complete Mental Health ("Flourishing in Life")

CHECKPOINT 3-2. UNDERSTAND THE FOUR CHARACTERISTICS ASSOCIATED WITH MENTAL HEALTH	
Characteristic	*Description*
Positive affect	Subjective sense of well-being, feeling happy
Positive psychological and social function	Self-acceptance, fulfilling relationships, self-control
Productive activities	Participation and engagement in meaningful occupations
Resilience in the face of adversity and the ability to cope with life stressors	Persistence, tenacity, perseverance, and determination in reference to life challenges

Mental health was defined in 1999 by David Satcher, the surgeon general at the time, as "a state of successful performance of mental function, resulting in productive activities, fulfilling relationships with people, and the ability to adapt to change and cope with adversity" (U.S. Department of Health and Human Services [USDHHS], 1999, p. 4). Four characteristics are associated with positive mental health. They include the following:

1. Positive affect

2. Positive psychological and social function

3. Productive activities

4. Resilience in the face of adversity and the ability to cope with life stressors

The four characteristics associated with positive mental health are further described in Checkpoint 3-2 (USDHHS, 1999; World Health Organization [WHO], 2001).

In summation, positive mental health refers to "feeling well" and "doing well" (Miles, Espiritu, Horen, Sebian, & Waetzig, 2010). Mental health must also be perceived as a dynamic state of functioning that can vary throughout a person's life based on a number of biological (e.g., genetics), environmental (e.g., abuse/neglect), or situational (e.g., death of a family member) factors (Barry & Jenkins, 2007). Occupational therapy practitioners must be vigilant for any marked changes in a child's affect, social functioning, and ability to adapt to daily challenges due to the dynamic nature of mental health and well-being. Additionally, when working with children and youth, it is important to consider developmental factors such as age-related changes in a number of areas, including cognitive, emotional, and behavioral abilities. It is typical for early adolescents to develop a strong peer group identity or to want to look and act like their peers, for example. Knowing this helps adults appreciate the behaviors of early adolescents. Competencies gained at one stage of development provide a foundation for future competencies as young people face new challenges and opportunities. Understanding the age-related patterns of competence and disorder is important for developing promotion and prevention interventions (National Research Council [NRC] & Institute of Medicine [IOM], 2009).

Mental Ill Health

Mental ill health is a broad term that includes a continuum from mild symptomatology to the most severe disorders of differing duration and intensity (Barry & Jenkins, 2007). The terms **mental illness** and *mental disorder* are commonly used to refer to diagnosable psychiatric conditions that significantly interfere with a person's functioning, such as schizophrenia, bipolar disorder, and dementia. The term *mental health problem* often refers to more common issues such as anxiety and depression, which may be less severe and of shorter duration, but may develop into more serious conditions if left unattended (Barry & Jenkins, 2007).

Demographics

Approximately one in five children ages 9 to 17 has a diagnosable behavioral or emotional disorder, with the most common being anxiety (8%), depression (5.2%), substance abuse disorder (10.3%), conduct disorders (3.5%), and attention deficit hyperactive disorder (ADHD) (4.5%) (Koppelman, 2004; NRC & IOM, 2009). About half are mildly impaired and half significantly impaired. Those who are mildly impaired often do not meet the criteria for a mental health diagnosis and go untreated (Masia-Warner,

Nangle, & Hansen, 2006). Serious emotional disturbances affect approximately 4% to 13% of the U.S. population of children ages 4 to 17 and refer to a range of diagnosable behavioral and mental disorders that severely impair daily functioning in the home, school, and community (Simpson, Bloom, Cohen & Blumberg, 2005). A greater number of children and youth in the child welfare (50%) and juvenile justice (67% to 70%) systems have mental health challenges (NRC & IOM, 2009). Children with disabilities are also at greater risk of experiencing mental health challenges when compared with their nondisabled peers. It has been reported that approximately 11.5% experience mental health challenges, with only about 42% actually receiving mental health services (Witt, Kasper, & Riley, 2003).

A major obstacle to care is the challenge of early identification and diagnosis of mental illness because many disorders share common symptoms (Koppelman, 2004). For example, difficulty concentrating, changes in sleep, and social withdrawal may occur in children experiencing depression or anxiety. Accurate identification relies on information obtained from multiple sources, including the child, family, teachers, and physicians. Unfortunately, the majority of children who need mental health care do not receive services (approximately 70% to 80%), and for those receiving care, less than half receive adequate care (Masia-Warner, Nangle, & Hansen, 2006). Without intervention, mental health issues tend to become more severe over time, causing further emotional pain, functional challenges, and increased risk of alcohol and drug abuse.

A Public Health Approach to Children's Mental Health in Occupational Therapy

Given what we know about mental health, a public health approach to mental health has been advocated by the WHO (2001) that emphasizes the promotion of mental health as well as the prevention of and intervention for mental illness. Promoting children's mental health for successful everyday functioning and positive emotional well-being is best achieved when providing a continuum of care that involves families, schools, and communities (Stiffman et al., 2010). This continuum of care is often referred to as a **Multi-Tiered System of Supports (MTSS)** and is illustrated in Figure 3-1 (Sugai & Horner, 2009). The MTSS can be envisioned as a three-tiered model focusing on mental health promotion, prevention, and intervention, which can be used to guide occupational therapy for children and youth in multiple types of settings. This framework supports a change in thinking from the traditional, individually focused, deficit-driven model of service provision to a whole-population, strength-based approach. This model acknowledges that addressing mental health issues is too

complex to relegate to a few professionals. Leaders in the field of school mental health, for example, are calling for a paradigm shift to better prepare *all* school personnel to proactively address the mental health needs of *all* students (Koller & Bertel, 2006). All school personnel includes teachers, administrators, psychologists, social workers, and related service providers.

The three major tiers of service in the MTSS include **universal** (tier 1), or whole population; **targeted** (tier 2) services for those at risk; and **intensive individualized** (tier 3) services for those diagnosed with mental illness (Bazyk, 2011). The left side of the pyramid represents occupational therapy services in school settings, and the right side represents occupational therapy services in community settings. Although the emphasis of occupational therapy varies depending on context, all efforts share a common belief in the positive relationship between participation in a balance of meaningful occupations and health. For example, in schools, the role of occupational therapy is to help children benefit from their education and function successfully in academic and nonacademic aspects of the school environment. In contrast, services provided in the community will likely occur during out-of-school time. This warrants attention to the development of meaningful hobbies, leisure interests, friendships, independent living skills, and beginning work skills.

Differentiating Promotion, Prevention, and Intervention

It is important to make distinctions between these various practices because a public health approach to mental health involves promotion, prevention, and intervention. **Promotion** efforts emphasize competence enhancement, which includes building on strengths and resources (Barry & Jenkins, 2007). Mental health promotion includes creating supportive school, home, and community environments. It also includes reducing stigma and discrimination and educating children on how to develop and maintain positive mental health (Barry & Jenkins, 2007). Mental health promotion is enhanced by having a skilled and informed interdisciplinary workforce drawing from various sectors to include health, education, and community organizations. **Prevention** efforts focus on reducing the incidence and seriousness of problem behaviors and mental health disorders. This is accomplished by diminishing risk factors such as easy access to underage drinking and enhancing protective factors such as social and emotional competencies (Barry & Jenkins, 2007; Catalano, Hawkins, Berglund, Pollard, & Arthur, 2002). **Intensive individualized interventions** are provided to diminish the effects of an identified mental health problem and restore the child to an optimal state of functioning and positive mental health. Intervention at this level is often dependent on the specific mental health problem and/or formal diagnosis.

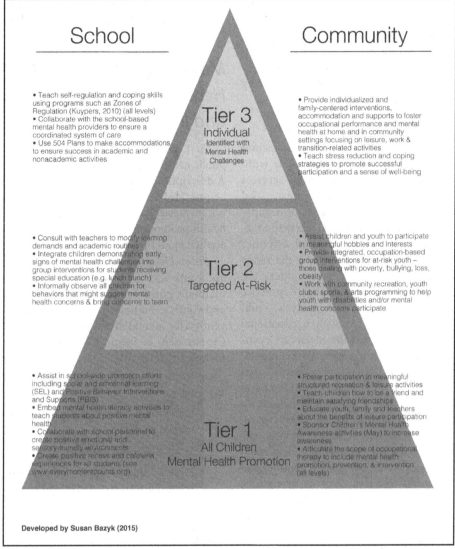

Figure 3-1. Multi-Tiered System of Supports (MTSS).

PART 2: THE OCCUPATIONAL THERAPY PROCESS

The occupational therapy process can be applied at each of the three tiers of the MTSS (Bazyk, 2011). The first step involves *gaining awareness, knowledge,* and *skills* necessary for addressing the mental health needs of children and youth at each tier. For example, at tier 1 in a school setting, it is important to obtain information about school-wide programs developed to promote positive behavior and support implementation in everyday practice. This may include applying positive behavioral interventions and supports. At tiers 2 and 3, the occupational therapy practitioner needs to become aware of the mental health continuum, including symptoms associated with various mental illnesses.

The second step involves *appraisal specific to each tier.* This may include observation, gathering information, or evaluations specific to each tier. At tier 1, appraisal might involve the use of various strategies to evaluate the mental health of children, as well as qualities of the physical and social environments. At the most basic level, occupational therapy practitioners should pay attention to every child's mental health by specifically observing emotions. One consideration is whether a child demonstrates periods of happiness, joy, and satisfaction throughout the day. Patterns of occupational participation should also be noted. Observe whether the child engages in a range of healthy and enjoyable occupations throughout the day, and explore if he or she has special interests and/or hobbies that foster a sense of joy and personal well-being. Finally, quality of the settings should be evaluated. Consider whether the settings involve caring adults who promote character strengths and positive emotions (Bazyk, 2011).

The third step involves *action,* indirect and direct intervention strategies that are specific to each tier. Actions are based on the appraisal process and refer to interventions and conditions that promote optimal mental health. An example of an action used to promote mental health at tier 1 is when the occupational therapy practitioner consults with teachers to understand behaviors associated with sensory defensiveness. This is followed by collaboration to modify interactions to enhance social interaction.

Occupation-Based Practice

There are a number of approaches specific to mental health that are important to know and be familiar with. Considering all approaches, occupational therapy services share a common commitment to the use of meaningful occupation to promote participation in a range of occupations. Education, play, leisure, work, social participation, activities of daily living (ADLs), instrumental activities of daily living (IADLs), and sleep/rest describe the range of occupations. Occupational therapy practitioners are uniquely qualified to provide occupation-based practice due to expertise in activity design, task analysis, child development, and group process… "As such, occupational therapy practitioners use activities as the means to 'occupation' and for participation within a variety of contexts" (Jackson & Arbesman, 2005, p. 31). In recent evidence-based reviews, the use of activity-based interventions such as arts and crafts, play, and games were supported in helping to improve peer and social interaction (Bazyk & Arbesman, 2013; Jackson & Arbesman, 2005). The suggested intervention strategies include using a variety of activities to teach and encourage skill development. They also recommended the use of peer models to foster practice of new skills, supportive adults to provide coaching, and a long enough intervention program to allow ample opportunity to practice emergent skills (Jackson & Arbesman, 2005). Activities should fit the child's interests and developmental level, as well as promote the desired social and emotional skills. The use of duos or small groups tends to be the most powerful form of intervention for promoting social competence. An effective occupational therapy practitioner assumes the role of activity designer and facilitator, as well as positive model, coach, and source of emotional support (Jackson & Arbesman, 2005).

All occupational therapy services emphasize competency enhancement. There are numerous opportunities for using occupation-based strategies in school, home, and community settings to promote mental health. Occupation-based services can be embedded in a number of natural contexts in schools to include recess, lunch, art, and physical education. In particular, game clubs can be used during recess, and lunch groups may be utilized in the cafeteria. Increased emphasis is being placed on participation in extracurricular activities. This opens the door for occupational therapy practitioners to help children and youth develop and participate in enjoyable hobbies and interests during after-school hours. Examples include activities such as arts, recreation, music, sports, and club activities (Bazyk, 2011).

Major Approaches Used in Mental Health Promotion, Prevention, and Intervention

First, an overview of the major approaches used in a public health approach to mental health will be introduced. A description of the occupational therapy process will then be provided for each of the three tiers of service. Although not inclusive, the following approaches are useful in mental health promotion, prevention, and intervention and can be applied at all three tiers of the MTSS.

Mental health literacy focuses on providing all children and youth with a working knowledge of how to develop and maintain positive mental health. It also provides children and youth a method to recognize, manage, and seek intervention for mental illness (Barry & Jenkins, 2007; Griffiths, Christensen, & Jorm, 2009). Examples of this approach include the following:

- Recognizing when a mental health disorder is developing
- Knowledge about effective self-help strategies for milder problems
- Where to seek assistance
- First aid skills to support others who are developing a mental disorder or are in a mental health crisis (Jorm, 2012).

Suggested strategies for promoting positive mental health are provided in Tables 3-1 to 3-5. The strategies are divided by their components. These components include positive affect/feeling happy, positive character traits, positive institutions, competencies and strengths, and coping abilities.

Social and emotional learning (SEL) refers to the process of helping children recognize and manage emotions, think about their feelings and how one should act, regulate behavior based on thoughtful decision making, and acquire important social skills for developing healthy relationships in life (Elias et al., 1997). It is believed that emotional and social skills must be developed to prevent feelings from "hijacking" thoughts and actions (Goleman, 1995). The five major skill areas viewed as essential include self-awareness, self-management, social awareness, relationship skills, and responsible decision making (Collaborative for Academic, Social, and Emotional Learning [CASEL], n.d.). A meta-analysis of 317 studies involving 424,303 participants of SEL programs indicated improvements in social–emotional skills, connection to school, academic performance,

	TABLE 3-1	
COMPONENT OF POSITIVE MENTAL HEALTH: POSITIVE AFFECT—FEELING "HAPPY"		
COMPONENT: POSITIVE AFFECT— FEELING "HAPPY"	**EVALUATION: GUIDING QUESTIONS**	**PROMOTION, INTERVENTION, AND STRATEGIES**
<ul><li>Joy, contentment, pleasure, optimism</li><li>Positive emotions reduce negative emotions and promote emotional resilience and psychological well-being (Fredrickson, 2004).</li><li>When we engage children in activities that are "fun," we are contributing to mental health. Explain this to others: "Having fun helps children feel good emotionally, which is a component of positive mental health."</li></ul>	<ul><li>Note the types of engagement that produce positive emotions in the child/youth. What is the child doing when he/she appears happy?</li><li>Does the child/youth demonstrate periods of joy/happiness throughout the day?</li><li>Note whether there has been an observable change in the child's overall disposition(e.g., from "sunny" disposition to withdrawn).</li><li>Tune into healthy occupations that a child appears to enjoy: Physical activities? Art? Music? Reading? Socializing?</li></ul>	<ul><li>Help children explore a range of occupations, and identify those that add meaning and joy to their lives.</li><li>Consciously design occupations for children and youth that lead to enjoyment and positive emotions and encourage continued participation. Why "enjoyment" matters – participating in enjoyable occupations can help promote mental health and foster resilience.</li><li>Recognize features of activities associated with positive emotions (e.g., those that utilize personal strengths, offer a just-right challenge, and allow choice).</li><li>Observe and articulate the mental health outcomes of participation in enjoyable occupations to children, families, and other health care providers.</li></ul>

attitudes about self and others, and positive social behavior while reducing conduct problems and emotional distress (Payton et al., 2008).

Positive behavioral interventions and supports (PBIS) provide a framework for preventing problem behaviors by proactively altering a situation before problems escalate. It has been suggested that concurrently teaching appropriate alternatives also aids in preventing problem behaviors (Bradshaw, Koth, Bevans, Ialongo, & Leaf, 2008). School-wide or universal PBIS interventions (SWPBS) are designed to create positive school environments for all students. This includes the majority of students who do not frequently present behavior problems, but would benefit from incentives that motivate them to follow school rules. Both the prevention of behavior problems and teaching pro-social behaviors is emphasized for the entire school (Freeman, et al., 2006). Other key features of SWPBS include the following:

- Clearly defined and communicated behavioral expectations written in positive terms, such as "Be respectful of others."

- Specific strategies for teaching appropriate behaviors
- Consistent application of procedures for correcting misbehavior to include consequences
- Acknowledgement of appropriate behaviors
- A support plan to meet the needs of students with chronic challenging behaviors

Schools reporting success in implementing SWPBS have identified multiple benefits. These include increased student attendance, student and teacher self-reports of a more positive and calm environment, and reduction in the numbers of behavioral disruptions (OSEP Center on Positive Behavioral Interventions and Support, 2013).

Participation in structured recreation and leisure activities is another important aspect of occupation-based practice when promoting mental health in children. Structured leisure activities are associated with many qualities present in paid work. They include regular participation schedules, rule-guided interaction, direction by one or more adult leaders, an emphasis on skill development that increases in complexity and challenge, performance that requires

TABLE 3-2
COMPONENT OF POSITIVE MENTAL HEALTH: POSITIVE CHARACTER TRAITS

COMPONENT: POSITIVE CHARACTER TRAITS	EVALUATION: GUIDING QUESTIONS	PROMOTION, INTERVENTION, AND STRATEGIES
<ul><li>Humor, love, kindness, artistic talent, curiosity, persistence, positive disposition, etc.</li><li>Nurturing</li><li>Creative</li><li>Sociable</li><li>Humorous</li><li>Inquisitive</li><li>Kind</li><li>Spiritual</li><li>Thoughtful</li><li>Cheerful</li><li>Flexible</li><li>Strong work ethic</li><li>Good listener</li><li>Energetic</li></ul>	<ul><li>What positive qualities are unique to each child? Look for qualities that reflect personality traits vs. specific skills such as having a sense of humor or a natural tendency to nurture others.</li><li>Identify the child's interests, which may fall outside of a traditional skill set, such as interests in trains, dolls, collecting rocks, painting, nurturing animals, etc.</li><li>Make a point of noting the child's unique character traits to the child and family (e.g., sense of humor, natural ability to nurture).</li></ul>	<ul><li>Help all children identify their unique signature strengths and engage in occupations that support and cultivate their expression (e.g., artistic talent, volunteer work)</li><li>Expose children to a variety of artistic, musical, and other creative activities in order to explore possible interests.</li><li>Avoid focusing solely on skills. Children with limited skills also have character strengths that must be acknowledged, celebrated, and fostered.</li><li>Guard against framing "intense interests" in a negative light (e.g., obsessions). Use intense interests to foster participation in a range of activities revolving around the intense interest. Example: Develop a book club focusing on reading books that involve trains for a child who has an intense interest in trains.</li></ul>

TABLE 3-3
COMPONENT OF POSITIVE MENTAL HEALTH: POSITIVE INSTITUTIONS

COMPONENT: POSITIVE INSTITUTIONS	EVALUATION: GUIDING QUESTIONS	PROMOTION, INTERVENTION, AND STRATEGIES
<ul><li>Environmental factors such as families, caring adults, and programs that foster character strengths and positive emotions</li></ul>	<ul><li>Do the settings where the child learns, socializes, and plays foster positive emotion and personal strengths?</li></ul>	<ul><li>Consult with teachers, administrators, and youth workers to create and/or adapt activities and the environment to promote positive experiences.</li><li>Advocate for programs to emphasize mental health promotion.</li><li>Modify the sensory environment to promote participation based on the child's unique sensory needs.</li></ul>

TABLE 3-4
COMPONENT OF POSITIVE MENTAL HEALTH: COMPETENCIES AND STRENGTHS

COMPONENT: COMPETENCIES AND STRENGTHS	EVALUATION: GUIDING QUESTIONS	PROMOTIONS, INTERVENTIONS, AND STRATEGIES
• Social and emotional skills • Skills needed for school, work, play, leisure, ADLs, and rest	• Use strength-based assessment tools such as the Devereux Student Strengths Assessment (K-8) (DESSA) (LeBuffe, Shapiro, & Naglieri, 2009). • Use a variety of functional assessments to evaluate skills needed for successful participation in home, school, and the community.	• Incorporate the child's strengths and interests into intervention activities. • Embed SEL goals into intervention activities. SEL areas include self-awareness, self-management, social awareness, relationship skills, and responsible decision making (www.casel.org). • Help children identify and talk about their feelings and think about how feelings influence behavior. • Help children become aware of how they can change how they feel by participating in enjoyable activities (i.e., occupational reflection); doing enjoyable activities can lessen feelings of depression; doing relaxation activities may help reduces stress; etc.

TABLE 3-5
COMPONENT OF POSITIVE MENTAL HEALTH: COPING ABILITIES

COMPONENT: COPING ABILITIES	EVALUATION: GUIDING QUESTIONS	PROMOTIONS, INTERVENTIONS, AND STRATEGIES
• Ability to cope with life stressors and challenges • Resilient • Adaptable • Flexible	• Observe how the child reacts to everyday challenges such as struggling with an assignment or losing a game. • Identify if the child uses problem-solving skills during the stressor. • Identify whether the child uses strategies to modify negative emotions during the stressor such as relaxation strategies or cognitive restructuring.	• Modify the environmental demands to match the child's capabilities. • Teach the child *problem-focused coping*, including efforts to change the source of stress (e.g., seeking support or assistance, modifying the environment). • Teach *emotion-focused coping*, including efforts to manage negative emotions associated with the stressor (e.g., emotional regulation, cognitive restructuring, cognitive distraction, thought stopping, etc.) (Pincus & Friedman, 2004).

sustained active attention, and the provision of feedback (Mahoney, Larson, Eccles, & Lord, 2005). Correlational research has demonstrated a positive relationship between participation in structured leisure and positive outcomes, including greater academic achievement, diminished delinquency, increased self-efficacy, and self-control (Larson, 2000). Given these benefits, it is important to pay particular attention to how children and youth spend time outside of school. Exposure to a range of potential leisure occupations and the availability of resources to support engagement are critical factors influencing the likelihood that children and adolescents will develop and maintain healthy leisure interests (Bazyk, 2011).

In terms of *sensory processing*, "[o]ccupational therapy practitioners recognize that well-regulated sensory systems can contribute to important outcomes in social-emotional, physical, communication, self-care, cognitive, and adaptive skill development" (American Occupational Therapy Association [AOTA], 2008, p. 1). This makes occupational therapy practitioners uniquely qualified to apply this knowledge and skill at the universal, targeted, and intensive levels to promote successful participation in school and community settings. All children and youth are sensory beings who respond to everyday sensation in individual ways. This results in sensory preferences that are reflected in the person's performance and interactions with others. Most people demonstrate moderate responses to sensory input, allowing for successful participation throughout the day. Individuals with certain disabilities (such as autism) or mental illness (such as psychosis) may respond to sensory input in a more intense manner, resulting in performance challenges (Dunn, 2007). Intense reactions to sensory input can negatively influence a person's emotions, causing irritability or tantrums. They may also impair social interaction, leading to withdrawal or aggressive behavior. Occupational therapy practitioners can play an important role in helping children, families, and professionals develop a working knowledge of sensory processing. This will help others to understand children's behaviors and modify everyday interactions and environments to foster success and well-being (Dunn, 2007).

At the universal level (tier 1), occupational therapy services can focus on educating relevant stakeholders about the impact of sensory processing on mental health (Dunn, 2007). Occupational therapy can also make environmental modifications to enhance performance (Champagne, 2008). An important goal is to help children and adults understand and respect sensory differences and as create environments that support a sense of comfort and emotional well-being. Applying our knowledge at each tier requires the use of a range of strategies, including direct and indirect services. Direct services include individual or group interventions, and indirect services include education, consultation with teachers and families, and environmental modifications.

Universal Services: All Children and Youth

Occupational therapy services at the universal level are geared toward the entire population. This includes children and youth with and without disabilities and/or mental health challenges. Tier 1 services reflect a dual commitment to promotion (the development of competencies) and prevention (a reduction of risk in the whole population, which includes the majority of children who do not demonstrate academic or emotional problems). At this level, the occupational therapy process focuses less on direct, individualized care and more on indirect services geared toward large groups of children and youth (Bazyk, 2011).

Awareness of school-wide and community-based promotion and prevention initiatives is critical. Examples include mental health literacy, SEL, and PBIS. Likewise, it is critical to become familiar with and use reputable online resources in order to develop and maintain information related to mental health promotion. Table 3-6 provides examples of useful online resources. Occupational therapy practitioners should appraise school and community settings for the presence and quality of their information related to mental health. Information should be based on a sound awareness of best practice related to mental health promotion and prevention. Initially, it is important to identify what educational policies and established programs exist. Then, systematic efforts or actions can be made to ensure that occupational therapy becomes an active and recognized team member within the system of care.

Universal services include informal observations of children in natural contexts, in-service education for school personnel and families, collaboration with school personnel to identify areas of need, and the provision of accommodations to enhance student functioning. Suggested tier 1 strategies aimed at promoting positive mental health and preventing mental health challenges include the following:

- *Informally observe all children* for behaviors that might suggest mental health concerns or limitations in social–emotional development. Occupational therapy practitioners should make note of the emotions of children while they participate in occupations and during interactions with children in school and community settings. The therapist may ask, "Does the physical and social environment support successful participation and enjoyment?" It may be important to bring any concerns to the educational team.

TABLE 3-6

MENTAL HEALTH INTERNET RESOURCES

AOTA: SCHOOL MENTAL HEALTH (SMH) TOOLKIT

Free, downloadable information sheets on a variety of topics, including depression, grieving, anxiety, obesity, etc.

Web address: www.aota.org/practice/children-youth/mental%20health/school-mental-health.aspx

CARING FOR EVERY CHILD'S MENTAL HEALTH

Substance Abuse and Mental Health Services Agency (SAMHSA) supports a comprehensive system-of-care approach to children's mental health. Sponsors an annual Children's Mental Health Awareness Day every May.

Web address: www.samhsa.gov/children/

NATIONAL INSTITUTE OF MENTAL HEALTH (NIMH)

The mission of NIMH is to diminish the burden of mental illness through research.

Web address: www.nimh.nih.gov

OFFICE OF THE U.S. SURGEON GENERAL

In 1999, Surgeon General David Satcher issued a comprehensive report on mental health. Chapter 3 covers children and adolescents.

Web address: www.surgeongeneral.gov/index.html

BAZELON CENTER FOR MENTAL HEALTH LAW

The Bazelon Center for Mental Health Law works on a broad array of children's mental health issues.

Web address: www.bazelon.org

CENTERS FOR SCHOOL MENTAL HEALTH—TECHNICAL ASSISTANCE CENTERS

In 1995 two national training and technical assistance centers focused on mental health in schools were established with partial support from the U.S. Department of Health and Human Services and the Center for Mental Health Services. One center is at UCLA and the other is at the University of Maryland at Baltimore. The websites include information and resources on school-based mental health programs.

Web address: www.smhp.psych.ucla.edu (UCLA)

Web address: www.csmh.umaryland.edu (University of Maryland at Baltimore)

SCHOOLMENTALHEALTH.ORG

This site offers school mental health resources for clinicians, educators, administrators, parents/caregivers, families, and students. The resources included in the site emphasize practical information and skills based on current research, including prominent evidence-based practices, as well as lessons learned from local, state, and national initiatives.

Web address: www.schoolmentalhealth.org

MINNESOTA CHILDREN'S MENTAL HEALTH ASSOCIATION

The mission is to promote positive mental health for all infants, children, adolescents, and their families through education and resources.

Web address: www.macmh.org

(continued)

Table 3-6 (continued)
Mental Health Internet Resources

BULLY PREVENTION

OSEP Technical Assistance Center on PBIS (free downloadable manuals): *Bully Prevention Manual: Elementary School Level; Bully Prevention Manual: Middle School Level* - Authors: Stiller, B., Ross, S., Horner, R.
Web address: www.pbis.org

STEPS TO RESPECT

Focuses on bully prevention and friendship development; developed by Committee for Children
Web address: www.cfchildren.org/steps-to-respect.aspx

EYES ON BULLYING TOOLKIT

What Can You Do? (free downloadable)
Web address: *www.eyesonbullying.org/pdfs/toolkit.pdf*

SOCIAL AND EMOTIONAL LEARNING AND BULLYING PREVENTION

Free downloadable
Web address: http://casel.org/wp-content/uploads/SEL-and-Bullying-Prevention-2009.pdf

PACER NATIONAL CENTER FOR BULLY PREVENTION

Free resources, information sheets, bookmarks, etc.
Web address: www.pacer.org/bullying/

PEER ADVOCACY GUIDE

How to address bullying of students with disabilities by engaging, educating, and empowering their peers with advocacy skills.
Web address: www.pacer.org/bullying/resources/activities/toolkits/pdf/PeerAdvocacyGuide.pdf

FRIENDSHIP SKILLS

Tony Attwood (www.tonyattwood.com) - Understanding and teaching friendship skills; friendship checklists
Web Address: www.tonyattwood.com.au/index.php?option=com_content&view=article&id=75:understanding-and-teaching-friendship-skills&catid=45:archived-resource-papers&Itemid=181

BIBLIOTHERAPY – USING BOOKS TO HELP CHILDREN LEARN ABOUT SEL:

- Carnegie Library of Pittsburgh
- **Web Address:** www.carnegielibrary.org/research/parentseducators/parents/bibliotherapy/

WORDS THAT HEAL

- Using Children's Literature to Prevent Bullying - Anti-defamation League
- **Web Address:** www.adl.org/education/curriculum_connections/winter_2005/

- *Clearly articulate the scope of occupational therapy practice* to include social participation, social–emotional function, and mental health promotion.
- *Promote mental health literacy* efforts offered in the school. Collaborate with health educators and school nurses to educate students about how to develop and maintain mental health and what to do if a person begins to feel mentally unstable. Make mental health a part of everyday conversation.
- *Collaborate with teachers and other school staff* to help them recognize the most effective learning styles of students. Ensure that students are able to meet classroom demands, and make accommodations as needed.

- *Assist in lunch and recess supervision.* Offer supports to help make lunch and recess enjoyable times of the day for all students with and without disabilities.

- *Support school-wide efforts to promote mental health literacy, SEL, and the use of PBIS.* Assist in the implementation of a variety of contexts to include the classroom, hallways, lunchroom, playground, and restrooms.

- *Learn about school prevention programs focusing on risk reduction.* This includes teen pregnancy, drug use, suicide, and bullying prevention initiatives. Encourage participation and reinforce the message.

- *Provide in-service education* to teachers and staff on the following topics:

  ○ Sensory processing: Adapt classroom practices based on the varying sensory needs of students to enhance emotional regulation and a sense of well-being (Williams & Shellenberger, 1996).

  ○ Enabling positive mental health and participation in enjoyable activities: Enjoyment is linked with a sense of emotional well-being and contributes to overall mental health.

- *Advocate* for inclusive structured leisure opportunities such as art, music, theater, sports, and clubs.

Targeted Services: Children and Youth at Risk of Mental Health Challenges

Targeted interventions are provided to support children and youth who have learning impairments and emotional challenges. Students of concern may also have life experiences that place them at risk for developing mental health challenges or engagement in problematic behavior. For example, children with developmental or physical disabilities might struggle with issues related to "feeling different," low self-esteem, or the stress associated with frequent medical appointments. Additionally, children with and without disabilities are likely to struggle with situational stressors such as friendship issues, bullying, parental divorce, the death of a family member, poverty, or academic challenges at some point in their lives (Bazyk, 2011). During such times, participation in enjoyable occupations, character strengths, coping strategies, and environmental supports can serve as important "buffers" in the prevention of mental ill health (Catalano, Hawkins, Berglund, Pollard, & Arthur, 2002). It is important for occupational therapy practitioners to remain vigilant to the presence of possible stressors. Occupational therapy practitioners should also advocate for and help develop services to counteract stressors and build competencies. Examples include grief support training for school personnel and promotion of participation in after-school clubs for students.

Appraisal efforts at this level need to emphasize efficient but careful screening for subtle changes in behavior and functional skills under the supervision of a registered occupational therapist (Bazyk, 2011). Children and youth at this level are generally not identified as having a mental or behavioral disorder, but often begin to show subtle changes in performance. A child who is mildly depressed, for example, might be quiet and withdrawn and underperform academically. A child with attention deficit disorder may have difficulty concentrating and getting homework completed. Anxiety might cause excessive stress for the child who is required to speak in front of the class. A variety of strategies can be used, including observations of performance and social interaction, informal interviews with the student or teacher, and screening assessments. The evaluation is followed by the development of a support plan that might include environmental modifications such as the reduction of expectations, modified interactions, and small group intervention.

Services need to emphasize both prevention of mental illness and the promotion of competencies to offset early symptoms, such as teaching relaxation strategies. Services also must involve a more direct role in evaluation and intervention compared with tier 1 services. At this level, occupational therapy practitioners might collaborate with teachers, social workers, or other mental health providers to develop and co-facilitate targeted interventions. Checkpoint 3-3 stresses the importance of services provided to both prevent mental illness and promote competencies.

Interventions at this level include a combination of modifications to the environment and/or the task. A modification to the environment might be providing color-coded folders for a student with ADHD. Another modification may be to encourage movement breaks throughout the day. A modification of a task might involve breaking down a homework assignment or giving one segment at a time to a student with anxiety. In addition to these services, the use of occupation-based groups is particularly appropriate at the targeted level. Purposeful activities such as arts and crafts, games, or cooking activities can be used to enhance skill development of various occupations, as well as to improve interpersonal and intrapersonal learning (Bazyk, 2011). The occupational therapy practitioner facilitates group processes targeting psychosocial abilities that are incorporated into an activity. Examples include the development of social skills, the identification and expression of feelings, and the development of a positive group identity. Research suggests that children who demonstrate personal or social difficulties benefit more from small groups. Small groups can provide a supportive environment and an opportunity to develop positive relationships with caring adults more than children who receive individual interventions (Shechtman, 2001).

CHECKPOINT 3-3. APPLY
Mental Health Promotion: Strategies for *optimizing* mental health before identification of a specific mental health problem   • Review Table 3-1. Brainstorm how occupational therapists can promote enjoyment during lunch and recess.   **Mental Health Prevention:** Strategies to *reduce* mental health *problems* before identification of a specific mental health problem   • Read AOTA's SMH Information Sheets on Obesity and Grieving Loss (www.aota.org/practice/children-youth/mental%20health/school-mental-health.aspx). For each at-risk population, plan a 1-hour occupation-based group applying intervention strategies suggested on these information sheets.

Specific targeted strategies include the following:

- *Learn about early signs of a variety of mental illnesses.* Mental illnesses can include depression, anxiety, obsessive-compulsive disorder, and schizophrenia as examples. Additionally, it is important to know how such symptoms might manifest themselves in the school and home settings.

- *Use both informal and formal evaluation strategies* to identify risk, changes in behavior, functional skills, and/or the early presence of mental health problems.

- *Evaluate social participation* with peers during all school activities, including recess and lunch.

- *Provide early intervening services or Section 504 accommodations* for students demonstrating behavioral or learning difficulties due to mild mental health disorders or psychosocial issues.

- *Consult with teachers* to modify learning demands and academic routines to foster successful participation and promote positive psychological functioning. Examples include breaking down school assignments and giving one part of an assignment at a time to minimize anxiety. Additionally, teaching relaxation strategies may be beneficial.

- *Contribute to school-wide bully prevention efforts.* Refer to www.pbis.org to find bully prevention manuals. Promote friendship development as a way to reduce the risk of bullying.

- *Provide parents with education* on how to adapt family routines or activities to support their children's mental health, especially with high-risk children.

- *Develop and run group programs to foster social participation* for students struggling with peer interaction.

Suggested tier 2 services geared toward children and youth at risk of developing mental health challenges are summarized in Table 3-7. More specific information on the treatment applications and occupational therapy process for children and youth in the early lifespan will be covered in Chapters 4 and 5.

Intensive Individualized Services: Children and Youth With Identified Mental Health Challenges

Tier 3 services are provided for children and youth with identified mental, emotional, or behavioral disorders that limit their participation in school, home, and community activities. Occupational therapy practitioners need to maintain in-depth knowledge of a range of mental health and behavioral disorders and current medical and psychosocial interventions for school and community settings. They also need to know how the disorders influence the person's functioning in a variety of occupational areas such as education, leisure, ADLs, and social participation. It is also important to become aware of the mental health disorders commonly present in children with various developmental disorders. Children with autism have a high risk of co-occurring anxiety disorders, for example. A variety of evaluation strategies such as observation, interviews, and formal assessment can be used in order to analyze factors limiting occupational performance.

Services provided at tier 3 are individualized to meet the specific needs of children and youth based on the mental health condition and presenting symptoms. Services at tier 3 will be described in more detail in Chapters 4 and 5. It is also important to work closely with the multiple providers likely to be involved. Systems-of-care approaches provide a framework for youth, families, schools, and community partners to provide individualized services and supports. This helps children and youth with serious emotional disturbances and their families achieve their desired goals (Sebian et al., 2007). Such approaches are necessary, as youth with serious mental health disorders typically receive services from two or more public agencies. Examples of services from public agencies include juvenile justice, child welfare, special education, and state and local mental health departments.

TABLE 3-7

TARGETED OCCUPATIONAL THERAPY SERVICES FOR CHILDREN AND YOUTH AT RISK OF MENTAL HEALTH CHALLENGES

AT-RISK CONDITION AND ASSOCIATED MENTAL HEALTH RISKS	OCCUPATIONAL PERFORMANCE RISKS	SUGGESTED OCCUPATIONAL THERAPY INTERVENTIONS
Obesity (~11% U.S. population) **Overweight** (~25%) Children at greatest risk of obesity are those living in poverty or with a disability (Bazyk, 2011) • Poor self-esteem and body image • Anxiety • Depression • May experience the negative effects associated with weight bias • Eating disorders (binge dieting and eating	• Social participation challenges. • Difficulty making and keeping friends due to weight bias • Higher risk of being bullied • Sleep/rest challenges due to risk of sleep apnea • Limited play/leisure. May find physical activities too challenging	• Emphasize "health at any size" versus weight loss. • Teach children about healthy food choices. • Work with school officials to decrease the availability of foods high in fat and sugar in the cafeteria and in vending machines. • Develop after-school programs that foster participation in enjoyable physical activities and healthy cooking. • Consult with school personnel to develop enjoyable physical activities during recess. • Work with school officials to prevent weight-biased bullying. • Embed SEL strategies to help children identify feelings and develop positive coping strategies.
Poverty (~16% U.S. population) **Low Income** (~37%) (Bazyk, 2011) • Depression • Anxiety • Substance abuse • Aggressive behavior	• Sleep problems due to stressful environment • Obesity due to limited access to fresh fruits, vegetables, and safe playgrounds • Limited opportunities to engage in extracurricular leisure activities resulting in boredom and participation in risky behavior	• Help parents consciously steer children away from street influences by monitoring free time and friendships. • Promote engagement in structured leisure activities outside of school such as sports, church groups, and creative arts in positive environments. • Foster SEL by identifying feelings and reflecting on how feelings influence behavior.

(continued)

TABLE 3-7 (CONTINUED)

TARGETED OCCUPATIONAL THERAPY SERVICES FOR CHILDREN AND YOUTH AT RISK OF MENTAL HEALTH CHALLENGES

AT-RISK CONDITION AND ASSOCIATED MENTAL HEALTH RISKS	OCCUPATIONAL PERFORMANCE RISKS	SUGGESTED OCCUPATIONAL THERAPY INTERVENTIONS
Grieving Loss The conflicted feelings caused by change due to loss (e.g., death of parent, friend, or pet; parental divorce; moving to a new home) (Bazyk, 2011) • Stress associated with loss may result in a range of behavioral changes (emotional withdrawal, regressive behaviors) • Anxiety • Depression • Difficulty concentrating at school • Psychosomatic complaints (headaches, stomach aches)	• ADL changes (altered eating patterns, bedwetting) • Altered sleep and rest, including excessive or limited sleep • Difficulty concentrating in school; drop in grades • Social withdrawal and friendship issues • Loss of interest in play/leisure activities	• Teach children how to provide support to friends who are grieving. • Help teachers recognize emotional and behavioral changes associated with grieving and suggest strategies for modifying expectations and providing support. • Encourage participation in enjoyable but low-stress activities with close friends to minimize feelings of isolation. • Use creative arts occupations to help children express feelings of loss either in small groups or individual sessions (e.g., journaling, making memory boards, scrapbooking, etc.). • Mention the person who died in everyday conversation to encourage the student to talk about what he or she valued in the relationship. • Be aware of "grief triggers" such as birthdays and holidays. Reassure children that heightened emotions during these times are a natural part of grieving.
Physical Disabilities (Petrenchik, King, & Batarowicz, 2011) • About 1 in 3 children with developmental disabilities are identified as having a co-occurring mental health condition such as anxiety and depression (Schwartz, Garland, Waddell, & Harrison, 2006) • Overemphasis on rehabilitation of physical impairments overshadows attention to social and emotional needs	• Social isolation may result in delayed social skills, lack of friends, and limited opportunities to develop extracurricular interests. • May have fewer opportunities to participate in extracurricular activities resulting in boredom and delayed skill development. • Poor self-esteem, depression, and/or anxiety may contribute further to social isolation.	• Encourage the child to express and process feelings related to reduced physical functioning. • Promote a balanced view of health, including attention to both physical and emotional needs of the child. • Foster sustained participation in enjoyable neighborhood- and community-based out-of-school activities to promote the development of interests and friends, and to build on strengths and talents. Such positive experiences help buffer the effects of life adversities and promote positive mental health. • Help create school and community environments that are inclusive, stimulating, satisfying, and enjoyable.

(continued)

TABLE 3-7 (CONTINUED)		
TARGETED OCCUPATIONAL THERAPY SERVICES FOR CHILDREN AND YOUTH AT RISK OF MENTAL HEALTH CHALLENGES		
AT-RISK CONDITION AND ASSOCIATED MENTAL HEALTH RISKS	OCCUPATIONAL PERFORMANCE RISKS	SUGGESTED OCCUPATIONAL THERAPY INTERVENTIONS
• More likely than typical peers to encounter negative social environments (stigmatized, marginalized, socially excluded, and bullied)		• Contribute to school-wide approaches emphasizing disability awareness and acceptance of differences.
Autism Spectrum Disorders (Crabtree & DeLany, 2011) • Higher rates of anxiety, depression, obsessive-compulsive, and ADHD disorder than the general population • Over 90% experience sensory processing challenges, which are associated with increased stress and social and communication challenges	• Challenges with social participation, making and keeping friends, and social isolation due to sensory modulation and communication difficulties • ADLs: May see restricted diets and clothing choices due to sensory modulation issues. • Delays in academic, independent living, and work skills due to social, cognitive, and sensory challenges	• Promote social participation in natural contexts with typically developing peers in order to foster generalization of skills. • Offer group-based sensorimotor play programs to foster language and social participation. • Foster participation in extracurricular activities to promote the development of interests and meaningful friendships. • Use Social Stories to teach the child how to respond in a specific situation. • Develop peer support programs such as Circle of Friends (Pallis, 2008), lunchtime clubs, and Best Buddies (Best Buddies International, 2010) to prevent isolation and bullying while fostering friendships.
ADHD, Learning Disabilities (LD), Developmental Coordination Disorder (Poulsen, 2011; Young, 2007) • Low self-esteem due to difficulties in school and home performance • Social exclusion • Anxiety • Depression	• School: Failure to attend to details, careless errors, avoids challenging academic tasks that require sustained mental effort, frequent shifts in attention, may have visual perception or reading problems (LD), difficulty organizing school materials in locker or desk, forgets homework • ADLs: Messy eating or drinking; irregular sleeping	• Encourage the identification and expression of feelings by applying SEL strategies. • Help children explore and successfully participate in extracurricular leisure interests based on areas of strength in order to enhance feelings of competence and autonomy. Provide leisure coaching if necessary (Ziviani et al., 2009). • Analyze the student's sensory needs and develop a sensory diet to successful function in home, community, and school contexts.

(continued)

TABLE 3-7 (CONTINUED)

TARGETED OCCUPATIONAL THERAPY SERVICES FOR CHILDREN AND YOUTH AT RISK OF MENTAL HEALTH CHALLENGES

AT-RISK CONDITION AND ASSOCIATED MENTAL HEALTH RISKS	OCCUPATIONAL PERFORMANCE RISKS	SUGGESTED OCCUPATIONAL THERAPY INTERVENTIONS
	• IADLs: Disorganized bedroom and study space, homework incomplete, poor follow-through with chores • Leisure: Inattention to instructions, performance erratic, difficulty waiting turn, may have coordination problems (Developmental Coordination Disorder) • Social participation: May be teased or bullied for poor performance.	• Help parents and teachers understand the reasons for the child's behaviors and offer support and solutions for changing and adapting the unwanted behaviors. • Modify the environment and tasks to foster organization and the development of routines (e.g., using color coding).
Children who have experienced trauma Examples of trauma: • Community, school, and domestic violence • Physical abuse, sexual abuse, and neglect • Natural disasters • Medical trauma Mental health challenges: • Post-traumatic stress disorder • Anxiety • Depression • Conduct disorder • Eating disorders • Oppositional defiant disorder	• Sleep disorders • ADLs: May demonstrate poor hygiene and self-care. • Social participation: Social withdrawal and isolation. May have difficulty trusting people. • School: Poor attendance, low grades, difficulty concentrating, and behavioral challenges • Play/leisure: Loss of interest in leisure activities and play	• Modify home and school environments to create safe, secure, and sensory-friendly spaces (e.g., weighted lap pads, fidget toys, rocking chairs, and soothing lights). • Apply the Sanctuary Model to help create collaborative and healing environments that promote recovery from trauma. Refer to www.sanctuaryweb.com. • Structure predictable routines in home and school. • Tune into the child's affect and emotional responses and triggers for problem behaviors. Develop strategies to modify them. • Offer small occupation-based groups to provide opportunities to share feelings, learn new coping strategies, and engage in enjoyable creative occupations.

(continued)

TABLE 3-7 (CONTINUED)

TARGETED OCCUPATIONAL THERAPY SERVICES FOR CHILDREN AND YOUTH AT RISK OF MENTAL HEALTH CHALLENGES

AT-RISK CONDITION AND ASSOCIATED MENTAL HEALTH RISKS	OCCUPATIONAL PERFORMANCE RISKS	SUGGESTED OCCUPATIONAL THERAPY INTERVENTIONS
• May engage in self-destructive and risky behaviors (Bloom, 1995; Stein et al., 2003)		• Provide leisure coaching to help children identify and participate in enjoyable extracurricular activities. • Teach relaxation skills, including yoga, deep breathing, and progressive relaxation.
Children at risk of psychosis and demonstrating signs of prodromal phase (Downing, 2011) • Subtle, experiential symptoms may ebb and flow in frequency and intensity up to 4 years before the onset of an illness. • Cognitive changes in functioning such as difficulty concentrating or remembering information. May experience jumbled thoughts or confusion. • May experience perceptual distortions such as hearing one's name called or increased sensitivity to sounds. • May demonstrate behavioral changes such as withdrawal or increased irritability.	• Social participation: Deteriorating social function. Altering relationships with family and friends. May become socially isolated. • School: Problems staying focused in class or during studies and may demonstrate a drop in grades. • Work: May demonstrate declining performance such as tardiness and a failure to complete work assignments. • Leisure: May drop out of extracurricular activities. • ADLs: May demonstrate dramatic changes in appetite and difficulty in dressing and/or hygiene. • Sleep/rest: May demonstrate dramatic changes in sleep, either difficulty sleeping or excessive sleep.	• Offer in-services to school personnel and families about sensory preferences and how to modify the environment to decrease stress and promote positive functioning. • Offer small group sessions to foster participation in enjoyable activities in order to reduce stress and promote socialization. • Consult with teachers and parents to make accommodations to reduce stress and enhance participation, such as decreasing activity demands; assisting with organization of a task; reducing environmental stimulation; and developing routines that include exercise, healthy nutrition, and good sleep hygiene.

Compiled from Bazyk, S. (2011). *Mental health promotion, prevention and intervention with children and youth: A guiding framework for occupational therapy.* Bethesda, MD: AOTA Press.; Best Buddies International. (2010). *Best buddies.* Retrieved from www.bestbuddies.org/best-buddies; Bloom, S. L. (1995). Creating sanctuary in the school. *Journal for a Just and Caring Education, 1*(4), 403-433.; Crabtree, L., & Delaney, J. V. (2011). Autism: Promoting social participation and mental health. In S. Bazyk (Ed.). *Mental health promotion, prevention and intervention with children and youth: A guiding framework for occupational therapy* (pp. 163-187). Bethesda, MD: The American Occupational Therapy Association, Inc.; Downing, D. (2011). Occupational therapy for youth at risk of psychosis and those with identified mental illness. In S. Bazyk (Ed.). *Mental health promotion, prevention and intervention with children and youth: A guiding framework for occupational therapy.* Bethesda, MD: The American Occupational Therapy Association, Inc.; Pallis, B. (2008). *Circle of friends: Testimonials.* Retrieved from www.circleoffriends.org.; Petrenchik, T. M., King, G. A., & Bartowicz, B. (2011). Children and youth with disabilities: Enhancing mental health through positive experiences of doing and belonging. In S. Bazyk (Ed.). *Mental health promotion, prevention and intervention with children and youth: A guiding framework for occupational therapy.* Bethesda, MD: The American Occupational Therapy Association, Inc.; Poulsen, A. (2011). Children with attention deficit hyperactivity disorder, and learning disabilities. In S. Bazyk (Ed.). *Mental health promotion, prevention and intervention with children and youth: A guiding framework for occupational therapy.* Bethesda, MD: The American Occupational Therapy Association, Inc.; Schwartz et al. (2006). *Mental health and developmental disabilities in children. Research report prepared for Children and Youth Mental Health.* Vancouver: British Columbia Ministry of Children and Family Development, Children's Health Policy Centre.; Stein, et al. (2003). A mental health intervention for school children exposed to violence: A randomized controlled trial. *JAMA, 290*(5), 603-611. Young, R. L. (2007). The role of the occupational therapist in attention deficit hyperactivity disorder: A case study. *International Journal of Therapy and Rehabilitation, 14*(10), 454-459.; Ziviani et al., (2009). Movement skills proficiency and physical activity: A case for Engaging and Coaching for Health (EACH) Child. *Australian Occupational Therapy Journal, 56*(4), 259-265.

CHECKPOINT 3-4. ANALYZE
Explain how an occupational therapy practitioner could contribute to tier 1, 2, and 3 services in a school setting. Give examples. Delineate the role of the occupational therapist and the occupational therapy assistant in each example.

Specific tier 3 services for children and youth with identified mental health challenges include but are not limited to the following:

- *Evaluate school function.* This includes classroom participation, ADL performance, play/leisure, social participation, and beginning work skills in a variety of natural contexts such as the classroom or lunchroom.

- *Collaborate with teachers.* This includes modifying classroom expectations based on student-specific behavioral or mental health needs.

- *Analyze students' unique sensory needs and develop intervention strategies* to promote sensory processing to enhance successful function in multiple school contexts such as the classroom or cafeteria.

- *Provide ways to modify or enhance school routines* to reduce stress and the likelihood of behavioral outbursts.

- *Provide tips for promoting successful functioning throughout the school day.* This may include transitioning to classes, organizing work spaces such as the desk and locker, handling stress, and developing strategies for time management.

- *Collaborate with the other school-based mental health providers, teachers, and administrators* to ensure a coordinated system of care for students needing intensive interventions.

- *Promote the development of individual interests* by exploring extracurricular activities. Provide the necessary supports to enhance successful participation.

- *Offer individual or group interventions* for students with serious emotional disturbances. This can be done through special education or Section 504 to enhance participation in education, social activities, play/leisure, and ADLs.

- *Use coaching models* to help youth with mental health and physical challenges participate in meaningful leisure occupations.

Anxiety and depression are the two most common mental health disorders present in children and youth. Therefore, occupational therapy practitioners should be well versed in recognizing symptoms associated with those conditions and providing interventions to help children feel good emotionally and function well throughout the day. Regardless of the condition, services need to focus on helping children engage in activities that promote feelings of emotional well-being and modifying environments to reduce stress. It is also important to help the child develop reasonable goals for maintaining participation and daily routines that include good nutrition and some physical exercise (Downing, 2011). Checkpoint 3-4 helps to differentiate the role of the occupational therapist and occupational therapy assistant with tier 1, 2, and 3 services in a school setting.

SUMMARY

This chapter provided a foundation for reframing occupational therapy's role in children's mental health. Content emphasized the promotion of positive mental health for all children and youth by building positive qualities and personal strengths in addition to remediating problems and impairments. A three-tiered MTSS model focusing on a public health approach to mental health was introduced. This model helps practitioners envision universal, targeted, and intensive services. Evaluation techniques and intervention strategies for each tier were suggested to the reader. Additional information on helpful strategies for working with children and youth with a variety of mental health disorders can be found at www.schoolmentalhealth.org as well as on the AOTA website (www.aota.org).

PART 3: APPLICATIONS

The following activities will help you identify key aspects of this chapter that were highlighted in this text. Activities can be completed individually or in a small group to enhance learning.

1. You are talking to a friend about mental health. In your own words, explain what positive mental health is and what you would observe to inform you about a child's mental health.

2. Brainstorm the kinds of strategies and activities you might offer to celebrate Children's Mental Health Awareness Day in May. Be creative.

3. Explore the Action for Happiness website (www.actionforhappiness.org/). Brainstorm everyday strategies that you could embed in practice to help children and youth experience happiness.

4. Identify children and youth who are at risk of developing mental health challenges (tier 2). Identify how you might help prevent mental health challenges in these populations.

5. Go to the AOTA website (www.aota.org) and download and print the School Mental Health toolkit. Read these information sheets. Plan to share these with your fieldwork supervisors.

REFERENCES

American Occupational Therapy Association. (2008). *Addressing sensory integration across the lifespan through occupational therapy.* Bethesda, MD: AOTA Press.

Barry, M. M., & Jenkins, R. (2007). *Implementing mental health promotion.* Edinburgh, Scotland: Churchill Livingstone/Elsevier.

Bazyk, S. (2011). *Mental health promotion, prevention, and intervention with children and youth: A guiding framework for occupational therapy.* Bethesda, MD: AOTA Press.

Bazyk, S., & Arbesman, M. (2013). *Occupational therapy practice guidelines for mental health promotion, prevention, and intervention for children and youth.* Bethesda, MD: AOTA Press.

Best Buddies International. (2010). *Best Buddies.* Retrieved August 13, 2010, from www.bestbuddies.org/best-buddies.

Bloom, S. L. (1995). Creating sanctuary in the school. *Journal for a Just and Caring Education, 1*(4), 403–433.

Bing, R. (1981). 1981 Eleanor Clark Slagle lecture: Occupational therapy revisited: a paraphrastic journey. *American Journal of Occupational Therapy, 35,* 499-518.

Bradshaw, C. P., Koth, C. W., Bevans, K. B., Ialongo, N., & Leaf, P. J. (2008). The impact of school-wide positive behavioral interventions and supports (PBIS) on the organizational health of elementary schools. *School Psychological Quarterly, 23,* 462-473.

Catalano, R. F., Hawkins, D., Berglund, M. L., Pollard, J. A., & Arthur, M. W. (2002). Prevention science and positive youth development: Competitive or cooperative frameworks? *Journal of Adolescent Health, 31,* 230-239.

Champagne, T. (2008). *Sensory rooms in mental health.* Retrieved from www.ot-innovations.com/clinical-practice/sensory-modulation/sensory-rooms-in-mental-health-3/.

Collaborative for Academic, Social, and Emotional Learning. (n.d.). *What is SEL? Skills and competencies.* Retrieved from http://casel.org/why-it-matters/what-is-sel/skills-competencies/.

Crabtree, L., & Delaney, J. V. (2011). Autism: Promoting social participation and mental health. In S. Bazyk (Ed.), *Mental health promotion, prevention, and intervention with children and youth: A guiding framework for occupational therapy* (pp. 163-187). Bethesda, MD: The American Occupational Therapy Association, Inc.

Downing, D. (2011). Occupational therapy for youth at risk of psychosis and those with identified mental illness. In S. Bazyk (Ed.), *Mental health promotion, prevention, and intervention with children and youth: A guiding framework for occupational therapy* (pp. 141-161). Bethesda, MD: The American Occupational Therapy Association, Inc.

Dunn, W. (2007). Supporting children to participate successfully in everyday life by using sensory processing knowledge. *Infants and Young Children, 20,* 84-101.

Elias, M. J., Zins, J. D., Weissberg, R. P., Frey, K. S., Greenberg, M. T., Haynes, N. M.,…Shriver, T. P. (1997). *Promoting social and emotional learning: Guidelines for educators.* Alexandria, VA: Association for Supervision and Curriculum.

Freeman, R., Eber, L., Anderson, C., Irvin, L., Horner, R., & Bounds, M., Dunlap, G.(2006). Building inclusive school cultures using school-wide PBS: Designing effective individual support systems for students with significant disabilities. *Research and Practice for Persons with Severe Disabilities, 31,* 4–17.

Fredrickson, B. L. (2004). The broaden-and-build theory of positive emotions. *Philosophical Transactions of the Royal Society B: Biological Sciences, 359,* 1367-1377.

Griffiths, K. M., Christensen, H., & Jorm, A. F. (2009). Mental health literacy as a function of remoteness of residence: An Australian national study. *BMC Public Health, 9,* 1-20. Retrieved from www.ncbi.nlm.nih.gov/pmc/articles/PMC2670295/

Goleman, D. (1995). *Emotional intelligence: Why it can matter more than IQ.* New York: Bantam Books.

Jackson, L. L., & Arbesman, M. (Eds.). (2005). *Occupational therapy practice guidelines for children with behavioral and psychosocial needs.* Bethesda, MD: AOTA Press.

Jorm, A. F. (2012). Mental health literacy: Empowering the community to take action for better mental health. *American Psychologist, 67,* 231-243.

Keyes, C. L. (2007). Promoting and protecting mental health as flourishing: A complementary strategy for improving national mental health. *American Psychologist, 62,* 95-108.

Koller, J. R., & Bertel, J. M. (2006). Responding to today's mental health needs of children, families, and schools: Revisiting the preservice training and preparation of school-based personnel. *Education and Treatment of Children, 29,* 197-217.

Koppelman, J. (2004). *Children with mental disorders: Making sense of their needs and systems that help them* (NHPF Issue Brief No. 799). Washington, DC: George Washington University, National Health Policy Forum.

Larson, R. W. (2000). Toward a psychology of positive youth development. *American Psychologist, 55,* 170–183.

LeBuffe, P. A., Shapiro, V. B., & Naglieri, J. A. (2009) The Devereux Student Strengths Assessment (DESSA). Lewisville, NC: The Kaplan Company.

Mahoney, J. L., Larson, R. W., Eccles, J. S., & Lord, H. (2005). Organized activities as development contexts for children and adolescents. In J. Mahoney, R. Larson & J. Eccles (Eds.), *Organized activities as contexts of development: Extracurricular activities, after-school and community programs* (pp. 3-23). Mahwah, NJ: Lawrence Erlbaum.

Masia-Warner, C., Nangle, D. W., & Hansen, D. J. (2006). Bringing evidence-based child mental health services to the schools: General issues and specific populations. *Education and Treatment of Children, 29,* 165-172.

Miles, J., Espiritu, R. C., Horen, N., Sebian, J., & Waetzig, E. (2010). *A public health approach to children's mental health: A conceptual framework.* Washington, DC: Georgetown University Center for Child and Human Development, National Technical Assistance Center for Children's Mental Health.

National Research Council and Institute of Medicine. (2009). *Preventing mental, emotional, and behavioral disorders among young people: Progress and possibilities.* Washington, DC: The National Academies Press.

OSEP Center on Positive Behavioral Interventions and Support. (2013). Positive behavioral interventions & supports. Retrieved from www.pbis.org

Pallis, B. (2008). *Circle of friends: Testimonials.* Retrieved from www.circleoffriends.org/.

Payton, J., Weissberg, R. P., Durlak, J. A., Dymnicki, A. B., Taylor, R. D., Schellinger, K. B., & Pachan, M. (2008). *The positive impact of social and emotional learning for kindergarten to eighth- grade students: Findings from three scientific reviews.* Chicago, IL: Collaborative for Academic, Social, and Emotional Learning.

Petrenchik, T. M., King, G. A., & Batarowicz, B. (2011). Children and youth with disabilities: Enhancing metal health through positive experiences of doing and belonging. In S. Bazyk (Ed.), *Mental health promotion, prevention, and intervention with children and youth: A guiding framework for occupational therapy* (pp. 189-205). Bethesda, MD: The American Occupational Therapy Association, Inc.

Pincus, D. B. & Friedman, A. G. (2004). Improving children's coping with everyday stress: transporting treatment interventions to the school setting. *Clinical Child and Family Psychology Review, 7(4)*, 223-240.

Poulsen, A. (2011). Children with attention deficit hyperactivity disorder, developmental coordination disorder, and learning disabilities. In S. Bazyk (Ed.), *Mental health promotion, prevention, and intervention with children and youth: A guiding framework for occupational therapy* (pp. 231-265). Bethesda, MD: The American Occupational Therapy Association, Inc.

Sebian, J., Mettrick, J., Weiss, C., Stephan, S., Lever, N., & Weist, M. (2007). *Education and system-of-care approaches: Solutions for educators and school mental health professionals.* Baltimore, MD: Center for School Mental Health Analysis and Action, Department of Psychiatry, University of Maryland School of Medicine.

Shechtman, Z. (2001). Prevention groups for angry and aggressive children. *Journal of Specialists in Group Work, 26*, 228-236.

Schwartz, C., Garland, O., Waddell, C., & Harrison, E. (2006). *Mental health and developmental disabilities in children. Research report prepared for Children and Youth Mental Health.* Vancouver: British Columbia Ministry of Children and Family Development, Children's Health Policy Centre.

Seligman, M. E. P., & Csikszentmihalyi, M. (2000). Positive psychology: An introduction. *American Psychologist, 55*, 5-14.

Simpson, G. A., Bloom, B., Cohen, R. A., & Blumberg, S. (2005). *U.S. children with emotional and behavioral difficulties: Data from 2001, 2002, and 2003 National Health Interview Surveys* (Advance Data From Vital and Health Statistics No. 360). Hyattsville, MD: National Center for Health Statistics. Retrieved from www.cdc.gov/nchs/products/ad.htm.

Stein, B.D., Jaycox, L. H., Kataoka, S. H., Wong, M., Tu, W., Eliot, M. N., & Fink, A. (2003). A mental health intervention for school children exposed to violence: A randomized controlled trial. *JAMA, 290*(5), 603-611.

Stiffman, A. R., Stelk, W., Horwitz, S. M., Evans, M. E., Outlaw, F. H., & Atkins, M. (2010). A public health approach to children's mental health services: Possible solutions to current service inadequacies. *Administration and Policy in Mental Health, 37*, 120-124.

Sugai, G., & Horner, R. H. (2009). Responsiveness-to-intervention and school-wide positive behavior supports: Integration of multi-tiered approaches. *Exceptionality, 17*, 223-237.

U.S. Department of Health and Human Services. (1999). *Mental health: A report of the surgeon general* (Executive Summary). Rockville, MD: U.S. Department of Health and Human Services, Substance Abuse and Mental Health Services Administration, Center for Mental Health Services, & National Institute of Mental Health.

Williams, M. S., & Shellenberger, S. (1996). *"How does your engine run?": A leader's guide to the alert program for self-regulation.* Albuquerque, NM: TherapyWorks.

Witt, W. P., Kasper, J. D., & Riley, A. W. (2003). Mental health services use among school-aged children with disabilities: The role of sociodemographics, functional limitations, family burdens, and care coordination. *Health Services Research, 38*, 1441–1466.

World Health Organization. (2001). The World Health Report: *Mental health: new understanding, new hope.* Geneva: Author.

Young, R. L. (2007). The role of the occupational therapist in attention deficit hyperactivity disorder: A case study. *International Journal of Therapy and Rehabilitation, 14*(10), 454-459.

Ziviani, J., Poulsen, A., & Hansen, C. (2009) Movement skills proficiency and physical activity: A case for Engaging and Coaching for Health (EACH) Child. *Australian Occupational Therapy Journal, 56*(4): 259-265.

Development and Participation in Occupation
The Early Lifespan
Tina Champagne, OTD, OTR/L

KEY TERMS

- Developmental Stages
- Evaluation
- Evaluation Process
- Lifespan Development Approach
- Occupational Participation

- Occupational Performance
- Occupational Performance Patterns
- Occupational Performance Skills
- Occupational Profile

- Occupations
- Recovery
- Sensory Diet
- Social Participation
- Strengths-Based Approach
- Trauma-Informed Care

CHAPTER LEARNING OBJECTIVES

After completion of this chapter, students should be able to:

1. Recall the general developmental stages of childhood.

2. Identify symptoms associated with mental health disorders that can occur in the early lifespan.

3. Recognize the reciprocal relationship between mental health and occupational participation.

4. Examine the impact of trauma on the physical, emotional, and cognitive development of a child.

5. Identify formal and informal methods used to evaluate health, well-being, and participation in life in the early lifespan.

6. Compare the roles of the occupational therapist and occupational therapy assistant in the occupational therapy process.

Manville, C.A., & Keough, J. L.
Mental Health Practice for the Occupational Therapy Assistant (pp 75-109).
© 2016 Taylor & Francis Group.

CHAPTER OUTLINE

INTRODUCTION

The potential possibilities of any child are the most intriguing and stimulating in all creation. (Wilbur, & Du Puy, 1932, p. 166)

The early lifespan is a time of rapid physical growth, ongoing exploration, and developmental maturation. During this critical period, self-concept, self-regulation, and relational capacities form. All of these aspects of the self continue to take shape over time and are influenced by genetic predispositions, as well as one's experiences. Thus, it is essential that children are sufficiently nurtured and well cared for across the early lifespan in order to foster an optimal developmental foundation from which greater capacities emerge. During the early lifespan, however, problems may be encountered, such as traumatic experiences, learning challenges, developmental delays, and physical injuries. At times, these problems may negatively influence the developmental process and a child's ability to participate in meaningful life roles and activities.

Each child and each family system has its own values, innate strengths, and occupational needs. Occupational therapy practitioners work with children and families to help foster health, the developmental process, and successful engagement in roles and occupations. This chapter provides an introduction to the general developmental milestones and occupations of the early lifespan and some examples of conditions and challenges to occupational participation that may occur. An overview of some of the assessment methods used by occupational therapy practitioners during the early lifespan as part of the evaluation process will also be explored.

PART 1: DEVELOPMENTAL PATTERNS INFLUENCING OCCUPATIONAL PERFORMANCE AND PARTICIPATION

Developmental Stages of Childhood

Within the literature, four broad categories of development are often referred to as the ***developmental stages*** (Checkpoint 4-1) of the early lifespan (Centers for Disease Control and Prevention [CDC], 2013a). These include early childhood (ages 0 to 5 years), kindergarten (5 to 6 years), middle childhood (6 to 12 years), and adolescence (13 to 18 years). The developmental stages are categorized by milestones that are typically expected to emerge within each given age range. They also serve as a guideline or road map to help identify and better understand the varied building blocks of growth and maturation in children and youth. Information related to developmental milestones is often categorized into physical, cognitive, communication, social, and emotional skills (CDC, 2013a). The American Academy of Pediatrics (2013) and the CDC (2013a) provide the following general examples of early childhood developmental milestones:

- *Infant (0 to 12 months)*
  - Raises head and chest when on stomach
  - Stretches and kicks on back
  - Opens and shuts hands
  - Brings hand to mouth
  - Grasps and shakes toys

CHECKPOINT 4-1. REMEMBER

List the four developmental stages and then identify six skills associated with each stage.

- Begins to develop social smile
- Begins to express emotion with face and body
- Imitates some movements and expressions
- Follows moving objects
- Recognizes familiar objects and people at a distance
- Rolls over
- Enjoys playfulness
- Starts using hands and eyes in coordination
- Prefers sweet smells and soft textures
- Sits up (Figure 4-1 displays a child sitting up in her development of early childhood.)
- Crawls
- Stands up

- *Toddler (1 to 3 years)*
  - Walks alone
  - Pulls toys behind when walking
  - Climbs onto and into furniture and objects
  - Climbs through jungle gyms
  - Runs and jumps with both feet
  - Kicks a ball
  - Imitates behavior of others
  - Demonstrates awareness of self as separate from others
  - Enjoys the company of other children
  - Finds objects even when hidden two or three levels deep
  - Sorts by shape and color
  - Plays make-believe

- *Preschooler (3 to 4 years)*
  - Climbs well
  - Walks up and down stairs, alternating feet
  - Begins to skip
  - Runs easily
  - Pedals tricycle
  - Bends over without falling
  - Engages in imaginary play
  - Shows affection for familiar playmates
  - Takes turns in games

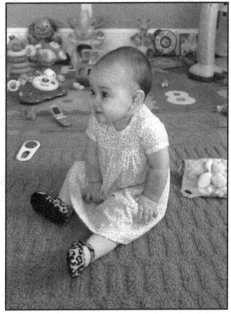

Figure 4-1. Child sitting up in the development of early childhood.

- Understands "mine" and "his/hers"
- Makes mechanical toys work
- Matches an object in hand to picture in book
- Plays make-believe
- Sorts objects by shape and color
- Colors within lines

- *Kindergartner (5 to 6 years)*
  - Prints name when provided with a sample to copy
  - Cuts with scissors
  - Completes up to 20-piece puzzle
  - Easily manipulates tiny objects
  - Hops for long distances with ease
  - Stands on one foot for 8 to 10 seconds
  - Good balance during hopping/skipping
  - Able to role-play and participate in organized, more complex group games
  - Play themes are increasingly more realistic

- *Middle Childhood (6 to 12 years)*
  - Increasing abstract reasoning and problem-solving skills
  - Improving precision and dexterity in sensory perceptual and motor skills

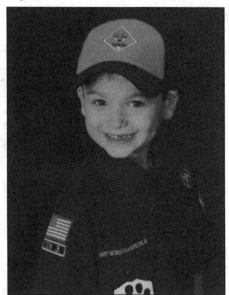

Figure 4-2. Child participating in Cub Scouts during the middle childhood phase.

- ○ Play includes humor such as jokes and comics
- ○ Able to play organized sports (cooperative and competitive)
- ○ May have collections and specific hobbies
- ○ Able to play card, board, and computer games that require more complex skills
- ○ Increasingly more cooperative/less egocentric
- ○ May join community groups or clubs (e.g., Girl/Boy Scouts; Figure 4-2 displays a child participating in Cub Scouts during the middle childhood phase.)
- • *Adolescence (12 to 18 years)*
  - ○ Growth spurts and acclimation to bodily changes
  - ○ Onset of puberty (girls 11 to 14 years; boys 12 to 15 years)
  - ○ May be self-conscious about appearance and body image
  - ○ Identity formation is occurring
  - ○ Highly influenced by peers
  - ○ Establishing distance of self from parents; increasing independence
  - ○ Exploratory sexual behavior; may become sexually active
  - ○ Cognition: Logical, hypothetical, abstract skills develop throughout adolescence
  - ○ Increased ability to perform instrumental activities of daily living (IADLs) independently

- ○ Engages in work or volunteer activities
- ○ Learns to drive; becomes more independent with transportation

Children grow, develop, and demonstrate occupational performance skills at different rates. An individual child may meet developmental milestones earlier or later than other children, which may subsequently affect occupational performance and participation. Occupational therapy practitioners use knowledge related to the developmental stages during the evaluation process as a guideline for the early detection of developmentally based strengths, concerns, and needs.

When developmentally based delays are identified, the child's pediatrician will usually recommend or refer the child and family to the specific health care service that is considered medically necessary. When problems affect occupational performance and participation, the pediatrician often refers the child for occupational therapy services. Occupational therapy practitioners work collaboratively with children in the early lifespan and their families to identify and achieve appropriate developmental needs and occupational goals. During the early childhood ages of birth to 3 years, if developmental concerns arise, children are usually referred by their physician for an early intervention screening. Early intervention programs offer a variety of services, including occupational therapy, when appropriate. During the preschool years, children may receive occupational therapy services through outpatient clinics and preschool programs such as Head Start. Children and youth in the middle childhood and adolescent years often obtain occupational therapy services in schools, outpatient clinics, and community-based programs; however, some children may also receive services in residential, inpatient, and juvenile justice programs. Occupational therapy services for young adults are typically provided in outpatient and community-based settings.

Over the years, in addition to incorporating knowledge of the developmental milestones and stages cited in the literature, theorists have increasingly employed a ***lifespan development approach*** to study development (Brandtsadter & Lerner, 1999; Lerner, 2002; Overton, 2010). The lifespan development approach incorporates the belief that development occurs across the lifespan and is affected by societal, cultural, psychological, and environmental variables. Roles, rituals, and routines also significantly affect the developmental process (Fiese et al., 2002; Segal, 2004). Within this comprehensive view, each individual's personal values and motivations are seen as significantly important factors. Occupational therapy practitioners investigate these variables and the impact of occupational participation on the developmental process across the lifespan (Humphrey & Womack, 2014).

Occupational Therapy Domain: Areas of Occupation and Participation

The Occupational Therapy Practice Framework (OTPF) provides definitions and guidelines to help occupational therapy practitioners understand the domain and process of occupational therapy practice (American Occupational Therapy Association [AOTA], 2014b). Mosey (1981) asserted that knowledge of one's practice domain helps to guide the professional when providing services to clients. Thus, it is important for practitioners to understand the occupational therapy domain when working with children, youth, and families during the early lifespan.

The occupational therapy domain includes performance in areas of occupation, occupation performance skills, occupation performance patterns, context, environment, client factors, and activity demands (AOTA, 2014b). During the evaluation process, occupational therapists work with children and families to help identify their values, needs, occupational goals, and where occupational performance and participation strengths and barriers exist. Occupational therapy assistants often help with the evaluation process under the supervision of the occupational therapist.

Throughout the early lifespan, children build the capacities and competence necessary to support engagement in meaningful life roles and occupations. The OTPF uses the term *occupations* to categorize the many occupations of daily living. **Occupations** can include activities of daily living (ADLs), IADLs, education, work, play, leisure, and social participation (AOTA, 2014b). Each area of occupation is described next in more detail.

Activities of Daily Living

Activities of daily living are tasks that involve caring for one's body. They include bathing/showering, bowel and bladder management, dressing, eating, feeding, functional mobility, personal device care, personal hygiene and grooming, sexual activity, sleep/rest, and toileting hygiene (AOTA, 2014b, p. 630). In infancy, total dependence on the primary caregiver(s) for all aspects of ADL management is expected, and some examples include feeding, bathing, changing diapers, and dressing. In contrast, toddlers and young children begin to develop the ability to actively perform ADL tasks with parental support and supervision. Some examples of ADL activities toddlers and young children begin to perform include self-feeding, dressing, brushing teeth, bathing, grooming, and hygiene. Figure 4-3 displays a child receiving assistance with grooming by getting a haircut.

The category of rest and sleep pertains to sleep preparation and participation (AOTA, 2014b). Rest and sleep are assessed during the evaluation process and are often areas in need of assistance for children and families. Rest and sleep may be disrupted when a child experiences mental health–related symptoms such as anxiety, depression, or

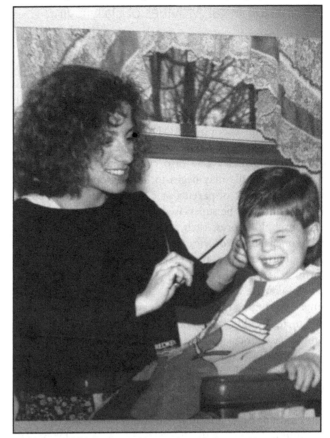

Figure 4-3. Child that is sensitive receives a haircut.

posttraumatic stress. Additional issues that may have a negative impact on rest and sleep include illness, racing thoughts, nightmares, an inconsistent sleep routine, and difficulty with feeling comfortable or safe. The caregiver's ability to rest and sleep is often affected when children have difficulty in this area, as they must remain awake or wake up often in order to attend to the child's fears, worries, and safety and needs. In adolescence and young adulthood, rest and sleep problems can negatively affect other areas of occupation (e.g., school and work performance) and affect overall health and wellness. Occupational therapy practitioners work with children and families to evaluate existing barriers and develop supports to rest and sleep. Some of these supports may include consistent bedtime habits, routines, and rituals that reinforce rest, sleep, and healthy biorhythms.

Children gradually become independent with ADL performance and management over time. By middle childhood (ages 6 to 12 years), ADL performance requires considerably less supervision. Occupational performance and participation in ADL tasks are typically evaluated by occupational therapists. Occupational therapy assistants often help with the evaluation process under the supervision of the occupational therapist by completing delegated observations and assessments and reporting assessment-related information back to the occupational therapist (AOTA, 2014a).

Instrumental Activities of Daily Living

Instrumental activities of daily living are tasks that support everyday living and include care of others, care of pets, child rearing, communication device use, community mobility, financial management, health management and maintenance, home establishment and management, meal preparation and clean-up, safety procedures and emergency responses, and shopping (AOTA, 2014b). In early childhood, ages 0 to 5 years, ADL performance and participation are often a primary area of occupational focus; however, some IADL skills may begin to be developed in children with the support of parents or caretakers. For example, a young child may be supervised to assist with select aspects of household chores, such as helping to clear the dinner table or placing groceries into a shopping cart. With support and supervision, they may assist with care of pets, performing activities like putting water into the pet's drinking bowl. Likewise, they may also help in the care of their siblings by bringing them a snack or drink with supervision.

During middle childhood, ages 6 to 12 years, there is an increased focus on participation in IADL participation. Examples of IADL activities that children at this stage may engage in include making a sandwich for lunch, cleaning one's bedroom, doing homework, and managing an allowance. It is typically a significant expectation of children in late childhood (adolescence) and young adulthood that they become independent in all aspects of IADL performance. Examples of IADL participation of adolescents and young adults include learning to drive or take the bus, obtaining a higher education, managing home care tasks, and financial management. In the evaluation process, occupational therapy practitioners evaluate the strengths of the client, as well as barriers to ADL performance and IADL participation.

Education and Work

Education and work are also included in the OTPF as areas of occupation. Education includes both formal educational participation, such as going to school, college, and taking a course, and informal educational interests, exploration, and needs identification (AOTA, 2014b). Education is a significant part of the early lifespan and, therefore, an area of occupation often explored and supported by occupational therapy practitioners with children and youth. Work includes activities required to identify, acquire, and maintain participation in both job- and volunteer-related roles and activities (AOTA, 2014b). In early childhood, young children may attend preschool programs if enrolled by their caregivers. In many countries, children are enrolled in kindergarten at about 5 years of age and then continue to attend school through their elementary school, middle school, and high school years. During junior high and high school, the focus of the educational experience may be geared toward a specific trade (i.e., carpentry, plumbing, cooking) or focus on preparation for higher education. Higher education may occur once a high school diploma or its equivalent is achieved; however, some college-level courses may be completed during high school at select schools. Occupational therapy practitioners evaluate strengths and barriers to education, work performance, and participation in education and work-related activities in order to assist clients with meeting related needs and goals.

Play

Play is defined as "any spontaneous or organized activity that provides enjoyment, entertainment, amusement or diversion" (Parham & Fazio, 1997, p. 252). Play, a primary area of childhood occupation, includes exploration and participation (AOTA, 2014b), and play is an area evaluated by occupational therapy practitioners.

Even during infancy, babies begin to interact playfully with family and caregivers. Play helps to facilitate attachment formation and relational engagement between parents, siblings, and other caregivers. Play also helps to develop fine and gross motor skills, sensory perceptual, cognitive, social, and emotional capacities.

During infancy, play often includes imitation, animated expressions, varied sights, sounds, and use of toys. As toddlers, children typically begin to play with others in the form of parallel play (side by side). Young children learn how to take turns and play more cooperatively over time. Sharing and taking turns are some of the basic social skills that emerge between the ages of 18 and 24 months. In addition, young children become increasingly able to perform multiple related play actions in a sequence. As toddlers, children may also demonstrate the emergence of symbolic play skills, using one object to represent another (e.g., sticks to represent people or blocks to represent food).

During the preschool years (ages 3 to 4 years), play is increasingly oriented toward engagement with other children. By the age of 5, children are typically more outgoing and are able to play cooperatively. During middle childhood (ages 6 to 12 years), children become increasingly more social and are able to engage in both cooperative and competitive games, demonstrate increased cognitive and emotional regulation capacities, and display more precision in skilled sensorimotor abilities. Figure 4-4 displays a girl playing hopscotch during middle childhood.

Occupational therapy assessment tools are often used to evaluate occupational performance during the preschool years. One example of an occupational therapy assessment tool used with preschoolers is the Miller Assessment for Preschoolers (Miller, 1988).

Social Participation

Social performance and participation are areas of occupation evaluated by occupational therapy practitioners when warranted. Areas of occupation may be assessed using informal methods like clinical observations, as well as through the formal assessment methods. **Social participation** includes interactions and activities that occur on peer, friend, family, and community levels (AOTA, 2014b). The ability to relate to others socially and demonstrate effective interpersonal skills is a critical occupational performance skill that is needed across the lifespan.

Social skills begin to develop in infancy during interaction with caregivers and family. They increase throughout early childhood alongside the development of language and articulation skills. Later, the ability to identify and appropriately communicate one's needs develops and continues to expand throughout the early lifespan. Finally, the capacity to perceive and appropriately respond to the needs of others and to understand verbal and nonverbal communication typically evolves across the early childhood years. Occupational therapy assistants collaboratively assist occupational therapists during the evaluation process and may perform portions of standardized evaluations. Importantly, occupational therapy assistants must develop service competency with standardized evaluations that are used with children and youth in the early lifespan. Some examples of evaluation tools often used by occupational therapy practitioners to assess areas of occupation during the early lifespan are outlined in Table 4-1.

Daily experiences serve to provide rich opportunities for growth; learning; and the development of increased capacities, interests, and skills. Occupational therapy practitioners understand the power of occupational participation and its role in fostering growth and maturation over time. Throughout the early lifespan, any number of difficulties may arise, however, and negatively affect mental health and occupational participation.

According to the OTPF, *occupational performance skills* are defined as observable "units of performance" that affect function and are demonstrated when people engage in actions, activities, and occupations (AOTA, 2014b, p. 612). Occupational performance skills include motor, process, communication, and social skills (AOTA, 2014b). Occupational therapy practitioners are aware that occupational performance skills are dynamic in nature and develop in context and over time (AOTA, 2014b). For instance, many different performance skills are needed in order to play a sport at school, participate in a birthday party at a friend's house, and complete homework.

Occupational performance skills are analyzed during the occupational therapy evaluation process, as these skills affect occupational participation. For example, poor fine motor skills may result in difficulty with managing clothing fasteners (buttons, zippers), handwriting, and opening containers (e.g., milk carton at school). Occupational therapy practitioners are skilled in evaluating occupational performance skills that are needed to fully engage in childhood occupations, such as play, education, and work. Intervention planning and implementation and its relationship to occupational performance skills will be explored in Chapter 5.

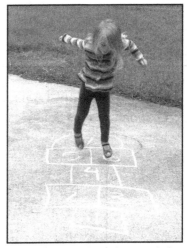

Figure 4-4. Girl playing hopscotch during middle childhood.

Occupational performance patterns are patterns of behavior that are specifically related to the daily life activities and occupations of clients (AOTA, 2014b). Occupational performance patterns include habits, routines, and roles (AOTA, 2014b). Table 4-2 provides examples of occupational performance patterns of the early lifespan.

The following clinical vignette shows how occupational therapy practitioners work collaboratively to assess client factors, occupational performance skills, patterns, and participation during the occupational therapy initial evaluation process. Spotlight 4-1 portrays Daniel, a 9-year-old boy who has a diagnosis of autism spectrum disorder. Although children with autism have many strengths, they may also demonstrate challenges in some of the following areas: verbal and nonverbal communication, social–emotional skills; inflexibility of behavior; difficulty coping with change and transitions; sensory processing challenges; and stereotypical, restrictive, or repetitive behaviors. These challenges can occur to such a degree (mild, moderate, or severe) that they negatively affect occupational performance and participation.

When working with children, it is particularly important that occupational therapy practitioners include the family in the evaluation process whenever possible and explore their values, strengths, needs, and goals. This information is then used to co-create a therapeutic intervention plan. In Daniel's referral, one of the primary requests from his parents was assistance in identifying a host of sensory supports that could be used to try to help decrease Daniel's behavioral outbursts and ease transition times to increase participation and quality of life. The initial assessment process included gathering the developmental history, initial sensory processing information based on parent reports, and the occupational therapist's observations. Daniel's assessment results revealed that he has difficulty with

	TABLE 4-1	
	ASPECTS OF OCCUPATIONAL THERAPY DOMAIN AND EARLY LIFESPAN ASSESSMENT	
OCCUPATIONAL THERAPY DOMAIN	**DOMAIN ASPECTS**	**ASSESSMENT TOOLS**
Areas of Occupation	• Activities of Daily Living • Instrumental Activities of Daily Living • Rest and Sleep • Education • Work • Play • Leisure • Social Participation	• Participation and Environment Measure (Coster et al.) • Assessment of Preschool Children's Participation (Law et al.) • School Function Assessment (Coster et al.) • Pediatric Interest Profiles (Henry) • Test of Playfulness (Bundy) • Leisure Diagnostic Battery (Witt et al.) • Occupational Performance History Interview II (Keilhofner et al.) • Canadian Occupational Performance Measure (Law et al.) • Self-Directed Search (Holland)
Client Factors	• Values • Beliefs • Spirituality • Body Functions • Body Structures	• Self-Perception Profile for Children (Harter) • Self-Perception Profile for Adolescents (Harter) • Family Environment Scale (Moos & Moos) • Occupational Circumstances Assessment- Interview Rating Scale (OCAIRS) (Forsyth)
Occupational Performance Skills	• Motor and Praxis Skills • Sensory Perceptual Skills • Emotion Regulation Skills • Cognitive Skills • Communication and Social Skills	• Assessment of Motor & Process Skills (Fisher & Jones) • Bruininks-Oseretsky Test of Motor Proficiency, 2nd Ed (BOT-2) (Bruininks & Bruininks) • Sensory Integration & Praxis Test (SIPT; Ayres) • Sensory Profiles (Dunn; Brown & Dunn) • Clinical Observation of Motor and Postural Skills (Wilson) • Revised Children's Manifest Anxiety Scale 2nd Ed. (Reynolds & Richmond) • Beck Depression Inventory (Beck et al.) • Coping Inventory (Zeitlin) • Functional Emotional Assessment Scale (Greenspan et al.) • Behavior Rating Inventory of Executive • Functioning (BRIEF) (Gioia et al.) • Social Profile (Donohue)

(continued)

TABLE 4-1 (CONTINUED)		
ASPECTS OF OCCUPATIONAL THERAPY DOMAIN AND EARLY LIFESPAN ASSESSMENT		
OCCUPATIONAL THERAPY DOMAIN	**DOMAIN ASPECTS**	**ASSESSMENT TOOLS**
Occupational Performance Patterns	• Habits • Routines • Roles • Rituals	• Assessment of Life Habits in Children (Noreau et al.) • Family Routines Inventory (Jensen et al.) • Home Observation for Measurement of the Environment (HOME)—Revised (Caldwell & Bradley) • Adolescent Role Assessment (Black) • Role Checklist (Oakely et al.) • Routines-based Interview (McWilliams et al.)
Context and Environment	• Cultural • Personal • Physical • Social • Temporal • Virtual	• Environmental Restriction Scale (Rosenberg et al.) • Home Observation for Measurement of the Environment (Caldwell & Bradley) • School Observation Environment (Hanft & Place) • Evaluation of Social Interaction (Fisher & Griswold) • School Situations Questionnaire (Barkley) • Test of Environmental Supportiveness (Bundy)
Activity Demands	• Objects Used and Their Properties • Space Demands • Social Demands • Sequencing and Timing • Required Actions • Required Body Functions • Required Body Structures	• Activity/Task Analysis

Compiled from American Occupational Therapy Association. (2014b). Occupational therapy practice framework: Domain and process (3rd ed.). *American Journal of Occupational Therapy, 68,* S1-S48.

tactile, oral, and auditory over-responsivity (hypersensitivity), somatosensory discrimination, motor coordination, and praxis skills. These different areas of difficulty contribute to Daniels's struggles with behavior and occupational participation. The assessment results were reviewed with Daniel's parents. Information was provided in order to help them better understand what the assessment results revealed and how both strengths and areas of difficulty affect Daniel and his family's ability to engage in meaningful life roles, routines, and activities.

As per the caregiver's request, the occupational therapist and occupational therapy assistant worked with Daniel and his parents initially to help identify sensory supportive strategies and to create a sensory diet for home implementation. A *sensory diet* is a daily routine that strategically incorporates specific, individualized sensorimotor strategies to utilize during key times of the day. Sensory diets support safety, adaptability, and occupational participation (Wilbarger, 1995; Wilbarger & Wilbarger, 2002).

Daniel's sensory diet included strategies that helped to target the transition times that his parents had identified as being the most difficult. These transition times included getting ready for school, coming home from school, mealtimes, and bedtime. The co-creation and use of a sensory

	TABLE 4-2

OCCUPATIONAL PERFORMANCE PATTERNS: EARLY LIFESPAN EXAMPLES

OCCUPATIONAL PERFORMANCE PATTERN	EARLY LIFESPAN EXAMPLES
Habits: "Automatic behavior that is integrated into more complex patterns that enable people to function on a day-to-day basis" (Neistadt & Crepeau, 1998, p. 869). Habits can interfere or support occupational participation and may be impoverished, dominating, or useful.	• Spontaneously buckles seat belt after getting into the car (useful habit) • Automatically changes out of school clothes and into play clothes after school (useful habit) • Self-harms when not within close proximity to mother (dominating habit) • Demonstrates the inability to complete hygiene and self-care tasks in adolescence (impoverished habit)
Routines: Regular, repetitive, observable patterns providing structure in daily living, involving a time commitment to perform. Routines may be promoting, satisfying, or damaging and are part of ecological and cultural contexts (Fiese et al., 2002; Segal, 2004).	• Follows the steps of the school routine throughout the day • Sequences through the steps of brushing teeth, bathing, putting on pajamas, getting into bed, and being read a nighttime story as part of the bedtime routine
Rituals: Actions that are symbolic and rich with cultural, spiritual, and/or social meaning that often represent a collection of events (Fiese et al., 2002; Segal, 2004). Rituals reinforce beliefs and values, and have a significant affective influence, affecting the client's identity.	• Wears a special locket with mother's picture when not able to be in close proximity to her • Helps to organize holiday celebrations • Goes to bed hugging a heart-shaped pillow, sprayed lightly with mother's perfume, in order to help fall asleep each night
Roles: Shaped by culture and society, roles are a set of behaviors defined and influenced by the client.	• Daughter/son • Sister/brother • Friend • Student • Worker

Compiled from American Occupational Therapy Association. (2014b). Occupational therapy practice framework: Domain and process (3rd ed.). *American Journal of Occupational Therapy, 68,* S1-S48.

diet requires the identification and practice of new strategies, rituals, and supportive routines that will be used to help support the development of new and useful habits. For Daniel and his family, these new habits will support safety and occupational participation. A few examples of the sensory supportive tools that were determined to be helpful include an organizational daily routine board with a checklist to be used throughout the day with support from his parents, an 8-lb. weighted lap pad to be used during car rides and at mealtimes at home, a half-hour of free play time at the local playground after school, and a bath and cuddle time while reading a story before bedtime.

The assessment process also revealed that Daniel has difficulty with praxis skills and sensory sensitivities that affect his ability to cope with transitions and engage in a variety of activities. Daniel and his parents collaborated with the occupational therapist and occupational therapy assistant in the decision to also target play, self-care, and praxis skills as part of occupational therapy treatment. These were areas of need that were not recognized as contributing to occupational barriers until the occupational therapy evaluation was conducted and reviewed with Daniel's parents. The occupational therapy process helped them to have a more

SPOTLIGHT 4-1. DANIEL

Daniel is a 9-year-old boy who likes cartoons, super heroes, and building things. He has been diagnosed with autism spectrum disorder. Daniel is initially referred for occupational therapy due to having many hypersensitivities. In particular, these hypersensitivities are related to the tactile and auditory systems. Daniel also displays difficulties with behavioral outbursts during transitions throughout the day and evening. Daniel's behavioral outbursts are severe at times. Cause for safety concerns include demonstrations of head banging and biting himself. These behaviors are negatively affecting the family's ability to participate in safe and meaningful routines and activities on a daily basis. The occupational therapy practitioner worked with Daniel and his parents to complete the occupational therapy evaluation process in order to collaboratively assess strengths and barriers to occupational participation.

Daniel's parents were well educated about autism, and were able to identify many of the antecedents to Daniel's behavioral outbursts. They were particularly interested in having the occupational therapist assess whether Daniel's sensory processing–related difficulties were playing a role in his outbursts and difficulty with transitions. As part of the evaluation process, Daniel's parents completed a developmental questionnaire and the sensory profile (Dunn, 1999). These tools are both caregiver questionnaires, and are used to begin to obtain the child's history, as well as the parent's perceptions of the child's strengths and sensory-processing challenges. Some of the information explored when using these questionnaires includes sensory processing; motor skills; and social, cognitive, and emotional capacities, as well as concerns related to safety and occupational participation. The occupational therapy assistant was able to help Daniel's parents complete the questionnaires and answer any questions that arose. The occupational therapist completed the initial interview, collaborated with the occupational therapy assistant, scored and reviewed the information the parents had provided, asked clarifying questions, and engaged directly in other assessment-related activities with Daniel.

The occupational therapy assistant introduced Daniel to the occupational therapy gym. This helped to decrease Daniel's anxiety about being in a new place. It also helped to build trust and develop the therapeutic relationship. The occupational therapy assistant reviewed the rules of the occupational therapy gym, and used a playful and empathic approach to help him feel more at ease within this playful, therapeutic space. Daniel was given the opportunity to explore and engage in activities in a client-directed manner. The occupational therapist and occupational therapy assistant used clinical observations of sensory integration (Blanche, 2002) during the session to identify Daniel's strengths, occupational performance skills, play preferences, and areas of difficulty throughout the initial evaluation session.

comprehensive understanding of Daniel's occupational strengths and needs.

Mental Health Applications

According to AOTA (2010), occupational therapists are qualified mental health practitioners. Chapter 3 explains how it is important for occupational therapy practitioners to reclaim their role in working with children and families as part of mental health service provision. In order to accomplish this goal, practitioners must consider ways of providing universal, targeted, and intensive services in a variety of contexts. Additionally, practitioners must be knowledgeable of state and national mental health initiatives, such as the public health framework (see Chapter 3), the recovery movement, and trauma- and attachment-informed care initiatives (Substance Abuse Mental Health Services Administration [SAMHSA], 2014a, 2014b; U.S. Department of Health and Human Services [USDHHS], 2003, 2011, 2012, 2013).

Mental Health Symptoms and Conditions

During the early lifespan, mental health is characterized by the development of effective coping skills, as well as cognitive, social, and emotional capacities (CDC, 2013a). According to the CDC (2013b, p. 2), "mentally healthy children have a positive quality of life and can function well at home, in school, and in their communities." Mental health problems and disorders are a significant public health concern that is typically identified when deviations from social and emotional development are recognized (CDC, 2013b). Genetic predispositions, developmental delays, and traumatic experiences all may contribute to the development of mental health–related symptoms and behaviors (De Bellis & Zisk, 2014; Liberzon et al., 2014; Stein, Lang, Taylor, Vernon, & Livesley 2002).

Children may be diagnosed with a mental health disorder when symptoms and behaviors continue over a specified period and interfere with safety and/or the ability to function (American Psychological Association [APA], 2013;

CDC, 2013b). Mental health symptoms and behaviors are evaluated as mild, moderate, or severe. In a recent study it was estimated that within the United States, 13% to 20% of children are diagnosed with a mental health disorder annually (CDC, 2013a), and mood disorders are the primary diagnosis of children admitted to inpatient treatment settings. Furthermore, inpatient admissions to mental health units increased by 80% in 2010 (CDC, 2013b). Suicide was reported as "the second leading cause of death" among children between ages 12 and 17 (CDC, 2010, p. 2). These data demonstrate the increasing rate of mental health concerns in the United States.

Mental health disorders are classified in the *Diagnostic and Statistical Manual of Mental Health Disorders* (DSM) (APA, 2013). Within the DSM, and under each general diagnostic category, there is a further breakdown of the related diagnoses, corresponding symptoms, and behavior patterns. Information related to age of onset and the timeframes in which symptoms are experienced is also included. For instance, although a child may demonstrate symptoms of anxiety, at least some of those symptoms must have been noted for more days than not for at least 6 months before an anxiety disorder can be diagnosed (APA, 2013).

Mental health and medical diagnoses are typically identified by physicians, psychiatrists, psychologists, neuropsychologists, and neurologists. Occupational therapists do not diagnose individuals; however, aforementioned professionals that conduct diagnostic evaluations may request information that is gathered during the occupational therapy evaluation process as part of the client's medical record review. In this way the occupational therapy evaluation provides information that may be used to inform the diagnostic process. Additionally, children may be prescribed medications by physicians or psychiatrists as part of medical and mental health treatment.

Some examples of common mental health diagnoses that may be identified during the early lifespan are as follows:

- Autism spectrum disorders
- Attention deficit hyperactivity disorder
- Anxiety disorders
- Mood disorders
- Oppositional defiant disorder and conduct disorders
- Substance-related disorders
- Eating disorders
- Trauma and stress-related disorders

Autism Spectrum Disorders

Autism spectrum disorders are neurodevelopmental in nature and are characterized by persistent difficulties in emotional and social interaction, restrictive and sometimes stereotyped behaviors, inflexibility in routine and high dependence on structure, hypersensitivity patterns, and restricted interests (APA, 2013). These problems may significantly affect occupational participation across contexts and often continue throughout the lifespan. Self-injurious behaviors are forms of harm inflicted toward the self. Head banging, hitting, pinching, and punching are examples of self-harming behaviors that may be seen in children with developmental delays, autism spectrum disorders, mental health, and traumatic stress–related disorders.

Attention Deficit Hyperactivity Disorder

Children and youth diagnosed with attention deficit hyperactivity disorder are commonly referred for occupational therapy services. In a recent correspondence from the CDC (2013b, p. 1), "attention-deficit/hyperactivity disorder (6.8%) was the most prevalent parent-reported diagnosis among children aged 3 to 17 years. This was followed by behavioral or conduct problems (3.5%), anxiety (3.0%), depression (2.1%), autism spectrum disorders (1.1%), and Tourette syndrome (0.2%) among children aged 6 to 17 years." Children with attention deficit disorder (ADD) may have problems with attention span, impulsivity, hyperactivity, and distractibility. They frequently have difficulty focusing and sustaining attention on tasks at home and school, become bored easily, and have difficulty with following through on and finishing tasks. Adolescents and young adults with ADD may have difficulty with school and work performance due to their symptoms and may impulsively participate in high-risk activities.

Anxiety Disorders

Children with anxiety disorders tend to have excessive feelings of worry, fearfulness, uneasiness, and dread that are not necessarily based on realistic appraisals. Anxiety is stressful and can become overwhelming, and consequently has a negative influence on occupational performance and participation. Children and youth with anxiety disorders may demonstrate isolative behavior from their peers, sleep disturbance, impairment with executive functioning, and low frustration tolerance during performance of everyday activities.

Mood Disorders

Mood disorders generally include depression and bipolar disorders (APA, 2013). General symptoms of mood disorders include feelings of irritability, fluctuations in attention/concentration levels, a change in interest and enjoyment of activities, increased or decreased appetite, and sleep disturbance. Symptoms of mood disorders often fluctuate and may be cyclical. With bipolar disorder, symptoms experienced may include mania or hypomania, grandiosity, decreased need for sleep, excessive involvement in activities, distractibility, pressured speech, and excessive talking (APA, 2013). Decreased activity levels, sadness, crying, decreased energy, irritability, and feelings of hopelessness often occur with depression (APA, 2013), and an increase in aggressive behavior may also be noted in children who are depressed. It is important to note that anxiety and depression sometimes occur together.

Oppositional Defiant Disorder and Conduct Disorder

Oppositional defiant disorder and conduct disorder are also diagnosed in the early lifespan. Oppositional defiant disorder is characterized by a pattern of anger and irritability, an argumentative stance, and vindictive or defiant behavior toward authority figures that lasts for at least 6 months (APA, 2013). Conduct disorder is diagnosed through the presence of persistent and repetitive behaviors that extend over time. Such behaviors may include aggression toward people or animals, property destruction, deceitfulness or theft, and serious violations of social norms or the basic rights of others (APA, 2013).

Substance-Related Disorders

Substance-related disorders may be diagnosed in young adults. Substance-related disorders are those that involve substances and may include, among others, alcohol, cannabis, hallucinogens, inhalants, opioids, sedatives, hypnotics, anxiolytics, and stimulants (APA, 2013). These substances typically produce feelings of pleasure or calm for the individual using them, although adverse effects may occur. Occupational therapy practitioners who work with young adults should always be on the lookout for symptoms and behaviors associated with these disorders and share any concerns with parents. Some symptoms and behaviors associated with drug use are as follows:

- Cold, sweaty palms or shaking hands
- Excessive sweating
- Extreme hyperactivity or excessive talkativeness
- Frequent rubbing of the nose
- Frequent back and forth twisting of the jaw
- Puffy face; pale or flushed face
- Red, watery eyes with pupils smaller or larger than usual
- Runny nose
- Changes in physical coordination
- Slowed or staggering walk
- Slurred speech
- Tremor in hands, feet, or head

Addiction is defined as the continued use of a mood-altering substance or behavior despite adverse consequences. Research has shown that individuals who begin to experiment at a young age have a higher chance of addiction later in life. This is why it is important to notice early the signs of substance abuse in teens and young adults. Recognizing the early signs of addiction may allow parents and caregivers to intervene before their teen moves from abuse to dependence. Prolonged and excessive use of substances may cause cognitive, behavioral, psychological, and physiological symptoms that affect the performance of valued activities and limit occupational engagement. Behavioral warning signs of drug abuse may include the following:

- Changes in appetite or sleep patterns
- Changes in friends
- Changes in personality or attitude
- Neglects responsibilities
- Chronic dishonesty
- Decreased focus on personal appearance
- General loss of energy
- Moodiness and irritability; mood swings
- Paranoia and aggression
- Secretive or suspicious behavior
- Unexplained silliness or giddiness
- Unexplained drop in grades; skipping school
- Unexplained need for money or reluctance or inability to describe spending habits
- Withdrawal from social activities or loss of interest in activities that the teenager enjoyed previously

Eating Disorders

Eating disorders are serious illnesses that affect both the physical and socioemotional health of young people. Recognizing and trying to address eating disorders often has a significant impact on the youth and the family system, and may cause significant mortality and morbidity. Although eating disorders are rare in the general population, they are relatively common in teenagers (male and female) and particularly in young women. They represent the third most common chronic illness (after asthma and obesity) in adolescent females. Eating disorders are also classified as self-injurious behavior; the early warning signs of an eating disorder include the following:

- A constant focus on dieting, food, and exercise
- Feeling stressed when unable to exercise
- Frequent weighing
- Visits to the bathroom after meals
- Insisting on having different meals from the rest of the family
- Increasing social withdrawal

Some examples of eating disorders include anorexia nervosa, bulimia nervosa, avoidant/restrictive food intake, and binge-eating disorders (APA, 2013). Occupational therapy practitioners working with youth with eating disorders

CHECKPOINT 4-2. UNDERSTAND
Go online to learn more about the symptoms associated with each of the mental illness diagnoses listed earlier. Consider how these symptoms would affect a child's ability to socialize with peers, learn in school, and perform everyday activities.

are often employed by schools, inpatient, residential, foster care, forensic, and outpatient programs.

Checkpoint 4-2 reviews the previously discussed diagnoses.

Trauma and Stress-Related Disorders

According to the U.S. Department of Health and Human Services (2012), 676,569 children were victims of child abuse or neglect, and approximately 1,570 American children died from abuse or neglect in 2011. Another recent study revealed that one in six children and their parent(s) develop symptoms of posttraumatic stress following the experience of physical injury, which affects the overall recovery process (Kassam-Adams, Marsac, Hildenbrand, & Winston, 2013). The pervasive effects of trauma, particularly when trauma occurs in childhood, are well researched (De Bellis & Zisk, 2014; Feletti et al., 1998; SAMHSA, 2014b; USDHHS, 2013).

There has been a national trauma-informed care initiative within the United States since 2003 (National Association of State Mental Health Program Directors [NASMHPD], 2009; SAMHSA, 2014a, 2014b; USDHHS, 2003). *Trauma-informed care* is a model of care that requires all practitioners working with clients with mental health concerns to be aware of the following:

- The high prevalence of trauma incidence among mental health service users

- The pervasive influence of trauma (particularly when trauma occurs in early childhood)

- The provision of services that address the pervasive impact of trauma (NASMHPD, 2009)

For occupational therapy practitioners, a trauma-informed care approach begins with having an understanding of how trauma affects children, youth, and families. Trauma history should be assessed and addressed in the occupational therapy process (Champagne, 2011a, 2011b; NASMHPD, 2009; SAMHSA, 2014b). Information about a child's trauma history may be obtained through a variety of methods, including chart reviews, caregiver report, the child's self-report, and records obtained from other service providers.

Standardized assessment tools help to identify whether a child has a trauma history. Three examples of standardized assessment tools used with children include the Trauma Symptom Checklist for Children (Briere, 1996), the Child PTSD Symptom Scale (Foa, Johnson, Feeny, & Treadwell, 2001), and the Child Trauma Screening Questionnaire

(Kenardy, Spence, & Macleod, 2006). Questionnaires are also available that have been developed by agencies and organizations to help explore trauma history, triggers, warning signs, and helpful coping strategies. The Massachusetts Department of Mental Health (MA DMH) has published trauma-informed screening tools that have been created in collaboration with occupational therapists. One example of a trauma-informed questionnaire is the safety tool, which is sometimes also referred to as a de-escalation tool (MA DMH, 2013). This and many other tools and resources on trauma-informed care are free, accessible on the internet, and may be used with children and youth (MA DMH, 2013; NASMHPD, 2015; SAMHSA, 2014b).

Van der Kolk (2005, 2006) helped to spearhead the broader recognition of the pervasive impact of complex trauma in early childhood across developmental domains, and referred to it as developmental trauma disorder. The definition of what events constitute a traumatic event has evolved and expanded over time. Examples of traumatic events now include physical, sexual, and emotional abuse; neglect; bullying; natural disasters; invasive medical procedures; divorce; incarceration of a caregiver; witnessing abuse; and ongoing challenges associated with physical, cognitive, and health disorders, among others. Bullying is another example of a type of traumatic experience that may occur during early childhood. Bullying is becoming more widely recognized and validated as a potentially traumatic experience. When trauma is experienced and not addressed, it can contribute to the development of mental health symptoms and concerns. In some instances, bullying has led to the engagement in maladaptive coping strategies, self-injurious behaviors, and even suicide.

The degree or extent to which traumatic stress affects human beings is very individual. Trauma experiences increase the risk for anxiety, posttraumatic stress, mood disorders, problems with attention and concentration, dissociation, and the dysregulation of stress hormones (APA, 2013; Klengel et al., 2013). The nervous systems of children who have experienced trauma are often in a hypervigilant state, which leads to the prioritization and processing of information from the environment, such as noxious sensory stimuli, in order to quickly detect threats and employ defense mechanisms (Croy, Schellong, Joraschky, & Hummel, 2010; Hendler et al., 2003). Traumatic experiences and problems with attachment formation have also been found to contribute to the development of anxiety and stress-related symptoms and behaviors. Further, for those with preexisting sensory overresponsivity (SOR) patterns, there is a higher risk of developing posttraumatic stress disorder (PTSD; Hendler et al, 2003).

Research has revealed that traumatic experiences that are prolonged, severe, and occur before the age of 5 can have pervasive effects. Trauma can affect the developing structure and function of the brain and affect the development of occupational performance skills. It may also lead to engagement in self-injurious behaviors, medical complications, inability to form healthy relationships, and engagement in risk-taking behaviors. Research further suggests some of the following may occur when trauma is encountered in early childhood (SAMHSA, 2014b; USDHHS, 2013):

- Diminished growth of the cortex and left hemisphere, creating a predisposition for depression

- Decreased connectivity in the corpus collosum, which may lead to symptoms of attention deficit hyperactivity disorder

- Irritability of the limbic system, which may set the stage for panic and PTSD

- Diminished growth of the limbic system and hippocampus, which may lead to memory problems and dissociation

The Adverse Childhood Experiences Study is a landmark study in the field of trauma. It demonstrated that, if left unaddressed, chronic and multiple traumatic events that occur prior to the age of 18 will lead to a variety of health risk behaviors, medical diseases, disability, and social and emotional problems in adulthood (Feletti et al., 1998).

Children and youth may struggle with significant distress and feelings of shame and grief associated with life events, such as the loss of a loved one, parental incarceration, domestic abuse, parental separation, and divorce. If these feelings are not recognized and addressed, the emergence of mental health symptoms and behaviors may occur and include avoidance of activities, behavioral outbursts, anxiety, depression, sleep disturbances, clinging to or rejection of caregivers, and self-injury (e.g., self-mutilation, substance abuse, eating disorders).

Environmental stressors may be time limited or longer term in nature (Davidson, 2005). Examples of time-limited stressors include temporary financial problems, family relocation, changing schools, changing child care providers, and marital distress of parents. Examples of longer-term stressors include divorce, death of a caregiver, chronic illness of a family member, chronic financial problems, homelessness, social discrimination, and prejudice. In addition, when repeatedly exposed to home environments that are unpredictable, chaotic, or traumatic, children may develop problems with filtering and processing of sensations, thereby increasing their risk of developing maladaptive coping strategies (Aron & Aron, 1997; Gouze, Hopkins, LeBailly, & Lavigne, 2009).

For those experiencing trauma symptoms, a wide range of challenging social environments may be difficult to manage, particularly during adolescence. Research demonstrates that for some adolescents, alcohol and marijuana may be used as maladaptive coping strategies (self-medication), and that substance abuse in adolescence is also associated with the severity of PTSD symptoms (Cornelius et al., 2010; Hovdestad, Tonmyr, Wekerle, & Thornton, 2011).

Occupational therapy practitioners who work with children throughout the early lifespan may play a critical role in helping to prevent or significantly decrease traumatic stress by providing trauma-informed care. According to Kassam-Adams, Marsac, Hildenbrand, and Winston (2013), all health care providers should become more trauma informed. Health care providers, including occupational therapy practitioners, must help to recognize trauma symptoms and behaviors; address traumatic stress reactions associated with the traumatic event(s); minimize potentially traumatic aspects of treatment delivery; and identify children and youth who need additional monitoring, interventions, or referral to additional services (e.g., psychologists, higher level of care).

Trauma-informed interventions require a supportive, nurturing, nonjudgmental approach that involves parents and caregivers. Trauma-informed care focuses on fostering the following:

- Feelings of safety and stability

- A cohesive sense of self; self-identity

- Adaptive, subjective appraisals by the child and family

- Developmental capacities

- Self-regulation skills

- Development of coping skills and strategies

Checkpoints 4-3, 4-4, and 4-5 outline some of the physical, cognitive, relational, and behavioral milestones that typically develop in early childhood, middle childhood, and adolescence. These checkpoints also provide examples of indicators that may be seen in children who have experienced traumatic stress at different developmental stages.

Attachment and Self-Regulation

Relational capacities are influenced by genetic predispositions and experiences over time. The primary caregiver's ability to attune to the needs of a child from infancy throughout childhood is critical to the development of healthy attachment formation, the capacity to self-regulate, and develop higher-order skills. Positive early bonding experiences help infants and young children develop a secure base and support the development of a positive internal working model (Bowlby, 1973; Schore, 2001). Bowlby (1973) suggested that a positive internal working model represents the healthy development of the following:

CHECKPOINT 4-3. UNDERSTAND EFFECTS OF TRAUMA IN EARLY CHILDHOOD		
Early Childhood (0 to 5 years)	Developmental Milestones	Effects of Trauma

Physical	• Rapid physical changes
	• Sensorimotor skills:
	  ○ Sit up
	  ○ Crawl
	  ○ Stand, walk, run
	  ○ Talk
	  ○ Use utensils, write, draw
	• Sleep: establish day/night routines; bio-rhythms
	• Toilet training
		• Regression to earlier behaviors (e.g., baby talk, bedwetting)
		• Developmental delays
		  ○ Speech delays
		  ○ Feeding/eating problems
		  ○ Slow or unable to achieve senso-rimotor skills
		• Sleep disturbances

Cognitive	• Develops the awareness that other people and things continue to exist even when out of site (object permanence) • Develops imitation, sorting, sequencing, and organizational skills (of self, objects, and space) • Develops attention and problem-solving skills • Develops impulse control	• Cognitive regression (e.g., difficulty with problem solving; poor impulse control; delays in ability to pay attention, sequence, and organize)
Relational (self and others)	• Develops feelings of safety, security, and trust that basic needs will be met; bonds with primary caregiver(s) • Autonomy and increased independence (e.g., learning to self-feed, dress, complete self-care tasks, explore the world) • Generally positive and optimistic sense of self and the world	• Afraid of being away from primary caregiver and of going to sleep. • Feelings of fearfulness and helplessness; cannot count on safety/needs being met • Difficulty being soothed • Core sense of shame and guilt • Unusually quiet or anxious, agitated and hyperactive; hypervigilant

Behavioral	• Separation anxiety (clingy, crying upon separation, difficulty being soothed by another adult) usually dissipates by age 2
	• Temper tantrums at times
	• Shows affection for familiar family members and playmates
	• Play stages:
	  ○ Parallel play (ages 2 to 3)
	  ○ Associative play (ages 3 to 4)
	  ○ Cooperative play (ages 4 to 5)
		• Separation anxiety and fearfulness beyond age 2 years
		• Increased power struggles
		• Temper tantrums more extreme and frequent; may become violent toward self, others, or animals
		• Continued dependence and/or avoidance with self-care activities (e.g., feeding, dressing, toileting, bathing)
		• Often behind in developmentally appropriate play stages

CHECKPOINT 4-4. UNDERSTAND EFFECTS OF TRAUMA DURING MIDDLE CHILDHOOD		
Middle Childhood (Ages 6 to 12 years)	*Developmental Milestones*	*Effects of Trauma*
Physical	• Fewer physical changes earlier in this stage; growth spurts later in this stage • Increasing motor coordination and precision • Up to 10 hours of sleep recommended	• Poor sleep and nightmares • Problems with eating and bowel/bladder control may be evident • Difficulty with sensorimotor skill development (e.g., shoe tying, riding a bike, playing sports) • Somatic complaints (e.g., headache, stomachache) • Sensory modulation problems (sensory overresponsivities and underresponsivities)
Cognitive	• Able to focus on academic skills development • Increasing understanding of cause and effect • Attention, concentration, and organizational skills further develop • Increasing understanding of concepts of time	• Poor attention span and concentration skills • Difficulty sequencing through tasks/activities • Learning problems • Misperception of information • Difficulty understanding concepts of time
Relational (self and others)	• Generally positive and optimistic sense of self and the world • Self-esteem increases • Sense of responsibility develops • Initiates and spends more time with peers • Increasing involvement in community groups or teams (e.g., scouts, sports) • Increasing ability to manage impulses • Learns to be aware of and able to maintain social boundaries • Develops pro-social skills	• Feels responsible for trauma(s) and fearful that trauma(s) will recur • Hyperreactivity to traumatic reminders (triggers) • Hypervigilant; irritable; mood swings negatively impact ability to create and maintain positive peer relationships • Poor impulse control • May be withdrawn and avoidant • Difficulty with being aware of and maintaining social boundaries • Difficulty with developing pro-social skills

Behavioral	• Able to follow established routines:
	  ○ Mealtimes
	  ○ School
	  ○ Play time
	  ○ Homework
	  ○ Bed time	

(continued)

CHECKPOINT 4-4. UNDERSTAND EFFECTS OF TRAUMA DURING MIDDLE CHILDHOOD (CONTINUED)		
Middle Childhood (Ages 6 to 12 years)	*Developmental Milestones*	*Effects of Trauma*

Behavioral	• Expanding curiosity:
	  ○ Questions caregivers more
	  ○ Explores activities without care-givers
	  ○ Tries new things and activities in different context
	• Increasing self-control, fewer tantrums
	• Cooperative and competitive play skills
	• Curious about opposite sex but understands and generally main-tains personal boundaries and appropriate behaviors
	• Does not vandalize the property of family or others
	• Does not harm animals
		• Difficult behaviors:
		  ○ Withdrawn
		  ○ Isolative
		  ○ Difficulty sharing
		  ○ Tantrum
		  ○ Aggression
		  ○ Violent outbursts
		  ○ Swearing
		  ○ Unsafe
		  ○ Oppositional
		• Regressive behaviors:
		  ○ Bedwetting
		  ○ Thumb sucking
		  ○ Baby talk
		  ○ Dependence on caregivers for self-care tasks
		• May refuse to attend school
		• Repetitive play themes related to traumatic events or with violent themes
		• May demonstrate sexualized behaviors (e.g., alone, in public, may attempt to engage others)
		• May harm animals
		• May set fires

Adapted from Bassuk, E.L., Konnath, K., & Volk, K. T. (2006). *Understanding traumatic stress in children*. The National Center on Family Homeless-ness. Retrieved from www.familyhomelessness.org/media/91.pdf.		

- A strong and positive sense of self-identify
- Clarity of boundaries between self and others
- Self-regulation
- A general sense of well-being
- Resiliency

Some examples of parental behaviors and techniques that contribute to the ability to bond (attunement) include swaddling, swaying and rocking in a loving manner, caring eye contact, communicating, singing, talking, neutral warmth, and timely, consistent responsiveness. Positive attachment behaviors also include appropriate adjustment of caregiver response according to situational needs and severity, and interactions that support ongoing feelings of safety and acceptance (Hughes, 2004; Schore, 2001). Figure 4-5 illustrates an attuned mother and her baby as they develop attachment.

Attachment styles emerge from a combination of variables and are often presented as being on a continuum. Variables that influence a caregiver's capacity to develop and maintain attunement with one's child include one's temperament, mental and physical health factors, developmental abilities and delays, one's own sensory processing patterns, and cultural and economic influences. Attachment styles have been identified in the literature, and may be influenced across the lifespan (Levy & Orlans,

CHECKPOINT 4-5. UNDERSTAND EFFECTS OF TRAUMA ON ADOLESCENCE

Adolescence (Ages 13 to 18 years)	Developmental Milestones	Effects of Trauma
Physical	• Growth spurts • Puberty • Sleep: more sleep is needed in adolescence	• Developmental delays may be evident • Puberty may be delayed • Sleep disturbances
Cognitive	• Able to maintain attention and concentration • Able to hypothesize and abstract reason at increasingly higher levels • Able to solve complex problems	• Difficulty with attention span and concentration • Difficulty with problem solving, particularly when experiencing relational problems • May have learning disabilities • Difficulty with impulse control
Relational (self and others)	• Identity formation: examines beliefs of others and organizes own perceptions, values, beliefs, and attitudes into a coherent sense of self • Generally positive and optimistic sense of self and the world • Able to create and maintain positive peer relationships • Able to repair relationships when there are problems • Increased awareness of the greater good	• May have poor body image • Identity confusion, difficulty trusting self, may be immobilized or without direction • Difficulty managing intense emotions, may be violent and have frequent mood swings • Poor self-esteem, feelings of inadequacy, sense of shame and guilt • May overcompensate for poor self-esteem with grandiosity or narcissism • Difficulty maintaining close peer relationships
Behavioral	• There may be rebellious behavior at times in early adolescence, but it is less extreme and generally resolves by late adolescence • Follows rules and laws • Engages in safe behaviors • Increasingly independent with IADLs	• Risk-taking behaviors • Outward rejections of parent's values and standards and relies on peers for support • Rebellious behaviors • May break rules and laws • Continued reliance on parents and others for assistance with some IADLs

Adapted from Bassuk, E. L., Konnath, K., & Volk, K. T. (2006). *Understanding traumatic stress in children.* The National Center on Family Homlessness. Retrieved from www.familyhomelessness.org/media/91.pdf.

1998; Liotti, 1999, 2009; Main & Solomon, 1990). Awareness of attachment styles helps caregivers and practitioners improve their understanding of the strengths and barriers in the parent/child relationship and provide appropriate interventions and recommendations that support healthy attachment experiences, increased capacity for growth, resiliency, and occupational participation (Champagne, 2011a). Table 4-3 provides a review of attachment styles and the potential influence on social participation.

It is also important to emphasize that insecure attachment styles do not always emerge due to a caregiver's difficulty with bonding or his or her regulatory capacity. For instance, children with developmental delays and difficulty with sensory processing may have caregivers who are highly attuned, but the child may have difficulty engaging with the caregiver(s) due to severe tactile, auditory, visual overresponsivity, or other difficulties. Thus, practitioners must not assume that insecure attachment styles are caused

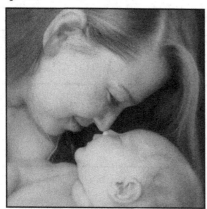

Figure 4-5. Attuned mother and her infant as they develop mother–infant attachment.

solely by lack of caregiver capacity or neglect. The occupational therapy evaluation process provides an opportunity to begin exploring the attachment styles and the developmental capacities of children, youth, and caregivers as they pertain to health, wellness, occupational performance, and participation.

Temperament

All people are born with their own unique combination of physical features such as skin tone, eye color, physique, and temperament traits. The nine temperament traits initially identified by Thomas, Chess, and Birch (1968) is outlined in Table 4-4. It is not recommended to use temperament traits to profile an individual. Rather, temperament trait information is useful in helping parents, caregivers, and practitioners consider a child's strengths and barriers in order to provide supports to help nurture children and youth according to their own unique needs and occupational goals. Different temperament dimensions may result in parents and caregivers having difficulty in understanding how to best parent their children. Understanding, patience, and consistency of response by primary caregiver(s) are essential to fostering feelings of safety, maturation, health, and resiliency throughout the early lifespan.

In addition to monitoring the physiological milestones during the early lifespan, it is important to identify and nurture strengths and positive mental health components of every child, as discussed in Chapter 3 (see Table 3-2). Occupational therapists use a **strength-based approach** to work with children and families. Using a strength-based approach does not include a sole focus on diagnoses, problems, or areas of difficulty. Rather, this approach emphasizes the client's abilities. Strengths are used in order to help foster increased safety, occupational performance skills, and participation. Having a strength-based approach is also part of what is expected by the recovery movement (USDHHS, 2003).

The evaluation process requires a focus not only on occupational performance skills and patterns, but also on each child's unique temperament, personality traits, strengths,

and interests. For instance, Bobby is a 12-year-old boy, and some of his primary character strengths are that he is very nurturing, kind, creative, inquisitive, and humorous. He loves and excels in science and math, builds different types of models, and likes animals. As noted earlier, occupational therapy practitioners must help children and their caregivers identify their unique abilities and engage in occupations that further support and cultivate their expression. In this case, they would help Bobby and his caregivers become more aware of his strengths, interests, and skills in order to expand upon them. There are multiple ways to help Bobby increase his occupational engagement and build upon his positive character traits and skills. Occupation-based examples include participating in science fairs, going to science museums, attending an after-school or summer camp program that fosters advancement in science and math, and creative exploration of the environment, all of which would further the expression of his strengths. His kind and nurturing qualities may be built upon by engagement in volunteer activities. Examples include helping to tutor children who struggle in math or science, taking care of the animals at a local animal shelter, or helping out at food kitchens or local community centers.

The Recovery Movement

Although the recovery movement is often thought of as pertaining to individuals in the middle and late lifespan, the recovery movement is applicable to the early lifespan as well. **Recovery** is defined as "a journey of healing and transformation enabling a person with a mental health problem to live a meaningful life in a community of his or her choice while striving to achieve his or her full potential" (USDHHS, 2003, p. 4). The recovery movement is a current national and international mental health initiative. This initiative calls for individualized and client-driven care that is strengths based, respectful, and trauma informed (USDHHS, 2003). Recovery-focused services are also relevant when working with children, youth, and families during the early lifespan.

PART 2: EVALUATION OF THE EARLY LIFESPAN

The Evaluation Process

Like all aspects of occupational therapy services, the evaluation process is collaborative and individualized. The **evaluation process** is used to foster the therapeutic relationship; it helps the client and the occupational therapy practitioner identify meaningful and important values, occupational needs and goals, and related strengths and barriers that affect occupational performance and participation (AOTA, 2014b). The client's strengths, interests, and

TABLE 4-3

ATTACHMENT STYLES

ATTACHMENT STYLE	CHILD'S VIEW AND RESPONSE
Secure	Caregiver is viewed and utilized as a secure base. Child is well adjusted and able to engage in generally healthy relational exchanges.
Insecure-avoidant	Child feels little to no attachment. Demonstrates very little or no distress when caregiver departs or returns. Child may become "rebellious" and have a low self-esteem and self-image.
Insecure-ambivalent	Child does not view or utilize the caregiver as a secure base. Child is highly distressed upon separation and demonstrates more extreme responses of anxiety, ambivalence, fear, and/or anger. Child is preoccupied with being within close proximity to caregiver. Often anxious or angry with caregiver when present.
Insecure-disorganized	Child demonstrates a significantly disorganized attachment to caregiver. May demonstrate highly fearful responses, become disoriented, and/or demonstrate stereotypical behaviors when in the presence of the caregiver.

Compiled from Levy, T. M., & Orlans, M. (1998). Attachment, trauma and healing: Understanding and treating attachment disorder in children and families. Washington, D.C.: Child Welfare League.; Liotti, G. (1999). Disorganized attachment as a model for the understanding of dissociative psychopathology. In J. Solomon & C. George (Eds.). *Attachment disorganization* (pp. 291-317). New York: Guilford Press.; Liotti, G. (2009). Attachment and dissociation. In P. F. Del & J. O'Neil (Eds.). *Dissociation: DSM-V and beyond* (pp. 53-65). New York: Routledge Press.; Main, M., & Solomon, J. (1990). Procedures for identifying infants as disorganized/disoriented during the Ainsworth Strange Situation. In M. Greenberg, D. Chichetti, & E. M. Cummings (Eds.). *Attachment in the preschool years: Theory, research and intervention* (pp. 121-160). Chicago, IL: Chicago University Press.

TABLE 4-4

TEMPERAMENT TRAITS

TEMPERAMENT TRAIT	DESCRIPTION
Activity level	Amount of movement and bodily activity
Biological regularity	Regularity of biological functions (e.g., hunger, sleep–wake cycles, bowel elimination)
Adaptability	How quickly or slowly the child adapts to a change in routine or overcomes an initial negative response
Approach/withdrawal	How the child initially reacts to a new person or an unfamiliar situation
Sensitivity threshold	How sensitive the child is to potentially irritating stimuli (e.g., scents, sounds, touch, taste, temperatures, crowds)
Intensity of emotional response	How strongly the child reacts to positive and negative situations; the energy level of mood expression, whether positive or negative
Distractibility	How easily the child is distracted by unexpected stimuli; degree of attention and concentration when not necessarily interested
Quality of mood	The amount of pleasant and cheerful behavior (positive mood), as contrasted with fussy, sad, and unpleasant behavior (negative mood)
Persistence/attention span	How long the child will keep at a given activity without giving up

Compiled from Thomas, A., Chess, S., & Birch, H. (1968). *Temperament and behavior disorders in children*. New York: University Press.

skills are identified and strategically emphasized, utilized, and built upon to help overcome barriers to reaching occupational goals.

Evaluation information may be gathered and contributed by an occupational therapy assistant under the supervision of an occupational therapist. Whenever appropriate, interdisciplinary staff (i.e., doctors, nurses, teachers, other therapists) is encouraged to provide any additional information that may contribute to the evaluation process.

Occupational therapy evaluations are conducted with children, youth, and families in order to do the following:

- Identify eligibility for occupational therapy services

- Substantiate insurance claims or address litigation

- Identify if further or more comprehensive assessments are warranted

- Provide information used to support the diagnostic process

- Help develop the intervention plan

- Provide information that may be useful in developing supportive recommendations; plans or placement in other programs; or contexts in home, schools, and residential programs

- Evaluate the progress of occupational therapy services over time, such as reevaluation

- Determine the outcomes of the services provided, such as developmental gains, functional outcomes, and participation outcomes

After receiving a referral, the occupational therapist may begin the evaluation process. The *evaluation* consists of the occupational profile and analysis of occupational performance. It usually starts with a review of background information. Caregiver questionnaires may be used to gather information about the child's developmental history, strengths, values, and areas of need or concern. The next step is typically the interview process, where it is important to begin with building a therapeutic relationship. The process of developing a trusting therapeutic relationship can be challenging for occupational therapy practitioners when working with children and families with a history of trauma. Individuals with trauma histories may have difficulty with trust and an insecure attachment style.

A trauma-informed approach should be utilized when interviewing clients. For instance, when inquiring about an individual's trauma history, ask "what happened" rather than inadvertently insinuating that something is "wrong" with him or her. It is important to be empathetic and nonjudgmental with clients, especially when inquiring directly about someone's trauma history (NASMHPD, 2009; SAMHSA, 2014). A nonjudgmental, trauma-informed approach helps children and caregivers foster the therapeutic relationship and supports the ability to engage in deeply personal conversations, such as those related to traumatic experiences. Spotlight 4-2 highlights a trauma-informed and recovery-focused approach.

Occupational Profile

The occupational therapy evaluation process consists of an interview, any other additional processes needed to develop the occupational profile (e.g., completing questionnaires, record review), and the analysis of occupation (AOTA, 2014b). Questions that must be answered in order to create the occupational profile include the following:

- Who is the client?

- Why is the client seeking service?

- What are the client's values and strengths?

- What occupations and activities are successful or causing challenges?

- What contexts and environments support or inhibit desired outcomes?

- What is the client's occupational history?

- What are the client's priorities and targeted outcomes?

The *occupational profile* is a summary of the information obtained during the occupational therapy evaluation. It includes the client's background information, needs, values, priorities, desires, outcomes, occupational history, patterns of daily living, strengths, and interests. The occupational profile also summarizes barriers to personal safety, health, wellness, and participation (AOTA, 2014b). Analysis of occupational performance is the direct observation of the client's performance and the process through which targeted needs and goal areas are identified (AOTA, 2014b). National and international mental health initiatives also affect the occupational therapy process. Spotlight 4-3 illustrates the clinical vignette of Randy, which is provided to help demonstrate how a trauma- and attachment-informed, recovery-focused approach is used by occupational therapy practitioners. This spotlight also demonstrates how to shift the focus off of what is "wrong with the individual" to empathically exploring "what happened" as part of the evaluation process when exploring one's trauma history.

Clinical Reasoning: Informing the Evaluation Process

Occupational therapy practitioners use professional experience, theories, frames of reference, and evidence-based practice guidelines to help foster clinical reasoning throughout the occupational therapy process (Cohn & Coster, 2014). Clinical reasoning helps the practitioner make sense of the information gathered (values, needs, and goals; developmental milestones; and areas of occupation).

A variety of occupational therapy practitioners have created frameworks that are used as a guide during the clinical process. Strengths and barriers to occupation are identified

SPOTLIGHT 4-2. RACHEL

Rachel's story demonstrates how a trauma-informed and recovery-focused approach is used with an adolescent during the evaluation process and informs the clinical reasoning and intervention planning process. Rachel is a 14-year-old girl with a history of being a very good student. She was highly active in sports and popular with her peers. Rachel also had a tendency, however, to be anxious at times and very self-critical. Her father was transferred to a new job prior to Rachel starting high school, which required the family to move to another state. Rachel had to leave her friends, school, and close-knit, small community due to this long-distance move. The family moved to a much larger town, and she attended the local public high school.

Rachel had significant difficulty with this transition. Within the first few weeks at the new school, she started to get bullied by some of the older high school girls. Rachel became increasingly depressed, exhibited increased symptoms of anxiety, and her self-esteem rapidly diminished by the end of the first month of school. She struggled not only with the traumatic stress related to the bullying, but also with the overall stress of the move. Additional stressors included the loss of her prior peer, teacher, and community relationships and lack of participation in school-based activities such as sports.

Rachel's preexisting problems with anxiety and self-criticism quickly exacerbated after the move. Over time, she began to withdraw, developed panic attacks, struggled with her schoolwork, and did not engage in any school-based or leisure activities. By the end of the first semester, she had started to develop an eating disorder by starving herself.

Rachel shared some of her fears, feelings, and concerns during the initial evaluation process. Her feelings included the following:

- Feeling fearful for her personal safety at school
- Severe self-loathing
- Extreme emotions
- Loneliness: missed old friends and had difficulty making new friends
- Feeling "not good enough" to try out for school sport teams
- Extreme difficulty focusing on and completing schoolwork

She was unable to identify any current strength. Her engagement and participation in a variety of occupational areas had plummeted. This included healthy self-care management tasks and social, emotional, leisure, and school performance skills.

The occupational therapist and occupational therapy assistant worked with Rachel to help her identify her strengths, values, and goals during the occupational therapy evaluation process. Rachel started to explore the functions or roots of her feelings and behaviors, rather than focusing solely on the behaviors themselves. The occupational therapist and occupational therapy assistant also worked with Rachel in identifying her occupational strengths and goals.

As part of the occupational evaluation process, the Beck Depression and Beck Anxiety Scales were used to help Rachel become more self-aware of the symptoms of depression and anxiety she experienced. It also was used to help her recognize the impact depression and anxiety were having on her life. Exploration of what was triggering her fears, depression, anxiety, and decreased self-esteem also helped Rachel realize that starving herself was largely a form of self-punishment. Rachel was blaming herself for not being accepted at her new school, for having no friends, and for doing poorly in school. The occupational therapy practitioners introduced Rachel to the wheel of life worksheet (Mind Tools, 2013). This helped Rachel to identify the different areas of life balance and satisfaction, to explore areas of strength and areas she wanted to prioritize working on.

Rachel was also supported in identifying what she needed in order to feel safe at school. Under the direction of the occupational therapist, the occupational therapy assistant provided Rachel with the assistance needed to help her address the bullying issues. They identified and practiced healthy anxiety reduction and coping strategies. Expressive art activities were used to help Rachel recognize her feelings of grief and loss for prior relationships through her love of art. They also helped her to identify and re-engage in some of the occupations that she highly valued. She was supported in identifying ways to stay in contact with past friends,

(continued)

SPOTLIGHT 4-2. RACHEL (CONTINUED)

develop new and supportive peer and teacher relationships, and locate other school-based supports. These were some of the initial collaborative occupational therapy evaluation and intervention approaches used with Rachel that are trauma informed and recovery focused in nature. The initial evaluation process helped Rachel identify her occupational strengths, needs, values, and goals and supported the co-creation of the initial occupational therapy intervention plan.

in collaboration with clients and then combined with the therapist's knowledge and use of theory. Propositions are established, which are explicit ideas about cause-and-effect relationships that can be tested. These propositions support assumptions or opinions about what areas need to be assessed and the therapeutic approaches that might help (Cohn & Coster, 2014).

Propositions and assumptions significantly affect clinical reasoning and, thereby, the occupational therapy process. Propositions and assumptions are also articulated and tested in theories and frameworks of practice. For instance, A. Jean Ayres (2005) was an occupational therapist and developmental psychologist. She was the first occupational therapist to publish a theoretical model on the influence of the sensory perceptual and motor systems on the developmental process, occupational performance, and participation (including attachment formation). Ayres created the framework of sensory integration, which is now referred to as *Ayres' Sensory Integration* (ASI) (Ayres, 1968, 1979). Figure 4-6 illustrates the Ayres' model of sensory integrative processes and how these processes affect development, occupational skills, performance, and participation.

Ayres proposed that children learn and build upon innate strengths and capacities through engagement in occupations. Engagement includes experiences with caregivers, people, different physical environments, other types of ongoing interactions, and experiences in the world. For example, an infant relies on his or her primary caregiver to feel safe, to learn to self-regulate, and to develop early motor skills, such as sitting up, crawling, and standing. A school-aged child engages with other children in order to practice sharing and playing cooperatively.

Ayres created propositions from which the assumptions of her frame of reference were established (Ayres, 1968, 1979, 1989, 2005). The five ASI propositions include the following:

1. *Neuroplasticity* occurs across the lifespan and supports the ability of the brain to change, adapt, and heal.

2. Dynamic interactions between lower- and higher-order cortical areas of the nervous system are fundamental to sensory integrative processes.

3. There is a natural and sequential order to the neurophysiological development of sensory integrative processes.

4. Each individual has the ability to adapt and adjust actions on the environment. This promotes an *adaptive response* as a natural response to the feedback of the central nervous system.

5. Each individual has an *inner drive* that supports the ability to meet and master challenges, and supports the development of sensory integrative processes.

ASI fidelity criteria outline the structural and process elements specific to the ASI framework (Parham et al., 2007, 2011). Thus, the propositions of any theoretical framework chosen and used by an occupational therapy practitioner influence clinical reasoning and how one will approach the evaluation and intervention process (e.g., evaluation tools selected, therapeutic interventions considered).

Analysis of Occupational Capacity and Dysfunction

The evaluation process requires the occupational therapist to use information gathered about the client in combination with clinical reasoning skills to conceptualize, communicate, and account for clinical decisions and outcomes that emerge over time. Occupational therapy practitioners are unique in that each client is viewed as an "occupational human being for whom access and participation in meaningful and productive activities is central to health and well being" (AOTA, 2014b, p. 613). The analysis of occupational performance is part of the evaluation process and involves the use of screening and assessment tools (Checkpoint 4-6) designed to assess the client's strengths, needs, concerns, and barriers to occupation (AOTA, 2014b). Occupational therapy assistants help occupational therapists with the analysis of occupational performance by helping to gather information that contributes to the overall evaluation process.

Assessment Tools and Types

Screening is a brief process that indicates areas of strengths and concerns. Assessments occur in context and consist of information gathering and engaging in the use of informal information, formal tools, standardized and nonstandardized instruments, and strategies. Informal approaches or tools are often simpler or intuitive in nature. Information gained cannot be generalized, and

SPOTLIGHT 4-3. RANDY

Randy is a 16-year-old boy and is currently living in a residential program due to difficulty with increased self-harming behaviors, isolation, and oppositional and aggressive behaviors toward his parents over the past 2 years. He has been having difficulty with sustaining attention on tasks during home and school performance, has had decreased social participation, and has been heavily experimenting with a variety of substances. There has been a heightened and prolonged focus on his areas of difficulty by parents and other caregivers. They are concerned due to the severity of his behaviors and growing frustrations and fears for his safety and health. His family members and the residential program staff requested an occupational therapy evaluation to assist with identifying ways to help Randy increase safe behaviors, school, leisure, and social participation. The diagnoses listed in Randy's medical record include attention deficit disorder, oppositional defiant disorder, and substance abuse disorder.

The occupational therapist asked Randy, his parents, and residential staff about his strengths, interests, and skills as part of the evaluation process. It was reported that he is very artistic, humorous, outgoing, and social. He also likes to skateboard and snowboard, enjoys amusement park rides, enjoys music, likes to draw, and plays the guitar. Over the past 2 years, however, there has been a significant change in his behaviors and decreased occupational participation. When discussing attachment history with his parents, it was reported that there was a strong and secure attachment history until these "difficult behaviors" started to occur "more recently" in adolescence.

Using trauma- and attachment-informed and recovery-focused approaches, the occupational therapist and occupational therapy assistant employed the use of art expression in a nonconfrontational manner to help explore some of Randy's self-perceived values, strengths, and needs as part of the interview process. The use of the interview process and the art activity also provided an initial opportunity for clinical observations of sensorimotor, cognitive, social, communication, and emotional performance skills. Randy began to draw a detailed picture that appeared to depict a significant degree of anger.

The occupational therapist started talking with Randy about his strong drawing skills. Randy had no difficulty with fine motor performance during the drawing activity. He was able to demonstrate the ability to pick up on social cues and to speak effectively when calm. The occupational therapy practitioner gently asked him why he had stopped engaging in activities that he is talented at and used to enjoy. The practitioner asked the question as part of the interview, and in a kind, empathic, and strength-based manner to maintain the progress started with developing a rapport.

Randy started to rip up his drawing and reported information to the occupational therapy practitioner related to a history of abuse. He went on to say that he feels like if he talks about the abuse to his parents, "they will tell everyone about what happened," and he believed that others would see him as "disgusting and damaged." He also talked about being angry with his parents because it was a friend of the family who abused him and they did not consider that this person would "do such a thing to him" or notice that something terrible had occurred. Although he was not ready to disclose the nature of the abuse just yet, Randy was able to begin to discuss some of what had happened to him and related his feelings.

In addition to shame and embarrassment, he felt a sense of guilt about the abuse. Randy was having difficulty fully realizing that his feelings of guilt were also part of what he was struggling with. This was a turning point for Randy that happened to come about during part of the evaluation process. A trauma- and attachment-informed and recovery-based approach helped to decrease the focus on the negative aspects of Randy's behaviors and thereby decreased the degree of defensive behaviors evidenced. A safer, strength-based, and supportive therapeutic approach was co-created. In this way, the occupational therapy practitioner was able to provide a therapeutic stance from which a supportive therapeutic relationship fostered the ability to help Randy feel less defensive, safer, and better able to talk about painful and difficult experiences.

Randy struggled primarily with the following occupational performance skills: emotion; regulation; and cognitive, social, and communication skills. Over time, Randy was able to begin to relate to how his feelings and difficulty communicating with his parents continued to negatively influence his quality of life and the ability to meet his occupational goals. The occupational therapy practitioners helped Randy identify and utilize supports for his attention and learning needs, as well as coping, problem-solving, and communication skills.

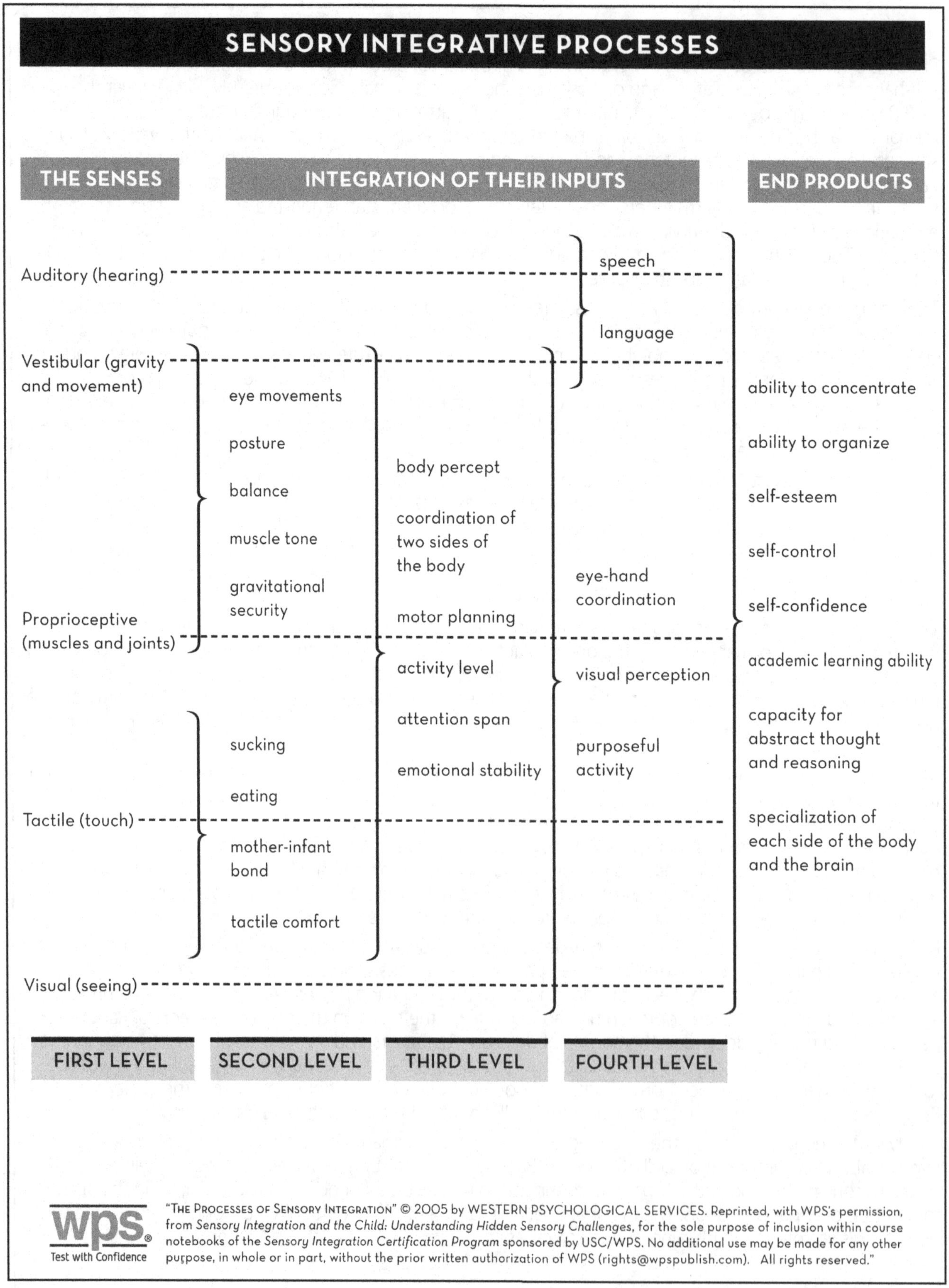
SENSORY INTEGRATIVE PROCESSES
THE SENSES
INTEGRATION OF THEIR INPUTS
END PRODUCTS
Auditory (hearing)
Vestibular (gravity and movement)
Proprioceptive (muscles and joints)
Tactile (touch)
Visual (seeing)
eye movements
posture
balance
muscle tone
gravitational security
sucking
eating
mother-infant bond
tactile comfort
body percept
coordination of two sides of the body
motor planning
activity level
attention span
emotional stability
speech
language
eye-hand coordination
visual perception
purposeful activity
ability to concentrate
ability to organize
self-esteem
self-control
self-confidence
academic learning ability
capacity for abstract thought and reasoning
specialization of each side of the body and the brain
FIRST LEVEL
SECOND LEVEL
THIRD LEVEL
FOURTH LEVEL
wps. Test with Confidence
"The Processes of Sensory Integration" © 2005 by WESTERN PSYCHOLOGICAL SERVICES. Reprinted, with WPS's permission, from Sensory Integration and the Child: Understanding Hidden Sensory Challenges, for the sole purpose of inclusion within course notebooks of the Sensory Integration Certification Program sponsored by USC/WPS. No additional use may be made for any other purpose, in whole or in part, without the prior written authorization of WPS (rights@wpspublish.com). All rights reserved."

Figure 4-6. Ayres Sensory Integrative processes.

CHECKPOINT 4-6. ANALYZE
Refer back to Table 4-1. Go online to research the assessment tools: Are they standardized or not? Are they normative or criterion referenced? According to the occupational therapy practice law in your state, which of these assessments (if any) could an occupational therapy assistant administer?

TABLE 4-5
ASSESSMENT TOOLS, AGE RANGES, AND STATED PURPOSE

TEST NAME	AGE RANGE	STATED PURPOSE
Assessment of Life Habits in Children (Noreau, Fougeyrollas, & Lepage, 2003)	Birth to 4 years and 5 to 13 years	Assess the level of performance of life habits and daily activities in various contexts
Beery–Buktenica Test of Visual-Motor Integration (6th Ed.) (Beery, Buktenica, & Beery, 2010)	2 to 100 years	Screen visual motor, visual perceptual, and motor coordination skills
Miller Assessment for Preschoolers (Miller, 1988)	2 years, 9 months to 5 years, 8 months	Assess for developmental delays and pre-academic skills
Pediatric Interest Profiles: Kid's Play Profile Preteen Play Profile Adolescent Leisure Interest Profile (Henry, 1998)	6 to 21 years	Assess play and leisure interests and participation
Revised Knox Preschool Play Scale (Knox, 1997)	Birth to 6 years	Observational assessment of play skills
School Function Assessment (Coster, Deeney, Haltiwanger, & Haley, 1998)	5 to 8 years	Evaluate and monitor a child's participation, task supports, and activity performance in elementary school
Sensory Profile (Dunn, 1999)	3 to 10 years	Assess how the child processes sensory information in everyday situations and link the results with functional performance

the interpretation of the results heavily relies on the skills of the clinician or observer. Formal assessment strategies and tools follow a specific procedure with an outline of what is assessed, how it is assessed, and how the information obtained is applied and communicated in the occupational therapy process. Standardized assessments are more sophisticated in design and are implemented according to specific criteria. They provide quantifiable, normative, and/or criterion-referenced results. Table 4-5 provides examples of standardized assessment tools often used with children and youth and the general purpose of each tool.

Normative-referenced instruments gather information to determine whether a person is functioning in a manner that is more or less similar to a particular sample population, such as age group and level of development. Criterion-referenced instruments use descriptors rather than normative variables to compare performance or participation.

The type of evaluation and its focus depend on the client's needs, values, and goals, as well as the practice setting in which it is administered. Practice settings may include the home, a school or after-school program, an outpatient clinic, an inpatient setting, and a forensic setting, among others. The length of time allotted for completion of an occupational therapy evaluation varies. In most settings, occupational therapists generally have a short time to complete an initial evaluation. Therapists may be allotted additional time by their employer to score completed assessment tools and write up the evaluation documentation. It is possible, however, for a parent, school, or other organization to hire an occupational therapist on a consultation basis.

Consultants may be asked to provide a highly comprehensive, independent evaluation that can take a significantly longer time to complete. Such comprehensive occupational therapy evaluations are not typically reimbursed by an individual's insurance benefit and are often paid for privately or by an organization (e.g., school system).

The following procedural checklist can help guide occupational therapists with their clinical reasoning when considering the methods and instruments to be used during the occupational therapy evaluation process:

- Review the reasons for the referral.
- Gather relevant medical, educational, and family histories.
- Collaboratively identify and consider the child and caregiver priorities.
- Identify and consider both the chronological and developmental age of the child.
- Determine the most appropriate theoretical frames of reference.
- Identify the purpose of the evaluation, and select and implement the most appropriate evaluation methods and tools
- Consider the evaluation requirements of the setting or agency
- Identify resources available to caregiver, interdisciplinary professionals, instruments and equipment available, time, and environment

A variety of questionnaires may be used to gather information about a child. Developmental questionnaires, sensory profiles (parent/teacher), attachment-related questionnaires, and interest checklists are some examples. It is important, however, to choose the most appropriate tools and not to overwhelm caregivers with too many questionnaires at once. Thoughtfulness and appropriateness in the selection of screening and assessment tools are part of the decision made by the occupational therapist using clinical reasoning skills. Although the occupational therapy assistant can help gather information related to the assessment process, the interpretation of all assessment information is completed by the occupational therapist (AOTA, 2014a).

Table 4-6 illustrates examples of screening and assessment tools that may be used by occupational therapy practitioners during the evaluation process when working with children.

Evaluation Structure: Clinical Applications

Spotlight 4-4 and Table 4-6 illustrate how the OTPF evaluation structure applies when conducting the initial evaluation process when working with children (AOTA, 2014b). This occupational profile example is not all-inclusive, but demonstrates how evaluation information may be initially gathered.

A more detailed example of the development of the occupational therapy profile is provided in Spotlight 4-5 for Karly and in Table 4-7. Again, this clinical example is not all-inclusive, but helps demonstrate how information initially obtained during the evaluation process helps to identify strengths and occupational performance and participation concerns.

Table 4-7 further outlines some of the initial information gathered throughout the evaluation process, which will be used to inform the occupational therapy goals, treatment planning, and implementation process.

Ultimately, all information obtained during the evaluation process is typically entered into initial evaluation documentation by the occupational therapist. Chapter 5 will provide a continuation of Karly's occupational profile by adding examples of interventions and outcomes.

Summary

Occupational therapists and occupational therapy assistants work collaboratively to provide occupational therapy services to children and families during the early lifespan. Evaluation is an essential component of the occupational therapy process. This chapter focused primarily on the initial evaluation as the starting point for occupational therapy service delivery. Occupational therapy practitioners exercise reflective and skilled clinical judgment when collaborating with clients and families during the evaluation process. Teachers, other interdisciplinary professionals, and key stakeholders may also contribute to providing information used during the evaluation process (teacher questionnaires, neuropsychological evaluation reports, interdisciplinary team discussions). Even after the initial evaluation process is completed, assessment continues throughout the occupational therapy process and includes all interactions, formal assessments, and informal observations over time. This cyclical process of assessment and decision making includes observation and reflection combined with action. A more formalized reassessment occurs after a period, which helps to identify whether occupational therapy goals have been met or if continued services are warranted.

During the early lifespan, positive mental health and wellness are supported by the development of a secure attachment with primary caregiver(s), effective self-regulation, and coping skills; this in turn supports the development of higher occupational performance capacities and occupational participation. Children may experience distressing mental health symptoms and may become diagnosed with mental health disorders when symptoms and behaviors exist and continue over a specified period (APA, 2013). Barriers to occupational participation may arise when mental health symptoms and challenges are evident.

A public health approach can be useful when working with children and families with mental health–related concerns because it focuses not only on mental health promotion, but also on prevention and intervention (Bazyk, 2011). Occupational therapy practitioners must utilize strength-based and trauma-informed approaches when providing services to children with mental illness. Recovery-focused services, although often associated with adults, are also relevant to working with children, youth, and their families during the early lifespan.

The occupational profiles of children in different developmental stages and with different mental health challenges were used to help demonstrate key points of this chapter.

TABLE 4-6

OCCUPATIONAL THERAPY EVALUATION PROCESS: MIDDLE CHILDHOOD APPLICATION

TIMOTHY'S INITIAL EVALUATION: AGE 8 YEARS, 10 MONTHS

CONTEXT: OUTPATIENT CLINIC

Occupational Therapy Practice Framework	Methods and Assessments
1. *Occupational Therapy Profile:* Initial step in the evaluation process *Analysis of Occupation:* More specific and direct assessment of what supports/hinders performance and participation	• Initial interview with parent and child. Gather history, values, interests, patterns of daily living, strengths, needs, and client's priorities for occupational therapy services • Direct observation of parent and child during the initial session within the clinical environment • Collaboratively discuss occupational concerns and priorities
a. Parent and Teacher Questionnaires	• Parent completion of the clinic's informational and developmental questionnaires • Sensory profiles: Caregiver and teacher questionnaires (Dunn, 1999)
b. Informal Play & Relational Observations	• Timothy's self-selected play activities in outpatient clinical spaces • Interactions with parents throughout the evaluation process
c. Formal Assessments	• Clinical observations based on sensory integration (Blanche, 2002) • Bruininks–Oseretsky Test of Motor Proficiency, Second Edition (BOT-2) (Bruininks & Bruininks, 2005)

Compiled from American Occupational Therapy Association. (2014b). Occupational therapy practice framework: Domain and process (3rd ed.). *American Journal of Occupational Therapy, 68,* S1-S48.

SPOTLIGHT 4-4. TIMOTHY

Timothy is 8 years, 10 months old. He lives at home with his biological family, who is very supportive of him. He is a very intelligent, kind, curious, and thoughtful child. Timothy has a diagnosis of autism and has been struggling at home and school due to what his parents and pediatrician identified as sensory processing, social, and anxiety-related difficulties, particularly during transitions. Timothy receives occupational therapy services at school for school-based concerns. His family is seeking outpatient services to target home and community-based concerns as well.

At a local outpatient clinic, the occupational therapist and occupational therapy assistant worked collaboratively with Timothy and his family to identify his strengths and any existing barriers to participation in the home and community-based activities. The occupational therapy assistant participated in helping the occupational therapist conduct the evaluation process. The occupational therapy assistant provided Timothy's parents with evidence-based caregiver questionnaires. The occupational therapy assistant also provided information about observations of Timothy's behaviors while interacting with a variety of sensory-rich experiences and social interactions with other children within the clinic setting.

SPOTLIGHT 4-5. KARLY

Karly is 4 years, 7 months old. She is a very sweet, curious, inquisitive, energetic, and humorous child. Karly enjoys music, likes learning about animals, and loves to play on the playground with her foster parents. She was removed from her home at age 3 due to ongoing abuse and neglect. This included severe emotional, physical, and sexual abuse throughout the first 3 years of her young life. Initially, Karly experienced multiple foster placements due to her symptoms and behaviors. These included severe tantrums, impulsivity, and self-injurious behaviors such as head banging and hitting herself. Currently, she continues to engage in self-injurious behaviors at times, and displays a high degree of assaultiveness when she becomes dysregulated, is overwhelmed, or experiences trauma triggers. Karly has difficulty with participation in daily life activities such as sleeping, eating, and bathing, and in the ability to engage in safe and developmentally appropriate interactions with other children and adults. She has lived in her current foster home since age 3.5 years. Karly has been able to develop a close bond with her foster mother in particular. Due to having a significant trauma history, Karly continues to fear that her foster mother will leave her, not return when she goes out on errands, stop loving her, and send her to a different foster placement, despite ongoing reassurance to the contrary. She carries these fears largely due to her past trauma history.

Karly has been diagnosed with posttraumatic stress disorder (PTSD) and has an insecure-disorganized attachment style, which has contributed to also receiving a diagnosis of reactive attachment disorder. Some of the primary symptoms of PTSD that affect Karly's safety and occupational participation include re-experiencing past events, nightmares, and avoidance of stimuli related to the traumatic history. She also has numerous sensory-processing difficulties. These include severe hypersensitivities to touch and sound; low registration; and difficulties with muscle tone, postural control, clumsiness, and fine motor coordination. Karly demonstrates extreme impulsivity at times and difficulty with communicating her needs, particularly when triggered, anxious, or fearful.

Some of the occupational performance areas directly affected by her early childhood trauma experiences include the following:

- Sleep (nightmares, fearfulness of her bedroom and bathrooms)
- Poor nutritional intake (does not like warm or hot food temperatures, avoids many food textures)
- Dressing and tooth brushing (resistance due to fearfulness of the bathroom; sensitivities to clothing, toothbrush, and toothpaste)
- Poor safety awareness (refusing seat belt use, tries to bolt from car when driving on highways, runs into the street without awareness of traffic)
- Difficulty playing with same-aged peers (parallel play only, often strikes out at same-aged peers, unable to attend birthday parties or other outings with same-aged children)
- Difficulty staying seated at school (seated work, arts/crafts activities) and home (mealtimes, coloring, watch movies)
- Difficulty when not in close proximity to foster mother (clingy, tantrums)
- Difficulty going into the community with her foster family (stores, restaurants)
- Difficulty with school performance (attention span, handwriting and coloring skills)
- Poor safety awareness (engages in self injurious behaviors, assaultive at times)

TABLE 4-7
OCCUPATIONAL PROFILE AND ANALYSIS OF OCCUPATION FOR KARLY

CLIENT INFORMATION

Child's First Name: Karly **Child's Age:** 4 years, 7 months

Child's Year in School: Preschool **Parent/Guardian's Name:** Joan (foster mother)

EVALUATION

Referred by: Pediatrician and child's social worker

Reasons for referral (information is initially provided by the referral source)**:** Difficulty with tantrums and hitting self and others, head banging when overwhelmed or triggered, resistant to activities of daily living, poor sleep, very clingy to foster mother, difficulty with becoming easily overstimulated and dysregulated in school and community environments (e.g., stores, restaurants, birthday parties), difficulty staying seated and attentive for even short periods at school and home during seated activities (e.g., coloring, eating, playing).

BACKGROUND INFORMATION

Background information was obtained through: interview and questionnaires completed with foster mother, communication with Karly's social worker, review of previous medical and mental health records provided by the social worker.

Strengths: Karly is very affectionate when she feels safe and secure. She feels curious and enjoys gross motor play activities, music, singing, swinging, and going to the park with her foster parents. She has developed a strong attachment to her foster mother.

Family history: Removed from her biological family's home at age 3 and has been in foster care since that time. Little information is available about the status of Karly's biological parents. She has no siblings. The foster family is very supportive and resourceful.

Medical history: Failure to thrive, microcephaly, fetal alcohol syndrome

Mental health diagnoses: Posttraumatic stress disorder and reactive attachment disorder (sometimes also referred to as *insecure-disorganized attachment style*)

Developmental history: Karly has met most gross motor milestones. Primary developmental concerns at this time are as follows:

- Difficulty with sleep, home, school, and social participation

- Safety awareness

- Problems with attention, emotion, and self-regulation

- Difficulty organizing herself in order to participate in daily routines

- Sensory hypersensitivities

- Sensory-seeking behaviors (use of too much force, need for constant movement)

- Poor body awareness, poor social boundaries

- Tantrums with transitions, particularly in moderate-to-high stimulus environments and when foster mother not within view

Educational history: Attends preschool

Occupational history/profile: (see the aforementioned narrative in Spotlight 4-5)

EVALUATION OF OCCUPATIONAL PERFORMANCE

Analysis of Occupation: Assessments Administered

- **Structured assessments:** Initially it was very difficult to engage Karly in structured assessments due to the degree of dysregulation she was experiencing; therefore, the following were used:

(continued)

TABLE 4-7 (CONTINUED)

OCCUPATIONAL PROFILE AND ANALYSIS OF OCCUPATION FOR KARLY

- ○ Clinical observations based on sensory integration theory (Blanche, 2002)
- ○ Child attachment checklist (caregiver questionnaire)
- ○ Sensory profile (Dunn, 1999) (caregiver questionnaire)
- **Unstructured observations:** Using more of an unstructured and playful approach and using client-directed play activities, the following areas of concern were directly observed:
  - ○ Required close proximity to foster mother at all times or she would tantrum or self-injure
  - ○ Hypervigilance
  - ○ Tactile and sound sensitivities
  - ○ Easily elicited startle response
  - ○ Seeks proprioception
  - ○ Continuously seeks vestibular and proprioceptive input
  - ○ Clumsy
  - ○ Uses too much force
  - ○ Has difficulty with transitions
  - ○ Very short attention span (>1 minute unless engrossed on task, but even then attention span >5 minutes)
  - ○ Difficulty organizing herself
  - ○ Difficulty with gravitational awareness
  - ○ Mildly low muscle tone
  - ○ Clumsy

Primary Areas of Concern Based on the Evaluation Process:

- Occupational participation concerns as outlined in Spotlight 4-5
- Other factors identified in the evaluation process:
  - ○ Significant separation anxiety
  - ○ Hypervigilance
  - ○ Very short attention span (>1 minute unless engrossed on task, but even then attention span >5 minutes)
  - ○ Significant difficulty with emotion identification and regulation
  - ○ Triggered by certain activities, places (bathing/bathroom, bed/bedroom, shopping)
  - ○ Prone to violent outbursts/aggressive behaviors toward self, caregivers, and others
  - ○ Difficulty with gravitational awareness, poor spatial and body awareness
  - ○ Low muscle tone (mild)
  - ○ Difficulty with fine motor skills
  - ○ Constantly seeking out movement (e.g., spinning, running, climbing, rocking)
  - ○ Seeks out self-initiated deep touch pressure (e.g., strong hugs at times, back massages by foster mother)

(continued)

TABLE 4-7 (CONTINUED)
OCCUPATIONAL PROFILE AND ANALYSIS OF OCCUPATION FOR KARLY

- Tactile, sound, and oral sensitivities:
  - ○ Difficulty tolerating most clothing types and fabrics/seams
  - ○ Difficulty with hair brushing, face washing, nail clipping
  - ○ Very picky eater
  - ○ Difficulty with moderate and high stimulus environments (stores, restaurants, lunch room at school)
  - ○ Highly distracted by sensory stimuli

Additional strengths identified: Wants to succeed and please adults; hard worker; highly energetic; she is inquisitive; enjoys and seeks out gross motor play activities; is more easily engaged using play, music, and sing-a-longs; likes stuffed animals and soft textures

*It will be important to emphasize and build upon strengths identified throughout the occupational therapy intervention sessions.

Some of these clinical examples will be expanded upon in Chapter 5 to demonstrate how occupational therapy practitioners collaboratively use the evaluation process and results to collaboratively plan and implement occupational therapy goals and therapeutic interventions as part of the occupational therapy process.

PART 3: APPLICATION

The following activities will help the student identify key aspects of this chapter that were highlighted in the text. These questions also highlight the objectives at the start of the chapter. Activities are suggested to be completed individually or in a small group to enhance learning.

Individually answer these questions:

1. Why is it important for occupational therapy practitioners to be knowledgeable of state and national mental health initiatives? Give an example.

2. What are some of the social, environmental, and economic variables that may influence the occupational engagement of children and youth? Identify two examples of each.

3. Give three reasons why evaluation is a critical part of the occupational therapy process.

4. Does the evaluation process only occur at the start of the occupational therapy process? Explain your answer.

In groups, complete these activities:

1. List activities that help support the development of a secure attachment style.

2. Create a list of activities that may be used in conjunction with the occupational therapist to evaluate a child–caregiver relationship as part of the evaluation process.

3. Identify three examples of how occupational therapy assistants can contribute to the evaluation process in the early lifespan.

REFERENCES

American Academy of Pediatrics. (2013). Healthychildren.org. Retrieved from www.healthychildren.org/english/ages-stages/teen/Pages/default.aspx.

American Occupational Therapy Association. (2010). Specialized knowledge and skills in mental health promotion, prevention, and intervention in occupational therapy practice. Retrieved from http://otmentalhealth.weebly.com/uploads/9/7/7/1/9771940/specialized_skills_in_mental_health.pdf.

American Occupational Therapy Association. (2014a). Guidelines for supervision, roles, and responsibilities during the delivery of occupational therapy services. *American Journal of Occupational Therapy, 68,* S16-S22.

American Occupational Therapy Association. (2014b). Occupational therapy practice framework: Domain and process (3rd ed.). *American Journal of Occupational Therapy, 68,* S1-S48.

American Psychological Association. (2013). *Diagnostic and statistical manual of mental health disorders* (5th ed). Washington, DC: Author.

Aron, E., & Aron, A. (1997). Sensory-processing sensitivity and its relation to introversion and emotionality. *Journal of Personality and Social Psychology, 73*(2), 345-368.

Ayres, A. J. (1968). Sensory integrative processes and neuropsychological learning disability. *Learning Disorders, 3,* 41-58.

Ayres, A. J. (1979). *Sensory integration and the child.* Los Angeles, CA: Western Psychological Services.

Ayres, A. J. (1989). *Sensory integration and praxis tests*. Los Angeles, CA: Western Psychological Services.

Ayres, A. J. (2005). *Sensory integration and the child: Understanding hidden sensory challenges* (Rev. ed.). Los Angeles, CA: Western Psychological Services.

Bassuk, E. L., Konnath, K., & Volk, K. T. (2006). Understanding traumatic stress in children. The National Center on Family Homlessness. Retrieved from www.familyhomelessness.org/media/91.pdf.

Bazyk, S. (2011). *Mental health promotion, prevention, and intervention with children and youth: A guiding framework for occupational therapy*. Bethesda, MD: AOTA.

Beery, K., Buktenica, N., & Beery, N. (2010). *The Beery-Buktenica Developmental Test of Visual-Motor Integration* (6th ed.). San Antonio, TX: Pearson.

Blanche, E. I. (2002). *Observations based on sensory integration theory*. Torrance, CA: Pediatric Therapy Network.

Bowlby, J. (1973). *Attachment and loss, Vol. 2: Separation*. New York: Basic Books.

Brandtsadter, J., & Lerner, R. M. (1999). *Action and self-development: Theory and research through the lifespan*. Thousand Oaks, CA: Sage.

Briere, J. (1996). *Trauma Symptom Checklist for Children (TSCC) professional manual*. Odessa, FL: Psychological Assessment Resources.

Brown, C., & Dunn, W. (2002). *Adolescent/Adult Sensory Profile*. Pearson Assessment.

Bruininks, R. H., & Bruininks, B. D. (2005). Bruininks-Oseretsky Test of Motor Proficiency, Second Edition (BOT-2). Minneapolis, MN: Pearson Assessment.

Centers for Disease Control and Prevention. (2010). Web-Based Injury Statistics Query and Reporting System (WISQARS). Retrieved from www.cdc.gov/ injury/wisqars/index.html.

Centers for Disease Control and Prevention. (2013a). Developmental milestones and stages. Retrieved from www.cdc.gov/ncbddd/child-development/index.html.

Centers for Disease Control and Prevention. (2013b). Mental health surveillance among children, 2005-2011. *Morbidity and Mortality Weekly Report, 62*(2), 1-35.

Champagne, T. (2011a). Attachment, trauma and occupational therapy practice. *OT Practice, 16*, CE1-CE8.

Champagne, T. (2011b). *Sensory modulation and environment: Essential elements of occupation* (3rd ed Rev.). Sydney, Australia: Pearson Assessment.

Cohn, E. & Coster, W. (2014). Unpacking our theoretical reasoning: Theory and practice in occupational therapy. In B. B. Schell, G. Gillen, & M. J. Scaffa (Eds.) *Willard & Spackman's occupational therapy* (12th ed., pp. 478-493). Philadelphia, PA: Lippincott, Williams & Wilkins.

Coster, W., Deeney, T., Haltiwanger, J., & Haley, S. (1998). *School function assessment*. San Antonio, TX: Pearson Assessment.

Cornelius, J., Kirisci, L., Reynolds, M., Clark, D., Hayes, J. & Tarter, R. (2010). PTSD contributes to teen and young adult cannabis use disorders. *Addictive Behaviors, 35*, 91-94.

Croy, I., Schellong, J., Joraschky, P. & Hummel, T. (2010). PTSD, but not childhood maltreatment, modifies responses to unpleasant odors. *International Journal of Psychophysiology, 75*, 326-331.

Davidson, D. (2005). Psychosocial issues affecting social participation. In J. Case-Smith (Ed.), *Occupational Therapy for Children* (pp. 449-480). St. Louis, MO: Elsevier Mosby.

De Bellis, M., & Zisk, A. (2014). The biological effects of childhood trauma. *Child and Adolescent Clinics of North America, 23*, 185-222.

Dunn, W. (1999). *Sensory Profile*. San Antonio, TX: Therapy Skill Builders.

Feletti, V., Anda, R., Nordenberg, D., Williamson, D., Spitz, A., Edwards, V.,...& Marks, J. (1998). Relationship of childhood abuse and household dysfunction to many of the leading causes of death in adults. The Adverse Childhood Experiences Study. *American Journal of Preventative Medicine, 14*(4), 245-258.

Fiese, B. H., Tomcho, T. J., Douglas, M., Josephs, K., Poltrock, S., & Baker, T. (2002). A review of 50 years of research on naturally occurring family routines and rituals: Cause for celebration? *Journal of Family Psychology, 16*, 381-390.

Foa, E. B., Johnson, K. M., Feeny, N. C., & Treadwell, K. R. H. (2001). The child PTSD symptom scale: A preliminary examination of its psychometric properties. *Journal of Clinical Child Psychology, 30*, 376-384.

Gouze, K., Hopkins, J., LeBailly, S., & Lavigne, J. (2009). Re-examining the epidemiology of sensory regulation dysfunction and comorbid psychopathology. *Journal of Abnormal Child Psychology, 37*, 1077-1087.

Hendler, T., Rotshtein, P., Yeshurun, Y., Weizman, T., Kahn, I., Ben-Bashat, D., & Bleich, A. (2003). Sensing the invisible: Differential sensitivity of visual cortex and amygdala to traumatic context. *Neuroimage, 19*, 587-600.

Henry, D. (1998). *Pediatric interest profiles*. Retrieved from, http://www.cade.uic.edu/moho/resources/files/assessments/PIPs%20Manual.pdf

Hovdestad, W., Tonmyr, L., Wekerle, C., & Thornton, T. (2011). Why is childhood maltreatment associated with adolescent substance abuse? A critical review of explanatory models. *International Journal of Mental Health Addiction, 9*, 525-542.

Hughes, D. (2004). An attachment-based treatment of maltreated children and young people. *Attachment & Human Development, 6*, 263-278.

Humphrey, R., & Womack, J. (2014). Transformations of occupations: A life course approach. In B. B. Schell, G. Gillen, & M. J. Scaffa (Eds.) *Willard & Spackman's occupational therapy* (12th ed., pp. 60-71). Philadelphia, PA: Lippincott, Williams & Wilkins.

Kassam-Adams, N., Marsac, M. L., Hildenbrand, A., & Winston, F. (2013). Posttraumatic stress following pediatric injury: Update on diagnosis, risk factors, and intervention. *JAMA Pediatrics*. Retrieved from http://archpedi.jamanetwork.com/article.aspx?articleid=1748357#Abstract.

Kenardy, J. A., Spence, S. H., & Macleod, A. C. (2006). Screening for posttraumatic stress disorder in children after accidental injury. *Pediatrics, 118*(3), 1002-1009.

Klengel, T., Mehta, D., Anacker, C., Rex-Haffner, M., Pruessner, J., Pariante, C. M.,...Binder, E. B. (2013). Allele-specific FKBP5 DNA demethylation mediates gene-childhood trauma interactions. *Nature Neuroscience, 16*, 33-41.

Knox, S. (1997). Development and current use of the Knox Preschool Play Scale. In L. D. Parham & L. S. Fazio (Eds.), *Play in occupational therapy for children* (pp. 35–51). St. Louis, MO: Mosby/Year Book.

Lerner, R. M. (2002). *Concepts and theories of human development* (3rd ed.). Mahwah, NJ: Lawrence Erlbaum Associates.

Levy, T. M., & Orlans, M. (1998). Attachment, trauma and healing: Understanding and treating attachment disorder in children and families. Washington, DC: Child Welfare League.

Liberzon, I., King, A., Ressler, K., Almli, L., Zhang, P., Ma, S., Galea, S. (2014). Interaction of the ADRB2 gene polymorphism with childhood trauma in predicting adult symptoms of posttraumatic stress disorder. *JAMA Psychiatry, 71*, 1174-1182.

Liotti, G. (1999). Disorganized attachment as a model for the understanding of dissociative psychopathology. In J. Solomon & C. George (Eds.), *Attachment disorganization* (pp. 291-317). New York: Guilford Press.

Liotti, G. (2009). Attachment and dissociation. In P. F. Del & J. O'Neil (Eds.), *Dissociation: DSM-V and beyond* (pp. 53-65). New York: Routledge Press.

Main, M., & Solomon, J. (1990). Procedures for identifying infants as disorganized/disoriented during the Ainsworth Strange Situation. In M. Greenberg, D. Chichetti, & E. M. Cummings (Eds.), *Attachment in the preschool years: Theory, research and intervention* (pp. 121-160). Chicago, IL: Chicago University Press.

Massachusetts Department of Mental Health. (2013). Resource guide: Creating positive cultures of care. Retrieved from www.mass.gov/eohhs/gov/departments/dmh/restraintseclusion-reduction-initiative.html.

Miller, L. (1988). *Miller Assessment for Preschoolers*. San Antonio, TX: Pearson.

Miller, L. J. (1988). *Miller Assessment for Preschoolers: MAP manual* (Rev. ed.). San Antonio, TX: Psychological Corporation.

Mind Tools. (2013). Wheel of life worksheet. Retrieved from www.mindtools.com/pages/article/newHTE_93.htm.

Mosey, A. C. (1981). *Occupational therapy: Configuration of a profession*. New York: Raven.

National Association of State Mental Health Program Directors. (2009). *Training curriculum for creation of violence-free, coercion-free treatment settings and the reduction of seclusion and restraint* (7th ed.). Alexandria, VA: National Association of State Mental Health Program Directors, Office of Technical Assistance.

National Association for State Mental Health Program Directors. (2015). National center for trauma informed care: Additional tools. Retrieved from www.samhsa.gov/nctic.

Neistadt, M. E., & Crepeau, E. B. (Eds.). (1998). *Willard & Spackman's occupational therapy* (9th ed.). Philadelphia, PA: Lippincott, Williams & Wilkins.

Noreau, L., Fougeyrollas, P., & Lepage, C. (2003). *Assessment of life habits for children*. Quebec, Canada: INDCP.

Overton, W. M. (2010). Lifespan: Concepts and issues. In R. M. Lerner, W. F. Overton, A. M. Freund, & M. E. Lamb (Eds.). *The handbook of lifespan development: Cognition, biology and methods.* (Vol. 1, pp. 1-29). Hoboken, NJ: John Wiley & Sons.

Parham, L. D., Cohn, E. S., Spitzer, S., Koomar, J., Miller, L. J., Burke, J. P., Brett-Green, B., Mailloux, Z., May-Benson, T., Smith Roley, S., Schaaf, R. C., Schoen, S., & Summers, C. A. (2007). Fidelity in sensory integration intervention research. *American Journal of Occupational Therapy, 61*, 216-227.

Parham, L. D., & Fazio, L. S., (1997). *Play for occupational therapy for children*. St. Louis, MO: Mosby.

Parham, L. D., Smith Roley, S., May-Benson, T., Koomar, J., Brett-Green, B., Burke, J. P., Cohn, E. S., Mailloux, Z., Miller, L. J., & Schaaf, R. C. (2011). Development of a fidelity measure for research on effectiveness of Ayres Sensory Integration intervention. *American Journal of Occupational Therapy, 65*(2), 133-142.

Schore, A. (2001). Effects of secure attachment on right brain development, affect, regulation, and infant health. *Infant Mental Health Journal, 22*, 7-67.

Segal, R. (2004). Family routines and rituals: A context for occupational therapy interventions. *American Journal of Occupational Therapy, 58*, 499-508.

Stein, M., Lang, K., Taylor, S., Vernon, P., Livesley, W. J. (2002). Genetic and environmental influences on trauma exposure and posttraumatic stress disorder symptoms: A twin study. *American Journal of Psychiatry, 159*, 1675-1681.

Substance Abuse Mental Health Services Administration. (2014a). *Leading CHANGE 2.0: Advancing the behavioral health of the nation 2015-2018*. HHS Publication No. (PEP) 14-LEADCHANGE2. Rockville, MD: Substance Abuse and Mental Health Service Administration.

Substance Abuse and Mental Health Services Administration. (2014b). *Trauma-informed care in behavioral health services*. Treatment Improvement Protocol (TIP) Series 57. HHS Publication No. (SMA) 13-4801. Rockville, MD: Substance Abuse and Mental Health Services Administration.

Thomas, A., Chess, S., & Birch, H. (1968). *Temperament and behavior disorders in children*. New York: University Press.

U.S. Department of Health and Human Services. (2003). *Achieving the promise: Transforming mental health care in America. Final Report*. New Freedom Commission on Mental Health, DHHS Publication Number SMA-03-3832 ed. Rockville, MD.

U.S. Department of Health and Human Services. (2011). Substance Abuse Mental Health Services Administration's (SAMHSA) Strategic Initiatives Fact Sheet. Retrieved from http://store.samhsa.gov/product/SAMHSA-Strategic-Initiatives-Fact-Sheet/SMA11-4666.

U.S. Department of Health and Human Services, Administration for Children and Families, Administration on Children, Youth and Families, Children's Bureau. (2012). Child maltreatment 2011 Retrieved from www.acf.hhs.gov/programs/cb/research-data-technology/statistics-research/child-maltreatment.

U.S. Department of Health and Human Services. (2013). Childhood maltreatment: Consequences. Retrieved from www.cdc.gov/violenceprevention/childmaltreatment/consequences.html.

Van der Kolk, B. (2005). Developmental trauma disorder: Toward a rational diagnosis for children with complex trauma histories. *Psychiatric Annals, 35*(3), 401-408.

Van der Kolk, B. (2006). Clinical implications of neuroscience research and PTSD. *Annals of the New York Academy of Science, 1071*, 277-293.

Wilbarger, P. (1995). The sensory diet: Activity programs based upon sensory processing theory. *Sensory Integration Special Interest Section Quarterly, 18*(2), 1-4.

Wilbarger, J., & Wilbarger, P. (2002). Clinical application of the sensory diet. In A. C. Bundy, S. J. Lane & E. A. Murray (Eds.), *Sensory integration theory and practice* (2nd ed., pp. 339-341). Philadelphia, PA: F. A. Davis.

Wilbur, R. L., & Du Puy, W. A. (1932). Continental conservation. In R. L. Wilbur & W. A. Du Puy (Eds.). *Conservation in the Department of the Interior* (pp. 152-167). Washington, D. C.: United States Government Printing Office.

RESOURCES

Administration for Children & Families: www.acf.hhs.gov

American Occupational Therapy Association: www.aota.org

American Psychological Association: www.apa.org

American Academy of Pediatrics: www.aap.org/en-us/Pages/Default.aspx

Centers for Disease Control and Prevention: www.cdc.gov/ncbddd/childdevelopment/index.html

Healthy Children: www.healthychildren.org/english/ages-stages/teen/Pages/default.aspx

International Society for Traumatic Stress Studies: www.istss.org

National Center for Learning Disabilities: www.ncld.org

National Child Traumatic Stress Network: www.nctsn.org

National Center for Trauma Informed Care: www.samhsa.gov/nctic

United States Surgeon General: www.surgeongeneral.gov/initiatives/prevention/strategy/mental-emotional-well-being.html

5

Occupational Therapy Intervention
Promoting Occupational Participation

Tina Champagne, OTD, OTR/L

KEY TERMS

- Activity Analysis
- Adaptability
- Adaptive
- Adaptive Response
- Attachment
- Client-Directed
- Co-Occupation
- Emotional Regulation
- Intervention Implementation
- Intervention Planning
- Occupation
- Occupational Analysis
- Occupational Identity
- Occupation-Based Interventions
- Purposeful Activity
- Resilience
- Self-Esteem
- Self-Regulation
- Sensory Modulation
- Therapeutic Use of Self

CHAPTER LEARNING OBJECTIVES

After completion of this chapter, students should be able to:

1. Identify key components of the occupational therapy intervention planning and implementation processes.
2. Summarize typical childhood occupations and the corresponding occupational performance skill.
3. Describe key factors necessary to providing client-centered, individualized care.
4. Outline occupational therapy interventions used during the early lifespan to help maximize health, safety, and occupational participation.
5. Compare evidence-based and promising occupational therapy interventions that may be utilized with children and families with varied mental health, trauma, and attachment-related needs.

Manville, C.A., & Keough, J. L.
Mental Health Practice for the Occupational Therapy Assistant (pp 111-155).
© 2016 Taylor & Francis Group.

CHAPTER OUTLINE

INTRODUCTION

The American Occupational Therapy Association (AOTA) emphasizes that occupational therapy practitioners are qualified mental health practitioners (AOTA, 2010). It is within the scope of practice of occupational therapy practitioners to provide integrative, promising, and evidence-based interventions that support mental health and participation (AOTA, 2010). A central tenant of occupational therapy is the understanding that participation in meaningful life roles, activities, and engagement in *occupation* fosters health, wellness, and quality of life (AOTA, 2014b). Occupation is dynamic in nature and is defined as

> activities ... of everyday life, named, organized, and given value and meaning by individuals as a culture. Occupation is everything people do to occupy themselves, including looking after themselves ... enjoying life ... and contributing to the social and economic fabric of their communities. (Law, Polatajko, Baptiste, & Townsend, 1997, p. 32)

Hocking (2014) further explains that occupation provides "the physical activity, mental stimulation, and social interaction we need to keep our bodies, minds and communities healthy. In addition, through participation in occupation, we express ourselves, develop skills, experience pleasure and involvement, and achieve things we believe to be important" (p. 79).

Occupational therapy intervention is defined as a skilled, therapeutic, and collaborative process between the client and occupational therapy practitioner that enables engagement in occupation to support the client's goals and priorities (AOTA, 2014b). It is important to emphasize that the identified *client(s)* vary, depending on the intervention,

scope, and focus. Client(s) may be individuals, which may include caregivers or family members in some instances, and also groups of individuals (e.g., organizations) and populations. Role competence, occupational performance, adaptation, prevention, health, wellness, quality of life, and client satisfaction are examples of client intervention priorities and outcome areas (AOTA, 2014b).

The national child mental health and World Health Organization (WHO, 2001) initiatives advocate for the adoption of a public health approach when working with children, adolescents, adults, and caregivers (National Executive Training Institute [NETI], 2009). A public health approach emphasizes the importance of interventions that foster the general promotion of mental health and the prevention of mental illness, and that specifically target the needs of children with mental illness (AOTA, 2010; Bazyk & Arbesman, 2013; Champagne, 2011b, 2014; Champagne & Stromberg, 2004; WHO, 2001). Occupational therapy practitioners are qualified mental health practitioners who integrate public health models and initiatives as part of occupational therapy services (AOTA, 2010).

When using a public health approach, occupational therapy interventions are provided in a manner that occurs across three major levels or tiers (Bazyk & Arbesman, 2013). The major intervention tiers include the following:

1. Tier 1: Universal mental health promotion and prevention services

2. Tier 2: Targeted or selective services

3. Tier 3: Intensive, individualized mental health services

Refer to Chapter 3 for more specific information on the use of the public health model in the school setting.

It is important to help increase the protective factors and decrease risk factors in support of mental health, wellness, adaptation, and participation when working with children and adolescents. To this end, the public health model advocates the use of *promotion, prevention,* and *intensive individualized* interventions. *Promotion-focused* interventions primarily target competency building when working with all client types (AOTA, 2013; Bazyk & Arbesman, 2013). *Prevention-focused* interventions are intended to accomplish the following:

- Reduce the seriousness and incidence of problem behaviors and mental health disorders

- Increase protective factors, such as social and emotional competence, feeling supported, and clarity of behavioral expectations

- Reduce the risk factors for developing a mental illness, such as poverty and trauma (AOTA, 2013a; Bazyk & Arbesman, 2013; Miles, Espiritu, Horen, Sebian, & Waetzig, 2010)

Intensive individualized interventions are those that specifically target particular mental health symptoms, problems, and behaviors, while supporting optimal functioning and mental health (AOTA, 2013; Bazyk & Arbesman, 2013; Miles et al., 2010). Early education is essential to increase mental health literacy and reduce stigma in children and youth.

The categories of intervention in the public health model are similar to the intervention approaches proposed in the Occupational Therapy Practice Framework (OTPF). The intervention approaches in the OTPF include create or promote; prevent, establish, or restore; maintain; and modify (AOTA, 2014b). Interventions occur across service delivery areas such as direct care, advocacy, and consultation. Mental health promotion requires building supports, relational and developmental competencies, and positive environments, which helps to reduce existing mental health symptoms and risk factors. This chapter will focus primarily on the public health intervention levels of targeted and selective (tier 2) and intensive, individualized interventions (tier 3) in fostering prevention of illness and promotion of health, adaptation, resilience and occupational participation.

PART 1: CO-CREATING AND IMPLEMENTING THE INTERVENTION PLAN

The Intervention Planning and Implementation Processes

Therapeutic *intervention planning* in occupational therapy refers to the process where the results of the occupational therapy evaluation are reviewed and the goals and

plan for provision of services are created in collaboration with the client(s). Part of the intervention planning process also includes the identification of potential discharge criteria, referral sources, and any other resources that may be helpful to the client and family. The *intervention implementation* process includes carrying out the intervention plan and reviewing the intervention goals and outcomes over time. Outcomes review helps determine the extent to which the client's goals are or are not being met, whether any changes to existing goals need to be made, and when discharge from occupational therapy services is warranted. The intervention planning and implementation processes are dynamic and individualized based upon the client's and caregiver's values, strengths, needs, and goals.

Occupational Therapy Intervention Planning

An important tenet of occupational therapy is that all aspects are client centered, which also applies to the development and implementation of the intervention plan. In a client-centered approach, the strengths, wishes, values, and goals of the client are central to the occupational therapy process. It is important to recognize, however, that some occupational therapy theories and frameworks take this one step further and require a client-directed approach. Ayres' Sensory Integration (ASI) is an example of an occupational therapy framework that promotes a client-directed approach; it also includes caregiver(s) when working with children. In a *client-directed approach*, the process is not only client centered, but the client also leads the therapeutic process, and the occupational therapy practitioner provides support. For instance, rather than the therapist selecting and instructing the child through a specific therapeutic activity, the child engages in activities that are self-selected while being supported by the occupational therapy practitioner. During the occupational therapy process, occupational therapy practitioners may use a client-centered or client-directed approach, depending on the needs of the client and the theoretical model(s) used (Checkpoint 5-1).

The development of the intervention plan is also influenced by input from involved team members such as social workers, pediatricians, and teachers. Thus, developing the intervention plan includes co-creating the therapeutic goals, identifying the intervention approaches, mechanisms for service delivery, potential discharge criteria, and outcome methods to be used in a collaborative manner (AOTA, 2014b). Discussion regarding future educational needs, recommendations for transition services, and additional referrals may also be warranted (AOTA, 2014b). Some questions to consider during the intervention planning and implementation process include the following:

- What is meaningful to the child and caregiver?

- What intervention activities would best support the client's occupational values, needs, and goals?

CHECKPOINT 5-1. UNDERSTAND

Explain the difference between client-centered and client-directed activities. Give a specific example of each type of activity that includes the role of the occupational therapy assistant.

- What interventions are promising and evidence informed and will support the client's goals?

- What are the environmental affordances and constraints involved in the practice setting(s)?

- Will the selected interventions support occupational participation?

The development and monitoring of the intervention plan is the responsibility of the occupational therapist. The occupational therapy assistant may provide input that is taken into consideration during the development of the intervention plan, which is directed and supervised by the occupational therapist (AOTA, 2014a). The occupational therapist is responsible for identifying the theories, frames of reference, models of practice, and evidence that will best support positive therapeutic outcomes when developing the intervention plan (AOTA, 2014a).

The chronological age and developmental level of the child also affect the intervention planning and implementation processes. Occupational performance skill areas include communication and interaction skills, process skills, and motor skills, all of which contribute to occupational participation (AOTA, 2014b). It is important to note that many children with mental health–related challenges, including those who have experienced trauma, often present at a lower developmental level than would be expected for their chronological age across many body structures, body functions, and occupational performance skill areas (Perry & Hambrick, 2008; van der Kolk, 2005, 2006).

Another variable that influences the intervention planning process includes the setting where the services are provided. Occupational therapy practitioners work with children and adolescents in a variety of practice environments. Examples of settings and programs can include the following:

- Homes
- School systems (mainstream and schools for children with behavioral challenges)
- After-school programs
- Outpatient clinics
- Partial hospitalization programs
- Inpatient hospitals
- Residential programs
- Juvenile justice programs (correctional)
- Day programs
- Early intervention programs

- Community-based settings and programs (e.g., camp programs)

The setting where the client receives services influences the intervention planning and implementation processes in many ways. For instance, occupational therapy practitioners working with infants and toddlers typically provide services as part of an interdisciplinary team through early intervention programs. Early intervention services are typically provided in the home and focus on helping the child and family identify strengths and barriers related to engagement in meaningful roles and occupations.

At times, services may not be able to adequately address safety needs if provided inside the home or at school. For instance, when safety is of significant concern, children and adolescents may be admitted to inpatient units, partial hospitalization programs, residential settings, and after-school programs that provide specialized services for children with mental health or behavioral concerns. Children and youth who face legal charges may be sent to a juvenile justice setting by the court. Typically, it is the recommendation or decision of the larger treatment team (which includes caregivers), child protection services, or the legal system that determines whether a child is admitted to a higher level of care or juvenile justice setting. In addition to the client(s) and occupational therapy practitioner(s), the treatment team may consist of teachers, nurses, social workers, psychologists, and psychiatrists.

Another variable that affects occupational therapy treatment planning and implementation process is the average length of stay or allowable amount of treatment time for the provision of occupational therapy services. Currently, the average length of stay in most acute care inpatient hospital settings is approximately 7 to 9 days. In residential programs, a child may be admitted for 3 to 12 months. In the school system, a child is generally enrolled for the school year and potentially for summer programs depending on the child's needs and educational goals. These timeframes, therefore, may influence the amount of occupational therapy services an individual receives. State and federal laws, third-party payers, and relevant organizational rules and regulations must also be considered when determining how to implement occupational therapy services across varied levels of care.

In addition to working directly with children and families, occupational therapy practitioners work with organizations and populations in the community, where they may provide consultation, education, and advocacy as warranted (AOTA, 2014b). Occupational therapy practitioners may also work on policy development and implementation and political advocacy, and many hold managerial, supervisory,

CHECKPOINT 5-2. APPLY

List the variables that should be considered in the intervention planning process, then illustrate each variable with an example.

and other positions in which they have the opportunity to help support mental health promotion. In these additional roles, occupational therapy practitioners can help support the ability to obtain access to occupational therapy services and manage and supervise existing services (Checkpoint 5-2).

Occupational Therapy Intervention Implementation

Implementation of the intervention plan occurs after the completion of the intervention planning process. The OTPF provides a guideline for how to proceed through the occupational therapy process, in which occupational therapy practitioners use the therapeutic use of self, occupations, and meaningful activities that support the client's occupational needs and goals (AOTA, 2014b). Therapeutic use of self is one of a practitioner's most important therapeutic tools. *Therapeutic use of self* is the skilled and strategic use of one's verbal and nonverbal communications, personality, attitude, ideas, and perceptions to help develop and maintain the therapeutic relationship and meet the occupational therapy goals (AOTA, 2014b). It is essential that the client feels safe with the occupational therapy practitioner when addressing mental health–related needs and goals. Attention to therapeutic use of self is particularly critical when working with people with trauma histories and different attachment styles. The skilled use of one's voice, body positioning, rhythm, energy level, and pace are examples of how occupational therapy practitioners modify the way they interact for therapeutic purposes. The ability to actively listen and attune to the client and caregiver is another critical element of therapeutic use of self. All of these skills contribute to the ability to develop a therapeutic relationship, and are described in more detail in Chapter 14.

Since the beginning of the profession, the therapeutic use of occupation has been promoted as a central tenet in occupational therapy. According to the AOTA (2014b), occupational therapy practitioners "recognize that health is supported and maintained when individuals are able to engage in occupations and in activities that allow desired or needed participation in home, school, workplace, and community life situation" (p. 611).

The occupational therapy assistant must be aware of the identified needs and goals of each client in order to engage him or her in therapeutic interventions that will help achieve positive outcomes (AOTA, 2014a). The occupational therapist delegates responsibility to the occupational therapy assistant to work on those areas of the treatment plan in which he or she has demonstrated competency (AOTA, 2014a). Each client's progress is continually monitored, documented, and revised as needed during the intervention implementation process (AOTA, 2014b).

As reviewed in Chapter 4, the child's age and developmental and mental health capacities are all considered when selecting the interventions that will be used. The occupational therapy practitioner must also determine whether the grading of activities or environmental modifications will be needed. For instance, a child may have difficulty with coordinating both sides of the body to the degree that it negatively affects the ability to meet occupational goals, such as dressing or playing. The occupational therapy practitioner would begin by facilitating engagement in graded activities and occupations that help to develop the underlying client factors, occupational performance skills, and the child's self-confidence. The occupational therapy practitioner may also help parents, teachers, and staff to consider helpful environmental modifications. An example of an environmental modification would be to reduce distractions in the physical environment if a client has difficulty with focusing attention or is easily overstimulated. The reduction of environmental stimulation may be helpful in fostering the ability to focus on homework in the home or class work and group participation at school. The occupational therapy practitioner might work with an adolescent to help identify and engage in positive, pro-social leisure activities in a community-based after-school program. These are just a few examples of some of the different ways occupational therapy practitioners provide services to help target specific occupational needs and goals in different contexts.

Occupational Therapy: Intervention Types

According to the OTPF, the therapeutic use of occupations and activities may include the use of occupation-based interventions, purposeful activities, and preparatory methods that match the client's specific values, needs, and goals (AOTA, 2014b). *Occupation-based interventions* are activities and occupations that are used to help meet the specific needs and goals of the client. The client-directed use of play on a playground that is used to target occupational goals is an example of an occupation-based intervention. *Purposeful activities* are interventions that are strategically selected and used to support the development of specific skills that promote occupational participation. Role playing with an adolescent in order to practice how to interview for a job is an example of a purposeful activity. The use of particular games or puzzles to help develop specific occupational performance skills is another example of a purposeful activity. *Preparatory methods* are specific therapeutic approaches that are used to help prepare the client for participating in meaningful roles and occupations. The use of a weighted blanket to help decrease feelings of anxiety in order to improve a child's participation in sleep, play, self-care, therapeutic, or educational activities is an example of a preparatory method. It is the responsibility of all occupational therapy practitioners to understand each category of occupational therapy intervention.

In addition to the occupational therapy intervention types described by the OTPF (AOTA, 2014b), the public health approach mentioned earlier in this chapter promotes the use of the three-tier model of interventions (Bazyk & Arbesman, 2013). Table 5-1 reviews the three-tier model of major interventions and provides examples of the client types and interventions that correspond to each level.

Occupational Analysis and Activity Analysis

Occupational analysis is a process that is individualized and embedded in the subjective perspective of the client, the client's occupational performance, and performance context(s) (Crepeau, Boyt Schell, Gillen, & Scaffa, 2014). Occupational analysis considers not only the activity in question, but also the client's values, client factors (body structures and functions), meaningful life roles and activities, occupational performance skills and patterns, and environmental and contextual variables (AOTA, 2014b). Occupational analysis is used to help understand each client as an occupational being and places the "person in the foreground" (Crepeau et al., 2014, p. 244).

Activity analysis is a process used when dissecting a given activity into its corresponding steps, activity demands, and component parts. The information obtained through activity analysis helps the occupational therapy practitioner identify whether an activity will need to be modified to meet the client's needs and abilities (AOTA, 2014b). Occupational therapy practitioners use activity analysis and occupational analysis throughout the occupational therapy process to help identify the client's strengths, values, needs, and where the barriers to activity and occupational participation exist (e.g., physical impairments, activity or environmental limitations affecting dressing, showering, doing homework, or engagement in cooperative play). The information obtained through activity analysis and occupational analysis is used to collaboratively identify and prioritize goal areas, interventions, and resources that may be useful to the client (Crepeau et al., 2014).

Grading Activities

Grading activities and occupations refer to the modification of an activity to match a client's specific needs and strengths in order to offer the "just right challenge." Activity, environmental, and/or contextual demands may be gradually modified to meet specific therapeutic goals of the client. Other examples of variables that are modified

to help the individual meet therapeutic goals include cognitive, social, emotional, and cultural elements. Some examples of how the therapeutic use of self may be graded is by changing the number of steps or verbal cues provided by the practitioner (e.g., going from maximum assistance to moderate), the amount of physical assistance (e.g., hand-over-hand assistance to set up), or through body positioning (e.g., being within close physical proximity to distant).

Intervention Intensity

The "just right" amount of intervention intensity can be difficult for an entry-level practitioner to initially identify, that is, when and to what degree to grade an activity or the environment. An activity may be "graded up" by increasing the activity demands when the client is able to complete the activity but further progress is desired. An activity may be "graded down" by decreasing the activity demands. Grading an activity down occurs when an activity is determined to be too difficult or there is concern that lack of progress will have a negative influence on factors such as motivation, social participation, performance, or self-esteem. It is essential to work collaboratively with clients to ensure the "just right challenge" occurs throughout the therapeutic implementation process.

Some of the variables to consider that are directly related to intervention intensity include frequency (how often), duration (how long), stimulus intensity (degree of the intensity of the stimulus), and the rhythm of the intervention (Champagne, 2011b). It is important to emphasize, however, that some clients may be able to tolerate more or less intervention intensity than others. In addition to intervention intensity, the client's age, needs, goals, and interests must all be considered when collaboratively selecting, grading, or adapting activities, equipment, and the physical environment. To illustrate, consider the example of the occupational therapy practitioner who is working with a child having difficulty with play participation due to problems with low extensor tone, bilateral coordination, and balance skills (demonstrating difficulty with vestibular discrimination). The occupational therapy practitioner will consider a variety of activity options that are age and culturally appropriate, safe to use in the setting, and specifically target the child's needs and goals. The ability to grade the intensity of the vestibular input is considered in the selection of activities and occupations. Linear movement, such as the movement provided by a glider rocker, is typically less intense than arcs, which is the type of movement experienced when swinging on a swing set. Linear and arc movements are typically less intense than the rotary movement experienced on a sit-and-spin or merry-go-round. Although each individual is unique, a person who is sensitive to vestibular stimulation may have difficulty tolerating activities that require having the feet off the ground (e.g., swinging), the experience of varying heights (climbing up a slide), navigating on unstable surfaces (e.g., hikes, going

TABLE 5-1

PUBLIC HEALTH INTERVENTION LEVELS

INTERVENTION LEVEL	TARGETED CLIENT	INTERVENTION FOCUS	INTERVENTION EXAMPLES	OCCUPATIONAL THERAPY PROCESS EXAMPLES	RESOURCE AND PROGRAM EXAMPLES

Tier 1: Universal	All children and adolescents with or without mental health or other occupational barriers	Indirect services focused on affecting larger populations targeting promotion and prevention goals	1. Work with key stakeholders to promote specific interventions to become part of public policy (e.g., integration of positive behavioral interventions and supports; mental health literacy programs for adolescents; sensory supportive interventions)
			
			2. Work with schools or school systems to implement prevention interventions (e.g., anti-bullying and social and emotional learning interventions, after-school programs)
				Evaluation:
				• Broad based, population specific (not focused on individual clients) (e.g., literature review, statistics, surveys)
				
				Intervention:
				• Promotion and prevention interventions to whole populations
					Intervention examples:
					Promotion:
					• Health promotion:
					  ○ Improve mental health literacy
					  ○ Increased participation in physical activity (McNeil et al., 2009)
					• Social skills promotion:
					  ○ SEL in school and after school programs (Durlak, Weissberg, Dymnicki, Taylor, & Schellinger, 2011)
					
					Prevention: problem behaviors, substance abuse, sexual activity)
					• Positive Action Program (grades K to 12) (Beets et al., 2009)
					• Positive adolescent life skills training
					• Anti-bullying prevention programs (Trofti & Farrington, 2009)

(continued)

TABLE 5-1 (CONTINUED)

PUBLIC HEALTH INTERVENTION LEVELS

INTERVENTION LEVEL	TARGETED CLIENT	INTERVENTION FOCUS	INTERVENTION EXAMPLES	OCCUPATIONAL THERAPY PROCESS EXAMPLES	RESOURCE AND PROGRAM EXAMPLES

Tier 2: Targeted	Children and adolescents with difficulty with learning, emotional, and/or developmental concerns, and those at risk for developing mental health or behavioral problems	Consultation, individual or group services (indirect and direct occupational therapy services)	1. Consultation with teachers to help create and integrate sensory diet strategies into the daily routine to support learning, social, and emotional capacities
			
			2. Provide direct group services to help target children and adolescents with specific risk factors (e.g., obesity, loss, bullying, life skills)
				Evaluation:
				• Specific to the needs of at-risk youth and families (e.g., early detection screenings, participation scales)
				
				Intervention:
				• Specific to the at-risk concerns and often target the following:
				  ○ Environmental modifications
				  ○ Task or activity modifications
				  ○ Increased opportunity for health-promoting occupational participation
				  ○ Education/training
					Assessment examples:
					• Children's Assessment of Participation (CAPE) and Enjoyment and Preferences for Activities of Children (PAC) (King et al., 2004)
					
					• Perceived Efficacy and Goals Setting System (Missiuna, Pollock, & Law, 2004)
					
					• School Function Assessment (SFA) (Coster, Deeney, Haltiwanger, & Haley, 1998)
					
					• Occupational Therapy Psychosocial Assessment of Learning (Townsend et al., 1999)
					
					Intervention program examples:
					• Fast Track Program: to reduce the risk for developing conduct and other mental health disorders
					
					• Parenting program for teenage mothers (Coren & Barlow, 2001)

(continued)

TABLE 5-1 (CONTINUED)

PUBLIC HEALTH INTERVENTION LEVELS

INTERVENTION LEVEL	TARGETED CLIENT	INTERVENTION FOCUS	INTERVENTION EXAMPLES	OCCUPATIONAL THERAPY PROCESS EXAMPLES	RESOURCE AND PROGRAM EXAMPLES
Tier 3: Intensive	Children and adolescents with identified mental health and/or behavioral challenges that limit participation in meaningful roles and occupations	Direct, intensive, and individualized interventions (individual and group services). Includes involved systems (e.g, family, school, providers)	1. Provide individualized services to help target specific mental health and/or behavioral health barriers to occupational performance and participation 2. Work with the client, family, and community-based providers to support "wraparound" services	• Referral: parent and physician refer a child due to sensory-processing barriers affecting occupational participation. • Occupational therapy evaluation: Co-creation of occupational profile, which includes evaluation of sensory processing • Individualized intervention planning and implementation: includes an emphasis on sensory-processing (home, school, community) supports to foster occupational participation • Education and resources provided: to client and family, includes information about sensory processing	Assessment examples (may be used during the evaluation process): • Sensory-processing measures (home and school contexts) (Miller-Kuhanek, Henry, Glennon, Parham & Ecker, 2008) • Sensory profiles (home and school contexts) (Brown & Dunn, 2002; Dunn, 1999) • Bruininks-Oseretsky Test of Motor Proficiency (Bruininks & Bruininks, 2005) • Sensory Modulation Screening Tool or Sensory Defensiveness Checklist (Champagne, 2011b) Intervention resources: • How Does Your Engine Run? (Williams & Shellenberger, 1994) • Sensory Modulation Program (Champagne, 2011b) • The Tool Chest (Henry, 2001) • BrainWorks sensory diet tools (Wild, 2014)

Adapted from Arbesman, M., Bazyk, S., & Nochajski, S. M. (2013). Systematic review of occupational therapy and mental health promotion, prevention and intervention in children and youth. *American Journal of Occupational Therapy, 67,* 120-130.; Bazyk S., & Arbesman, M. (2013). *Occupational therapy practice guidelines for mental health promotion, prevention and intervention for children and youth.* Bethesda, MD: AOTA; McNeil, D. A., Wilson, B. N., Siever, J. E., Ronca, M., & Nah, J. K. (2009). Connecting children to recreational activities: Results of a cluster randomized trial. *American Journal of Health Promotion, 23,* 376-387.

for a boat ride), or engaging in activities requiring rotary movement such as spinning (e.g., amusement park rides). Conversely, a person who seeks out activities affording more intense vestibular input may enjoy and need more of the intensity provided by the activity types mentioned. In this way, the client factors (e.g., sensory and perceptual), occupational performance skills (e.g., motor, communication, and process skills), and patterns factor significantly into the intervention planning process.

The intensity of input also relates to the other sensory systems as well. Using taste as an example, sweet tastes are often less intense than spicy, which are often less intense than sour, bitter, or smoky flavors (Champagne, 2011b). When considering the intensity of body positioning, being upright is often perceived as less intense than being out of straight planes (diagonals). Diagonals are considered less intense than bending over forward or arching backward (Champagne, 2011b). Again, everyone is different and therefore, the examples provided are not to be viewed as a rigid protocol; rather, they may be used as a guideline to help occupational therapy practitioners develop clinical reasoning skills related to understanding and grading intervention intensity.

In terms of movement, occupational therapy practitioners also take into account the type and degree of movement required by any given task. For example, some activities are more sedentary than active in nature. Sedentary activities may include watching a movie, reading a book, rocking in a rocking chair, sitting, and listening to music. Active activities may include cleaning, riding a bicycle, showering, playing on the playground, playing a game, and cooking. Everyone is different. Thus, a person's perception of the degree of intensity of any given stimulus, activity, or occupation is very individual and must be considered when grading or modifying activities, equipment, and physical environments.

Chaining and Levels of Assistance

Chaining is an approach used by occupational therapy practitioners when clients have difficulty with self-esteem, frustration tolerance, attention span, organizational skills, emotion regulation skills, sequencing, praxis, or other occupational performance skills. The overall goal of chaining is to provide the amount of support needed to help clients increase frustration tolerance and improve feelings of self-esteem, competence, and success. Forward chaining provides the opportunity for a child or an adolescent to start engagement in a given activity or task and sequence through to the point where assistance is needed. The occupational therapy practitioner can then provide the level and type(s) of supports needed for successful completion. When using backward chaining, the therapist completes much of the activity or task and the client completes the remaining portions while receiving positive reinforcement. With both forward and backward chaining, the goal is to provide the "just right" amount of support needed for successful participation. The amount of support needed is faded as developmental capacities are developed and outcomes are achieved.

Occupational therapy practitioners also help identify the level of assistance needed to participate in meaningful life roles and occupations. Levels of assistance include the following:

- Independent
- Independent with setup
- Supervision
- Minimal assistance
- Moderate assistance
- Maximal assistance
- Dependent/total assistance

For instance, a child may need total assistance to open containers, or only set-up assistance and verbal cues for support. How much assistance a client requires to complete any given activity or occupation can be used as an outcomes measure to determine if the therapeutic goals have been met. If goals have not been met, additional occupational therapy services and other supports are considered. Spotlight 5-1 describes safety and social participation in the clinical vignette of Jorge.

Intervention Review and Outcomes

Under the supervision of the occupational therapist, the occupational therapy assistant consistently monitors the ability level of the client and progress made toward treatment goals. Occupational therapy practitioners are able to provide modifications to interventions as needed to provide the "just right challenge" in order to help the client meet his or her goals (AOTA, 2014a). The occupational therapy assistant must also document the treatment interventions used, the client's response to those interventions, and progress made over time. The information provided by the occupational therapy assistant is used by the occupational therapist on an ongoing basis to supervise the occupational therapy process. A more formalized intervention review is the responsibility of the occupational therapist and is conducted to help determine whether the implementation plan should continue with or without modifications and when discharge is warranted. Key questions that are considered during the intervention review process include the following:

- What can the client specifically do, and what are the remaining challenges and barriers?

- Has the client's ability to participate in the identified meaningful occupations increased and, if so, to what degree?

SPOTLIGHT 5-1. CLINICAL VIGNETTE. JORGE: SAFETY AND SOCIAL PARTICIPATION

Jorge, a 6-year-old boy, is residing at a residential program and struggling with safety, social, emotional, and sensorimotor skills. Some of his strengths include that he is inquisitive, intelligent, energetic, and has a variety of interests. A chart review revealed that Jorge has been diagnosed with pervasive developmental disability (American Psychological Association, 2013), difficulty with anxiety and unsafe behaviors, and he has had a significant early childhood trauma history.

The occupational therapist worked collaboratively with Jorge, his foster parents, and the staff in order to create the occupational therapy intervention plan. Jorge demonstrated difficulty with safety awareness, social boundaries, sensorimotor performance, emotion, and behavioral regulation. He was initially admitted to a residential program due to the severity of his self-injurious behaviors, poor safety awareness, and aggressive outbursts toward his parents and family members. Currently, he is unable to talk to peers without physically touching or bumping into them, which worsens when he is excited or upset. He often becomes aggressive, impulsive, and uses too much force with staff or when playing with peers at the residential program. Difficulty with these occupational performance skills negatively affects safety, both Jorge's and his family's. The ability to live at home, attend school, make and keep friends, and other aspects of occupational participation are affected.

Occupational therapy services are part of the residential services offered to Jorge and his foster family while he is part of the program. He will reside at the program for a minimum of 6 to 9 months until Jorge and his foster family are ready to start the transitional process toward discharge home. This is to support the transfer of skills learned at the program to home. The following example demonstrates some of the initial occupational therapy interventions. These targeted his ability to become more self-aware and to recognize and maintain boundaries, both with peers and within the physical environment.

Long-Term Goal: Jorge will demonstrate the ability to maintain body boundaries with peers at the residential program with moderate assistance of verbal and environmental cues within 6 weeks.

- Intervention and activity examples
  - Increase self-awareness (body awareness, boundaries)
    - Play games that require adjustments in the amount of physical force used: Don't Break the Ice, Ants in the Pants, Operation
    - Assist with setting the table for dinner: requires considerations for personal space, adjustment of force of movements, navigation of personal space with others who are helping (staff and peers)
    - Provide ongoing activity choices that will help Jorge increase body awareness (e.g., play activities providing increased proprioceptive and tactile stimulation)
  - To improve emotion regulation skills, Jorge will:
    - Identify his emotions and learn how to verbalize how he is feeling
    - Create and utilize a self-rating tool
    - Identify strategies to help with modulating his emotions and behaviors that will be available at different times of day (use of weighted lap pad, deep belly breathing, playing on the playground)
    - Integrate the use of self-rating into the residential program routine with all children and staff
    - Create places and guidelines with positive reinforcement to be able to take "breaks"
    - Play games with peers that help him to increase social and emotion regulation skills
  - Help Jorge to identify and sit on his carpet square during house meetings and groups
    - Help Jorge choose and decorate his own carpet square
    - Discuss why carpet squares are used until he is able to explain to therapist, staff, or other peers
  - Help Jorge identify what areas in his bedroom are his and where he can and cannot go (shares a bedroom with one other child)
    - Use visual cues (colorful tape, signs)

(continued)

**SPOTLIGHT 5-1. CLINICAL VIGNETTE. JORGE: SAFETY AND
SOCIAL PARTICIPATION (CONTINUED)**

¤ Assist the children who are sharing the bedroom to develop a short list of "rules" for their space that is sensitive to each child's needs and goals

○ Collaboratively develop and consistently use a positive behavioral reward system with the child and staff, as well as consequences:

¤ Educate the child and staff about how to use the positive behavioral reward system

¤ Co-create a clear plan for appropriate consequences when problems occur

---

- What has been instrumental to the client and family in making gains?

- Should the client's goals be modified?

Outcomes are evaluated by the occupational therapist, who identifies the specific methods and tools to be used for that process. The occupational therapist is also responsible for the measurement and interpretation of the outcomes. In the instances where the occupational therapist and occupational therapy assistant have identified that the assistant is competent in administering the outcome measure selected by the therapist, the occupational therapy assistant may help in collecting the outcome data and documenting them accordingly (AOTA, 2014a). The methodology used to evaluate outcomes helps to answer the following questions:

- Has the client met the goals established?

- If not, to what degree have the goals been met or not met?

- Should the client continue with services or be discharged?

  ○ Does the client want to continue occupational therapy services?

  ○ Is there sufficient justification for continued services?

- What additional education, advocacy, resources, or referrals are needed?

PART 2: MENTAL HEALTH, OCCUPATIONAL PERFORMANCE, AND PARTICIPATION

Fostering Adaptability and Resiliency

When assessing occupational performance and participation throughout the intervention process, occupational therapy practitioners look at how the child is able to explore the environment; engage in meaningful relationships, roles, and tasks; and demonstrate competency in performance skills during occupational participation. Occupational therapy practitioners work with children and families to help identify contextual factors affecting the ability to engage in occupations. They identify what is satisfactory (achievement) and any necessary modifications, enhancements, or resources required to help support occupational participation. It is important to understand that what is meaningful and important to one person may or may not be meaningful and important to another. A client will not be intrinsically motivated to explore or engage in an occupation or intervention if it is not meaningful to him or her. Additionally, a person may become more intrinsically motivated to participate in an intervention if the occupational therapy practitioner helps him or her to understand the reasoning behind it.

Understanding the child's current abilities helps occupational therapy practitioners utilize abilities as strengths during the intervention process to help conquer occupational barriers and meet goals. For example, a sense of competence when exploring and engaging in meaningful life roles and activities can help a child achieve personal goals and feel a sense of accomplishment. Focusing on a child's strengths and not solely on the problems is critical to helping children and families develop a positive sense of self. Self-esteem is influenced by the ability to be successful in individual roles and everyday life activities across the lifespan. Self-esteem helps children cope with and mediate feelings of shame, embarrassment, and a negative self-concept when encountering occupational barriers. A person's occupational identity is shaped, in part, by one's perceptions of competence and achievement.

Children and adolescents may miss opportunities for developing performance skills due to mental health symptoms, as well as a variety of other factors. Some examples of additional variables that can affect the achievement of developmental and educational goals include neglect, poverty, ongoing traumatic experiences and stressors, frequent moves (e.g., multiple foster care placements), and repeated hospitalizations. Difficulty with attention and concentration, emotion regulation, social and communication skills, and problematic behaviors may also affect the ability to meet occupational goals. Role-play that includes the opportunity for children to take on new roles and engage in activities that they may have missed out on can help foster occupational competence, satisfaction, and quality of life. The sense of accomplishment and competence that results from occupational participation increases the child's motivation to perform and improves occupational satisfaction. Consider a young child who is being bullied and is afraid to play with peers on the playground during recess. Imagine being in high school and struggling to meet educational goals. Over time, a child's occupational identity and self-esteem can be seriously compromised if he or she does not receive assistance to target these occupational barriers and develop feelings of self-esteem, self-worth, and developmental competence.

Adaptability and the Adaptive Response

In everyday life, individuals receive feedback and information from within their bodies, as well as the physical environment, as they engage in meaningful roles, activities, and social interactions. The ability to change behavior in accordance with the variety of occupational demands needed in different life roles and activities requires **adaptability**. A person's degree of adaptability influences role performance, social and emotional responses, behaviors, the personal satisfaction experienced when engaging in roles and occupations, and ultimately, quality of life. A child who experiences difficulty coping with transitions is demonstrating challenges with adaptability. Examples of transitions include the following:

- Waking up in the morning and getting ready for the day
- Going to school (e.g., leaving the house and getting on the bus)
- Transitioning in and out of breaks and different classes throughout the day
- Leaving school and coming home; after-school hours
- Transitioning from play to homework time
- Getting ready for bed and being able to fall asleep

Many children with mental health and behavioral problems have difficulty with transitions. Occupational therapy practitioners help children, families, teachers, and staff to manage transitions by using some of the following strategies and resources. They include the following:

- Helping to identify what transitions are most difficult and why
- Helping clients and caregivers learn how to prepare for transitions
- Providing education and resources on transitional supports

- Evaluating for and recommending the use of supports that assist with and ease transitions. Examples include technology, sensory strategies, educational, and vocational supports
- Helping clients develop skills to support transitions and improve occupational participation. Examples include self-determination, functional mobility, education, and employment-related skills
- Collaborating with interdisciplinary professionals to help coordinate services and resources needed.

Another basic concept in occupational therapy is **adaptation**. Adaptation is related to adaptability and refers to the ability to adjust to occupational demands. What is considered to be a "successful" adaptation often differs for each client. Adaptation affects a person's perceptions, attitudes, values, behaviors, and quality of life. The effectiveness of the therapeutic process is measured, in part, "by the child's ability to respond successfully to previously difficult or disorganizing challenges" (Ayres, 2005, p. 143). Evidence of increased adaptability is demonstrated when the child and family are able to change in the face of stress and adversity. **Resilience** is the ability to cope with stressors and face vulnerability factors. Adaptability and resiliency can be considered different manifestations of a person's capacities to experience and respond to stress, problems, or changes within and/or outside of the individual and the physical environment.

The **adaptive response** is best understood as a dynamic process, and it is often evidence to occupational therapy practitioners that an intervention is providing the "just right challenge." Many occupational therapy theories and frames of reference specifically explain the centrality of adaptation and the adaptive response within occupational therapy. In ASI, Ayres defined the **adaptive response** as "an appropriate action in which the individual responds successfully to some environmental demand" (2005, p. 199). Ayres (2005) proposed that the more intrinsically motivated and self-directed the engagement of the child in meaningful occupation (e.g., play), the higher the probability that the child will achieve the neurobiopsychosocial developmental integration that leads to higher-order occupational performance skills and participation.

Think back to when you were a child and you wanted to learn how to ride a bicycle. Because you were intrinsically motivated to succeed, you worked hard to develop the multiplicity of occupational performance skills required for the occupational goal of riding your bike. The many performance skills required to ride a bike were not likely to have been a part of your conscious awareness at that time. The client factors and occupational performance skills needed to ride a bike include some of the following: physical strength and endurance, dynamic balance, motor coordination, visual-perceptual-motor integration, frustration tolerance, the ability to sequence through the steps of

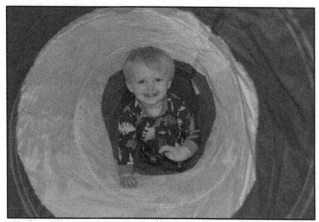

Figure 5-1. Child playing in tunnel.

the activity, and the motivation to keep trying until you succeed! Each adaptive learning experience contributes to the ability to meet the next set of occupational performance challenges involved in learning how to ride a bike. Ayres also asserted that neuroplasticity is enhanced through occupational participation (e.g., engagement in self-care activities, play), whereby developmental and foundational skills increase in complexity. Each adaptive experience helped to support your ability to achieve the goal of learning how to ride a bike. Imagine how much more difficult the process of learning to ride a bike would have been if this goal was being pushed upon you by someone else and if you did not particularly care to learn how to ride a bicycle at the time, or were fearful due to problems with balance or motor coordination.

Occupational therapy practitioners use a variety of theories to help clients meet their occupational goals. When working with children with mental health challenges, childhood occupations are used to help foster adaptability, development, resiliency, and occupational participation. Occupational therapy practitioners use childhood occupations to target specific occupational goals, promote mental health, and prevent mental illness and behavioral problems. Figure 5-1 demonstrates a child engaged in play during part of an occupational therapy intervention process.

Childhood Occupations and Mental Health Applications

Children and families live, learn, and play together in context and over time. These experiences help to lay the foundation for bonding, relationship formation, *self-regulation*, development, occupational participation, and overall health and wellness across the lifespan (Blaustein & Kinninburgh, 2010; Feletti et al., 1998; Perry & Hambrick, 2008; van der Kolk, 2005, 2006). Childhood occupations take place at home, school, and within the community and are used as therapeutic interventions by occupational therapy practitioners. Activities of daily living (ADLs)

(self-care), instrumental activities of daily living (IADLs) (home care and community living skills), play, school, and work occupations constitute some of the primary occupations of childhood and adolescence. Research supports the importance of the provision of occupational therapy interventions within the person's natural context and with the family system whenever possible. Refer to Chapter 4 for more information about each of these areas of occupation.

Occupational therapy interventions may be provided to help establish or restore, create or promote, adapt or modify, maintain, and prevent (AOTA, 2014b). An understanding of childhood development and occupational therapy theories and frames of reference are used to help guide the clinical reasoning process. Table 5-2 provides examples of how occupational therapy theories and frames of reference are correlated with intervention by using an example of a child who is having difficulty with buttoning, which is affecting his ability to dress independently.

Childhood occupations require the ability to sequence through the steps of each activity involved. Using the processes of occupational analysis and activity, occupational therapy practitioners identify the steps required of each activity, environmental and contextual supports, barriers, and other activity demands involved. Occupational analysis in particular helps the occupational therapy practitioner identify and explain the dynamic nature of the occupational strengths and barriers experienced by the child and the family system in context and over time. Some common childhood occupations include the ability to play and attend social events with peers (e.g., birthday parties, community events). According to the OTPF (AOTA, 2014b), the following are examples of occupational performance skills:

- Motor skills: mobility, coordination, postural control, strength, endurance, effort, and energy

- Process skills: one's fund of knowledge, attention, temporal organization, adaptation, organization of space and objects

- Communication/interactional skills: the ability to recognize social cues and norms, express affect, use gestures, ask for information, share personal information appropriately, develop a rapport with others, demonstrate respect for others, maintain personal boundaries, and demonstrate reciprocity

Occupational performance skills support social participation, such as cooperative play and engagement in group activities.

The following list provides examples of interventions that an occupational therapy practitioner may consider to help facilitate play and social participation with a child who is having difficulty:

- Play a game of choice with just one person before engaging in larger group activities

- Play games of increasing difficulty with one person initially

TABLE 5-2

OCCUPATIONAL BARRIER TO DRESSING: ABILITY TO BUTTON CLOTHING

OCCUPATIONAL THERAPY: INTERVENTION APPROACHES	OCCUPATIONAL THERAPY: THEORIES AND FRAMES OF REFERENCE	OCCUPATIONAL THERAPY: INTERVENTION EXAMPLES
Establish, restore, and maintain	Person-Environment-Occupation (PEO) Developmental Neurodevelopmental Ayres Sensory Integration (ASI)	Use specific interventions to help establish, restore, or maintain skill: • Play games that require the use of small or thin pieces to help work on fine motor manipulation and strength before working up to buttoning (preparatory intervention) • Engage in client-directed, occupation-based activities that develop or increase body functions and improve dexterity and sensorimotor skills in order to increase occupational participation (playing at the playground; playing with Play-Doh; finding and removing small objects from Theraputty; write or draw with a vibrating pen; engaging in occupational therapy services in a sensory integration gym) • Maintain current fine motor performance skills and occupational participation by engaging in play activities as part of the daily routine (e.g., arts and crafts class, insert coins into piggy bank)
Modification, adaptation	PEO Developmental Neurodevelopmental ASI	Make modifications to the activity demands or environment: • Modify the task: child wears clothing with larger or fewer buttons, or only completes some of the buttoning and a caregiver completes the remainder of the task • Adapt the clothing: May have/use clothes without buttons or have other types of fasteners (Velcro) • Modify the environment: Practice buttoning in a quiet place with minimal distractions and with additional time *(continued)*

TABLE 5-2 (CONTINUED)

OCCUPATIONAL BARRIER TO DRESSING: ABILITY TO BUTTON CLOTHING

OCCUPATIONAL THERAPY: INTERVENTION APPROACHES	OCCUPATIONAL THERAPY: THEORIES AND FRAMES OF REFERENCE	OCCUPATIONAL THERAPY: INTERVENTION EXAMPLES
Prevention, education	PEO Developmental Neurodevelopmental ASI	Prevent the potential for failure or difficulty with meeting the occupational goals; prevent occupational barriers; provide education • Occupational therapy practitioner provides education to caregivers, therapist, and school staff to help the team understand the barriers to occupational performance and intervention plan • Occupational therapy practitioner provides modeling of how to work with the child in a graded manner to reduce the potential for behavioral outbursts and to support occupational goals • Occupational therapy practitioner reviews interventions with parents in order to help identify other activities that will help the child develop buttoning skills over time • Encourage parents to have child participate in activities that encourage regular, active fine and gross motor movement (swimming, playground use)

- Collaboratively explore, identify, and plan ways to use sensory supports in order to fully participate in social and play activities with peers (small and large group considerations)
- Help parents, teachers, staff, and clients identify the warning signs that indicate when the child may be getting overwhelmed or triggered
- Identify a plan for how to cope when overwhelmed or when triggers occur
- Create a social story to help explore specific social scenarios and corresponding skills
- Role-play specific ways to be assertive in small or large social situations
- Attend a noncompetitive social activity with a group
- Co-create a daily or weekly schedule or routine board to help the child plan and follow the specific sequence of activities and expectations

Play and leisure participation are often referred to as *primary childhood occupations*. Occupational therapy practitioners use play and leisure activities to help work toward occupational and mental health goals, such as increased self-esteem and pro-social behaviors. Playgrounds, games, toys, and a host of other play and leisure activities are used in occupational therapy in order to help achieve client goals. The following list demonstrates examples of play activities that might be used to work on therapeutic goals with children of different ages. They include the following:

- 0 to 12 months: rattles, stuffed toys, play mats, manipulatives, mobiles, musical toys
- 1 to 3 years: blocks, books, Crayola Beginnings, dressing dolls, musical instruments, large-sized puzzles, tops, tricycle, sand and water play (Figure 5-2 illustrates a 2-year-old child coloring)
- 4 to 6 years: Coloring/drawing/cutting activities, charades for kids, dancing, LEGOs (The LEGO Group),

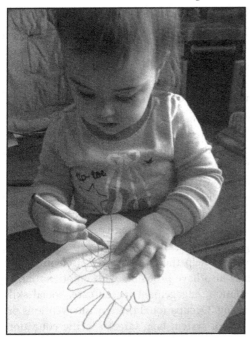

Figure 5-2. Coloring hand picture.

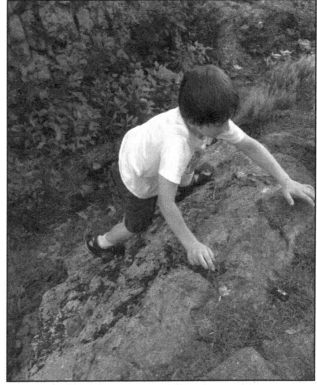

Figure 5-3. Climbing.

musical instruments, Play-Doh (Hasbro), puzzles, train set, sit and spin, soccer, swimming

- 7 to 12 years: Arts and crafts, biking, hiking (Figure 5-3), 3-dimensional puzzles, games (Ants in the Pants [Milton Bradley], Don't Break the Ice [Hasbro], Don't Spill the Beans [Hasbro], Hungry Hungry Hippos [Hasbro], I Spy games [Young Explorers], Operation [Hasbro], Perfection [Hasbro]), card games, K'NEX [K'NEX Industries Inc.], model building, pet care, skateboard, sports (baseball, basketball, gymnastics, soccer, skiing, swimming), skating, Wii (Nintendo) games

- 13 to 18 years: Arts and crafts, beading, games (Boggle [Hasbro], Twister [Hasbro]), card games, dance, fishing, knitting, painting, pet care, playing sports, riding a bike, Scrabble (Hasbro), sewing, skateboard, playing sports, and Wii games

IADLs include occupations that help individuals support themselves at home or in the community (e.g., home care, money management, child care). As children develop, it is important that they are increasingly able to complete IADLs in an age-appropriate manner in preparation for adulthood. Chore charts may be used to help parents recognize age-appropriate chores for young children through adolescence. For example, an occupational therapy assistant might work on having a latency-aged child help to set the table or put groceries away, whereas an adolescent may engage in meal preparation and cooking. Some of the occupational performance skills used when making a meal include the following:

- Motor skills: grasp, release, strength, and dexterity needed to open/close containers, bilateral coordination, postural control, and mobility

- Process skills: initiation, attention, organization of food and cooking equipment/utensils, and sequencing skills

- Communication/social skills: ability to ask for help and for items appropriately and as needed

When grading the intervention, the long-term goal for the adolescent might address the ability to prepare an entire meal. Occupational therapy practitioners could work with the client to progress toward this goal by assisting the adolescent to first plan and then make a simple snack. As meal preparation skills develop, additional and/or more complicated meals may be considered. Examples of graded skills and activities associated with a long-term goal of making a larger meal such as spaghetti dinner may include the following:

- Create a list of items needed to prepare the meal

- Shop for the items needed

- Organize the workstation

- Make the meal (with attention to safety, cleanliness, and detail)

- Serve and eat the meal

- Clean up

Occupational therapy practitioners help clients work on a variety of life skills such as meal preparation in both individual and group sessions.

Sleep and Rest

Getting enough sleep and rest throughout the early childhood and adolescent years is critical to health promotion. Occupational therapy practitioners are instrumental in helping to educate clients about the importance of sleep and rest. The ability to fall asleep, stay asleep, and have restful sleep is often difficult for clients with mental health–related symptoms and behaviors. Barriers to sleep and rest for children can include nightmares, problems with bladder and bowel control, difficulty with controlling worrying thoughts and fears, and symptoms related to mental health diagnoses such as hyperactivity, anxiety, and trauma triggers.

Although it is important to respect the diversity of each family's routines, common recommendations for promoting sleep include helping the client to do the following:

- Identify any barriers to falling or staying asleep (fears and worrying thoughts, discomfort, nightmares).

- Establish specific bedtime rituals and a routine (read a bedtime story, provide reminders and ample time prior to bedtime to wind down, avoid alerting activities prior to bedtime).

- Ensure the child feels and is safe.

- Identify ways to help the child relax and decrease environmental stimulation (use quiet and soothing music, dim lighting, reduce distractions in the home environment).

- Identify ways to help the child feel comfortable (nightlight, cotton sheets and pajamas with no seams, white noise to drown out sounds [fan, sound machine], ultra soft and/or weighted blanket).

- Teach child to be increasingly independent about sleep hygiene.

School

Children and adolescents with mental health–related challenges may become overwhelmed by school-based expectations and occupations. As a child ages, some activities may become increasingly difficult to navigate at school. They include the following:

- The ability to follow the school's pace and routine

- Cope with academic and learning challenges

- Concentrate and pay attention throughout the day

- Coordinate bodies to perform occupations efficiently (e.g., gym class, handwriting, self-care tasks)

- Understand social cues and norms

- Use organizational and sequencing skills

- Regulate emotions

- Cope with stress or trauma related to a variety of variables (e.g., sensory processing challenges, re-experiencing, hypervigilance, trauma triggers, and any other stressors and problems at school and home may be on the child's mind)

Children with mental health symptoms and behavioral problems that interfere with educational participation may receive occupational therapy services in school as part of the education plan. A child with attention deficit hyperactivity disorder (ADHD), for example, may benefit from occupational therapy services to help increase school performance and participation. The occupational therapy practitioner often helps identify strategies to increase self-organizational skills, to manage or decrease distractions, and to help the child stay focused in school. This child may also have problems with emotional and behavior regulation, engagement in self-care, social skills, and handwriting. Occupational therapy interventions provided in the school system help target specific educational and occupational goals that influence school performance and participation. Although there are a variety of ways to write goals, an example of a school-based occupational therapy goal may include the following, "The child will accurately and consistently copy assignments from the board independently in 3 to 5 minutes within 9 months." It is understood that in order to meet this educational goal, the child will need to be able to initiate and terminate the activity, remain attentive and on task, maintain postural control, modulate the amount of force used, and exhibit other fine motor dexterity and organizational skills necessary to complete the task in a consistent and timely manner.

The occupational therapy practitioner must also consider mental health needs when working with children who are experiencing barriers to participating in meaningful roles and occupations. Let's assume the aforementioned goal is for a child with ADHD, who is having difficulty with distractibility, impulsivity, attention span, and emotion regulation to the degree that it is negatively affecting the ability to complete his school work (school participation). Examples of some of the common sensory supportive and preparatory interventions often used with children with ADHD to assist with self-regulation include the following:

- Frequent movement breaks

- Fidget tools

- Pencil grips

- TheraBand (TheraBand Brand) around the legs of the chair

- Weighted/compression vest

- Organizational tools

- Environmental modifications/adaptations

Additional occupational therapy interventions may be used with the child as needed to help target postural control and fine motor skills necessary for legible handwriting. Interventions frequently used with children to support development of handwriting include molding clay or Play-Doh, cutting shapes, drawing with templates, sorting coins and putting them through slots, sewing, using tweezers or chopsticks to pick up and sort small items, lacing and building projects, arts and crafts, and computer and board games. These different activities help to promote hand strengthening, dexterity, and eye–hand coordination for the purpose of meeting this child's specific school-based occupational therapy goals. Social skills groups may be used to teach pro-social skills, including active listening and maintenance of personal space. Therapeutic groups also help children to develop emotion regulation skills, self-control, and the ability to follow directions.

In order to help address the regulatory, behavioral, and organizational challenges associated with ADHD, occupational therapy practitioners may provide recommendations to teachers, staff, and caregivers. According to the American Academy of Pediatrics (AAP) (2014), examples of common recommendations for use with children with ADHD in both school and home settings include the following:

- Provide clear, well-defined expectations, rules, and routines.

- Modify the environment to have reduced stimulation and distractions (not near high-traffic or busy areas [windows, walkways, doors]).

- Do not isolate or single out the child.

- Create a self-rating tool to chart areas of progress and further need; cue the child to use as needed.

- Encourage the child to use a graphic organizer; offer support for ongoing use and organization.

- Help break down goals, assignments, and instructions to smaller and more manageable steps; celebrate successes.

- Provide immediate rewards and consequences for behavior (emphasize effort made, as well as goals met).

- Emphasize and utilize positive behavioral rewards whenever possible.

- Identify and provide an opportunity for use of the child's preferred learning style (often multisensory approaches are helpful).

- Allow the child frequent movement breaks.

- Assist the child with maintaining an organized workspace and school bag.

- Integrate the use of sensory support tools.

- Closely supervise child with friends. Child may need help with learning appropriate social behavior.

- Use lists, reminders, and alarms (e.g., timer, watch, or phone alarms) to help with memory.

- Keep language positive.

- Ensure a healthy lifestyle: well-balanced diet, enough rest/sleep, and regular exercise (playground, gym, sports participation).

- Provide a supportive homework environment and use a homework schedule.

- Support engagement in activities facilitating pro-social skills: play dates or noncompetitive group activities (i.e., swimming, karate, dance, music, art groups or lessons).

- Promote what the child is good at by integrating participation in that activity into weekly routine.

- Limit choices.

- Use a calm approach to discipline: kind words, redirection when needed; talk with children about problematic behaviors when all are calm.

- Spend time with child doing activities that help promote mutual fun and bonding experiences and help the child to feel good about himself or herself.

Many of these recommendations are also used by occupational therapy practitioners working with children diagnosed with a variety of mental health conditions and learning disabilities, particularly when it is evident that organizational and behavioral supports are needed. As with all interventions, however, recommendations must be individualized to the specific needs and goals of the child and family.

Work

Work is an occupation that is typically targeted as an intervention when working with older children in the adolescent stage of development. Work capacities are acquired in a variety of ways, but prevocational skills are initially developed through participation in leisure and social activities. Such activities promote the acquisition of interpersonal skills, the ability to make and follow through on commitments, time management, and self-control. The ability to identify a job that is appropriate and then to acquire and maintain that job requires self-knowledge and a variety of occupational skills and capacities in order to be successful (Kielhofner, 2002). Occupational therapy practitioners help target the prevocational and vocational skills to help clients succeed at work-related goals. Some examples of therapeutic interventions used with adolescents include prevocational activities such as helping the youth with: identifying strengths and areas of volunteer or work interest; creating a resume; establishing or enhancing interview and social skills through role-play; identifying common work-related expectations; and completing, submitting, and following up on job applications. Occupational therapy services may also be used to help develop other occupational performance skills needed to obtain and maintain employment. Table 5-3 highlights childhood occupations, performance skills that may be used in each occupation, and examples of intervention goals.

The clinical vignette of Jacob in Spotlight 5-2 demonstrates how occupational therapy practitioners might engage with an adolescent when addressing work-related goals.

Trauma and Attachment-Informed Care

As discussed in Chapters 3 and 4, national initiatives have been underway since 2003 to help promote mental health and to transform the culture of mental health care settings to become recovery focused, trauma and attachment informed, and more nurturing and healing (United States Department of Health and Human Services [USDHHS], 2011, 2012, 2013). Trauma-informed care requires (1) the awareness that many clients in need of mental health care services have had some degree of trauma; (2) the understanding of the profound neurobiological, psychological, and social impact of trauma; and (3) the provision of care that recognizes and addresses trauma sequelae (NETI, 2009; USDHHS, 2013). An exhaustive review of the varied trauma and attachment-informed care interventions used across mental health settings is not the intent of this section. Some of the evidence-based and promising practices used by occupational therapy practitioners with children and families with trauma and attachment-related needs and goals are identified next.

One of the common approaches to trauma treatment includes a three-phase model. These three phases include (1) stabilization; (2) processing and grieving; and (3) reconnection, integration, and transformation (Luxenberg, Spinazzola, Hidalgo, Hunt, & van der Kolk, 2001). Part of the stabilization process is working with the client to ensure that the individual is feeling safe and is as stabilized as possible in order to begin to engage in other treatment services. This is not a linear model; this is evidenced when individuals begin the processing and grieving phase and they become destabilized and require the focus of treatment to go back to fostering stabilization. The process is much like a dance in that there can be a back and forth with these phases, or they may occur together during a session, and it is important to be aware of the complexity of this process in order to support the therapeutic process. Occupational therapy practitioners assist clients in identifying and using strategies to assist not only with the stabilization phase, but with the others as well. In addition to the three-phase model of trauma treatment, a component-based approach

has been promoted for use with children (Cooke et al., 2005). This approach includes an emphasis on the following general areas:

- Safety
- Skill building
- Positive attachment formation
- Meaning making
- Trauma processing
- Development of positive sense of self

Additionally, Levy and Orlans (1998) introduced three focal points of trauma-informed treatment: revisit, revise, and revitalize. *Revisit* refers to identifying the developmental level of the individual when the attachment and trauma-related experiences occurred in order to help identify any related symptoms, triggers, and subsequent developmental areas of need. *Revise* refers to the process of collaborating with the client to identify strengths, needs, and concerns (e.g., beliefs, strengths, attachment pattern, triggers, helpful coping strategies). *Revitalization* refers to the process of recognizing and celebrating skill development and positive change over time, while continuing to support hope, continued goal setting, and occupational participation (Champagne, 2011a; Levy & Orlans, 1998). Occupational therapy practitioners use these and other trauma and attachment-focused models to help identify ways to become more trauma informed in order to provide integrative services to clients with trauma and attachment-related needs and goals (Champagne 2011a, 2011b; LeBel & Champagne, 2010; Massachusetts Department of Mental Health [MA DMH], 2014). As clients engage in these different phases or work on any of the component areas reviewed, they may begin to feel more safe and organized; it is also possible, however, for people to become dissociative and to have flashbacks, intense memories, nightmares, and discomfort with feeling more self-aware (e.g., bodily sensations, thoughts, memories, intense emotions). When these vulnerable experiences occur, it is important to continue to assist individuals in a skilled and responsible manner, as it is often a significant part of the recovery process.

Attachment

As discussed in Chapter 4, when working with children with trauma and mental health–related barriers to health, wellness, and occupational participation, it is common to find that many of them have developed insecure **attachment** styles. For more information on attachment and attachment styles, refer back to Chapter 4. When a child or adolescent has developed an insecure attachment style, he or she may experience difficulty with self-awareness (including body awareness), emotion identification, and self-regulation, and many encounter problems with the ability to develop and maintain healthy relationships. A variety of deficits in occupational performance skills is

TABLE 5-3

CHILDHOOD OCCUPATIONS: OCCUPATIONAL BARRIERS AND GOAL EXAMPLES

AREAS OF OCCUPATION	OCCUPATIONAL BARRIERS	OCCUPATIONAL GOAL EXAMPLES
ADL: Sleep/Rest	Sequencing and problem-solving skills Organizational skills Time management Emotion regulation Sensory modulation	Child/youth will independently follow the bedtime routine and utilize sleep strategies 5 out of 7 days per week within 1 month.
ADL: Social	Self-expression and communication skills Impulse control Problem-solving skills Emotion regulation Sensorimotor skills	Child/youth will resolve conflicts with peers during sports activities with minimum assistance of one to two verbal cues within 2 weeks.
IADL: Home care	Memory Sequencing Attention span Emotion regulation Sensorimotor skills Time management	Child/youth will complete chores independently two times per week with minimum assistance of verbal cues.
Play: Safety	Sensorimotor skills: • Praxis • Bilateral coordination • Spatial relations Sensory modulation Emotion regulation Self-expression Social and communication skills	Child/youth will safely navigate playing on the playground without acquiring an injury, harming self or peers, in two out of three opportunities, with moderate assistance of verbal cues, within 4 weeks.
Education/Work	Sensorimotor skills: • Praxis • Bilateral coordination • Spatial relations • Visual-perceptual-motor skills Emotion regulation Attention span Social and communication skills	Child/youth will use a dynamic tripod grasp during homework in two out of three trials per week within 4 weeks.

SPOTLIGHT 5-2. CLINICAL VIGNETTE: JACOB

Jacob is 18 years old and will be graduating from high school in 1 year. He likes to read, is a hobbyist, goes to the gym two times per week, is skilled in using computers, and is interested in technology. He has made significant strides in understanding and managing his symptoms of bipolar disorder. Occupational barriers that were identified include the following:

- Continued difficulty with social skills and boundaries at times
- Difficulty coping with being told what to do/oppositionality (especially when spoken to in an authoritative tone)
- Difficulty with identifying work values, strengths, and interests
- Difficulty with grandiosity, irritability, and rapid speech patterns

His symptoms are currently fairly well managed. Jacob and his treatment team (providers) believe he is ready to start exploring work interests.

The Canadian Occupational Performance Measure (COPM) was used to help identify, summarize, and prioritize occupational performance strengths and barriers as part of the evaluation process. He is currently doing well with self-care and school performance. Jacob lives at home with his family and completes his chores regularly. The use of the COPM helped to identify the following occupational barriers to obtaining and maintaining a job:

- Although Jacob wants a "real job," he is concerned about the following:
  - His ability to continuously take orders from a boss
  - His ability to cope with coworker and customer attitudes in the workplace on an ongoing basis
  - His ability to continue to manage his symptoms in a manner that will support his physical, social, and emotional work performance
- Jacob wants to be able to develop positive work relationships, but has difficulty with self-confidence. He fears that people will become aware that he has bipolar disorder and the potential repercussions due to stigma.

Jacob's interventions take into consideration his person-environment-occupation–based performance strengths and needs using the Person-Environment-Occupation Model (Law et al., 1996). Jacob felt he needed the most assistance from occupational therapy with his ability to find, secure, and maintain a "real job." He also identified that he needed help with strengthening his ability to create and maintain work relationships. Some of the initial intervention recommendations included the following:

- Complete values clarification and work interest checklists.
- Help identify two to four different types of jobs and work environments that best match Jacob's interests, strengths, and needs.
- Of the positions identified, apply for and schedule interviews in order to secure a job that best matches Jacob's interests, strengths, and needs:
  - Complete job applications
  - Follow up on applications as needed
  - Schedule interview(s)
  - Plan for the interview and role-play
- After obtaining and starting a new job, complete the Work-Environment Impact scale (Moore-Corner, Kielhofner, & Olson, 1998) to help identify potential person-environment-occupation–related barriers in the workplace.
- Keep a work journal about his experiences, confidence level, work performance, social interactions, and environmental considerations. This will help to increase self-awareness, log and track progress, and identify areas to continue addressing in therapy.

(continued)

SPOTLIGHT 5-2. CLINICAL VIGNETTE: JACOB (CONTINUED)

- Use an app (e.g., Optimism [Optimism Apps Pty Ltd], My Mood [Aspyre Solutions Pty Ltd], or T2 Mood Tracker [The National Center for Telehealth and Technology]) to track how he is feeling to support the ability to manage symptoms and use of coping strategies.

- Practice pro-social behaviors in the community and work contexts.

- Identify and practice positive social skills and boundaries when at the gym and when visiting hobby shops and the local bookstore.

- Identify and practice positive social skills at work with his boss and co-workers.

- Monitor progress and modify interventions as needed over time.

A critical component to working with Jacob included ongoing support of his desire and motivation to get a job as part of his overall recovery process. Another critical component included helping to establish the "just right fit" with the person-environment-occupation elements in a manner that supported getting a job and increasing occupational performance fit and participation over time.

Although Jacob was able to meet his occupational goals over time, individuals are often not able to obtain and maintain competitive employment goals. In these instances, supported employment may be an option (Substance Abuse and Mental Health Services Administration [SAMHSA], 2014). If Jacob displayed less occupational readiness, some of the following interventions may have been suggested:

- A comprehensive vocational assessment

- Increased focus on stress and symptoms identification, self-awareness, and stress and symptoms management techniques

- Social skills group for older teens or young adults

- Join a club related to his hobbies or areas of work related to his interests

- Starting off with engaging in volunteer or part-time work opportunities in settings that would help Jacob practice specific skills

- Vocational rehabilitation referral

- Increased family support

- Identify and recommend attending a support group for teens/young adults with bipolar disorder

---

usually present in these individuals as well, which may have a negative impact on safety, health and wellness, and occupational participation. Within the attachment literature, it is recommended that practitioners assist clients and caregivers in developing a more secure attachment base, which helps to foster relationship formation, increased self-awareness and self-regulation skills, and other higher-order competencies (occupational performance and participation; Blaustein & Kinninburgh, 2010).

Helping a parent and child to become more attuned to each other and teaching them to play and have fun together (co-occupation) are often occupational therapy goals that help to foster a secure attachment base (Figure 5-4). *Co-occupation* is when two or more individuals are involved in an occupation together (Zemke & Clark, 1996). Another area of occupational therapy intervention is helping parents learn how they can co-create and utilize rituals and routines to promote feelings of safety and security in their children and family system. Structure

and consistency are critical elements across all contexts when working with children with attachment, trauma, and other mental health–related needs and goals (Blaustein & Kinniburgh, 2010; Champagne, 2011a, 2011b; Kinniburgh & Blaustein, 2005).

Specific therapeutic interventions used to help foster relational, self-regulation, and other developmental skills in children with an insecure attachment style (e.g., attachment disorders) are intervention areas targeted by occupational therapy practitioners. One example includes occupational therapy interventions based on sensory integration and processing frameworks, which are often used as trauma and attachment-informed treatment approaches to help foster engagement in meaningful roles, activities, and occupations (Ayres, 2005; Champagne, 2011a, 2011b; 2012; Williams & Shellenberger, 1994). Sensory-based approaches can be used during individual or group sessions to help foster some of the following:

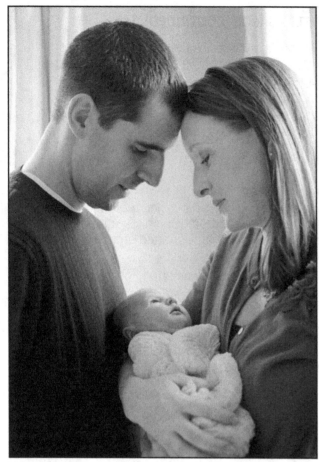

Figure 5-4. Parents with child.

- A sense of safety and stability
- The developmental process
- Organizational skills and emotion regulation
- A more coherent and positive sense of self
- The ability to have fun
- Self-nurturance and self-care
- Coping and social skills enhancement
- Trauma processing
- Occupational participation

Sensory-based approaches are part of the interventions promoted in trauma and attachment-informed mental health initiatives, due to the positive outcomes observed when offered in a skilled and individualized manner (MA DMH, 2014; NETI, 2009). Even equipment that is classically used when implementing an occupational therapy services using an ASI framework can be used to facilitate engagement in play-based, positive relational (attachment) occupations. Figure 5-5 illustrates an occupational therapist and another family member using a play activity with a young child to help foster a positive connection. This activity was

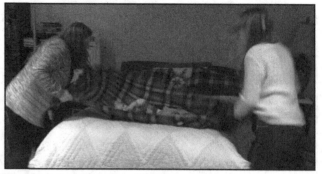

Figure 5-5. Parents playing with child.

used to promote feelings of safety, attachment, body and spatial awareness, and fun!

Interventions are used to foster a more secure attachment relationship when occupational therapy services focus on trauma and attachment-related needs and goals. Helping to enhance the attachment relationship provides a foundation from which higher-level social and relationship skills can develop.

A variety of attachment-based practice models are utilized by occupational therapy practitioners when working with clients and families with attachment-related needs and goals. These models help occupational therapy practitioners by providing the clinical rationale and resources needed to enhance the occupational therapy evaluation and intervention processes. Some attachment theorists have even integrated occupational therapy–related interventions within their frameworks, such as the Attachment, Self-Regulation, and Competency (ARC) framework (Blaustein & Kinninburgh, 2010). The ARC framework is intended to be used with children and families who have experienced multiple or prolonged traumatic stress. The ARC framework includes three fundamental domains targeted during the intervention process to help foster the relational process:

1. Attachment: developing a safe caregiving system (trauma informed) that supports the child's developmental, emotional, and relational needs

2. Self-regulation: developing the ability to regulate and tolerate one's experiences

3. Competency: nurturing and supporting developmental capacities and resiliency

Table 5-4 outlines the three primary domains of ARC, broken down into 10 building blocks for intervention (Blaustein & Kinninburgh, 2010).

Later in this chapter, the clinical vignette of Karly and her foster parent, Joan, demonstrates how the ARC model is used in combination with ASI as part of occupational therapy services.

Attachment-Based Family Therapy (ABFT) is another model that has been identified as promising; it is used to

TABLE 5-4
ATTACHMENT, SELF-REGULATION, AND COMPETENCY FRAMEWORK: 10 BUILDING BLOCKS
1. **Caregiver attunement:** Provide support and education to the caregiver to foster the ability to recognize and attend to his or her own emotional responses and needs
2. **Attunement:** Loving, empathic, and attentive responses; use of active listening
3. **Consistent responses:** Timely and reliable caregiver responses
4. **Routines and rituals:** Increase feelings of safety and predictability through routines and rituals
5. **Affect identification:** Foster self-awareness of one's emotions and of what influences different types of changes in emotional states
6. **Affect modulation:** Help identify safe and effective strategies to help manage emotional experiences and different degrees of autonomic nervous system arousal
7. **Affect expression:** Assist in developing the ability to express emotions effectively
8. **Developmental tasks:** Foster the child's ability to meet developmental milestones
9. **Executive functions:** Support the use of problem-solving skills, the ability to make healthy choices, and the ability to control one's impulses
10. **Self-development and identity:** Foster the development of a coherent, positive, and future-oriented sense of self

help repair the parent–child relationship and build competence (Diamond et al., 2010). The ABFT approach can be used with children and families across age ranges. For instance, therapeutic sessions with adolescents can foster the adolescent's identity, autonomy, and attachment style, while parents work on developing their own attachment capacities and enhancing their parenting skills and personal supports. When both parties are ready, family therapy sessions are used to identify and resolve both past and existing problems, and to practice new *emotion regulation* and interpersonal effectiveness skills. As trust develops and developmental competencies grow, therapy shifts to focus on supporting the adolescent's continued self-management and interpersonal competencies and vocational and educational goals.

Other trauma and attachment models that are being used to inform the occupational therapy evaluation and intervention processes include some of the following:

- Neurosequential Model of Therapeutics (Perry & Hambrick, 2008)
- Dyadic Developmental Psychotherapy (Hughes, 2006)
- Somatic Experiencing (Levine, 2014)

These and other models can be used in combination with occupational therapy theories and frames of reference, as appropriate and with proper training. In some instances, occupational therapy practitioners have worked with professionals from other disciplines to create or enhance existing psychotherapeutic models. An example of this collaboration is the SAFE PLACE Model by Daniel Hughes and Jane Koomar (2010). The SAFE PLACE Model combines elements from Hughes' (2006) Dyadic Developmental Psychotherapy model and ASI (Ayres, 2005).

In addition to working with children and families who have attachment-related needs and goals, occupational therapy practitioners may work with teenage parents. Working with teenage parents promotes mental health for both the parent and child.

Coren and Barlow (2001) revealed that parenting programs for adolescent mothers and their young children have achieved a variety of positive outcomes in the following areas:

- Enhanced mother–infant interaction
- Increased parental knowledge and attitudes
- Improved maternal self-confidence
- Enhanced maternal identity

Positive Parenting, Discipline, and Learning Models

Occupational therapy practitioners teach positive parenting and discipline techniques in order to assist parents to provide clear, consistent, and supportive rules and boundaries. General recommendations for positive parenting approaches include the following:

- Model self-care, self-regulation, positivity, and proactive behaviors.

- Focus on and reward the child's strengths and positive behaviors.

- Validate the child's feelings.

- Help the child problem solve, but do not do it for him or her.

- Help the child engage in self-care activities (e.g., sleep hygiene, taking care of one's body).

- Help the child engage in and practice self-regulation strategies.

- Reward for positive behaviors.

- Help the child learn how to identify and face fears.

- Tell the child that it is okay to be different and impossible to be "perfect."

A gentle or moderate form of correction is often necessary when disruptive behaviors emerge. A strong correction, however, in the form of the use of an authoritative stance with firm limit setting is sometimes needed when a child's behavior is escalating or there are safety concerns (Davidson, 2005). For more specific recommendations on positive parenting for each of the different stages of development (infant through age 17), refer to the Centers for Disease Control and Prevention (CDC) website (CDC, 2014a). The CDC also has a Web page devoted to how to raise safe and healthy kids (CDC, 2014b). More resources to assist parents in developing a positive parenting style include 1, 2, 3, Magic (Phelan, 2010), Collaborative and Proactive Solutions (Greene, 2014), and a host of free resources available on the Child Welfare League of America (CWLA) and the AAP websites.

The Positive Parenting Program (also known as Triple P) is an example of an evidence-informed, promising practice that provides adults with tools to help manage stress, problem behaviors (e.g., tantrums, aggression, anxiety, hyperactivity, and disobedience), and other family concerns (de Graaf, Speetjens, Smit, de Wolff, & Tavecchio, 2008). One of the primary goals of the Triple P program is to prevent severe emotional and behavioral problems in children by fostering nurturing and positive relational supports and enhancing parenting competence and confidence. The five steps that are considered the key to the Triple P program include the following:

1. Create an interesting and safe environment

2. Have a positive learning environment

3. Use assertive discipline

4. Have realistic expectations

5. Take care of yourself as a parent

Why is it important to be aware of attachment, positive parenting, and discipline models and approaches? When working with children and adolescents, occupational therapy practitioners also work with families, caregivers, teachers, mental health staff, and other providers. Occupational therapy practitioners help advocate for clients and families and often provide education and modeling for how to interact and work with children and families in a variety of contexts. Occupational therapy practitioners may also introduce environmental modifications, sensory supportive tools, adaptive equipment, and other forms of assistive technology as part of the occupational therapy process.

In addition to parent and caregiver education, occupational therapy practitioners often provide education to staff who work with children and adolescents with emotional and behavioral problems. Educational topics may include behavioral symptoms associated with problems in sensory processing, how to increase a child's body awareness, and how to help children and adolescents develop emotion regulation skills in order to meet safety and occupational goals. Occupational therapy practitioners also help staff understand the therapeutic use of self when working with children. Techniques that are often reviewed include the following:

- Modeling appropriate behavior and a calm affect

- Altering the environment

- Redirecting

- Cuing appropriate behavior

- Discussing and modeling the use of alternatives/skills

- Providing reassurance

- Providing validation

- Providing explanations

- Helping the child sequence through activities

- Demonstrating kindness and assertiveness skills

- Making healthy choices

The manner in which adults talk to and teach children about feelings, skill development and utilization, and problem solving directly affects the child's ability to understand, express and regulate emotions, and use skills (CWLA, 2014; National Center for Learning Disabilities [NCLD], 2014). Occupational therapy practitioners often assist caregivers and staff to understand the variables that underlie emotion regulation and to provide services that directly assist in this process. Some additional examples of interventions that can be used when working with children who demonstrate aggressive behaviors include the following:

- Help the child identify his or her triggers and warning signs.

- Help the child identify helpful strategies, and have these strategies readily available (e.g., self-soothing and distraction techniques).

- Be clear about what is appropriate, what is not, and what the consequences will be if aggressive behaviors occur.

- Model the behavior you would like to see and do not overreact.
- Limit the amount of violent and aggressive behavior to which the child is exposed (e.g., video games, music, television, movies).
- Provide opportunities for active movement and stretching throughout the day.
- Provide opportunities for children to release their emotions in ways that do not harm others.
- Provide reassurance and redirection as needed.

Sensory approaches have also been utilized for prevention purposes and de-escalation purposes in order to help reduce the use of violent and traumatic interventions such as seclusion and restraint (Champagne, 2011b; Champagne & Stromberg, 2004; LeBel & Champagne, 2010; MA DMH, 2014; NETI, 2009).

In this era of evidence-based practice, it is important to be aware that evidence-based approaches currently exist (CWLA, 2014; NCLD, 2014) and are being used in mental health and educational settings to help support the development of emotional literacy and pro-social behaviors. Emotional literacy is the ability to identify, understand, and manage one's own emotions; develop empathic social awareness and pro-social behaviors; and manage challenging situations with self-control (Goleman, 1996). Social and emotional learning (SEL) is an evidence-based program that is used to enhance emotional literacy. Some examples of interventions used in the SEL model include adult role modeling; expressing emotions; labeling a child's feelings; and playing games, singing songs, and reading stories with new feeling words (Durlak et al., 2011). The SEL model uses a student-centered approach that is strength based. This approach helps to build core competencies in students using academic methods that are developmentally and culturally sensitive (Bradshaw, Bottani, Osher, & Sugai, 2014).

Positive behavioral supports (PBS) is an evidence-based approach that uses functional behavior assessment in an effort to replace challenging behaviors with pro-social skills within school systems (Horner, Sugai, & Anderson, 2010; Sugai et al., 2000). The PBS program is used to address the needs of individual students as well as the entire school body and facility (i.e., the physical environment, activity demands, instructional pace, general behavioral reinforcement, and curriculum design). The PBIS model is used by school administrators, teachers, and staff to make changes to the school's organizational structure. Examples of such changes include enhancing or eliminating existing systems and procedures, and using outcome data to guide future decisions related to academic performance and behavioral performance within the student body.

Bradshaw et al. (2014) explain that, although both the PBS and SEL models aim to promote positive, pro-social behavior and academic achievement, they differ in very fundamental ways. Occupational therapy practitioners must understand how these evidence-based models are currently being used with children with mental health and behavioral challenges and explore how they can be integrated with occupational therapy frames of reference to support the best possible outcomes for students. For example, schools incorporating PBS and SEL may benefit from integrating the use of sensory-based and other occupational therapy interventions with these models.

Sensory Processing, Coping, and Social Skills Interventions

The application of sensory-processing approaches is increasing in mental health and educational settings. Including a sensory-processing lens helps to provide a more developmental, humanistic, and public health approach to trauma and attachment-informed care in order to help support people with mental health, behavioral, and occupational participation challenges in achieving recovery goals (NETI, 2009). Further, whether or not an individual has problems with sensory processing, sensory modulation-focused approaches are often useful to everyone in the promotion of mental health, wellness and for stress management purposes (Champagne, 2011b). Occupational therapy practitioners are viewed as instrumental to the ability to safely and responsibly implement the use of sensory approaches in mental health practice, given that sensory-processing knowledge is more within the occupational therapy scope of practice than most other disciplines working in mental health settings.

Sensory Processing

Sensory-processing patterns have been recently classified as sensory modulation, sensory discrimination, and sensory-based motor abilities (Bundy, Lane & Murray, 2002; Miller & Lane, 2000). Problems with sensory modulation are regulatory in nature and include sensory overresponsivity and underresponsivity to stimuli (neurological threshold continuum), which may be evidenced and observed behaviorally (e.g., active and passive strategies to regulate) (Brown & Dunn, 2002; Dunn, 1999; Miller & Lane, 2000). Problems with sensory discrimination—the ability to perceive or detect stimuli in a manner that supports safety, self-regulation, and occupational participation—may occur in any one or multiple sensory systems. Sensory discrimination skills significantly support a variety of client factors, occupational performance skills, and occupational participation. Problems with sensory-based motor abilities can affect postural control and praxis skills (dyspraxia). For more information on sensory processing, refer to Chapter 4. Table 5-5 demonstrates areas of occupational performance that may be affected by having a sensory processing problem such as dyspraxia. Corresponding interventions are also presented that may be helpful when working with children with dyspraxia in schools or residential programs.

Sensory modulation is the regulatory component of sensory processing. Sensory modulation approaches are strategies used to calm, alert, and organize the nervous system; they may be used by anyone, whether there are problems with sensory processing or not. Sensory modulation tools can be used to specifically enhance one's stress management and coping skills repertoire and for general health and wellness purposes. When a person has difficulty with sensory modulation, it is often helpful to assist the client in becoming more self-aware and to identify additional strategies to help cope with and potentially change sensory-related discomforts, challenges, and occupational barriers.

Sensory approaches may be used with individuals or applied programmatically across different settings (e.g., home, educational, hospital, mental health, and forensic settings). Sensory modulation–related interventions are often taught by occupational therapy practitioners to interdisciplinary staff in order to help institute and help follow through with the skilled and responsible use of sensory modulation–related approaches across mental health and educational settings. Resources created by occupational therapy practitioners are available that help to operationalize the use of sensory modulation–related approaches on both individual and programmatic scales. Two of these programs are the Sensory Modulation Program (SMP) (Champagne, 2011a, 2011b, 2012) and *How Does Your Engine Run?* (Williams & Shellenberger, 1994). The SMP may be adapted for use with clients across a variety of age ranges, and the general components include the following:

- Therapeutic use of self
- Sensory diet (e.g., sensory-supportive routines infused with sensory strategies and tools)
- Sensorimotor activities and occupations
- Sensory modalities (e.g., weighted items, sound therapy programs, clinical aromatherapy)
- Environmental modifications (e.g., home modifications, sensory rooms, sensory gardens, environmental enhancements)
- Caregiver education

A sensory diet is a daily routine that strategically includes sensory-supportive prevention and de-escalation strategies that is created and used to help target the child's and family's specific needs and goals (Wilbarger, 1995). Sensory diets may also be created and implemented programmatically (strategic plan of interventions worked into the program or classroom routine). After the evaluation process, if the client and family are interested in including sensory approaches as part of the occupational therapy intervention planning and implementation process, the specific needs of the client are reviewed, goals are collaboratively established, and interventions that will help meet the occupational needs and goals of the client are identified. The process often begins with helping clients and caregivers with increasing self-awareness, identifying sensory-related and other resources that may be helpful, and often includes the creation and implementation of a home program (e.g., sensory diet) in addition to occupational therapy sessions (e.g., individual, group).

The SMP provides a variety of resources to help implement individual and group sessions for children through adult populations (Champagne, 2011a, 2011b, 2012). For instance, with the SMP groups for children and adolescents, a variety of activities is individualized for the group participants, but a general format is used to target some of the following areas to help support occupational performance and participation: emotion identification and regulation activities, the creation and use of self-rating tools, sensorimotor exploration and challenges, sensory modulation tools and kits, and social skills education and practice (e.g., role-play).

The *How Does Your Engine Run?* program also provides a host of intervention resources to help occupational therapy practitioners implement sensory strategies as part of the occupational therapy process (Williams & Shellenberger, 1994). Other occupational therapy resources providing information and tools that can be used during individual and group sessions include the following:

- BrainWorks (Wild, 2014)
- SticKids (Community Therapy Associates, 2014)
- Modulation Modes (Champagne, 2011b)
- Zones of Regulation (Kuypers, 2011)
- *The Tool Chest: For Teachers, Parents, and Students* (Henry, 2001)

In addition to sensory modulation strategies, other techniques—including narrative therapy, social and sensory stories, and other sensory-supportive interventions (e.g., expressive arts, animal-assisted therapies, and complementary therapies)—are used to help increase self-awareness and self-esteem and to promote a positive self-narrative. The DIR Floortime Model (developmental, individual differences, relationship-based) is a therapeutic program used by occupational therapy practitioners, as well as other professionals who have obtained additional training in the intervention (Greenspan & Wieder, 2006). Central to the DIR Floortime Model is a focus on the client's emotions, interests, and relationships and the impact on providing graded learning opportunities to build upon higher-level skills such as emotional, relational, and intellectual capabilities. When occupational therapy practitioners are on interdisciplinary teams implementing DIR Floortime, sensory approaches are part of the occupational therapy focus provided, when applicable.

When addressing the full complement of sensory-processing skills (modulation, discrimination, and motor skills), rehabilitation professionals (occupational therapy, physical therapy, and speech and language pathologist) have the educational background necessary to target all

TABLE 5-5

DYSPRAXIA: COMMON CHALLENGES AND INTERVENTIONS FOR SUPPORTING PERFORMANCE AND PARTICIPATION IN SCHOOL AND RESIDENTIAL SETTINGS

DYSPRAXIA: COMMON CHALLENGES	SCHOOL AND RESIDENTIAL CHALLENGES	SCHOOL AND RESIDENTIAL SUPPORTS
Gross motor coordination Difficulty with: • Maintaining bodily boundaries • Performing coordinated motor movements (hopping, jumping, skipping, catching, kicking objects, jumping jacks) • Walking in a straight line • Bumping into things/people • Clumsiness	May have difficulty with: • Transitioning between classes • Gym class performance • Self-care and dressing performance (zipping coat, fastening pants after toileting, tying shoes) • Getting into and standing in lines • Playing games with peers on the playground or at the residence (sports, hopscotch, jump rope) • Using playground equipment • Riding a bike, scooter, or skateboard	• Use a graded approach and encouragement to assist with participation in daily activities that foster daily, active, full-body movement (playground use, Wii games, swimming). • Use a noncompetitive approach and foster an inclusive/supportive learning atmosphere. • Remind/help prepare the body for action (e.g., cue to put hands out to catch ball; postural cues; engage in activities that are rich in proprioceptive and deep touch pressure input). • Provide visual cues to help understand how to position the body when needed (e.g., pictures and/or demonstration of yoga poses). • Use hand-over-hand assistance when needed. • Provide assistance to use playground equipment and sensorimotor-related activities at the residence. • Provide reassurance and positive reinforcement as appropriate.
Fine motor coordination Difficulty with: • Fine motor coordination and dexterity (e.g., use of hands) • Eye–hand coordination • Bilateral coordination • Difficulty with modulating the amount of force to use (e.g., may not use enough force to open containers, or may accidentally break things by being too rough)	May have difficulty with: • Using writing, cutting, and art-related tools (pencil, scissors) • Handwriting, drawing, coloring • Arts/crafts performance • Using utensils at mealtimes (knife and fork) • Opening containers (milk carton, paint) • Using fasteners, dressing (zipping coat or pants) • Copying (from board, when trying to draw or write)	• Practice the use of utensils, opening containers, and the use of fasteners in a graded manner. • Play games that require the use of fine motor skills and the modulation of force (e.g., Operation, Don't Break the Ice, Ants in the Pants, Barrel of Monkeys [Milton Bradley]). • Play with items and activities that promote fine motor coordination (e.g., LEGOs, cat's cradle, use of stress balls, Play-Doh, clay, crafts, cooking/baking). • Provide pencil grips, triangular-shaped writing utensils, vibrating writing utensils. • Provide Velcro fasteners when appropriate. • Provide multisensory fine motor and tactile supports (e.g., raised line paper, sandpaper letters to learn letter formation, different textured fine motor manipulatives). • Provide reassurance and positive reinforcement.

(continued)

TABLE 5-5 (CONTINUED)		
DYSPRAXIA: COMMON CHALLENGES AND INTERVENTIONS FOR SUPPORTING PERFORMANCE AND PARTICIPATION IN SCHOOL AND RESIDENTIAL SETTINGS		
DYSPRAXIA: COMMON CHALLENGES	**SCHOOL AND RESIDENTIAL CHALLENGES**	**SCHOOL AND RESIDENTIAL SUPPORTS**
Spatial relationships Difficulty with: • Bodily orientation/ body map • Directionality (over, under, in, out, behind) • Concepts of time • Understanding and following directions related to spatial relationships	May have difficulty with: • Staying in own seat • Understanding the schedule (difficulty understanding and being oriented to the schedule) • Maintaining personal boundaries (bumping into others, difficulty with the awareness of personal space) • Writing letters and sentences • Performing gym activities • Using playground or sports equipment • Following verbal directions to complete motor tasks (writing, art work, gym activities)	• Play games or use sing-a-longs that teach space and time concepts/orientation (e.g., If you're happy and you know it, Simon says, create and go through obstacle courses, Wii games). • Use of timers, alarms, visual schedule, checklists to sequence through activities/expectations (e.g., watch alarm, liquid or visual timer, daily schedule/routine checklist). • Use visual cues for boundary awareness and to foster awareness of bodily boundaries (e.g., marking boundaries with visual cues [color code], use of chairs with arms, carpet squares, or individual bean bag or rocking chairs). • Use activities and equipment that help to increase body awareness (e.g., those that provide increased proprioception and deep touch pressure). • Provide reassurance and positive reinforcement.
Attention/concentration Difficulty with: • Staying alert • Getting and staying focused • Sticking to one task at a time until completed • Processing multistep directions or large amounts of information at a time • Transitions	May have difficulty with: • Following the staff's or teacher's instructions • Staying on task • Finishing school work and homework • Processing all of the directions provided • Having a fragmented understanding of information being taught • Performing timed tests or other time-related expectations (e.g., transitions)	• Be sure to get the attention of the child before giving instructions. • Use concrete/simple language. • Allow extra time to process information. • Help the child get started on tasks and provide cues for sequencing and follow through as needed (e.g., visual checklists, verbal cues). • Reduce distractions. • Avoid interruptions when on task. • Allow/provide an area to take space when overwhelmed. • Provide reassurance and positive reinforcement.

(continued)

Table 5-5 (continued)		
Dyspraxia: Common Challenges and Interventions for Supporting Performance and Participation in School and Residential Settings		
DYSPRAXIA: COMMON CHALLENGES	**SCHOOL AND RESIDENTIAL CHALLENGES**	**SCHOOL AND RESIDENTIAL SUPPORTS**
Communication and social-emotional skills Difficulty with: • Self-expression (e.g., asking for or explaining needs, answering questions, explaining what happened) • Needing extra time to communicate (wants, concerns, feelings) • Recognizing and understanding social norms • Frustration tolerance, anxiety, and depression • Self-esteem due to multitude of challenges • Judging how to behave in social situations • Forming and maintaining friendships • Impulse control	May have difficulty with: • Answering the staff, teacher, or peers when questioned • Responding in a timely manner (needs extra time) • Making and keeping friends • Initiating when confused or needs help from teacher or peers • Poor awareness and maintenance of social and physical boundaries with staff, teachers, and peers	• Use closed rather than open-ended questions. • Use visual supports to help remember and explain personal experiences (e.g., social stories, sensory stories, feelings pictures). • Engage in role playing. • Teach concrete social skills. • Teach emotion identification and regulation skills. • Use simple self-rating scales. • Identify coping strategies and ensure access in the school environment. • Anticipate areas/situations that may be challenging and provide prompts to help use coping skills. • Provide counseling support as needed. • Offer reassurance and use a positive behavioral reward system. • Use clear, concrete rules, consequences, and reminders.

aspects of sensory processing within their scope of practice. It is recommended, however, that additional training be obtained for development of more advanced clinical reasoning and practice skills. Occupational therapy practitioners must recognize the specific sensory-processing strengths and needs of the clients with whom they work in order to provide interventions and recommendations that will support positive outcomes. When targeting all areas of sensory processing as part of occupational therapy practice, ASI is an occupational therapy frame of reference used by occupational therapy practitioners to help guide their learning and clinical practice. A systematic review conducted by May-Benson and Koomar (2010) suggested that the skilled use of the ASI approach may result in positive outcomes

in sensorimotor skills and motor planning; socialization, attention, and behavioral regulation; reading-related skills; participation in active play; and achievement of individualized goals. In a recent randomized, controlled research study, the use of ASI was reported to be a promising intervention for people with autism spectrum disorder (Schaaf, Benevides, Maillouz, Faller, Hunt, van Hooydonk, et al., 2013). For more information on the variables indicating fidelity to ASI, refer to Chapter 4.

Children with trauma histories who exhibit insecure attachment styles and mental health symptoms and behaviors often have a combination of developmental challenges (Checkpoints 5-3 and 5-4). The clinical vignette in Spotlight 5-3 builds upon the evaluation of Karly and Joan

---

CHECKPOINT 5-3. ANALYZE

Refer back to the discussion of mental health diagnoses and their symptoms found in Chapter 4. Analyze how the symptoms associated with autism spectrum disorder, attention deficit activity disorders, and mood disorders might affect sensorimotor, cognitive, and communication skills.

CHECKPOINT 5-4. EVALUATE

Review your responses from Checkpoint 5-3. Now evaluate them, based on the new information discussed in the paragraphs earlier. What tasks, if any, were missing from your analysis?

---

presented in Chapter 4 and illustrates the use of a combination of trauma, attachment, and sensory-based frameworks as part of the occupational therapy intervention process.

Coping, Stress Management, and Relaxation Skills

Occupational therapy practitioners work with children, adolescents, and their families to enhance coping and stress management skills across a variety of settings. In addition to sensory approaches, a variety of other strategies are used to help teach stress management and coping skills. Stress management and coping skills can help people become more self-aware, prevent and reduce symptoms of stress, increase self-control, and further develop resiliency (Kraag, Zeegers, Kok, Hosman, & Abu-Saad, 2006). *Relaxation techniques* are often considered coping and stress management interventions because they are used to help interrupt and decrease the stress response. Relaxation techniques include a wide range of therapeutic strategies that are also used to self-calm, self-soothe, improve mood, and increase one's mind–body and reality orientation (Alvord & Grados, 2005). Some examples of common relaxation techniques that may be modified for use with children and people of all ages include the following:

- *Deep breathing:* There are many different types of deep breathing exercises. Some of these techniques used with children may include blowing bubbles, use of a contest to see who can exhale the longest with each breath to promote deeper breaths, deep belly breathing, and others.

- *Progressive muscle relaxation:* Requires focusing on a specific part of the body in sequence, alternately tensing and then relaxing each part (e.g., face, jaw, shoulders, arms, hands, stomach, back, legs, feet).

- *Visualization* (also known as *guided imagery*): Use of one's imagination to focus on and mindfully experience pleasant thoughts and experiences, such as a favorite activity; a safe place; an appealing sound, taste, or aroma; eating a favorite food; a feeling of warmth from the sunshine on your face; etc. The use of a voice, picture, music, story, or other media can help "guide" the visualization experience.

- *Mindfulness or meditation:* Helps to decrease the stress response and ground and center the mind and body. It is often helpful to use a sensory cue as part of mindfulness practice to help children with difficulty with attention, concentration, and behavioral problems (e.g., focus on a specific sensory aspect of a tactile manipulative, the musical instruments playing while listening to a song, guess the sounds presented using a sound machine or between different scents using essential oils, the feeling of one's muscles during an isometric exercise).

- *Exercise and stretching:* Helps to decrease stress, improve mood, strengthen, and release tension in the body (e.g., yoga, dance, walks, hikes, sports, karate, Brain Gym exercises).

- *Humor or laughter:* Helps by serving as a significant stress and tension reliever.

- *Listening to music or playing an instrument:* Helps to relieve stress, improve focus, and improve mood.

- *Cuddling:* It is often helpful to cuddle with a loved one, a pet, a favorite blanket, or even a stuffed animal.

- *Sensory tools:* Help to foster feelings of safety and security; to become more self-aware, modulate emotions, and be more in control of feelings and behaviors.

- *Biofeedback:* The use of physiological measures (e.g., heart rate, blood pressure, electroencephalograph monitoring) while using a specific intervention (e.g., deep breathing) to demonstrate the physiological impact. Used to help teach the mind–body connection and the ability to change its patterns (e.g., stress, anxiety, inattention).

There are many examples of creative ways to use these and other relaxation techniques with children; these resources can be found on the Internet and in publications on relaxation, stress management, mindfulness practices, and coping techniques.

The ability to use strategies to cope with stressors and to support the ability to self-regulate, which includes the ability to calm and relax, as well as uplift when needed (sensory modulation), is considered a prevention approach

SPOTLIGHT 5-3. CLINICAL VIGNETTE: KARLY AND JOAN

Karly is 4 years, 7 months old and lives with a very caring and dedicated foster family. She was removed from her biological parents' home at age 3 because she had experienced repeated, severe, and multiple forms of trauma. She attended preschool, but due to the severity of her symptoms and behaviors, she had sporadic attendance. She was referred to outpatient occupational therapy services by her pediatrician and social worker, who reported that Karly was having difficulty with stabilizing her trauma-based symptoms and concerns that she had additional sensory processing–related challenges that limited her ability to engage in daily activities and routines. Karly was unable to go into the community with her foster family without tantrums (e.g., restaurants, birthday parties, shopping malls, grocery stores), and her foster parents had difficulty helping her participate in a variety of activities (bathing, dressing, brushing her teeth, playing). She had numerous trauma triggers and had been having nightmares about "monsters" trying to get her.

Some of Karly's strengths include that she is affectionate, is curious, has a strong attachment to her foster mother, and enjoys a variety of activities, such as, singing, listening to music (e.g., nursery rhymes), swinging on swings, playing at the park, a variety of gross motor play activities (e.g., climbing, running), and loves animals. Her praxis skills are also developmentally appropriate for her age range. She tends to avoid fine motor–related play activities (e.g., coloring, crafts, games that require fine motor skills).

From her medical history, her diagnoses include failure to thrive, microcephaly, fetal alcohol syndrome, post-traumatic stress disorder, and reactive attachment disorder.

Primary concerns at this time: problems with emotion and self-regulation; very short attention span; sensory overresponsivities that negatively affect ADLs rest, sleep, school, and social participation; sensory-seeking behaviors affecting home, school, and social participation (use of too much force, need for constant movement), poor body awareness (clumsy, poor awareness of physical boundaries); difficulty with fine motor skills; oppositional behaviors; tantrums with transitions, especially in moderate-to-high stimulus environments (stores, restaurants, birthday parties); and tantrums when her foster mother is not within view.

Taken from Chapter 4, the following were identified (in collaboration with Karly's foster mother) as occupational barriers that negatively affected safety and occupational participation (based upon the evaluation process):

- Trauma and attachment related:
  - Significant separation anxiety
  - Hypervigilance
  - Very short attention span (>1 minute)
  - Significant difficulty with sleep and nightmares
  - Significant difficulty with emotion regulation
  - Triggered by certain activities, places (bathing/bathroom, bed/bedroom)
  - Violent outbursts/behaviors toward self, caregivers, and others
- Sensorimotor processing related:
  - Difficulty with sustained sitting (postural control)
  - Difficulty with gravitational awareness (affecting safety awareness)
  - Poor spatial and body awareness
  - Low muscle tone (extensor muscles)
  - Difficulty with fine motor control and precision
  - Difficulty with transitions
- Tactile, oral, and sound sensory overresponsivity:
  - Difficulty tolerating clothing
  - Difficulty with hair brushing, face washing, nail clipping
  - Very picky eater

(continued)

SPOTLIGHT 5-3. CLINICAL VIGNETTE: KARLY AND JOAN (CONTINUED)

- ○ Difficulty with moderate and high stimulus environments (stores, restaurants, lunch room at school)
- ○ Startles easily
- Proprioception, vestibular, and tactile (deep pressure) sensory underresponsivity:
  - ○ Constantly seeking out movement (e.g., spinning, running)
  - ○ Seeks out self-initiated deep touch pressure (e.g., weighted blanket use, hugs)

In the Clinic

The occupational therapy practitioners working with Karly and her foster mother employed the use of the Attachment, Regulation, and Competency (ARC) model and Ayres' Sensory Integration (ASI) to begin the therapeutic intervention process.

The ARC Model

The ARC model requires the central participation of Karly and her foster mother in the intervention process to continue to develop and build upon their attachment relationship, which will also support the development of self-regulatory and other developmental capacities over time. Enhancing these developmental skills will help support occupational performance and participation. The ARC model also requires working directly with the primary caregiver(s) and Karly in sessions to help her foster parent(s) understand more about the impact of her trauma history and attachment needs on her safety concerns and occupational needs and goals. In addition, the centrality of the identification and use of co-occupations to foster the attachment process (to support attachment and self-regulatory capacities), as well as Karly's other occupational performance goals, is a primary focus of each session.

The occupational therapy practitioners demonstrated in sessions (through modeling) different ways to engage with Karly when she was struggling in session (e.g., with anxiety, safety, and behavioral challenges) and how to foster occupational participation. Karly's foster mother was encouraged to actively participate in the therapy sessions, and reassurance was used to help her gain confidence and increase knowledge in her parenting skills. The occupational therapist and the occupational therapy assistant worked with both Karly and her foster mother to provide education, modeling, and a therapeutic environment that was nonjudgmental, empathic, nonconfrontational, and fun.

ASI Model

The use of a sensory integration–style occupational therapy gym space was used during most of the initial occupational therapy sessions. This therapeutic gym space provided a safe, sensory-rich, and fun play space to use with Karly and her foster mother in a client-driven manner. The creative use of suspended swings, hammocks (e.g., cuddle swing), climbing equipment, and the ball pit are some examples of Karly's favorite play equipment and activities when she initially began occupational therapy services. Her foster mother was centrally included (through co-occupation) during sessions in the sensory integration gym space. The ability to engage in self-initiated play activities that offered the intensity of proprioceptive, tactile, and vestibular stimulation she needed helped Karly to have fun interactions with her foster mother and her occupational therapy practitioners, and also helped her to acquire other developmental capacities (e.g., self-regulation, self-awareness, and sensorimotor skills). Over time, she also increased her curiosity and participation in activities that helped to foster fine motor skill development (e.g., coloring, craft activities) and frustration tolerance for trying different types of fine motor tools (e.g., scissors, vibrating pen, tweezers, crayons, markers) in creative ways.

Throughout the first several sessions, sensory supportive strategies were also explored to integrate into an initial home program.

Initial Home Program

In addition, a strong emphasis on routines and rituals at home, which included sensory interventions and supports, became part of the home program. The occupational therapy practitioners worked with Joan and Karly to help them create home-based routines and supportive tools to foster their targeted occupational outcomes. For example, one of the most difficult times of day was the evening because Karly had anxiety and difficulty tolerating bathing, tooth and hair brushing, and dressing into her pajamas due to her sensory overresponsivity patterns, sensorimotor challenges, and her trauma history. Bathing and bedtime were *(continued)*

SPOTLIGHT 5-3. CLINICAL VIGNETTE: KARLY AND JOAN (CONTINUED)

believed to be some of the primary times when Karly's trauma was experienced prior to coming into her foster home; therefore, these activities were highly triggering and anxiety producing.

Additionally, having sensory sensitivities and sensorimotor challenges added to her anxiety, as well as the difficulty experienced around performing these daily activities.

Over the course of occupational therapy services, Karly and her foster mother identified a variety of sensory-supportive tools and approaches. One of the first tools created and integrated into her morning routine was the use of a daily schedule board, with pictures that Karly could move indicating the day of the week and what activities she was going to do throughout the day. This activity helped her to feel more organized and gave her a sense of the plan for the day. The occupational therapy practitioner and foster mother also created a positive behavior reward system, where Karly was able to earn stars for each activity on her board that she completed each day. Each star earned her one point, and she was able to earn different "rewards" with the different amounts of points that she saved up.

She also benefitted from a variety of other sensory supportive tools. Karly was able to find a vibrating toothbrush and particular toothpaste that she was able to tolerate more easily (e.g., a fruit-flavored paste versus mint-flavored gel). The occupational therapy practitioner provided Karly's foster mother with examples of vendors of children's clothing that made undergarments and clothing with soft materials without seams that Karly was much more able to tolerate (decreased some of the tantrums and oppositional behaviors during dressing; increased dressing participation). Joan was able to find bed sheets that Karly felt more comfortable in and a nightlight for her bedroom. Karly also benefitted from and used a weighted blanket and weighted doll at home, which her foster mother reported helped her to feel less anxious, fall asleep, and stay asleep more at night. Karly also really liked the smell of lavender, which reminded her of her foster mother, who used many lavender-scented products. Thus, Karly and the occupational therapy practitioner made lavender soap and sprays with lavender essential oils to use as part of her bath and bedtime rituals and routine. After identifying all of these tools that were helpful, all were integrated into her evening rituals and routine as follows:

- Prior to bath: singing songs while preparing for bath
- Brushing teeth: vibrating toothbrush and preferred toothpaste
- For taking bath: use of lavender soap, soft scrub brush, rubbing dry with soft towel
- Putting on pajamas: soft cotton without seams
- Cuddle time: cuddling with foster mother in rocking chair while reading bedtime stories
- Safety check: Karly and foster mother would go into her room and use her lavender spray to "spray away" any "monsters" from her room (under bed, closet, on her bed)
- Relax/quiet time in bed: Karly would put on her nightlight and soft music and would lie down with her weighted blanket and weighted doll

In addition, more scheduled time at the park after school and increased access to play equipment at home (e.g., mini-trampoline, sit-and-spin, swing, arts and crafts) helped to meet the intensity of her sensory needs. These additional activities became part of her positive behavioral reward system as well. The occupational therapy practitioners collaborated with her in-home therapist to help Karly's foster mother with implementing the new routine and the positive behavioral reward system at home. Within 3 months, Karly's symptoms and behaviors were more stabilized, she demonstrated more adaptability, and the occupational therapy practitioners were able to focus on other occupational needs and goals as well.

It is important to add that as Karly began to feel safer, more secure, and stabilized, she also began having an influx of trauma-related memories during occupational therapy sessions and at home, and the occupational therapy practitioners used play activities and ongoing reassurance with her and her foster mother to help identify and verbalize her feelings, thoughts, and worries so that they could be recognized and addressed. The occupational therapy practitioners shared this information with her therapeutic team and reported the statements Karly made (e.g., abuse allegations) to the child welfare authorities. It is common for clients with trauma histories to have increased access to traumatic memories once they feel more stabilized; therefore, occupational therapy practitioners must understand how to work with children and families that have trauma and attachment-related needs and goals.

to help reduce risk factors for mental illness and foster resiliency. Resiliency in children and adolescents is linked to the promotion of coping skills, parenting skills, and social supports. Research demonstrates that the use of massage, yoga, and relaxation techniques with children diagnosed with emotional and behavioral disturbance helps to increase self-confidence, communication, and social confidence (Powell, Gilchrist, & Stapley, 2008). Additionally, relaxation techniques used within 30 days of experiencing a traumatic stressor were found to help prevent the development of posttraumatic stress disorder among children and adolescents (Berkowitz, Stover, & Marans, 2010).

Other evidence-based and promising practices may also be used by occupational therapy practitioners when helping children learn how to cope more effectively, such as the Coping with Stress (CWS) course (Lynch, Hornbrook, Clarke, Perrin, Polen, O'Connor, & Dickerson, 2005). The CWS course is a 15-week group program that helps adolescents learn new coping strategies and increase the use of existing stress management skills. The program utilizes a variety of therapeutic activities, such as role-play, cartoons, group discussions, and parent education. Research demonstrates that increased knowledge and use of coping skills serves as a prevention approach for at-risk youth by increasing their resiliency and reducing vulnerability to the emergence of mood disorders later in life (Lynch, et al., 2005).

Other examples of interventions that are evidence based and used to target mental health promotion include school-based stress management, emotion regulation, and coping skills programs. Evidence supports that school programming used to teach emotion identification, communication, and emotion regulation skills to young children is effective (Joseph & Strain, 2003). A meta-analysis of existing research where children in grades 3 to 8 engaged in stress and coping skills programs identified that such programs help the children to reduce stress and increased coping skills (Kraag et al., 2006). The Coping Koala Program (Tomb & Hunter, 2004) is another example of a group program that can be used in a variety of settings to help reduce stress, anxiety, worrying thoughts, and fears and develop coping skills. When working with children and adolescents who have problems with aggression and anger management, the Coping Power Program is another evidence-based curriculum to consider. It addresses a combination of target areas that include pro-social skills, emotion regulation, stress and relaxation training, problem identification and problem-solving skills, and ways to handle peer pressure (Lochman & Wells, 2003).

Yoga

Yoga has been used in occupational therapy practice with a wide variety of populations. Research supports that yoga is helpful in improving cardiorespiratory functioning, flexibility, grip strength, body composition, physical fitness, and spatial and verbal memory. It also helps to reduce mental health symptoms (Birdee et al., 2009; Case-Smith, Sines, & Klatt, 2010; Manjunath & Telles, 2004). Research has demonstrated that the implementation of a yoga program as part of a school-based health promotion program helped students feel calmer and more focused, taught strategies to help control behaviors when feeling stressed, and helped to foster self-esteem (Case-Smith et al., 2010). Many resources are available to help occupational therapy practitioners incorporate yoga into occupational therapy practice. One organization that provides a wealth of yoga trainings and intervention tools for professionals is YogaKids, and it is the mission of YogaKids to promote peace, health, empowerment, and education (Wenig, 2005).

Creative and Expressive Arts

Creative and expressive arts are often used as therapeutic interventions to target a variety of occupational therapy goals, such as stress management, emotion regulation, and social participation. Creative and expressive arts are also used to help address traumatic stress, grief, and loss (Edgar-Bailey & Kress, 2010). Creating stories, books, and videos; drawing; making cartoons; knitting; crocheting; sewing; and the use of arts and crafts are some of the ways occupational therapy practitioners help incorporate the use of creativity and expressive arts into the occupational therapy intervention process. According to the National Endowment for the Arts, children and adolescents from low socioeconomic status who engage in the arts during school or after-school programs achieve higher rates of academic success (Catterall, Dumais, & Hampden-Thompson, 2012).

Research also supports that the performing arts (particularly drama) help facilitate emotion regulation, social skills development, and social participation. Dance and movement-related activities have been shown to decrease symptoms of anxiety and to improve mood, affect, body image, and feelings of well-being and to promote quality of life (Koch, Kunz, Lykou, & Cruz, 2014). Music-related interventions are used in a variety of ways with children and adolescents. Music-based interventions have proved to be effective in developing verbal and nonverbal communication skills while decreasing problematic behaviors in children and adolescents with developmental and behavioral disorders (Gold, Voracek, & Wigram, 2004). Writing music, creating beats, playing instruments, performing in a band, recording music, and singing in a chorus or a play are examples of ways to use music as an occupational therapy intervention. Sound therapy is another therapeutic modality that incorporates the use of music and sound that is filtered, gated, and spectrally activated to help strengthen auditory processing and decrease hypersensitivity in order to foster occupational participation. Sound therapy requires additional training and equipment, however, before it may be used as part of one's practice.

Social Skills and Participation

Children and adolescents with mental health and behavioral barriers to occupation can benefit from social skills interventions provided in individual and group formats (Champagne, 2012; Cook et al., 2008). According to Arbesman, Bazyk, and Nochajski,

[T]he evidence is strong that social and life skills programs are effective for a wide range of at-risk children and youth such as aggressive or rejected youth and teenage mothers. In addition, the evidence is strong that children with intellectual impairments, developmental delays, and learning disabilities benefit from social skills programming and play, leisure, and recreational activities." (2013, p. 125)

Social skills training helps to decrease problematic behaviors and increase communication, pro-social, and functional skills in children diagnosed with ADHD and behaviors related to conduct problems. There is also a strong foundation of evidence to support social and friendship skills training when working with children with developmental and autism spectrum disorders (Mackay, Knott, & Dunlop, 2007; Tse, Strulovitch, Tagalakis, Meng, & Fombonne, 2007). One example of a resource created by an occupational therapist to help identify levels of social participation in groups is the Social Profile (Donohue, 2005).

Bullying is another common social problem often seen when working with children and adolescents with differences. Occupational therapy practitioners may develop and help children engage in anti-bullying programs. Research recommends that some of the most important elements of an anti-bullying program include parent involvement and education, increased playground supervision, and classroom management (Trofti & Farrington, 2009).

Additional Evidence-Based Mental Health Interventions

When working in mental health settings, it is important to be educated in evidence-based practices that are used across professions and with varied populations. Occupational therapists working with clients with mental health needs and goals often receive further training in some of the following models and integrate these and other evidence-based approaches as part of occupational therapy practice when appropriate: cognitive behavior therapy (CBT), trauma-focused CBT, dialectical behavior therapy (DBT), and multisystemic therapy (MST; Bazyk & Arbesman, 2013).

Cognitive Behavior Therapy

CBT is an evidence-based practice combining cognitive psychology and behavioral approaches. It is often used with individuals who have been diagnosed with trauma, depression, ADHD, autism, obsessive-compulsive disorder, and anxiety and phobic disorders (Beck, 2011). According to Ginsburg and Kingery (2007), cognitive behavioral approaches include the following:

- Emotion and thoughts identification
- Cognitive reframing (restructuring) to help challenge and change faulty thoughts and emotional patterns
- Graded exposure to fears and contingency planning/rewards
- Emotion/affect regulation education and skills training
- Psychoeducation and relaxation techniques

Evidence demonstrates that combining therapeutic models is often useful when working with clients with mental health concerns. Occupational therapy practitioners often obtain additional training in CBT in order to skillfully utilize related strategies during the occupational therapy intervention process, and also to help support the carryover of the CBT interventions implemented as a member of the interdisciplinary team. Waddell, Hua, Garland, Peters, and McEwan (2007) found that the combination of social skills, parent training, and CBT interventions helped prevent conduct disorder, anxiety, and depression in children ages 0 to 18 years old. Cognitive behavioral techniques are often part of intervention programs created and implemented by occupational therapists (Champagne, 2011b). See Figures 5-6 through 5-8 for examples of emotion identification and rating scales created and used with children and families as part of the occupational therapy intervention process.

Trauma-Focused Cognitive Behavior Therapy

Trauma-focused CBT is an evidence-based practice used with children ages 3 to 18 who have had traumatic experiences leading to the development of significant emotional and behavioral problems (Cohen, Mannarino, & Deblinger, 2006). It includes the participation of both the child and caregiver. The intent of trauma-focused CBT is to assist both parties in identifying thoughts and feelings that are related to the traumatic event(s) and in working together to process those thoughts and feelings to explore the impact they have had on emotions and behaviors. The overarching goal is to help foster safety and healing, promote resiliency, and support the parent–child relationship.

Dialectical Behavior Therapy

Although initially researched and utilized with adult populations (Linehan, 1993), DBT has been modified and used with children and adolescents across a variety of mental health settings such as inpatient, residential, juvenile justice, and school programs (MacPherson, Cheavens, & Fristad, 2013). DBT integrates the theory and practices of CBT and Zen Buddhism and includes four primary

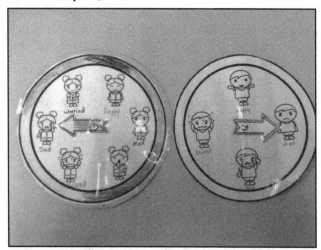

Figure 5-6. Feelings clock.

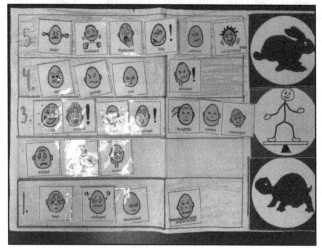

Figure 5-8. Feelings chart.

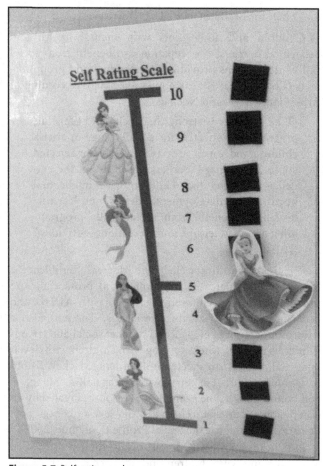

Figure 5-7. Self-rating scale.

teaching modules (Linehan, 1993). A core skill set taught as part of DBT is mindfulness, and it is also the first module. The other three modules of DBT include emotion regulation, interpersonal effectiveness, and distress tolerance skills (Linehan, 1993). Sensory approaches have also been used in combination with CBT and DBT by occupational therapists to enhance what these evidence-based programs offer (Champagne, 2011b).

Multisystemic Therapy

Another intensive therapeutic approach that integrates elements of cognitive behavioral and family therapy principles is MST. MST is an evidence-based therapeutic approach used with children between the ages of 12 and 17 years with severe emotional disturbance, antisocial and conduct behaviors, and/or engagement in substance abuse (MST Institute [MSTI], 2012). It specifically targets variables related to each youth and the natural environment, including the family system, social networks, school, and community (Henggeler, Sheidow, & Lee, 2007). The

overarching goals of the MST interventions generally include the following:

- Increasing the parent/caregiver skills and confidence to effectively discipline

- Improving family relationships

- Decreasing deviant peer contact and increasing pro-social peer relationships and contact

- Enhancing participation in school or vocational skills

- Engaging youth in pro-social leisure and recreational interests

- Co-creating a community-based support network to help caregivers achieve and maintain goals

MST has demonstrated positive outcomes in the reduction of hospitalization rates and improvements in child, adolescent, and family functioning, and in juvenile justice systems with youth with mental health problems and deviant behaviors (MSTI, 2012). Eight randomized trials have been conducted with MST and showed lower reoffending rates and a reduction in out-of-home placements (MSTI 2012). It is important to also mention that research in MST indicates that a system-based approach is required for successful outcomes (e.g., skilled therapist training, supervision, and institutional support of the MST program).

Research has shown differences in witnessing versus experiencing victimization in childhood; children who witnessed victimization had a positive correlation with the development of anxiety and depression, whereas those experiencing victimization were more likely to develop anxiety, depression, delinquency, and conduct problems (Ward, Martin, Theron, & Distiller, 2007). It has also been shown that children who receive significant supports after exposure to victimization tend to have a more resilient response than those who do not. Similar to the studies conducted on the MST approach, research indicates that interventions helpful in supporting resiliency include supportive after-school activities and enrichment programs, increased school supports and peer activities, and supports to help foster supportive family relationships and home environments (Ward et al., 2007). Occupational therapy practitioners work across all of the aforementioned contexts and are qualified to help develop and provide interventions for children, youth, and families that have witnessed or experienced victimization. Occupational therapy practitioners are also qualified to offer educational trainings to staff, organizations, communities, and populations on effective interventions.

SUMMARY

When working with children with trauma, attachment, and mental health–related barriers to occupational participation, it is necessary to be knowledgeable about the different types of mental health concerns that can emerge during the childhood and adolescent years. The occupational therapy assistant must understand a variety of occupational therapy frames of reference and mental health care models that are used as a foundation for intervention planning to support mental health, wellness, and the occupational participation of children and adolescents. Further, the occupational therapy assistant must possess the knowledge and skills necessary to collaboratively and skillfully implement therapeutic interventions under the supervision of an occupational therapist. Occupational therapy practitioners are qualified mental health practitioners who provide valuable services to children and families, as well as organizations and populations. Occupational therapy interventions provided by occupational therapy practitioners have been classified as intensive individualized services, targeted interventions, or universal interventions (Bazyk & Arbesman, 2013). Engagement in advocacy efforts, the implementation of promising and evidence-based therapeutic interventions, and working to help change public policy related to mental health are some of the many ways that occupational therapy

assistants may contribute to advancing the services offered to people with mental health needs and goals.

PART 3: APPLICATION

Fostering Positive Identity Formation

Although it is a lifelong process, an individual's self-esteem, values, and occupational identity are formed significantly during childhood and adolescence. ***Occupational identity*** refers to a person's sense of who he or she is and wants to become. ***Self-esteem*** is the degree of self-confidence and core beliefs a person has about him- or herself. Values are one's beliefs, standards, and qualities about what is right, good, and important and the degree of commitment the person has to these beliefs (AOTA, 2014b).

Depending on the age, strengths, and abilities of the child or adolescent, occupational therapy interventions are used to help foster identity formation and a more coherent and positive sense of self. Areas to explore when evaluating identity formation in a child or adolescent include the following:

- Values, strengths, likes, dislikes
- Degree of self-esteem
- Family structure, status of family relationships
- Rituals, routines, daily activities
- Friendships
- School and vocational interests
- Cultural ideation
- Spiritual ideation
- Sexual orientation

When a client is struggling in any of the aforementioned areas, occupational therapy practitioners may work with the child or adolescent to target occupational identity–related needs and goals. Although this list is not all-inclusive, some examples of activities and occupations that may be used to help children and adolescents with enhancing self-esteem and fostering identity formation include the following:

- Art expression
- Journaling
- Social stories
- Sensory stories
- Creating an "all about me" book (craft/art expression activity)
- Completing self-questionnaires related to this area of exploration
- Engaging in educational or vocational experiences

- Completing leisure or work interest checklists
- Exploring and engaging in different social groups or clubs (e.g., Girl and Boy Scouts, LGBT groups/clubs)
- Identifying and utilizing positive affirmations
- Alateen groups

When a child or adolescent has difficulty with occupational identity or self-esteem, he or she may demonstrate anxiety and behavioral problems when participating in occupations, particularly when engagement is related to the client's specific area(s) of perceived weakness. In such scenarios, occupational therapy interventions may include a combination of preparatory, purposeful, and occupation-based approaches, such as increasing self-awareness, occupational skill practice and development, and teaching coping skills to aid in the reduction of the mental health symptoms (e.g., anxiety) or behavioral concerns (e.g. perseveration, outbursts) evidenced when engaging in challenging occupations. An example of an occupational goal area for a child with a learning disability struggling with taking timed tests may be: *Charlie will complete an untimed test in school independently, without verbalizing or demonstrating symptoms of anxiety, within 3 months.* Some of the ways the occupational therapy practitioner may provide therapeutic supports to Charlie in order to help him meet this goal include the following:

- Offer validation of how hard it may be to complete tests at school
- Assist Charlie to identify his educational strengths and goals
- Assist Charlie to identify specific fears, areas of difficulty, and needs related to test taking
- Provide feedback and suggest potential support strategies for emotion regulation
- Identify potential educational support strategies (e.g., untimed tests)
- Provide education to Charlie's teachers on the topic of support strategies
- Support Charlie in continued participation in his education
- Engage in graded exposure activities to increase the ability to become more calm and successful in test taking

Clinical Vignettes

Three additional clinical vignettes are provided to demonstrate how occupational practitioners work with children and adolescents with mental health–related needs and goals.

Clinical Vignette: Owen

Owen is a 2-year-old boy living at home with his parents. He receives occupational therapy as part of his early intervention services at home. The occupational therapist working with Owen and his parents is also trained in the DIR Floortime approach (Greenspan & Wieder, 2006). Owen has been diagnosed with autism spectrum disorder and is not yet speaking or using verbalizations to communicate. His parents have been very distressed about their difficulty with understanding Owen and want to learn ways to better communicate with him. The occupational therapist used a combination of traditional occupational therapy services and the DIR Floortime approach to comprehensively assess developmental skills and to foster attachment and relational dynamics between the child and parents, and play was used as one of the primary intervention modalities. Like occupational therapy, DIR Floortime aims to meet each child and family where they are at and help them to relate and engage in meaningful childhood occupations.

Case-Smith and Arbesman (2008) identified six categories of research in the literature related to working with people with autism: (1) relationship-based, interactive interventions; (2) developmental skill–based programs; (3) sensory integration and sensory-based interventions; (4) social cognitive skill training; (5) parent-directed or parent-mediated approaches; and (6) intensive behavioral intervention. The DIR Floortime approach targets many of these areas in a manner specific to young children that can also be modified for working with older children. The occupational therapist targeted the building blocks of development and helped Owen's parents learn ways to interact and start picking up more on his nonverbal cues. As a result, Owen and his family were able to increase their ability to bond by co-creating ways to relate and engage in meaningful occupations. In addition to DIR Floortime, the occupational therapy practitioner provided evaluation and interventions related to sensory processing and occupation-based concerns such as eating, dressing, and playing.

Clinical Vignette: Rachel

Rachel is a 13-year-old girl living with her parents and 6-year-old brother. Rachel is friendly and artistic, and she plays the piano. She is an excellent student but struggles with getting up and going to school each day, and she reports that she is uncomfortable around her peers. She was diagnosed recently as having a general anxiety disorder. Some of the symptoms that Rachel experiences each day include the following:

- Extreme symptoms of anxiety
- Irritability
- Difficulty with attention and concentration in school
- Muscle tension

- Difficulty falling and staying asleep

- Feeling restless

- Feelings of impending doom when thinking about school and when actually attending classes (non-specific in origin/not related to a specific trigger at school)

Rachel is isolative while at school, and she does not participate in any form of social or after-school activities. She reports feeling exhausted all of the time, but is unable to fall asleep or stay asleep at night. She acknowledges experiencing frequent panic attacks, and has extreme fear of being asked questions in class. She does not eat at lunchtime and withdraws into the bathroom during lunch breaks. She reports that the stimulation in the hallways during the transitions between classes is too much. She complains of frequent body aches, stomachaches, and headaches.

Some examples of occupational therapy interventions that may be used to support Rachel's ability to participate in school-based occupations include the following:

- Assisting with creating a self-rating tool, which Rachel can utilize to track her progress

- Teaching and then practicing anxiety reduction techniques and strategies targeting muscle tension and other bodily symptoms she is experiencing (e.g., yoga, warm baths, aromatherapy, massage, creation and use of a sensory kit)

- Completing the Adolescent/Adult Sensory Profile and reviewing the results

- Identifying and utilizing sensory support strategies targeting Rachel's specific sensory patterns and needs

- Creating a sensory diet along with strategies to help Rachel manage difficult times of the day (complete with prevention and crisis de-escalation techniques)

- Exploring and implementing sleep hygiene strategies

- Identifying ways to engage with peers that are less anxiety producing

- Working with school staff to identify areas where Rachel can eat during lunchtime that are less over-stimulating and anxiety producing

- Collaborating with Rachel and her teachers to identify ways to lessen her anxiety when in class (e.g., seating placement, sensory strategies, a system to be able to communicate the need to take breaks)

- Assist with utilization of a school counselor and referral to a psychiatrist

After Rachel utilizes these interventions, it is important to periodically explore and review her progress with her and discuss with the occupational therapist whether continued occupational therapy services are warranted.

Clinical Vignette: Brock

Brock is a 16-year-old male with major depression who is living at home with his mother and father. His parents recently announced that they would be getting a divorce due to his father's alcoholism. Brock is a very intelligent young man who has many friends, likes to draw, and plays a variety of team sports. He periodically experiences overwhelming feelings of sadness accompanied by episodes of irritability and frequent body aches. Lately he has had a poor attention span and difficulty with concentration. He is also experiencing very low energy, loss of interest in meaningful activities and roles, problems with sleep, and a loss of appetite. When he is feeling this way, it is very difficult for him to get out of bed to go to school. He often avoids social events because he does not want his peers to know that he is depressed.

Brock currently receives occupational therapy services in school (primarily working on handwriting) and shared with the occupational therapy assistant that since his parents announced their divorce, he has been having increased feelings of depression and suicidal ideation (thoughts of suicide). The occupational therapist validated Brock's experience, then discussed the severity of Brock's symptoms and the possibility that he may need to get more help. Brock and the occupational therapist met together with the guidance counselor, where Brock shared that he was experiencing increased symptoms of depression accompanied by suicidal ideation. Brock was able to get increased support from his outpatient mental health providers and continued to attend school. During his occupational therapy sessions, Brock and the occupational therapy assistant continued to discuss Brock's feelings of grief and loss. Art expression activities were used to target both his mental health and handwriting goals. Brock was encouraged to use sensory support strategies to help identify and use both self-soothing and uplifting strategies. Under the supervision of the occupational therapist, Brock and the occupational therapy assistant worked together to create a sensory diet to help Brock use coping and sensory skills throughout the day in order to engage in occupations more easily. The occupational therapy assistant introduced him to an app called Optimism that allowed him to track how he was feeling each day, the strategies he was using to cope with his depression, and the effectiveness of these strategies over time. Brock was initially surprised to discover that his depression was improving and that he was increasingly engaging in meaningful roles and occupations. Brock became increasingly able to see his progress and continued to enhance his sensory diet.

Over time, Brock's guidance counselor and the occupational therapy assistant encouraged him to join a therapeutic group at school. When one of his friends disclosed he also was in the group, Brock reluctantly decided to give it a try. Brock was able to meet peers who were struggling with similar issues of grief and loss, divorce, and alcohol and substance abuse within the family. After a few weeks of participating in the group, Brock became increasingly more comfortable talking to others about his feelings. Over time, he began to offer suggestions to other students regarding strategies and supports that were helpful to him.

QUESTIONS AND LEARNING ACTIVITIES

The following questions and suggested learning activities are provided to help continue to enhance the development of clinical reasoning skills related to the information covered in this chapter.

1. Outline the key components of the occupational therapy intervention process.

    a. What is the role of the occupational therapy assistant during the intervention planning and implementation processes?

    b. In Spotlight 5-3, which parts of the interventions discussed could be provided by an occupational therapy assistant?

2. List the key factors necessary to provide client-centered and family-centered care.

    a. Why is it important to individualize occupational therapy interventions?

    b. Why is it important to include caregivers when providing occupational therapy services across the early lifespan?

3. Identify two different types of playground equipment. Create a list of examples of how the playground equipment might be used as an occupational-based intervention to help maximize health, safety, and occupational participation.

4. Name three to five evidence-based practices used by occupational therapy practitioners when working with children and adolescents with mental health–related barriers to occupational participation.

REFERENCES

Alvord, M. K., & Grados, J. J. (2005). Enhancing resilience in children: A proactive approach. *Professional Psychology: Research and Practice, 36*, 238-245.

American Academy of Pediatrics. (2014). Healthy Children: ADHD. Retrieved from, www.healthychildren.org/English/health-issues/conditions/adhd/Pages/default.aspx.

American Occupational Therapy Association. (2010). Specialized knowledge and skills in mental health promotion, prevention, and intervention in occupational therapy practice. Retrieved from www.aota.org/Practitioners/Official.aspx.

American Occupational Therapy Association. (2013). Mental health promotion, prevention and intervention in mental health for children and youth. Retrieved from www.aota.org/-/media/Corporate/Files/Practice/Children/CATCAPS/CMHCAT.ashx.

American Occupational Therapy Association. (2014a). Guidelines for supervision, roles, and responsibilities during the delivery of occupational therapy services. *American Journal of Occupational Therapy, 68*, S16-S22.

American Occupational Therapy Association. (2014b). Occupational therapy practice framework: Domain and process (3rd ed.). *American Journal of Occupational Therapy, 68*, S1-S48.

American Psychological Association. (2013). *Diagnostic and statistical manual of mental health disorders* (5th ed). Washington, DC: Author.

Arbesman, M., Bazyk, S., & Nochajski, S. M. (2013). Systematic review of occupational therapy and mental health promotion, prevention and intervention in children and youth. *American Journal of Occupational Therapy, 67*, 120-130.

Ayres, A. J. (2005). *Sensory integration and the child: Understanding hidden sensory challenges* (Rev. ed.). Los Angeles, CA: Western Psychological Services.

Barnes, K. J., Vogel, K. A., Beck, A. J., Schoenfeld, H. B. & Owen, S. V. (2008). Self-regulation strategies of children with emotional disturbance, *Physical & Occupational Therapy in Pediatrics, 28*(4), 369-387.

Bazyk, S., & Arbesman, M. (2013). *Occupational therapy practice guidelines for mental health promotion, prevention and intervention for children and youth*. Bethesda, MD: AOTA.

Beck, J. (2011). *Cognitive behavior therapy: Basics and beyond*. New York, NY: Guilford Press.

Beets, M. W., Flay, B. R., Vuchinich, S., Snyder, F. J., Acock, A., Li, K.,…Durlak, J. (2009). Use of a social and character development program to prevent substance use, violent behaviors, and sexual activity among elementary-school students in Hawaii. *American Journal of Public Health, 99*, 1438-1445.

Berkowitz, S. J., Stover, C. S., & Marans, S. R. (2010). The child and family traumatic stress intervention: Secondary prevention for youth at risk of developing PTSD. *Journal of Child Psychology and Psychiatry, 52*, 676-685.

Birdee, G. S., Yeh, G. Y., Wayne, P. M., Phillips, R. S., Davis, R. B., & Gardiner, P. (2009). Clinical applications of yoga for the pediatric population: A systematic review. *Academic Pediatrics, 9*, 212-220.

Blaustein, M., & Kinniburgh, K. (2010). *Treating traumatic stress in children and adolescents. How to foster resilience through attachment, self-regulation and competency.* New York: Guilford Press.

Bradshaw, C., Bottani, J., Osher, D., & Sugai, G. (2014). The integration of positive behavioral Interventions and supports and social and emotional learning. In M. D. Weist, N. Lever, C. Bradshaw, J. Owens (Eds.) *Handbook of School Mental Health: Issues in Clinical Psychology,* 101-118. New York, NY: Springer.

Brown, C., & Dunn, W. (2002). *Adolescent/Adult Sensory Profile.* San Antonio, TX: Pearson Assessment.

Bruininks, R. H., & Bruininks, B. D. (2005). *Bruininks-Oseretsky Test of Motor Proficiency, Second Edition (BOT-2).* Minneapolis, MN: Pearson Assessment.

Bundy, A., Lane, S., & Murray, E. (2002). *Sensory integration theory and practice* (2nd ed.). Philadelphia, PA: F. A. Davis.

Case-Smith, J., & Arbesman, M. (2008). Evidence-based review of interventions for autism used in or of relevance to occupational therapy. *American Journal of Occupational Therapy, 62,* 416-429.

Case-Smith, J., Sines, J., & Klatt, M. (2010). Perceptions of children who participated in a school-based yoga program. *Occupational Therapy, Schools & Early Intervention, 3,* 226-238.

Catterall, J. S., Dumais, S. A., & Hampden-Thompson, G. (2012). *The arts and achievement in at-risk youth: Findings from four longitudinal studies.* Washington, DC: National Endowment for the Arts. Retrieved from www.nea.gov/research/ arts-at-risk-youth.pdf.

Centers for Disease Control and Prevention (CDC). (2014a). Positive parenting tips. Retrieved from www.cdc.gov/ncbddd/ childdevelopment/positiveparenting/index.html.

Centers for Disease Control and Prevention (CDC). (2014b). Safe and healthy kids. Retrieved from www.cdc.gov/family/kids/.

Champagne, T. (2011a). Attachment, trauma and occupational therapy practice. *OT Practice, 16,* CE1-CE8.

Champagne, T. (2011b). *Sensory modulation and environment: Essential elements of occupation* (3rd ed Rev.). Sydney, Australia: Pearson Assessment.

Champagne, T. (2012). Creating groups for children and youth in community-based mental health occupational therapy practice. *OT Practice, 17,* 13-18.

Champagne, T. (2014). Sensory approaches. In Massachusetts Department of Mental Health (MA DMH). *Resource guide: Creating positive cultures of care.* Retrieved from www.mass.gov/eohhs/gov/ departments/dmh/restraintseclusion-reduction-initiative.html.

Champagne, T. & Stromberg, N. (2004). Sensory approaches in inpatient psychiatric settings: Innovative alternatives to seclusion and restraint. *Journal of Psychosocial Nursing, 42,* 35-44.

Child Welfare League of America. (2014). Positive parenting discipline tips. Retrieved from http://66.227.70.18/positiveparenting/ tipsdiscipline.htm

Cohen, J. A., Mannarino, A. P., & Deblinger, E. (2006). *treating trauma and traumatic grief in children and adolescents.* New York: The Guilford Press.

Community Therapy Associates (2014). SticKids. Retrieved from www. stickids.com.

Cook, C. R., Gresham, F. M., Kern, L., Barreras, R. B., Thornton, S., & Crews, S. D. (2008). Social skills training for secondary students with emotional and/or behavioral disorders: A review and analysis of the meta-analytic literature. *Journal of Emotional and Behavioral Disorders, 16,* 131-144.

Cooke, A., Spinazzola, J., Ford, J., Lanktree, C., Blaustein, M., Cloitre, M.,...van der Kolk, B. (2005). Complex trauma in children and adolescents. *Psychiatric Annals, 35*(5), 390-398.

Coren, E., & Barlow, J. (2001). Individual and group-based parenting programmes for improving psychosocial outcomes for teenage parents and their children. *Cochrane Database of Systematic Reviews, 101*(3).

Coster, W. J., Deeney, T., Haltiwanger, J. T., & Haley, S. (1998). *School Function Assessment.* San Antonio, TX: Psychological Corporation/ Therapy Skill Builders.

Crepeau, E. B., Boyt Schell, B. A., Gillen, G. & Scaffa, M. E. (2014). Analyzing occupational and activity. In B. A. Boyt Schell, G. Gillen, G., & M. E. Scaffa, *Willard & Spackman's Occupational Therapy* (12th ed., pp. 234-248). New York, NY: Lippincott Williams & Wilkins.

Davidson, D. A., (2005). Psychosocial issues affecting social participation. In J. Case-Smith (Ed.), *Occupational Therapy for Children* (5th ed., pp. 449-480). St. Louis, MO: Elsevier/Mosby.

de Graaf, I., Speetjens, P., Smit, F., de Wolff, M., & Tavecchio, L. (2008). Effectiveness of the Triple P positive parenting program on parenting: A meta-analysis. *Family Relations, 57,* 553-566.

Diamond, G. S., Wintersteen, M. B., Brown, G. K., Diamond, G. M., Gallop, R., Shelef, K., & Levy, S. (2010). Attachment-based family therapy for adolescents with suicidal ideation: A randomized controlled trial. *Journal of the American Academy of Child and Adolescent Psychiatry, 9,* 122-131.

Donohue, M. V. (2005). Social Profile: Assessment of validity and reliability in children's groups. *Canadian Journal of Occupational Therapy, 62,* 164-175.

Dunn, W. (1999). *Sensory Profile.* San Antonio, TX: Therapy Skill Builders.

Durlak, J. A., Weissberg, R. P., Dymnicki, A. B., Taylor, R. D., & Schellinger, K. B. (2011). The impact of enhancing students' social and emotional learning: A meta-analysis of school-based universal interventions. *Child Development, 82,* 405-432.

Edgar-Bailey, M. & Kress, M. (2010). Resolving child and adolescent traumatic grief: Creative techniques and interventions. *Journal of Creativity in Mental Health, 5,* 158-176.

Feletti, V., Anda, R., Nordenberg, D., Williamson, D., Spitz, A., Edwards, V....Marks, J. (1998). Relationship of childhood abuse and household dysfunction to many of the leading causes of death in adults. The Adverse Childhood Experiences Study. American Journal of Preventative Medicine, *14*(4), 245-258.

Ginsberg, G. S., & Kingery, J. N. (2007). Evidence-based practice for childhood anxiety disorders. *Journal of Contemporary Psychotherapy, 37,* 123-132.

Gold, C., Voracek, M., & Wigram, T. (2004). Effects of music therapy for children and adolescents with psychopathology: A meta-analysis. *Journal of Child Psychology and Psychiatry, 45,* 1054-1063

Goleman, D. (1996). *Emotional intelligence: Why it can matter more than IQ.* New York: Bantam Books.

Greene, R. W. (2014). *The explosive child: A new approach for understanding and parenting easily frustrated, "chronically inflexible" children* (5th ed. Rev.). New York: Harper Collins.

Greenspan, S., & Wieder, L. (2006). *Engaging autism: Using the Floortime approach to help children, relate, communicate and think.* Cambridge, MA: Perseus Books.

Henggeler, S. W., Sheidow, A. J., & Lee, T. (2007). Multisystemic treatment (MST) of serious clinical problems in youths and their families. In D. W. Springer & A. R. Roberts (Eds.), *Handbook of forensic mental health with victims and offenders: Assessment, treatment, and research* (pp. 315-345). New York: Springer Publishing.

Henry, D. (2001). *The tool chest: For teachers, parents and students.* Glendale, AZ: Henry OT.

Hocking, C. (2014). Contribution of occupation to health and wellbeing. In B. A. Boyt Schell, G. Gillen, & M. E. Scaffa, *Willard & Spackman's Occupational Therapy* (12th ed., pp. 72-81). New York, NY: Lippincott Williams & Wilkins

Horner, R. H., Sugai, G., & Anderson, C. M. (2010). Examining the evidence base for school-wide positive behavior support. *Focus on Exceptional Children, 42,* 1-14.

Hughes, D. (2006). *Building the bonds of attachment* (2nd ed.). New York: Jason Aronson.

Hughes, D., & Koomar, J. (2010). SAFE PLACE — Parenting strategies for facilitating attachment and sensory regulation (DVD). Boston: Spiral Foundation.

Joseph, G. E., & Strain, P. S. (2003). Helping young children control anger and handle disappointment. *Young Exceptional Children, 7*(1), 21-29.

Kielhofner, G. (2002). *A model of human occupation: Theory and application* (3rd ed.). Baltimore, MD: William and Wilkins.

King, G., Law, M., King, S., Hurley, P., Hanna, S.,...Young, K. (2004). Children's assessment of participation and enjoyment (CAPE) and preferences for activities of children (PAC). San Antonio, TX: Harcourt Assessment.

Kinninburgh, K. & Blaustein, M. (2005). Attachment, self-regulation and competency: A comprehensive intervention framework for children with complex trauma. *Psychiatric Annals, 35*, 424-430.

Koch, S., Kunz, T., Lykou, S., & Cruz, R. (2014). Dance movement therapy and dance on health-related psychological outcomes: A meta-analysis. *The Arts in Psychotherapy, 41*, 46-64.

Kraag, G., Zeegers, M. P., Kok, G., Hosman, C., & Abu-Saad, H. H. (2006). School programs targeting stress management in children and adolescents: A meta-analysis. *Journal of School Psychology, 44*, 449-472.

Kuypers, L. (2011). Zones of regulation. Retrieved from www.zonesof-regulation.com/the-zones-of-regulations-book.html

Law, M., Cooper, B., Strong, S., Stewart, D., Rigby, P., & Letts, L. (1996). The person-environment-occupation model: A transactive approach to occupational performance. *Canadian Journal of Occupational Therapy, 63*, 9-23.

Law, M., Polatajko, H., Baptiste, W., & Townsend, E. (1997). Core concepts of occupational therapy. In E. Townsend (Ed.), *Enabling occupation: An occupational therapy perspective* (pp. 29-56). Ottawa, ON: Canadian Association of Occupational Therapists.

LeBel, J., & Champagne, T. (2010). Integrating sensory and trauma-informed interventions: A Massachusetts state initiative, part 2. *Mental Health Special Interest Section Quarterly, 33*(2), 1-4.

Levine, P. (2014). *About somatic experiencing*. Retrieved from www.traumahealing.com/about-se.php.

Levy, T. M., & Orlans, M. (1998). *Attachment, trauma, and healing: Understanding and treating attachment disorder in children and families*. Washington, DC: Child Welfare League of America.

Linehan, M. (1993). *Cognitive-behavioral treatment of borderline personality disorder*. New York, NY: Guilford Press.

Lochman, J. E., & Wells, K. C. (2003). Effectiveness of the Coping Power program and of classroom intervention with aggressive children. Outcomes at a 1-year follow-up. *Behavior Therapy, 34*, 493-515.

Luxenberg, T., Spinazzola, J., Hidalgo, J., Hunt, C., & van der Kolk, B. (2001). Complex trauma and disorders of extreme stress (DESNOS) diagnosis, part two: Treatment. *Directions in Psychiatry, 21*, 373-392.

Lynch, F. L., Hornbrook, M., Clarke, G. N., Perrin, P., Polen, M. R., O'Connor, E., & Dickerson, J. (2005). Cost-effectiveness of an intervention to prevent depression in at-risk teens. *Archives of General Psychiatry, 62*, 1241-1248.

Mackay, T., Knott, F., & Dunlop, A. W. (2007). Developing social interaction and understanding in individuals with autism spectrum disorder: A groupwork intervention. *Journal of Intellectual and Developmental Disability, 32*, 279-290.

MacPherson, H. A., Cheavens, J. S., & Fristad, M. A. (2013). Dialectical behavior therapy for adolescents: Theory, treatment adaptations, and empirical outcomes. *Clinical Child and Family Psychology Review, 16*, 59-80.

Manjunath, N. & Telles, S. (2004). Spatial and verbal memory test scores following yoga and fine arts camps for school children. *Indian Journal of Physiology Pharmacology, 48*, 353-356.

Massachusetts Department of Mental Health. (2014). *Seclusion/restraint reduction initiative resources*. Retrieved from www.mass.gov/eohhs/gov/departments/dmh/restraintseclusion-reduction-initiative.html.

May-Benson, T. A., & Koomar, J. A. (2010). Systematic review of the research evidence examining the effectiveness of interventions using a sensory integrative approach for children. *American Journal of Occupational Therapy, 64*, 403-414.

McNeil, D. A., Wilson, B. N., Siever, J. E., Ronca, M., & Nah, J. K. (2009). Connecting children to recreational activities: Results of a cluster randomized trial. American Journal of Health Promotion, 23, 376-387.

Miles, J., Espiritu, R. C., Horen, N., Sebian, J., & Waetzig, E. (2010). *A public health approach to children's mental health: A conceptual framework*. Washington, DC: Georgetown University Center for Child and Human Development, National Technical Assistance Center for Children's Mental Health.

Miller Kuhaneck, H., Henry, D., Glennon, T., Parham, D., & Ecker, C. (2008). *The Sensory Processing Measure*. Los Angeles: Western Psychological Services.

Miller, L. J., & Lane, S. J. (2000, March). Toward a consensus in terminology in sensory integration theory and practice: Part 1: Taxonomy of neurophysiological processes. *Sensory Integration Special Interest Section Quarterly, 23*(1), 1-4.

Missiuna, C., Pollock, N., & Law, M. (2004). *Perceived efficacy and goal setting system* (PEGS). San Antonio, TX: Psychological Corporation.

Moore-Corner, R., Kielhofner, G., & Olson, L. (1998). *Work Environment Impact Scale*. Chicago, IL: Model of Human Occupation. Chicago Clearinghouse, University of Illinois at Chicago.

Multisystemic Therapy Institute. (2012). Data report. Retrieved from www.mstinstitute.org/MST-DataReport-2012-final.pdf.

National Center for Learning Disabilities. (2014). Tips to talk to your child about being distracted and unfocused. Retrieved from www.ncld.org/types-learning-disabilities/adhd-related-issues/adhd/how-to- talk-to-child-about-focus-distraction.

National Executive Training Institute. (2009). *Creating nurturing and healing cultures of care: Training curriculum for the reduction of seclusion and restraint*. Alexandria, VA: National Association of State Mental Health Program Directors.

Perry, B. D., & Hambrick, E. (2008). The neurosequential model of therapeutics. Reclaiming children and youth. *The Journal of Strengths-Based Interventions, 17*, 38-43.

Phelan, T. (2010). *1 2 3 magic: Effective discipline for children 2-12* (4th ed. Rev). Glen Ellyn, IL: Parent Magic.

Powell, L., Gilchrist, M., & Stapley, J. (2008). A journey of self-discovery: An intervention involving massage, yoga, and relaxation for children with emotional and behavioral difficulties attending primary schools. *European Journal of Special Needs Education, 23*, 403-412.

Schaaf, R. C., Benevides, T., Mailloux, Z., Faller, P., Hunt, J., van Hooydonk, E.,...Kelly, D. (2013). An intervention for sensory difficulties in children with autism: A randomized trial. *Journal of Autism and Developmental Disorders, 44*(7), 1493-1506.

Substance Abuse and Mental Health Services Administration. (2014). Supported employment: Evidence-based practices kit. Retrieved from http://store.samhsa.gov/shin/content//SMA08-4365/HowtoUseEBPKITS-SE.pdf.

Sugai, G., Horner, R. H., Dunlap., G., Hieneman, M., Lewis, T., Nelson, C. M.,...Wilcox, B. (2000). Applying positive behavioral support and functional behavioral assessment in schools. *Journal of Positive Behavior Intervention, 2*, 1-25.

Tomb, M., & Hunter, L. (2004). Prevention of anxiety in children and adolescents in a school setting: The role of school-based practitioners. *Children and Schools, 26*, 87-101.

Townsend, S., Carey, P. D., Hollins, N. L., Helfrich, C., Blondis, M., Hoffman, A.,...Blackwell, A. (1999). *The occupational therapy psychosocial assessment of learning (OT PAL)*. Version 2.0. Chicago, IL: Model of Human Occupation Clearing House. Department of Occupational Therapy, University of Illinois.

Trofti, M. M. & Farrington, D. P. (2009). What works in preventing bullying: Effective elements of anti-bullying programs. *Journal of Aggression, Conflict and Peace Research, 1*, 13-24.

Tse, J., Strulovitch, J., Tagalakis, V., Meng L., & Fombonne, E. (2007). Social skills training for adolescents with Asperger syndrome and high functioning autism. *Social Journal of Autism and Developmental Disorders, 37*, 1960-1968.

U.S. Department of Health and Human Services. (2011). Substance Abuse Mental Health Services Administration's Strategic Initiatives Fact Sheet. Retrieved from http://store.samhsa.gov/product/SAMHSA-Strategic-Initiatives-Fact-Sheet/SMA11-4666.

U.S. Department of Health and Human Services. (2012). Administration on Children, Youth and Families, Children's Bureau. Child Maltreatment 2011. Retrieved from www.acf.hhs.gov/programs/cb/research-data-technology/statistics-research/child-maltreatment.

U.S. Department of Health and Human Services. (2013). Childhood maltreatment: Consequences. Retrieved from www.cdc.gov/violenceprevention/childmaltreatment/consequences.html.

van der Kolk, B. (2005). Developmental trauma disorder: Toward a rational diagnosis for children with complex trauma histories. *Psychiatric Annals, 35*(3), 401-408.

van der Kolk, B. (2006). Clinical implications of neuroscience research and PTSD. *Annals of the New York Academy of Science, 1071,* 277-293.

Waddell, C., Hua, J. M., Garland, O. M., Peters, R. D., & McEwan, K. (2007). Preventing mental disorders in children: A systematic review to inform policy-making. *Canadian Journal of Public Health, 98,* 166-173.

Ward, C. L., Martin, E., Theron, C., & Distiller, G. B. (2007). Factors affecting resilience in children exposed to violence. *South African Journal of Psychology, 37,* 175-187.

Wenig, M. (2005). *YogaKids: Tools for Schools Teacher's Manual.* LaPorte, IN: YogaKids.

Wilbarger, P. (1995). The sensory diet: Activity programs based upon sensory processing theory. *Sensory Integration Special Interest Section Quarterly, 18*(2), 1-4.

Wild, G. (2014). *BrainWorks.* Retrieved from www.sensationalbrain.com.

Williams, M., & Shellenberger, S. (1994). *"How does your engine run?": A leader's guide to the alert program for self-regulation.* Albuquerque, NM: TherapyWorks.

World Health Organization. (2001). *International classification of functioning, disability and health.* Geneva, Switzerland: Author.

Zemke, R., & Clark, F. (1996). *Occupational science: The evolving discipline.* Philadelphia: PA: F. A. Davis.

6

Occupational Environment
of the Mid-Lifespan

Lee Ann Fallet, MA, CRC, OTR/L

KEY TERMS

- Americans With Disabilities Act
- Assertive Community Therapy
- Behavioral Approach
- Behavioral Health Care
- Cognitive Behavior Therapy
- Cognitive Therapy
- Community Mental
- Community Mental Health Act
- Community Mental Health Settings
- Developmental Frame of Reference
- Developmental Theory
- Dialectical Behavior Therapy
- Existential Therapy
- Gestalt Therapy

- Hierarchy of Needs
- Humanistic Perspective
- Intensive Outpatient Programs
- Medicaid
- Medicare
- Mental Health Parity Act
- Mindfulness
- Model
- Model of Human Occupation
- Motivational Interviewing
- National Alliance on Mental Illness
- Occupational Performance History Interview
- Partial Hospitalization Programs
- Patient Protection and Affordable Care Act

- Person-Centered Approach
- Psychoanalytic Theory
- Psychodynamic Approach
- Psychosocial Rehab Centers and Clubhouses
- Rational Emotive Therapy
- Recovery Movement
- Rehabilitation Act of 1973
- Sensory Integration Frame of Reference
- Shelters
- Social Model of Care
- Supported/Transitional Residential Services
- Theory
- Wellness Recovery Action Plan

Manville, C.A., & Keough, J. L.
Mental Health Practice for the Occupational Therapy Assistant (pp 157-174).
© 2016 Taylor & Francis Group.

CHAPTER LEARNING OBJECTIVES

After completion of this chapter, students should be able to:

1. Identify cultural, societal, and legislative factors affecting occupational therapy mental health services in the mid-lifespan.
2. Review how occupational therapy services transitioned to community-based services.
3. Describe the different settings where occupational therapy services are provided.
4. Examine how health care reform and legislation affect the provision of mental health occupational therapy services.
5. Compare and contrast nonoccupational therapy theories and models.
6. Compare and contrast occupational therapy frames of reference used in mental health.

CHAPTER OUTLINE

INTRODUCTION

American Occupational Therapy Association (AOTA) Centennial Vision:

> We envision that occupational therapy is a powerful, widely recognized, science-driven, and evidenced-based profession with a globally connected and diverse workforce meeting the society's occupational needs. (2014a)

AOTA Vision Statement:

> The American Occupational Therapy Association advances occupational therapy as the pre-eminent profession in promoting the health, productivity, and quality of life of individuals and society through the therapeutic application of occupation. (2014a)

AOTA Mission Statement:

> The American Occupational Therapy Association advances the quality, availability, use, and support of occupational therapy through standard-setting, advocacy, education and research on behalf of its members and the public. (2014a)

PART 1: CULTURAL, LEGISLATIVE, AND SOCIETAL FACTORS AFFECTING THE MID-LIFESPAN

The early evolution of mental health care was presented in Chapter 1. Chapter 1 also identified contextual factors affecting early mental health services provided by occupational therapists. These same factors apply in the provision of occupational therapy services to adults who have been diagnosed with a mental illness. They include cultural, societal, and legislative factors. In order to discuss the current status of mental health care in the United States, it is important to look back at how the transition to community-based services occurred. It is also important to explore how this transition affected the provision of occupational therapy services to individuals diagnosed with and at risk for mental illness.

The Transition to Community-Based Services

Deinstitutionalization and community mental health movements significantly helped to shape current mental health occupational therapy services. In the early 1960s, President John F. Kennedy signed the **Community Mental Health Act** (CMHA) of 1963. The CMHA was enacted to obtain federal funding for the development of community mental health centers in the United States. It provided grants to states to establish those centers, which were under the purview of the National Institute of Mental Health. The purpose of the CMHA was to provide for community-based care as an alternative to institutionalization. As a result, the number of individuals receiving treatment in state inpatient hospitals dropped from 600,000 in 1955 to fewer than 70,000 individuals currently (National Council for Behavioral Health, 2013). Although it was hoped that the passage of the CMHA would improve care for those with mental illnesses, many feel it has fallen short of its goal with lack of funding and adequate planning to provide effective services (Gutman, 2011; Peters, 2011).

As the amount of community-based services available to the mentally ill began to expand, the need to offer treatment for addiction disorders was identified as another way to help individuals function at optimum levels. These coordinated services became known as **behavioral health care.** They are provided by government, state, county, nonprofit, and for-profit organizations (National Council for Behavioral Health, 2013). The CMHA reversed the stance of the federal government to remain uninvolved in state care of the mentally ill, which had been established by the Indigent Insane Bill of 1854. However, it was soon discovered that deinstitutionalization outpaced funding available for community-based services and supports (Gutman, 2011).

Mental Health and Disability-Related Legislation

Federal legislation related to mental health care traces back to the 19th century. As stated earlier, the CMHA was an important piece of legislation that led to significant changes in the care of the mentally ill population. Along with the CMHA, federal involvement in health care was highlighted in the 1960s with the passage of amendments to Social Security that established Medicare, Medicaid, and the supplemental security income program.

The **Rehabilitation Act of 1973** was an influential piece of legislation that was signed by President Richard M. Nixon. This act redirected vocational rehabilitation

to make the most severely disabled its first priority. It stressed consumer involvement in rehabilitation planning and program evaluation, and supported rehabilitation research (Colorado State University, 2014). It was also the first "rights" legislation to prohibit discrimination against people with disabilities, including individuals diagnosed with mental illness. Title V of this legislative act prohibited discrimination on the basis of disability in programs conducted by federal agencies. This included programs receiving federal financial assistance, federal employment, and employment practices of federal contractors. Standards for determining employment discrimination under this act are the same as those that would be used in Title I of the Americans with Disabilities Act (Boston University College of Health & Rehabilitation Sciences Sargent College, 2014).

The **Americans With Disabilities Act** (ADA) of 1990 was signed by President George H. W. Bush. This act was a wide-ranging civil rights law that prohibited discrimination based on disability under certain circumstances. It afforded similar protections against discrimination to Americans with disabilities as did the Civil Rights Act of 1964. This made discrimination based on race, religion, sex, national origin, and other characteristics illegal (United States Department of Justice [USDOJ], Civil Rights Division, 2014a). In 2008, President George W. Bush signed the ADA Amendments Act. This act was intended to give broader protections for disabled workers and to "turn back the clock" on court rulings that Congress deemed too restrictive (USDOJ, Civil Rights Division, 2014b).

The **Mental Health Parity Act** (MHPA) was signed by President Bill Clinton in 1996. It required that annual or lifetime dollar limits set on mental health benefits be no lower than the limits set on medical and surgical benefits offered by a group health plan or health insurance. This act, however, was largely superseded by the Mental Health Parity and Addiction Equity Act (MHPAEA; United States Department of Labor [USDOL], Labor Employee Benefits Security Administration, 2010). The MHPAEA was signed by President George W. Bush in 2008. The law requires insurers who offer group health plans that include coverage for mental illness and substance abuse disorders to administer that coverage in a manner that is no more restrictive than provision of coverage offered for medical and surgical procedures. It is important to note that the MHPAEA did not require all group health plans to include mental health and substance use disorder benefits. It merely stated that when a plan *does* cover these benefits, they must be covered at levels that are no lower and with treatment limitations that are no more restrictive than would be the case for other medical and surgical benefits offered by the plan (USDOL, Labor Employee Benefits Administration, 2010).

The **Patient Protection and Affordable Care Act** (PPACA) was signed by President Barack Obama on March 23, 2010, and the Health Care Education and Reconciliation Act was signed by him on March 30, 2010. These legislative

---

CHECKPOINT 6-1. LIST

Chronologically list the legislation that has had a significant impact on the quality of life and services available to individuals with mental illness.

---

acts represented the most significant government expansion and regulatory overhaul of the U.S. health care system since the passage of Medicare and Medicaid in 1965. The PPACA aimed at increasing the rate of health insurance coverage for all Americans and reducing the overall cost of health care. It provides a number of mechanisms to increase the coverage rate to include mandates, subsidies, and tax credits to employers and individuals. Additional reforms aim to improve health care outcomes and streamline the delivery of health care. The PPACA requires insurance companies to cover all applicants and offer the same rates, regardless of pre-existing conditions or sex. On June 28, 2012, the U.S. Supreme Court upheld the constitutionality of most of the PPACA in the case of *National Federation of Independent Business v Sebelius* (American Public Health Association, 2013).

The primary reason for the debate over American health care is that the United States spends a higher percentage of its gross national product on this type of care than any other developed country. Despite this, millions of Americans go without access to health care, and the spending has not produced comparably high measures of health status (Institute of Medicine of the National Academies, 2004). On key measures such as life expectancy and infant mortality rate, the United States does not measure up to its peers in the developed world, most of which have some form of nationalized health care coverage available to 100% of their total populations (Random History and Word Origins for the Curious Mind, 2009).

With changes in health care coverage, delivery, and reimbursement in the United States as the result of the PPACA, Brown and McKenna (2013) discussed an emerging role for occupational therapists in the health care delivery system:

> The healthcare delivery system is expected to undergo dramatic changes in the coming years as a result of the need to control public and private expenditures on health care services. There is also recognition that patient outcomes and experiences can and should be improved. These goals have been coined the "Triple Aim" by the Institute for Healthcare Improvement. A key strategy to achieve the Triple Aim involves transforming and enhancing primary care service delivery, so that interprofessional teams of providers work together with patients to coordinate all their care. AOTA believes occupational therapy professionals can make a valuable contribution to these emerging primary care teams. (p. 5)

Checkpoint 6-1 will help learners identify legislation that has had a significant impact on individuals with mental illness.

Societal Factors and Advocacy

Societal factors associated with mental illness can include negative perceptions on the part of the public that come from a general lack of understanding. This lack of understanding may be based on preconceived stereotypes that people have regarding symptoms and behaviors associated with brain disorders that are biologically based and beyond the control of the individual who is exhibiting them. Individuals with a mental illness may be perceived, among other things, to be lazy, violent, or weak willed. This labeling can lead to discrimination in health care delivery, funding, and housing, and lead to bias aimed toward these individuals in social and recreational settings.

Hampton and Zhu (2011) found that, although attitudes toward people with psychiatric disabilities (PWPD) are improving, the primary source of difficulties encountered by PWPD is still the public's negative attitudes rather than the person's emotional/behavioral limitations. They also found that these attitudes correlated with demographic variables, including age, ethnicity, gender, education, and degree of contact that individuals had with PWPD. For example, it was found that, in general, individuals who were younger had received more education about PWPD. In addition, it was discovered that people who have had more contact with PWPD were more likely to have positive attitudes toward these individuals than those who were older, had less education, and experienced less contact. Hampton and Zhu expressed the sentiment that it is crucial that researchers continue to investigate the attitudes that people express toward PWPD in order to improve access to education, employment, health care, and rehabilitation. Improvements in medical technology, ongoing research, and advocacy efforts of organizations like the National Alliance on Mental Illness (NAMI) are helping to educate the public and increase community understanding and acceptance of individuals who have been diagnosed with a mental illness (NAMI, 2013).

NAMI is the nation's largest grassroots mental health organization, dedicated to building better lives for those affected by mental illness. Since its inception in 1979, NAMI has established itself as a formidable mental health advocacy organization. It has been the driving force behind a national investment in research, parity for mental health care, and increased availability of housing for individuals with mental illness. It has also worked to ensure that treatments and services are available to those in need when they need them most. NAMI provides free education, advocacy, and support programs to consumers and their parents, siblings, adult children, spouses, civil and domestic partners, and other involved relatives. It promotes the prevailing scientific judgment that "severe mental illness" is a brain disorder, which, at the present time, is neither preventable nor curable. The belief is that it is treatable, manageable, and recoverable with a combination of medication, supportive counseling, and community support services. These services include education and vocational training. NAMI's awareness efforts have successfully addressed the stigma of mental illness and helped to decrease the barriers to treatment and recovery (NAMI, 2014b).

Reimbursement for Services

Medical and rehabilitative psychiatric services provided in the inpatient or outpatient clinical setting are generally reimbursed by public or private insurance. Once a patient has attained and maintained a level of functioning where no further "improvement" in functioning can be demonstrated, psychotherapy and rehabilitative services are no longer considered to be medically necessary and are not covered by insurance. The general exception to this is ongoing medication management. Services provided in community-based settings, which may be considered habilitative, rely on grant, block grant, or private funding.

Insurance Reimbursement

The U.S. health care system relies heavily on private health insurance, which is the primary source of coverage for most Americans. According to the Centers for Disease Control and Prevention (CDC), approximately 61% of Americans under the age of 65 years have private health insurance (CDC, 2014). Public programs provide the primary source of coverage for most senior citizens and for low-income families who meet certain eligibility requirements. The primary public programs are Medicare, Medicaid, and the State Children's Health Insurance Program. Other public programs include military health benefits provided through TRICARE and the Veterans Health Administration, and benefits provided through the Indian Health Service. Some states have additional programs for low-income individuals (U.S. Census Bureau, 2014).

Private Insurance

Private insurance developed significantly in the mid-20th century. With the help of the American Hospital Association, hospitals joined together under the name of Blue Cross in order to decrease competition among hospitals offering prepaid plans. Consequently, to protect themselves from competition from Blue Cross, physicians created their own framework of prepaid plans that included coverage of physician services. Using the principles established by the American Medical Association, these physicians created Blue Shield, which offers medical and surgical benefits to hospitalized members. Some plans covered office visits as well (Thomasson, 2003).

With the success of Blue Cross and Blue Shield, commercial health insurance companies decided to enter the market. Employee-based plans improved with the power of labor unions, and in 1954, employer and employee contributions to health plans became exempt from taxes under the Internal Revenue Code (Thomasson, 2003).

Public Insurance

As mentioned earlier, Medicare and Medicaid were enacted in 1965 as amendments to the Social Security Act. *Medicare* is a federally funded program. It was originally established to provide coverage to Americans aged 65 years or older who were receiving retirement benefits from Social Security or the Railroad Retirement Board. In 1972, Medicare eligibility was extended to individuals under age 65 years with long-term disabilities and to individuals with end-stage renal disease (Centers for Medicare and Medicaid Services [CMS], 2013b). *Medicaid* is a program funded jointly by the federal government and the states, but it is administered at the state level. It was established to provide health care services to low-income children deprived of parental support, and their caretaker relatives, the elderly, the blind, and individuals with disabilities (CMS, 2013b).

Reimbursement for occupational therapy services that are provided to individuals who are diagnosed with a mental illness depends on the treatment setting, the sources of reimbursement (private insurance, public insurance, grants, or private funding), and the type of service being provided. The potential for expanded reimbursement for occupational therapy services under the PPACA will be discussed later in this chapter. Reimbursement for occupational therapy evaluation and treatment in specific settings will be discussed in Chapters 7 and 8.

This section of the chapter addressed the cultural, societal, and legislative factors that have affected the provision of mental health care in the United States, as well as the transition of service provision from inpatient to community-based settings. The next section will address the impact these factors have had on the evolution of mental health occupational therapy services, describe different service settings, discuss the potential impact of the PPACA on occupational therapy service provision, and identify opportunities for advocacy.

PART 2: OCCUPATIONAL THERAPY SERVICE SETTINGS IN THE MID-LIFESPAN

The Evolution of Occupational Therapy in Service Settings

Schwartz (2013) has stated that "the history of mental health treatment in the twentieth century provides a backdrop from which to view the evolution of psychosocial occupational therapy. It is important to remember that the profession did not develop in a vacuum" (p.. 113). Occupational therapy responded to changes in mental health treatment by developing its own innovative ideas about care and services. These ideas blended work in occupations and activities with new ideas about the treatment of the mentally ill.

Mental health treatment in the early 20th century was based on the principles of **moral treatment** and the psychobiological approaches of Adolph Meyer. The profession of occupational therapy (Peloquin, 1989), therapeutic communities (Hollander, 1981), and the Recovery Model (Shepherd, Boardman, & Slade, 2008) all have ties to the Moral Treatment Movement. As an early supporter of occupational therapy, Meyer believed there was a link between an individual's activities and activity patterns and his or her physical and mental health. Treatment in the early 20th century was generally provided in institutional settings; however, in his vision for the mental hygiene movement, Meyer advocated for community-based services to help people develop skills to cope with the demands of everyday living outside of the institution.

At the same time, Eleanor Clark Slagle began training occupational therapists. She taught them to create patient treatment goals that were based on three possible outcomes: (1) remaining in the institution, (2) returning to the community, and (3) preventing relapse for those already discharged to the community (Tiffany, 1978).

During the 1930s and 1940s, occupational therapists worked closely with psychiatrists in providing treatment to individuals diagnosed with a mental illness. Occupational therapy services were not initiated until a written prescription was received from the psychiatrist or physician treating the individual. The prescription would include information about the patient, precautions to be followed, and specific information about services being requested. Then, as now, occupational therapy focused on the whole person. Activities focused on the individual's life within the institution and included work, arts and crafts, recreation, and music (Hopkins & Smith, 1978).

In the 1940s and 1950s, the psychoanalytic object relation approach was added as part of mental health occupational therapy treatment, with Gail Fidler being one of the major proponents. She recommended that occupational therapy activities incorporate objects and object relations (the relationship with the nonhuman environment) as the primary treatment method. The 1950s also saw psychopharmacology shift from being used primarily for sedation to being used to target specific symptoms associated with psychosis, mania, and depression. This allowed patients to more fully participate in occupational therapy activities (Clauer & Wise, 1978).

The 1960s and 1970s were a time of questioning for those providing treatment in the field of mental health. Some occupational therapists believed that psychosocial occupational therapy would flounder because it was unable to articulate its uniqueness within the field of mental health. Woodside (1971) stated, "Society may lose a profession with a vibrant history and the potential for a healthy future. What are you doing to prevent this?"

In response, Shannon and Snortum (1965) described the use of activity or task-oriented groups as a complement to psychotherapy groups led by other professionals. In these groups, which would be led by an occupational therapist, the clients would have an opportunity to learn and practice new skills. Fidler (1969) envisioned a task-oriented group context in which a "laboratory for living" could take place. Reilly (1966) created a model occupational therapy treatment program and developed theory and research to substantiate its effectiveness. The model that Reilly and her colleagues developed was called *Occupational Behavior*. This would later evolve into the **Model of Human Occupation** (MOHO; Kielhofner, 2002)

It was also proposed at that time that the best environment for psychosocial occupational therapy might be within the community. Watanabe (1967) identified the client's home as the logical place to provide treatment. Howe and Dippy (1968) suggested that occupational therapists explore new practice sites such as community mental health centers or the psychiatric day hospitals. Bockoven (1971) strongly encouraged occupational therapists to provide services in the community based on moral treatment.

The 1980s and 1990s saw the development and refinement of several occupational therapy theoretical models and assessments that focused on the elements of occupation, context, and client-centered practice. These included the MOHO and the **Occupational Performance History Interview (OPHI)** developed by Kielhofner (1988; 2002); the Ecology of Human Performance Framework by Dunn, Brown, and McGuigan (1994); and the Canadian Occupational Therapy Performance Measure (COPM) by Baptiste and colleagues (1993). Their content reflected that of the Occupational Therapy Practice Framework (OTPF), which was published by AOTA in 2002 and revised in 2008 and 2013.

Psychosocial rehabilitation centers and clubhouses (non-hospital-based programs that provide restorative activities focused on an individual's strengths) were an environment where Fidler's "laboratory for living" took shape (Clubhouse International, 2013). A major focus of psychosocial rehabilitation is training in life skills (Hayes & Halford, 1993), including social skills, independent living, prevocational skills, stress management, and assertion (Schwartz, 2013). Other areas of psychosocial practice were identified. They included helping people cope with AIDS (Schindler, 1988), the need for development of cultural sensitivity and competence in therapists (Dillard et al., 1992), and women's mental health issues (Nahamias & Froelich, 1993). Psychosocial occupational therapists adhered closely to the humanistic principles of moral treatment, even when working within the medical model of inpatient psychiatric hospitals. The 1980s and 1990s were particularly significant for occupational therapy in that the profession began to focus on expanding and detailing the concept of occupation.

Continued advances in the efficacy of psychotropic medications drastically reduced the average length of stay for inpatient hospitalizations. Unfortunately, the decreased lengths of stay also reduced the number of occupational therapists working in inpatient settings. In 1973, 13.8% of all occupational therapists worked in an inpatient setting, whereas in 1990, that number declined to 4.6%. This percentage continued to shrink as the loss of occupational therapy positions in inpatient settings was not offset by an increase in community mental health positions. By the 1980s, it was apparent that the deinstitutionalization movement that began in the 1970s had not succeeded (Mollica, 1983). Sufficient funding was never provided to hire the necessary mental health professionals; community mental health centers were never built; residential homes were scarce and thus those with mental illnesses returned home to be cared for by their families, or were shifted from state institutions to nursing homes, or joined the ranks of the homeless (Schwartz, 2013, p. 120).

However, the move from inpatient to community-based care did provide the impetus for a treatment model shift from the medical model to a social model of care. The *Social Model,* which emphasizes the power of individuals with mental illnesses to direct and participate in their own recovery, ultimately developed into the *Recovery Movement* (Swarbrick, 2009). The fundamental concepts of the Recovery Movement include a holistic, individualized, and person-centered approach to treatment provision.

Another challenge faced by mental health professionals has been the managed care approach to reimbursement for services (VanLeit, 1995). In this approach, insurance companies scrutinize all of the services provided to the patients that they insure in an attempt to control costs. This has resulted in shortened lengths of stay, challenges to providing effective treatment, extensive paperwork and bureaucracy to justify treatment, and the loss of control of professional decision making. Despite these challenges, VanLeit

(1995) proposed that "at its best, managed care may actually support innovations and diversity of treatment approaches as long as empirical evidence supports the effectiveness of these approaches. It is even possible that mental health and substance abuse practices and outcomes may be improved" (p. 433). She argued that occupational therapists need to become visible, proactive, and accountable in the process of defining and developing a cost-effective continuum of programs and services. In addition, VanLeit encouraged therapists to emphasize community practice settings, identify effective treatment methods to measure outcome, and develop flexible guideline and implementation protocols.

Friedland and Renwick (1993) felt that voicing the belief that psychosocial occupational therapy practice was declining would possibly become a self-fulfilling prophecy. Consequently, they proposed that therapists get more involved in prevention and health promotion. "We should be involved in developing appropriate environments for housing the homeless … in facilitating adaptation in daily tasks for new immigrants … and in reducing stress and increasing well-being of persons in work and school environments" (p. 470).

Trickey and Kennedy (1995) conducted a survey of the agencies in South Carolina with mental health units. They examined why only a small percentage of occupational therapists worked in mental health. The researchers found that salary demands, turnover, lack of available applicants, and an inability to generate revenue were among the reasons facilities did not hire occupational therapists. On the other hand, Cottrell (1990) found that, despite the concerns voiced in the occupational therapy literature about a decline in psychosocial practice, there was a high level of perceived competence among the psychosocial occupational therapists that she surveyed. She reported that "90% of the 95 respondents perceived their ability to adapt their role to a changing practice and mental health system as good or excellent" (Cottrell, 1990, p. 122). In an article about the state of mental health practice, Bonder (1987) quoted Duhl (1982), who asserted, "mental health practitioners can influence the new paradigms that emerge by the ways they choose to work with their patients and in their communities. Thus, through our visions, we can create the future" (Bonder, 1987, p. 698).

Occupational Therapy Service Settings

Having reviewed the evolution of mental health treatment from an occupational therapy perspective, let us now review two approaches to mental health service delivery and settings in which mental health occupational therapy services can be provided. "As services for individuals with mental illnesses have shifted from the hospital to the community, there has also been a shift in the philosophy of service delivery. In the past, there was an adherence to

CHECKPOINT 6-2. REMEMBER	
• Community mental health settings	• Community support programs
• Community mental health centers (CMHCs)	• Outpatient treatment settings
• Assertive community treatment (ACT)	• Partial hospitalization programs (PHPs)
• Psychosocial rehabilitation centers/clubhouses	• Intensive outpatient programs (IOPs)
• Shelters	• Outpatient clinics
• Supported or transitional residential services	• Inpatient treatment settings

the medical model; now the focus is on incorporating the recovery model" (Castaneda, Olson & Cargill-Radley, 2013, p. 34).

The medical model and recovery models offer different approaches to providing mental health services. The medical model approach to service delivery often has the psychiatrist as the primary decision maker and overall coordinator of care. The focus is symptom management. These services can include medication management, group psychotherapy, and individual psychotherapy. The recovery model, on the other hand, has the consumer as the primary decision maker. The focus is individual choice and reintegration into community life. These services can include securing housing, managing finances, obtaining paid or volunteer employment, developing and maintaining supportive relationships in the community, skill training and resource development, and social role valorization (Anthony, Cohen, Farkas, & Gagne, 1990). Most consumers require both medical and recovery services to support their overall mental health and well-being.

> Rehabilitation is the learning process by which a person who has suffered physical, intellectual, and/or personality changes (secondary to injury or disease) recovers functioning to the extent possible, develops compensatory skills in areas where deficits persist, and adjusts emotionally to the level of functioning attained. Thus, rehabilitation is concerned with the patient's optimal physical recovery, reestablishment of skills, and achievement of a satisfactory quality of life. (Grief & Matterazo, 1982, p. 3)

The settings in which medical intervention and recovery approaches to treatment are offered can be found in Checkpoint 6-2. Each of these settings is described in more detail next.

Community Mental Health Settings

Community mental health settings provide services to adults who have been diagnosed with a mental illness. These settings can include, but are not limited to, CMHCs, *assertive community treatment (ACT)* teams, psychosocial rehabilitation centers/clubhouses, homeless shelters and

women's shelters, correctional facilities, senior centers, after-school programs, homes, and work sites (Brown & Stoffel, 2011; Castaneda, Olson, & Raley, 2013; Scheinholtz, 2010). Community mental health agencies can provide services to include supported or transitional residential services and community support programs.

Community Mental Health Centers

The CMS (2013a) define the core services offered by *community mental health centers*. These core services include the following:

- Outpatient services for children, the elderly, and individuals who are chronically mentally ill

- Residents of the CMHC's service area who have been discharged from inpatient treatment at a mental health facility

- 24-hour-a-day emergency care services

- Day treatment or other partial hospitalization or psychosocial rehabilitation services

- Screenings for patients being considered for admission to state mental health facilities to determine the appropriateness of such admissions

Assertive Community Treatment

The NAMI defines *ACT* as a service-delivery model that provides comprehensive, locally based treatment to people with serious and persistent mental illnesses. Unlike other community-based programs, ACT is not a linkage or brokerage case management program that connects individuals to mental health, housing, rehabilitation agencies, and services. Rather, ACT provides highly individualized services directly to consumers. ACT recipients receive multidisciplinary services and around-the-clock staffing of a psychiatric unit within the comfort of their own homes and communities. ACT team members are trained in the areas of psychiatry, social work, nursing, substance abuse, and vocational rehabilitation in order to have the competencies and skills necessary to provide for a client's multiple treatments, rehabilitation, and support needs. The ACT team provides these services 24 hours per day, 7 days per week, and 365 days per year.

Psychosocial Rehabilitation Centers/Clubhouses

Psychosocial rehabilitation centers and clubhouses provide a comprehensive dynamic program of supports for individuals with severe and persistent mental illnesses. Participants are called *members*. The restorative activities focus on a member's strengths rather than his or her impairments or illnesses. Participation in all activities is voluntary (Clubhouse International, 2013).

Shelters

Shelters describe living facilities providing temporary shelter to individuals who are homeless or victims of domestic violence. Structured programming may or may not be provided, and length of stay is variable.

Supported or Transitional Residential Services

Supported or transitional residential services are generally provided in a group home or apartment setting. They are designed to assist an individual in transitioning to a more independent living situation. They also help an individual remain stable in his or her current residential setting.

Community Support Programs

Community support programs are case management services provided by a team of mental health professionals. They focus on skill building and are generally provided to the individual outside of a facility, within the community (State of Connecticut Department of Mental Health and Addiction Services, 2014).

Partial Hospital Programs

A *partial hospital program (PHP)* provides services to individuals who, without those services, would likely require an inpatient level of care. Partial hospital programs are also used for clients who require further stabilization following an inpatient admission. These programs resemble short–term inpatient programs in that most of the treatment is offered in groups; however, the clients in a PHP return home at the end of the day. The services provided in a PHP differ from those offered in outpatient day treatment programs and psychosocial rehabilitation clubhouses in that any group activities that are considered to be social, recreational, and/or diversionary are not utilized for treatment.

Occupational therapy services provided in a PHP are covered by third party payers if it can be demonstrated through documentation that provision of such services required the skills of a qualified occupational therapist, and they were performed by an occupational therapist or occupational therapy assistant who was under the supervision of an occupational therapist (CMS, 2014).

Intensive Outpatient Programs

Intensive outpatient programs (IOP) are similar to PHPs. Patients in these programs, however, do not meet the criteria of being at risk for immediate hospitalization if the services were not provided. Therapeutic services are generally provided 3 to 5 days per week for an average of 3 hours per day. Lengths of stay are 2 to 6 weeks, and most services are provided in a group setting.

Outpatient Clinic

Outpatient clinics can be hospital or nonhospital based. They can provide a range of services such as medication management, individual psychotherapy, group psychotherapy, and case management services. These services are often provided in combination.

Outpatient Treatment Settings

Outpatient treatment can be provided in a variety of settings based on the needs of the individual. When the services are provided in a hospital based setting, the psychiatrist evaluates the client and remains actively involved throughout treatment. He or she provides direct supervision to the treatment team, including occupational therapy practitioners. All occupational services must be deemed reasonable and necessary to treat the patient's condition. In addition, improvement and/or stabilization of the patient's condition is expected (CMS, 2014).

Inpatient Treatment Setting

Inpatient treatment can be provided in a private inpatient setting, in for-profit or nonprofit community settings, or in public facilities sponsored by the state and federal government. Inpatient mental health units may be located within general hospitals, as well as hospitals that provide care exclusively to persons with a mental illness. Inpatient units can be either open or closed. The term *closed* refers to units in which the main entrance remains locked, preventing individuals from walking out of the hospital. Patients admitted to such settings are usually in an acute phase of their mental illness. They may be considered gravely disabled or a danger to themselves or others. Inpatient treatment is short term, which is usually less than 30 days; however, most inpatient admissions last less than 1 week.

With occupational therapists providing services across the mental health treatment continuum, it is important to examine how the PPACA might have an impact on the provision of occupational therapy services, especially as it relates to occupational therapy assistants. As discussed earlier in this chapter, the PPACA was designed to increase access to health care, increase quality of health care, and reduce health care costs. Included in the PPACA are 9 essential health benefits that must be offered at no dollar limits on every plan. These benefits are as follows: (1)

ambulatory patient services (outpatient care); (2)emergency services (trips to the emergency room); (3) hospitalization (treatment in the hospital for inpatient care); (4) maternity and newborn care; (5) mental health and addiction treatment; (6) prescription drugs and rehabilitative and habilitative services and devices; (7) laboratory services; (8) preventative services, wellness services, and (9) chronic disease treatment; and pediatric services (Obama Care Facts, 2014).

In an article entitled "Mental Health: Emphasizing Function and Performance," Tim Nanof (2012), director of public affairs at the AOTA, discussed the decline in occupational therapy practitioners working in mental health and the potential to increase these numbers under the PPACA. He stated that since the deinstitutionalization that followed the CMHA, the number of AOTA members working in mental health dropped from a high of 30% in the 1950s and early 1960s to less than 3% in 2012. He went on to point out that, with an estimated 32 million additional Americans expected to be covered by the PPACA, potentially 6 to 10 million would require mental health or substance abuse services. Citing a World Health Organization expectation, he stated that behavioral health disorders could surpass all physical causes of disability. With this increased demand, the community mental health system will need the services of occupational therapy practitioners.

Health Care Reform and the Occupational Therapy Assistant

The AOTA was active during the legislative process leading to the passage of the PPACA. AOTA worked to achieve victories such as inclusion of rehabilitation and habilitation with the 10 essential health benefits. One key focus of these efforts was to ensure that occupational therapy is a core component of the habilitation benefit. Habilitation includes services that are designed to help a person attain and maintain function. In contrast, rehabilitation has been limited to services that are designed to restore an individual to a previous level of function (Nanof, 2012).

As a vital part of the occupational therapy team, occupational therapy assistant practitioners in every state may see an increase in the number of potential clients in the future. Formerly uninsured persons who gain access to health insurance that covers occupational therapy services may seek services. In states that elect to expand Medicaid eligibility, even more people may have access to occupational therapy services, as occupational therapy will have to be covered as an essential health benefit. This could increase the demand for occupational therapy assistants to provide cost-effective services. Occupational therapy assistant practitioners will be able to provide habilitation services, which will have to be covered to some degree for most of the newly insured population, even if such coverage has often been excluded by private health insurance in the past.

Occupational therapy assistants may also have new opportunities to participate in care delivery models of the future such as Accountable Care Organizations (ACOs) and Patient-Centered Medical Homes (PCMHs). ACOs exist with different structures, but are generally systems of health care providers designed to improve patient outcomes, lower costs, and share in the resulting savings. PCMHs similarly can vary in terms of their structures, but generally consist of teams of health care providers coordinating an array of health care services across the care continuum, also with the goals of improving patient outcomes and lowering costs. (AOTA, 2014b, p. 1)

An increased emphasis on integrated, team-based, coordinated, and interdisciplinary care models will present new opportunities for occupational therapy assistants. Practitioners will be able to demonstrate the value of occupational therapy services and produce improved patient outcomes at lower cost. "New health care delivery models will create opportunities to promote the value and role of occupational therapy services in prevention, wellness, chronic disease management, and other areas" (AOTA, 2014b, p. 1). Occupational therapy practitioners can advocate for the use of their services to potential health care providers, employers, clients, and public policy decision makers. They can use the fact they are already recognized as educated, nationally credentialed, and highly skilled health care practitioners who are regulated by the state and recognized by major public and private payers as providers in order to promote themselves (AOTA, 2014b).

In addition to advocating for the profession, occupational therapy practitioners need to advocate for the individuals whom they serve. Advocacy is everyone's responsibility. An example of this comes from an individual who served in the Connecticut legislature and is the father of a boy who was diagnosed with schizophrenia. He offered the following comments with regard to the way mental health services are currently delivered and funded:

If I were a legislator today, I'd mandate—and provide funding to ensure—that every teacher receive training in recognizing symptoms of mental illness. I'd see that pediatricians are trained to make screening for mental health concerns a regular part of well-child exams. I'd require school administrators to incorporate recommendations from pediatricians and mental health professionals into students' IEPs. I'd put much more money into community mental health services. I'd integrate how services are delivered by funding collaborative community mental health programs and have them run by mental health professionals. I'd include services for chronically homeless people under this collaborative umbrella. And I'd make

CHECKPOINT 6-3. RESPOND
As you learn about each of these theories, respond to the following questions: 1. What is the name of the theory? 2. Who is the individual associated with its development? 3. What are the key points associated with this model? 4. Provide an example of a client who would benefit from treatment based on this model.

sure that there was supportive short-term and long-term community housing and treatment for everyone needing them. My son is schizophrenic. The "reforms" that I worked for have worsened his life (AOTA, 2012).

This section of the chapter examined the evolution of occupational therapy in various service settings, current occupational therapy service settings, health care reform, and the occupational therapy assistant and advocacy. In the final section of this chapter, occupational therapy and nonoccupational therapy theories and practice models will be discussed.

PART 3: MID-LIFESPAN PRACTICE MODELS AND THEORY

"A theory is a way of thinking about something" (Miller, 1988, p. 2). Gail Fidler, Anne C. Mosey, A. Jean Ayres, and Lena A. Llorens each used the term *theory* to refer to a conceptual framework when trying to explain, describe, or predict phenomena of concern to occupational therapy (Miller, 1988).

The term *model* was used by Mosey and Gary Kielhofner, although both used it in different ways. Kielhofner used the term to describe a conceptual framework or theory that was at the broad and complex end of the theory continuum, whereas Mosey used it to define the typical way in which a profession perceives itself, its relationship to other professions, and its association with the society to which it is responsible (Miller, 1988).

Miller (1988) stated that practice theories and frames of reference are two approaches that are used to relate theoretical systems to intervention. Both are systematic ways of organizing and applying knowledge to effect change, and are similar in that they share a common goal and use components of a theory. They serve as linking structures between theory and practice. Examples in the field of

occupational therapy would be Ayers, who used *theory*, and Mosey, who used *frames of reference* (Miller, 1988).

Nonoccupational Therapy Practice Models and Theories

In this section, nonoccupational therapy practice models, theories, and approaches to treatment will be described first, as some of these have formed foundations for occupational therapy theories, models, frames of reference, and treatment approaches. These will be followed by occupational therapy theories, practice models, and approaches to treatment. Checkpoint 6-3 provides questions to ask yourself as you learn about each of the following theories, practice models, and approaches to treatment.

Psychoanalytic Therapy

Sigmund Freud (1856-1939) was a neurologist and the originator of an approach to psychotherapy known as *psychoanalytic therapy*. The Freudian view of human nature is deterministic. According to Freud, the behavior of people is determined by irrational forces, unconscious motivations, biological and instinctual drives, and certain psychosexual events during the first 6 years of life (Cory, 1986, p. 12). Most theories of counseling and psychotherapy have been influenced in some way by psychoanalytic theory.

Adlerian Therapy

Alfred Adler (1870-1937) was a major contributor to the psychodynamic approach to therapy. Although he believed that the first 6 years of life largely determines who an individual becomes in adult life, unlike Freud, he believed that humans are motivated by social urges, that behavior is purposeful and goal directed, and that consciousness is the center of the personality (Cory, 1986). His theory stressed choice and responsibility, meaning in life, and self-realization. He proposed a subjective approach to psychology that focused "on internal determinants of behavior such as values, beliefs, attitudes, goals, interests, and the individual

TABLE 6-1

ERICKSON'S PSYCHOSOCIAL STAGES OF DEVELOPMENT

PERIOD OF LIFE	STAGE	PSYCHOSOCIAL TASK TO BE MASTERED
Infancy (0 to 1 years)	Trust vs. mistrust	To develop trust in others, especially in interpersonal relationships
Early childhood (1 to 3 years)	Autonomy vs. shame and doubt	To develop a sense of self-reliance
Preschool (3 to 6 years)	Initiative vs. guilt	To achieve a sense of competence and initiative
School age (6 to 11 years)	Industry vs. inferiority	To achieve a sense of being able to set and achieve personal goals
Adolescence (12 to 18 years)	Identity vs. role confusion	Clarification of self-identity, life goals, and life's meaning
Young adulthood (18 to 35 years)	Intimacy vs. isolation	To form intimate relationships
Middle ages (35 to 64 years)	Generativity vs. stagnation	To develop a sense of productivity
Later life (65 years and up)	Integrity vs. despair	To develop a sense of feeling personally worthwhile

Adapted from Cory, G. (1986). *Theory and practice for counseling and psychotherapy.* Pacific Grove, CA: Brooks/Cole Publishing Company.; Kaluger, G., & Kaluger, M. F. (1979). *Human development: The span of life.* St. Louis, MO: C. V. Mosby Company.

perception of reality" and that was "holistic, social, goal oriented, and humanistic" (Cory, 1986, p. 46).

Rational Emotive Therapy

Albert Ellis (1913-2007) "developed rational-emotive therapy (RET) after finding that his training as a psychoanalyst was inadequate in dealing with his clients" (Cory, 1986, p. 209). *RET's* basic hypothesis is that our emotions come from irrational beliefs, evaluations, interpretations, and reactions to life situations. In therapy, clients learn skills that give them the tools to identify and dispute irrational beliefs. They learn how to replace ineffective ways of thinking with effective and rational thoughts. As a result, they change their emotional reactions to situations (Cory, 1986).

Developmental Theory

Erik Erickson (1902-1994) was a developmental psychologist and psychoanalyst known for his theory on the psychosocial development of human beings. Erickson built on Freud's ideas and extended his theory by stressing the psychosocial aspects of development beyond early childhood. Erickson's *developmental theory* holds that psychosexual growth and psychosocial growth take place together. Individuals face the task of establishing equilibrium between themselves and their social world during each stage of life. Erickson described development in terms of the entire lifespan divided by specific crises to be resolved.

Table 6-1 depicts the stages of life and the crisis associated with each of them. According to Erickson, a crisis is equivalent to a turning point in life when people have the potential to move forward or regress. People either achieve successful resolution of conflicts or fail to resolve them at these turning points in development. To a large extent, life is the result of the choices we make at each of these stages.

Maslow's Hierarchy of Needs

Abraham Maslow (1908-1970), a psychologist, created a *hierarchy of needs* represented by five levels. Table 6-2 depicts the levels in this hierarchy.

The lower level is composed of "deficiency" or survival-based needs that include physiological, safety, and social needs. As a person moves up the hierarchy, the needs become less survival driven and more focused on components of happiness and personal success. Among the higher-level needs is the need for esteem. Self-actualization, the point at which the individual has realized his or her full potential, is at the top of the hierarchy. According to Maslow, lower-level needs have to be met before a person is able to concentrate on meeting higher-level needs.

Existential Therapy

Existential therapy was not founded by one particular person or group. It arose spontaneously in different parts of Europe. Rollo May and Irvin Yalom are the two men most associated with existential therapy in the United States.

TABLE 6-2
MASLOW'S HIERARCHY OF NEEDS

Self-Actualization	Morality, creativity, spontaneity, problem solving, lack of prejudice, acceptance of facts
Esteem Needs	Self-esteem, confidence, achievement, respect of others, respected by others
Social needs (Love/ Belonging)	Friendship, family, sexual intimacy
Safety Needs	Security of body, employment, resources, morality, family, health, property
Physiological Needs	Air, water, food, clothing, shelter, sex, sleep, excretion

Adapted from Andonian, L., Cara, E., & MacRae, A. (2013). Psychological theories and their treatment methods in mental health practice. In E. Cara & A. MacRae (Eds.). *Psychosocial occupational therapy: An evolving practice* (3rd ed., pp. 128-164). Clifton Park, NY: Delmar.; Maslow, A. (1943). Hierarchy of needs. Retrieved from www.abraham-maslow.com/m_motivation/Hierarchy_of_Needs.asp.

The existential view is grounded in the here and now and is based on a growth model that conceptualizes health rather than sickness. Existential therapy is considered an intellectual approach to therapeutic practice or a philosophy on which a therapist operates. It stands for a respect for the person, for exploring new aspects of human behavior, and for divergent methods of understanding people. It uses numerous approaches to therapy based on its assumptions about human nature (Cory, 1986).

Humanistic Perspective

The *humanistic perspective* focuses on the value, worth, and potential of the individual, with an emphasis on the integrity of the client–therapist relationship. Humanism developed as an alternative to psychodynamic and behavioral perspectives. English Quaker Samuel Tuke (1732-1819) took humanistic theory into clinical practice when he developed moral treatment, which was discussed earlier in this chapter. Moral treatment focused on the humane treatment of individuals with mental illness. Patients were encouraged to participate in a variety of work, leisure, and self-care activities that Tuke found had a positive, reality-orienting impact as it focused on the inherent worth of each individual (Andonian, Cara, & MacRae, 2013).

Person-Centered Approach

The *person-centered approach* is a humanistic branch of the existential perspective. It was developed by Carl Rogers (1902-1987), a psychologist, and is based on the belief that humans can develop in a positive and constructive manner if a climate of respect and trust is established. The person-centered approach aims for a greater degree of independence and integration of the individual, with the focus being on the person rather than the person's presenting problem. The goal of therapy is not to simply solve problems, but to also assist the client in his or her growth

process so that he or she can better cope with current and future problems (Cory, 1986).

Gestalt Therapy

Gestalt therapy is a form of existential therapy that was developed by Frederick Perls (1893-1970), a psychiatrist and psychotherapist. It is "based on the premise that people must find their own way in life and accept personal responsibility if they hope to achieve maturity. The basic goal is for clients to gain awareness of what they are experiencing and doing and thus to learn that they are responsible for what they are feeling, thinking, and doing" (Cory, 1986, p. 120). Perls took a holistic approach to personality, as he believed that every element of the person is connected to the whole. He was more concerned with exploring the here and now and the importance of examining one's present situation, as the past is gone and the future has not arrived. Perls felt that focusing on the past was a way of avoiding coming to terms with the full experience of the present (Cory, 1986).

Behavioral Therapy

The *behavioral approach,* originated in the 1950s and early 1960s, and was a radical departure from the psychoanalytic perspective. In behavioral therapy, there is an emphasis on cognition and action-oriented methods to help the individual take steps to change his or her behaviors. There were three major areas of development in the behavioral movement: classical conditioning, operant conditioning, and cognitive therapy.

In classical conditioning, behaviors are elicited from a passive organism. Examples of classical behaviors would include a knee jerk or salivation. In operant conditioning, behaviors are emitted from an active organism. Operant behaviors are those actions that operate on the environment to produce consequences.

Examples of operant behaviors include reading, writing, driving a car, and eating with utensils—the types of behaviors we perform in everyday life. When environmental change brought about by a behavior is reinforcing (provides a reward or avoids a negative consequence), the behavior is likely to occur again. If the behavior produces no reinforcement, then the behavior is less likely to recur (Cory, 1986).

Classical conditioning and operant conditioning models do not generally include insight-oriented concepts such as thinking, attitudes, and values. The cognitive trend in behavior therapy took these factors into consideration and used them in the therapeutic process.

Current behavioral therapy encompasses a variety of conceptualizations, research methods, and treatment approaches to explain and change behavior. It is grounded in a scientific view of human behavior that implies a systematic and structured approach to counseling where the person is the producer and the product of his or her environment (Cory, 1986).

Cognitive Therapy

Aaron T. Beck (b. 1921) is a psychiatrist who developed an approach known as *cognitive therapy*, which is similar to RET in that it assists the client in recognizing and discarding self-defeating thoughts. Beck was interested in his clients' automatic thoughts, particularly negative thoughts that persist even though they are contrary to objective evidence. He concluded that a client's internal dialogue plays a major role in behavior because the ways in which clients monitor and instruct themselves, give themselves praise or criticism, interpret events, and make predictions can provide insight into emotional disorders such as depression. Cognitive therapy can involve homework assignments to record self-defeating thoughts and then review them to form alternative observations (Cory, 1986)

Cognitive Behavior Therapy

Cognitive behavior therapy (CBT) is an approach to treatment that focuses on examining the relationship between thoughts, feelings, and behaviors. CBT combines basic behavioral and cognitive principles to assist individuals in exploring patterns of thinking that lead to self-destructive actions and the beliefs that direct these thoughts. Common features of CBT include the focus on the here and now and a directive or guidance role of the therapist. CBT is thought to be effective in the treatment of mood, anxiety, personality, eating, substance abuse, tic, and psychotic disorders (NAMI, 2014a).

Dialectical Behavior Therapy

Dialectical behavior therapy (DBT) was developed by Marsha M. Linehan (b. 1943), a psychologist and researcher. DBT is a comprehensive cognitive behavior treatment for complex, difficult-to-treat mental disorders such as borderline personality disorder (BPD) (Dimeff & Linehan,

2001). "BPD is a pattern of instability in interpersonal relationships, self-image, and affects, marked by impulsivity" (American Psychiatric Association, 2013, p. 645). DBT combines standard cognitive behavior techniques with Eastern mindfulness practices. DBT is an evidenced-based practice for treating BPD, and has also been effective in treating patients who present with mood disorders and self-injury and those with chemical dependency. DBT involves individual and group skill training and psychotherapy focusing on mindfulness, distress tolerance, emotion regulation, and interpersonal effectiveness (Dimeff & Linehan, 2001).

Motivational Interviewing

Motivational interviewing (MI) was developed by clinical psychologists William R. Miller and Stephen Rollnick, and utilizes a directive, client-centered counseling style that assists clients in exploring and resolving their ambivalence about changing problematic behavior (Rollnick & Miller, 1995). Prochaska, Norcross, and DiClemente (1994) identified six distinct stages of change: precontemplation, contemplation, preparation, action, maintenance, and termination. Ambivalence is a natural state of uncertainty that clients experience as they approach the change process due to conflicting feeling about the process and the outcomes of the change (Center for Evidenced-Based Practices, 2011). MI helps the client to examine and resolve this ambivalence (Rollnick & Miller, 1995).

MI recognizes that clients who need to make a change in their lives approach counseling at different levels of readiness. During counseling, some patients may have considered, but not initiated, steps to change behaviors. Other clients, especially those voluntarily seeking counseling, may be actively trying to change their behavior and may have been doing so unsuccessfully for years.

MI is nonjudgmental, nonconfrontational, and nonadversarial. It attempts to increase the client's awareness of the potential problems caused, consequences experienced, and risks faced as a result of the behavior in question. Alternatively, therapists help clients envision a better future and become increasingly motivated to achieve it. The strategy seeks to help clients think differently about their behavior and ultimately to consider what might be gained through change. It is critical to meet clients where they are (Prochaska, 1983) and not force clients toward change when they have not expressed a desire to do so.

Wellness Recovery Action Plan

Wellness Recovery Action Plan (WRAP) is a self-management and recovery system. It was developed by a group of people who had a variety of psychiatric symptoms and were trying to incorporate wellness tools and strategies into their lives so that they could feel better and move forward. WRAP is designed to decrease and prevent intrusive or troubling feelings and behaviors, to increase personal empowerment, to improve quality of life, and to assist people in achieving their own life goals and dreams (Copeland Center for Wellness and Recovery, 2012). WRAP was designed as a structured system to help the individual monitor uncomfortable and distressing feelings and behaviors. It focuses on reducing, modifying, or eliminating them through planned responses. The person experiencing symptoms is the one who develops his or her personal WRAP. The person may choose to have supporters and health care professionals help create the WRAP.

WRAP is being utilized in formal and informal recovery programs in all 50 states, as well as around the world. It has been recognized as an evidence-based practice approach in the field of mental health recovery. Researchers from the Department of Psychiatry at the University of Illinois recently conducted a study of 80 individuals who participated in WRAP programs. The research revealed significant improvements in symptoms and many psychosocial outcome areas associated with the recovery. Other research studies have validated the fact that significant numbers of people with mental health problems and substance abuse disorders have been able to self-manage their conditions with positive outcomes for over 2 decades (Onken et al., 2007).

Mindfulness

Jon Kabat-Zinn defined *mindfulness* as "the awareness that emerges through paying attention on purpose, in the present moment, and nonjudgmentally to the unfolding of experience moment by moment" (Kabat-Zinn, 2003, p. 145). Through mindfulness, the individual maintains a moment-by-moment awareness of thoughts, feelings, bodily sensations, and the surrounding environment. One pays attention to thoughts and feelings without judging them. When practicing mindfulness, the individual's thoughts tune into what is in the present moment rather than rehashing the past or imagining the future. Mindfulness has its roots in Buddhist meditation, but a secular practice of mindfulness entered the American mainstream through the work of Jon Kabat-Zinn and his Mindfulness-Based Stress Reduction (MBSR) program (Greater Good, 2014). Research on mindful meditation identifies that it improves emotional regulation and cognitive functioning, including memory, decision making, and focus. Mindful meditation also decreases the fear response, impulsive behavior, and mood disturbances. Research into meditation and its health benefits has been widely accepted. A mindfulness-based program is beneficial to those suffering from chronic illness, anxiety, and depression, as well as a variety of other problems.

Occupational Therapy Theories and Models of Practice

The principles of moral treatment formed the basis for psychiatric practice and the use of activity in occupational therapy treatment (Tiffany, 1978). At its inception, occupational therapy was part of the humanistic movement, and Adolph Meyer is often viewed as its philosophical founder (Peters, 2011).

The 1930s, 1940s, and 1950s saw occupational therapists working within the psychoanalytic frame of reference and exploring psychodynamic principles for treatment and activity analysis (Tiffany, 1978). With passage of the CMHA in 1963, new approaches to mental health treatment emerged with an emphasis on returning individuals to community functioning more rapidly, which resulted in a shift from the long-term, deep methods of psychoanalysis. This greatly expanded the service settings and approaches to treatment used by mental health occupational therapists. As new theories emerged in psychiatry, mental health occupational therapists developed theories and approaches reflective of the current trends. It has seemed, however, that the profession's theoretical approaches eventually returned to its humanistic roots (Tiffany, 1978). Having examined nonoccupational therapy theories, practice models, and approaches to treatment, let us now review some of those related to the field of occupational therapy.

As has been mentioned, Gail Fidler recommended that occupational therapy activities use the psychoanalytic object and objects relations approach as a primary treatment method. She sought to develop a rationale for the behavior of her patients in occupational therapy and to find a way to determine if that behavior was useful. She viewed purposeful activity as the core of occupational therapy and saw the use of activity as a communication process whereby thoughts and feelings were expressed nonverbally. She also stressed that object relationships are important for human development and functioning, and therefore used activities to facilitate the group process and development of interpersonal relationships. Training in communication, coping, social, and assertiveness skills were incorporated into occupational therapy treatment programs where the aforementioned "laboratory for living" could take place (Andonian et al., 2013).

Anne Mosey was influenced by Gail Fidler. She described activities therapy as being based on the assumption that psychosocial dysfunction is a lack of understanding of the self, or the inability to participate in the varied and complex tasks of everyday life, or both (Mosey, 1973). As a treatment, activity therapy was a here-and-now, action-oriented model, and involved learning through doing. There was an emphasis on the mastery of the nonhuman environment, with nonhuman objects being utilized in activities designed to enhance self-awareness and interpersonal relationships. Activities therapy was concerned with growth through action (Mosey, 1973).

Lela A. Llorens was another early occupational therapy practitioner who influenced theory development. She selected preoccupational therapy theorists, including Gesell, Piaget, Havighurst, Erickson, and Freud, and systematically applied their theories to occupational therapy practice in formulating her ***developmental frame of reference***. In this frame of reference, activities are used to facilitate human growth and development by enabling one to explore the environment, establish relationships, acquire knowledge, and adapt successfully to one's world.

When the University of Southern California questioned whether psychosocial occupational therapy should remain in the university curriculum, Mary Reilly created a model occupational therapy treatment program. It was based on a developmental framework that assumed old behaviors could be restored and new behaviors could be learned. There was an emphasis on the importance of work and the development of an individual's capacity for self-direction and decision making, thus giving the client the ability to take responsibility for his or her own decisions. Each client had a structured schedule that provided more normal living experiences. This schedule drew on Adolph Meyer's thoughts regarding the importance of habits, routine, temporal adaptation, and the balance of work and play. The program became the foundation for a theoretical model developed by Reilly and her colleagues called *Occupational Behavior*. Gary Kielhofner, who was a student of Reilly, further developed this model into what later became known as the *MOHO* (Schwartz, 2013).

MOHO grew out of Dr. Gary Kielhofner's master's thesis and occupational practice in the mid-1970s. It seeks to explain how occupation is motivated, patterned, and performed, and provides a broad and integrative view of human occupation. The individual is seen as being made up of three interrelated components: volition, habituation, and performance capacity. Volition is the motivation for occupation, habituation is the process by which occupation is organized into patters or routines, and performance capacity is the physical and mental abilities that underlie skilled occupational performance. MOHO also emphasizes the importance of the physical and social environments in which occupation takes place. It aims to understand occupation and to explain problems of occupation that occur in terms of the primary concepts of volition, habituation, performance capacity, and environmental context. It is intended for use with any person experiencing problems in his or her occupational life, and is designed to be applicable across the lifespan (University of Illinois at Chicago, 2014). With its focus on occupation, habits, routines, and motivation, it is a strong model for psychosocial practice (Schwartz, 2013). MOHO will be addressed further in Chapters 7 and 8.

SUMMARY

In this chapter, the transition of mental health occupational therapy treatment from being primarily an inpatient-based service to a primarily outpatient-based service was exemplified from three different perspectives. The first discussed the cultural, legislative, and societal factors affecting the treatment of adults in the mid-lifespan; the second examined occupational therapy service settings; and the third looked at the evolution of both nonoccupational therapy and occupational therapy theories and practice models. Chapters 7 and 8 will examine occupational therapy assessment and treatment of adults in the mid-lifespan.

PART 4: APPLICATIONS

1. Explore one of the pieces of legislation discussed in Part 1 and identify its impact on mental health occupational therapy service provision.

2. NAMI is often one of the first organizations a family member turns to for education and support when a loved one has been diagnosed with a mental illness. Explore the NAMI website (www.nami.org) from the perspective of a family member.

3. Select one of the treatment settings from Part 2 with which you are the least familiar and explore it further from the perspective of mental health occupational therapy service provision.

4. DBT, MI, CBT, WRAP, and mindfulness are all nonoccupational therapy models/approaches that are familiar to most mental health professionals. Select one and explore it further from both an occupational therapy and nonoccupational therapy perspective.

5. The MOHO is familiar to most occupational therapy professionals and was designed for use with any person experiencing problems in his or her occupational life. Explore it further from both a mental health and non–mental health occupational therapy perspective.

REFERENCES

American Occupational Therapy Association. (2012). The Pulse: The reforms I fought for worsened the life of my son with schizophrenia. Retrieved from www.washingtonpost.com/national/health-science/my-son-is-schizophrenic-the-reforms-that-i-worked-for-have-worsened-his-life/2012/10/15/87b74a98-eadd-11e1-b811-09036bcb182b_story.html

American Occupational Therapy Association. (2014a). About AOTA. Retrieved from www.aota.org/en/About AOTA.aspx.

American Occupational Therapy Association. (2014b). Health care reform and the occupational therapy assistant. Retrieved from www.aota.org/-/media/Corporate/Files/Advocacy/Health-Care-Reform/HCR-OTA.pdf.

American Psychiatric Association. (2013). *Diagnostic and statistical manual of mental disorders* (5th ed.). Washington, DC: American Psychiatric Publishing.

American Public Health Association. (2013). Health reform resources. Retrieved from https://www.apha.org/topics-and-issues/health-reform/health-reform-resources.

Andonian, L., Cara, E. & MacRae, A. (2013). Psychological theories and their treatment methods in mental health practice. In E. Cara, & A. MacRae (Eds.), *Psychosocial occupational therapy: An evolving practice* (3rd ed., pp. 128-164). Clifton Park, NY: Delmar.

Anthony, W. A., Cohen, M., Farkas, M., & Gagne, C. (1990). *Psychiatric rehabilitation.* Boston, MA: Boston University, Center for Psychiatric Rehabilitation.

Baptiste, S., Law, M., Pollock, N., Polatajko, H., McColl, M. A., & Carswell, A. (1993). The Canadian Occupational Performance Measure. *World Federation of Occupational Therapy Bulletin, 28,* 47-51.

Bockoven, J. S. (1971). Legacy of moral treatment: 1800s to 1910. *American Journal of Occupational Therapy, 25*(5), 223-225.

Bonder, B. (1987). Occupational therapy in mental health: Crisis or opportunity? *American Journal of Occupational Therapy, 41,* 495-499.

Boston University College of Health & Rehabilitation Sciences: Sargent College. (2014). The Rehabilitation Act of 1973. Retrieved from http://cpr.bu.edu/resources/reasonable-accommodations/the-rehabilitation-act-of-1973.

Brown, C., & Stoffel, V. (2011). *Occupational therapy in mental health: A vision for participation.* Philadelphia, PA: F. A. Davis.

Brown, D. & McKenna, T., (2013). Capital briefing: Identifying new roles for occupational therapy professionals in primary care. *OT Practice, 18*(13), 5.

Castaneda, R., Olson, L. M., & Radley, L. C. (2013). Occupational therapy's role in community mental health. Retrieved from www.aota.org/en/About-Occupational-Therapy/Professionals/MH/Community-Mental-Health.aspx.

Center for Evidence-Based Practices. (2011). Practices: Motivational interviewing. Retrieved from www.centerforebp.case.edu/practices/mi.

Centers for Disease Control and Prevention. (2014). Health insurance coverage. Retrieved from www.cdc.gov/nchs/fastats/health_insure.htm.

Centers for Medicare & Medicaid Services. (2013a). Community mental health centers. Retrieved from www.cms.gov/Medicare/Provider-Enrollment-and-Certification/CertificationandCompliance/CommunityHealthCenters.html.

Centers for Medicare & Medicaid Services. (2013b). History. Retrieved from www.cms.gov/About-CMS/Agency-Information/History/index.html?redirect=/history/.

Centers for Medicare & Medicaid Services. (2014). Medicare benefit policy manual. Chapter 6—Hospital services covered under Part B. Retrieved from www.cms.gov/Regulations-and-Guidance/Guidance/Manuals/downloads/bp102c06.pdf.

Clauer, C., & Wise, K. (1958). Tranquilizing drug effects on the schizophrenic patient in occupational therapy. *American Journal of Occupational Therapy, 12,* 69-73.

Clubhouse International. (2013a). About us: Mission and history. Retrieved from www.iccd.org/history.html.

Colorado State University. (2014). A brief history of legislation. Retrieved from http://rds.colostate.edu/history-of-legislation.

Copeland Center for Wellness and Recovery. (2012). The Wellness Recovery Action Plan (WRAP). Retrieved from http://copelandcenter.com/wellness-recovery-action-plan-wrap.

Cory, G. (1986). *Theory and practice of counseling and psychotherapy.* Pacific Grove, CA: Brooks/Cole Publishing Company.

Cottrell, R. F. (1990). Perceived competence among occupational therapists in mental health. *American Journal of Occupational Therapy, 44,* 69-73.

Dillard, M., Andonian, L., Flores, O., Lai, L., MacRae, A., & Shakier, M. (1992). Culturally competent occupational therapy in a diversely populated mental health setting. *American Journal of Occupational Therapy, 46,* 721-726.

Dimeff, L. & Linehan, M. M. (2001). Dialectical behavioral therapy in a nutshell. *The California Psychologist, 34,* 10-13. Retrieved from www.dbtselfhelp.com/DBTinaNutshell.pdf.

Duhl, L. (1982). New paradigms for mental health. *Hospital and Community Psychiatry, 33,* 693.

Dunn, W., Brown, C., & McGuigan, A. (1994). The ecology of human performance: A framework for considering the effects of context. *American Journal of Occupational Therapy, 48,* 595-607.

Fidler, G. S. (1969). The task oriented group as a context for treatment. *American Journal of Occupational Therapy, 23,* 43-48.

Friedland, J., & Renwick, R. M. (1993). The issue is psychosocial occupational therapy: Time to cast off the doom and gloom. *American Journal of Occupational Therapy, 47,* 467-471.

Greater Good: The Science of a Meaningful Life. (2014). *What is mindfulness?* Retrieved from http://greatergood.berkeley.edu/topic/mindfulness/definition.

Grief, E. & Matarazzo, R. G. (1982). *Behavioral approaches to rehabilitation: Coping with change.* New York: Springer Publishing Company.

Gutman, S. S. (2011). From the desk of the editor – Special issue: Effects of occupational therapy services in mental health practice. *American Journal of Occupational Therapy, 65*(3), 235-237. doi: 10.5014/ajot.2011.001339.

Hampton, N. Z. & Zhu, Y. (2011). Gender, culture, and attitudes toward people with psychiatric disabilities. *Journal of Applied Rehabilitation Counseling, 42*(3), 12-19.

Hayes, R., & Halford, W. K. (1993). Generalization of occupational therapy effects in psychiatric rehabilitation. *American Journal of Occupational Therapy, 47,* 161-167.

Hollander, R. (1981, Summer). Moral treatment and the therapeutic community. *Psychiatric Quarterly, 53*(2), 132-138.

Hopkins, H. L., & Smith, H. D. (Eds.). (1978). *Willard and Spackman's occupational therapy* (5th ed.). Philadelphia, PA: Lippincott

Howe, M., & Dippy, K. (1968). The role of occupational therapy in community mental health. *American Journal of Occupational Therapy, 22,* 521-524.

Institute of Medicine of the National Academies. (2004). *Insuring America's health: Principles and recommendations.* Washington, D.C.: The National Press. Retrieved from http://iom.nationalacademies.org/en/Reports/2004/Insuring-Americas-Health-Principles-and-Recommendations.aspx

Kabat-Zinn, J. (2003). Mindfulness based interventions in context: Past, present, and future. *Clinical Psychology Science and Practice, 10,* 144-156.

Kaluger, G. & Kaluger, M. F. (1979). *Human development: The span of life.* St. Louis, MO: C. V. Mosby Company.

Kielhofner, G. (2002). *Model of human occupation* (3rd ed.). Philadelphia, PA: Lippincott Williams and Wilkins.

Kielhofner, G., & Henry, A. D. (1988). Development and investigation of the Occupational Performance History Interview. *American Journal of Occupational Therapy, 42*(8), 489-498.

Law, M., Baptiste, S., Carswell, A., McColl, A., Polatajko, H., & Pollak, N. (2005). *The Canadian occupational performance measure* (4th ed.). Ottawa, Ontario: Canadian Occupational Therapy Association.

Maslow, A. (1943). Hierarchy of needs. Retrieved from www.abrahammaslow.com/m_motivation/Hierarchy_of_Needs.asp.

Miller, B. R. J. (1988). What is theory, and why does it matter? In *Six Perspectives on Theory for the Practice of Occupational Therapy* (pp. 1-16). Rockville, MD: Aspen Publishers.

Mollica, R. F. (1983). From asylum to community. The threatened disintegration of public policy. *New England Journal of Medicine, 308,* 367-372.

Mosey, A. C. (1973). *Activity therapy.* New York, NY: Raven Press.

Nahamias, R., & Froelich, J. (1993). Women's mental health: Implications for occupational therapy. *American Journal of Occupational Therapy, 47,* 35-41.

Nanof, T. (2012). Capital briefing: Mental health: Emphasizing function and performance. *OT Practice 17*(3), 5.

National Alliance on Mental Illness. (2013). Assertive community treatment fact sheet reviewed by Duckworth, K. & Freedman, J. Retrieved from http//ww.nami.org.

National Alliance on Mental Illness. (2014a). Cognitive behavioral therapy fact sheet reviewed by Duckworth, K. & Freedman, J. Retrieved from http//ww.nami.org.

National Alliance on Mental Illness. (2014b). About NAMI. Retrieved from www.nami.org/template.cfm?section+About_NAMI.

National Council for Behavioral Health. (2013). Community Mental Health Act. Retrieved from www.thenationalcouncil.org/about/national-mental-health-association/overview/community-mental-health-act/.

Obama Care Facts. (2014). Obama Care essential health benefits. Retrieved from http://obamacarefacts.com/essential-health-benefits.php.

Onken, S. J., Craig, C. M., Ridgway, P., Ralph, R. O., & Cook, J. A. (2007). An analysis of the definitions and elements of recovery: A review of the literature. *Psychiatric Rehabilitation Journal, 31*(1), 9-22.

Peloquin, S. M. (1989). Moral treatment: Contexts considered. *American Journal of Occupational Therapy, 43*(8), 537-544.

Peters, C. (2011). History of mental health: Perspectives of consumers and practitioners. In C. Brown & V. C. Stoffel (Eds.) & J. P. Munoz (A. Ed.), *Occupational therapy in mental health: A vision for participation.* Philadelphia, PA: F. A. Davis Company.

Prochaska, J. O., Norcross, J. C., & DiClemente, C. C. (1994). *Changing for good: A revolutionary six-stage program for overcoming bad habits and moving your life positively forward.* New York, NY: Avon Books.

Random History and Word Origins for the Curious Mind. (2009). In sickness and in health: The history of health insurance. Retrieved from www.randomhistory.com/2009/03/31_health-insurance.html.

Reilly, M. (1966). A psychiatric occupational therapy program as a teaching model. *American Journal of Occupational Therapy, 20,* 61-67.

Rollnick, S. & Miller, W. R. (1995). What is motivational interviewing? *Behavioral and Cognitive Psychotherapy, 23,* 325-334. Retrieved from www.motivationalinterview.net/clinical/whatismi.html.

Scheinholtz, M. (2010). *Occupational therapy in mental health: Considerations for advanced practice.* Bethesda, MD: AOTA Press.

Schindler, V. (1988). Psychosocial occupational therapy with AIDS patients. *America Journal of Occupational Therapy, 42,* 507-512.

Schwartz, K. B. (2013). The history and philosophy of psychosocial occupational therapy. In E. Cara, & A. MacRae (Eds.), *Psychosocial occupational therapy: An evolving practice* (3rd ed., pp. 100-102). Clifton Park, NY: Delmar.

Shannon, P., & Snortum, J. (1965). An activity group's role in intensive psychotherapy. *American Journal of Occupational Therapy, 19,* 344-347.

Shepherd, G., Boardman, J., & Slade, M. (2008). Making recovery a reality. Retrieved from http://imroc.org/wp-content/uploads/Making_recovery_a_reality_policy_paper.pdf

State of Connecticut Department of Mental Health and Addiction Services. (2014). Redefining case management: The Community Support Program (CSP) and the Recovery Pathways (RP) Initiative. Retrieved from www.ct.gov/dmhas/cwp/view.asp?q=457094.

Swarbrick, M. (2009). Historical perspective: From institution to community. *Occupational Therapy in Mental Health, 25,* 201-233.

Tiffany, E. G. (1978). Psychiatry and mental health. In H. H. Hopkins, & H. D. Smith (Eds.), *Willard and Spackman's occupational therapy* (5th ed., pp. 269-334. Philadelphia, PA: J. B. Lippincott Company.

Thomasson, M. (2003). Health insurance in the United States. In Whaples, R. (Ed), *EH.Net Encyclopedia.* Retrieved from http://eh.net/encyclopedia/health-insurance-in-the-united-states

Trickey, B. A., & Kennedy, D. B. (1995). Use of occupational therapists in mental health settings in North Carolina. *American Journal of Occupational Therapy, 49,* 452-455.

United States Census Bureau. (2014). Health insurance main. Retrieved from https://www.census.gov/hhes/www/hlthins/.

United States Department of Justice, Civil Rights Division. (2014a). Information and technical assistance on the Americans with Disabilities Act –Introduction to the ADA. Retrieved from www.ada.gov/ada_intro.htm.

United States Department of Justice, Civil Rights Division. (2014b). Questions and answers about the Department of Justice's Notice of Proposed Rulemaking to Implement the Americans with Disabilities Act Amendments Act of 2008. Retrieved from www.ada.gov/nprm_adaaa/adaaa-nprm-qa.htm.

United States Department of Labor, Employee Benefits Security Administration. (2010). Fact sheet—The Mental Health Parity and Addiction Equity Act of 2008 (MHPAEA). Retrieved from www.dol.gov/ebsa/newsroom/fsmhpaea.html.

University of Illinois at Chicago. (2014). Model of Human Occupation: Theory and application. Retrieved from www.uic.edu/depts/moho/intro.html.

VanLeit, B. (1995). Managed mental health care: Reflections in a time of turmoil. *American Journal of Occupational Therapy, 50,* 428-434.

Watanabe, S. G. (1967). The developmental role of occupational therapy in a psychiatric home service. *American Journal of Occupational Therapy, 21,* 353-356.

Woodside, H. (1971). The development of occupational therapy 1910-1929. *American Journal of Occupational Therapy, 25*(5), 226-230.

7

Development and Participation in Occupation
The Mid-Lifespan
Christine A. Manville, EdD, OTR/L

KEY TERMS

• Client Factors	• Expansive Mood	• Panic Attack
• Cultural Factors	• Generalization	• Performance Patterns
• Delusion	• Grandiosity	• Performance Skills
• Development	• Hallucination	• Psychosis
• Disorganized Behavior	• Illusion	• Relapse
• Disorganized Thinking and Speech	• Lability of Mood	• Role
	• Manic Episode	• Substance Use
• Euphoria	• Negative Symptoms	• Tolerance
• Exacerbation	• Occupational Identity	• Withdrawal

CHAPTER LEARNING OBJECTIVES

After completion of this chapter, students should be able to:

1. Discuss the development of occupational identity and the factors that contribute to it.

2. Identify the major tasks and primary life roles of individuals in the mid-lifespan.

3. Describe the symptoms associated with mental health disorders (schizophrenia and other psychotic disorders, depressive disorders, generalized anxiety disorder, bipolar and related disorders, substance-related disorders, personality disorders).

4. Recognize the potential impact of these symptoms on performance of occupations.

5. Formulate questions to gather information for the occupational profile.

6. Analyze the role of the occupational therapy assistant in the evaluation process.

7. Contribute to the creation of an occupational profile.

Manville, C.A., & Keough, J. L.
Mental Health Practice for the Occupational Therapy Assistant (pp 175-191).
© 2016 Taylor & Francis Group.

CHAPTER OUTLINE

INTRODUCTION

The lifespan development approach states that development occurs across the lifespan and is affected by societal, cultural, psychological, and environmental variables. Human development is a scientific discipline, with goals that include the description, explanation, prediction, and modification of behavior. Various theorists, including but not limited to, Abraham Maslow, Erik Erickson, and Robert Havighurst have created models of human development that define specific periods, tasks, and/or stages of growth (Craig & Baucum, 2002). Occupational therapy practitioners take developmental expectations into account when they collaborate with a client to create meaningful treatment goals. In order to achieve these goals, occupation-based interventions are selected that facilitate the change or growth in client factors and performance skills (motor, process, and social interaction) that are needed for successful participation in life roles and occupations. Within the area of mental health, participation has been identified as essential in the recovery process and in the achievement of quality of life (Drapalski et al., 2012). Participation is demonstrated by clients when they are carrying out occupations or daily life activities they find purposeful and meaningful. Quality of life is defined by each individual; thus, occupational therapy practitioners work with the client to create an individualized treatment plan that is intended to enhance the individual's occupational identity. This is known as *client-centered treatment*. **Occupational identity** is defined in the Occupational Therapy Framework (American Occupational Therapy Association [AOTA], 2014) as the "composite sense of who one is and wishes to become as an occupational being generated from one's history of occupational participation" (p. S43).

As stated earlier, the term **development** refers to changes that occur over time in an individual related to a number of variables, including but not limited to, client factors and context. **Client factors** "include an individual's values, beliefs, and spirituality; body functions; and body structures" (AOTA, 2014, p. S7). These factors primarily influence *how* an individual performs an activity. Context, as described earlier in this text, includes the interrelated conditions found within and around the client that influence performance (AOTA, 2014). Context determines, in large part, *when* and *whether* a client will attempt to perform that activity, if at all.

PART 1: DEVELOPMENT OF ROLE IDENTITY

In the Occupational Therapy Framework, culture is described as an important factor that surrounds a person and influences his or her behavior. The authors go on to state that the **cultural context** includes "customs, beliefs, activity patterns, behavioral standards, and expectations accepted by the society of which a client is a member" (AOTA, 2014, p. S9). Therefore, the cultural context influences the client's identity and activity choices. Useem and Useem (1963) define culture differently. They state, "Culture has been defined in a number of ways, but most simply … it is the learned and shared behavior of a community of interacting human beings" (p. 169). Using this definition, culture is described as it pertains to ways of thinking, behaving, or working that exist among a group of individuals who belong to a community. A **community** is defined as the people who live in a particular area, or a group of people who are considered a unit because of their shared interests or background (Cambridge Dictionary Online, 2014). A community may be created in any number of ways. The members of an organization such as the National Alliance on Mental Illness, people who reside in the same housing complex, employees who work in a small business, instructors at a specific college, occupational therapy assistant students who attend a particular school, employees of a large corporation, residents of a group home, and consumers of mental health services are just a few examples of different communities.

The culture in which an individual functions defines expectations for the emergence of certain roles at each stage in adult development. A *role* is a set of behaviors that has a socially agreed-upon function for which there is an accepted code of norms (Kielhofner, 1995). Every life role is structured by the perceptions, values and beliefs, and personal experience of the person who is assuming it, as well as the expectations of others in the social system and the community in which the culture is located. Take, for example, the role of a new occupational therapy assistant instructor walking for the first time into a classroom at a community college. The instructor was once a student, but had more recently functioned in the role of an occupational therapist who worked on a psychiatric unit in a local hospital. The students expect that this instructor knows about occupational therapy and mental health and will provide them with a syllabus, follow that syllabus during the semester, and teach them the information and skills needed to successfully complete the course. Likewise, the instructor has expectations of the occupational therapy assistant students that are based on her personal experience in the student role. These expectations include, among other things, how they will behave in the classroom setting, the type of assignments they should complete, the level of effort that they will put into those assignments, and what they will learn from completing them. The occupational therapy assistant program director expects that this instructor will follow accreditation standards when creating course content and institutional procedures in designing and teaching the mental health course. The administrator of the community college in which the occupational therapy assistant program is located expects that the instructor will follow institutional guidelines for teaching the course and evaluating student performance. Finally, the instructor expects that course evaluations and student success on the national certification examination for occupational therapy assistants will indicate her success in transitioning into the role of a teacher. This example illustrates how an occupational therapist learns what is expected of her in the new role of "occupational therapy assistant instructor" and outlines the explicit and implicit expectations of individuals from three different but related communities (i.e. the classroom, the occupational therapy assistant program, and the college in which the instructor is employed).

As described earlier, role identity includes the ability to perform activities and acquire skills that are needed to be successful within a particular life role. The life roles that individuals assume become part of their occupational identity. Occupational identity is demonstrated through occupational performance and is part of the occupational profile, which will be discussed in Part 2. Exactly how and when an individual acquires the skills for occupational participation depends, in part, on the social system that is in place to support him or her during the learning process, the physical environment in which he or she lives, and the culture in which he or she functions. In regard to mental health, culture in particular determines what behavior is considered typical versus atypical and when an individual may need to be evaluated for mental illness.

In the study of lifespan development, the successful completion of age-appropriate activities, assumption of typical life roles, and/or the utilization of certain performance skills associated with specified developmental stages are considered measures of mental wellness. To view more information on developmental theories, please refer to Table 6-1 for an outline of Erickson's stages of development and Table 6-2 for a list of Maslow's hierarchy of needs. A summary of Robert Havighurst's developmental tasks is found in Table 7-1.

In lifespan development, the terms *developmental milestones* and *major life tasks* are frequently used to describe attainment of performance skills, growth in self-awareness, and achievement of the ability to successfully interact with others. This focus resonates with the domain of occupational therapy, which is described as "achieving health, well-being, and participation in life through engagement in occupation" (AOTA, 2014, p. S4). Occupational therapy practitioners acknowledge the significance of engagement in occupations and participation in meaningful life roles on the developmental process across the lifespan (Humphry, 2009). In the practice area of mental health, occupational therapists and occupational therapy assistants focus on the ability of clients to successfully function in their chosen environment and effectively perform daily occupations that are meaningful to them. In the next section of this chapter, the primary roles associated with individuals in the mid-lifespan will be discussed, along with the occupations, developmental tasks, and performance skills expected to be demonstrated by individuals within that age group. Checkpoint 7-1 helps the student identify how culture affects the development of role identity.

Roles, Occupations, Tasks, and Skills in the Mid-Lifespan

Legally, one becomes an adult at the age of 18. However, as Kaluger and Kaluger (1974) pointed out, "the point in

TABLE 7-1
HAVIGHURST'S DEVELOPMENTAL TASKS

Tasks Associated With Young Adulthood	• Assuming civic responsibilities • Affiliating with social groups • Selecting a life partner • Managing a home • Learning to cohabit with a life partner • Selecting a career • Starting a family • Rearing children
Tasks Associated With Middle Adulthood	• Achieving civic responsibility • Developing adult leisure activities • Establishing and maintaining a budget/financial standard of living • Relating to one's spouse as a person • Adjusting to aging parents • Accepting the physiologic changes in one's body associated with aging
Tasks Associated With Older Adulthood	• Meeting social and civic responsibilities • Adjusting to diminishing health • Adjusting to the death of a life partner • Adjusting financially to retirement • Establishing an explicit affiliation with one's age group • Establishing an appropriate physical living arrangement

Note: the shaded areas denote tasks associated with the mid-lifespan.

CHECKPOINT 7-1. DESCRIBE
Describe how culture affects the development of role identity. List the life roles that are currently part of your identity.

time when people become adults cannot be designated in years, but rather as that point when they begin to assume the responsibilities of adulthood and take on the roles of adults." Using a sociological definition, individuals may be considered adults when they move out of their childhood home and begin their own household, become self-supporting or have selected a career, marry or reside with a life partner, start a family, and make significant contributions to the communities in which they function (Havighurst, 1972). For the average American adult in the early part of the mid-lifespan, these events typically occur from the 20s to 40s, which is termed *young adulthood*.

The latter part of the mid-lifespan is termed *middle adulthood* and includes individuals from the 40s through 50s. In this stage of development, it becomes more difficult to delineate milestones, as significant roles and activities are not the same for everyone. Kaluger and Kaluger (1979) describe this period as a time "when the traditional roles of parenting and family provider are nearing completion or have already ended … a time of more personal freedom, less economic stress, greater availability of leisure time and fewer demands for material growth" (p. 398). However, in reality, some individuals become parents for the first time during this timeframe, whereas their peers become grandparents. Others are changing careers, returning to college, and perhaps even retiring early. More commonly, significant developmental tasks at this stage of adulthood include relating to the spouse or lifelong partner as an individual, adjusting to aging parents, and accepting changes in physical appearance (Papalia, Olds & Feldman, 2002).

CHECKPOINT 7-2. UNDERSTAND
Describe the life roles and tasks associated with individuals in the mid-lifespan. Explain how roles affect the development of occupations. Provide examples to illustrate your explanation.

TABLE 7-2
BODY FUNCTIONS FREQUENTLY AFFECTED BY MENTAL ILLNESS

• Higher-level cognitive functions	• Orientation
• Attention	• Temperament and personality
• Memory	• Energy and drive
• Perception	• Sleep
• Thought	• Proprioceptive
• Functions of sequencing complex movement	• Vestibular
• Emotions	• Pain
• Experience of self and time	• Touch
• Consciousness	

Checkpoint 7-2 helps students identify life roles and tasks associated with the mid-lifespan.

Roles guide the selection of occupations. Occupations are defined as "[t]he things that people do that occupy their time and attention; meaningful, purposeful activity; the personal activities that individuals choose or need to engage in and the ways in which each individual actually experiences them" (Boyt Schell, Gillen, & Scaffa, 2014, p. 1237). When an individual presents with problems in completing significant tasks that are associated with typically developing life roles, the occupational therapist will begin to explore how the individual performs occupations in everyday life. In the Occupational Therapy Practice Framework, occupations are placed into categories. These categories include daily living skills (activities of daily living [ADLs]), instrumental activities of daily living (IADLs), rest and sleep, education, work, play, leisure, and social participation (AOTA, 2014, p. S6). Successful engagement in occupations is a key element to the development of a client's occupational identity and self-esteem.

Occupations must have purpose and meaning to the client, or he or she will not participate in them. Learning how to independently perform and engage in occupations occurs over the lifespan and incorporates the use of client factors, performance skills, and performance patterns. *Performance skills* are goal-directed, observable actions demonstrated by the client, and are key elements of successful occupational participation. They are categorized into motor skills, process skills, and social interaction skills. A multitude of body functions and body structures underlie each performance skill. *Performance patterns* are the habits, routines, roles, and rituals that can support or hinder occupational performance. These will be discussed in more detail in Chapter 8.

Client factors, described earlier in this chapter, affect performance skills. In order for a person to successfully execute an activity or occupation, these factors may need to be present in whole or in part. In regard to mental health practice, the need for evaluation of body functions and, in particular mental and sensory functions, is viewed as especially important, as dysfunction in these areas is associated with mental illness (American Psychiatric Association [APA], 2013). A list of body functions that are frequently affected by mental illness is contained in Table 7-2.

PART 2: MENTAL HEALTH DYSFUNCTION IN THE MID-LIFESPAN

Client factors are affected by the presence or absence of illness, disease, deprivation, disability, and life experiences (AOTA, 2014). According to Brown (2012), adults with a mental illness may neglect to perform or may demonstrate deficits in any of the areas of occupation due to the symptoms of their illness. In this section, the symptoms associated with six diagnostic categories of mental illness from the *Diagnostic and Statistical Manual of Mental Disorders* (DSM-5) will be described, along with their potential impact on performance of occupations. Although symptoms of these disorders may start at a much younger age, these diagnoses are typically diagnosed in the mid-lifespan and therefore are included in this chapter.

Schizophrenia and Other Psychotic Disorders

Schizophrenia has been diagnosed in people in all races, socioeconomic groups, and cultures. The term *schizophrenia* means "split mind." Over the centuries, this disorder has been attributed to possession by demons, multiple personalities residing within the same person, and even punishment by a higher power for evil done. None of these claims have proven to be true, although they have added to the stigma associated with the disease. What research has shown, however, is that genetic factors (Dempster, Viana, Pidsley, & Mill, 2013), environmental factors (Prasad et al., 2010), childhood trauma (Thompson et al., 2014), and physical disease may all contribute to this disease. In summary, it appears that schizophrenia has multiple causes.

Despite the potential number of causes, one thing is certain—an individual who is diagnosed with schizophrenia will experience psychosis. That is not to say that every person who becomes psychotic will eventually be diagnosed with schizophrenia. During the second half of the 20th century, one of the major advances in mental health was the recognition that psychosis has many causes. Psychotic disorders, including schizophrenia, are defined by the presence of one or more of the following: delusions, hallucinations, disorganized speech, disorganized behavior, and negative symptoms. Each of these symptoms is described next.

Delusions

A **delusion** is a false belief that cannot be explained by the patient's culture or education; the patient cannot be persuaded that the belief is incorrect, despite evidence to the contrary or the weight of the opinion. There are many types of delusions. Some of the more commonly known are as follows:

- *Grandeur*: Patients believe they are persons of exalted station, for example, God, Satan, or a movie star.
- *Guilt*: Patients feel that they have committed an unpardonable sin or grave error.
- *Ill health*: Patients believe they have a terrible disease, such as AIDS.
- *Jealousy*: Patients are convinced that their spouses or partners have been unfaithful.
- *Passivity*: Patients believe they are being controlled or manipulated by some outside influence, such as radio waves or the television.
- *Reference*: Patients feel they are being talked about, perhaps in the press or on television.

- *Thought control*: Patients believe ideas are being put into their minds by others.

Hallucinations

A **hallucination** is a false sensory perception that occurs in the absence of a related sensory stimulus. Hallucinations can affect any of the five senses, but auditory and visual hallucinations are the most common. To count as psychotic symptoms, hallucinations must occur when the person is fully conscious. This means that hallucinations that occur during delirium cannot be taken as evidence as one of the psychotic disorders. The same can be said for hallucinations that occur when someone is going to sleep or waking up; these can be regarded as normal experiences.

Illusions are experiences that must be discriminated from hallucinations. Illusions are simply misinterpretations of actual sensory stimuli. They usually occur in conditions of decreased sensory input, such as during the night. For example, a person awakens to the belief that someone is in her bedroom; when the light is turned on, what appeared to be a person crouching down is only a pile of clothes on the chair.

Disorganized Thinking and Speech

Even without delusions or hallucinations, a psychotic patient may have **disorganized thinking or speech**, in which mental associations are governed by rules not apparent to the observer or by no clear rules at all. Table 7-3 provides examples of disorganized thinking and speech.

Disorganized Behavior

Disorganized behavior refers to physical actions that do not appear to be goal directed (e.g., taking off one's clothes in public, repeatedly making the signs of the cross as you walk down the road, assuming and maintaining odd postures) and that may indicate psychosis. Note that it is important to distinguish what constitutes the term *bizarre*, as this is affected by the culture in which an individual functions.

Negative Symptoms

Negative symptoms include reduced range of expression of emotion (flat or blunted affect), markedly reduced amount or fluency of speech, and loss of will or motivation to do things (avolition). They are called negative because they give the impression that something has been taken away from the client, not added, as is the case with hallucinations and delusions.

The existence of psychosis is usually not hard to determine. Delusions, hallucinations, and disorganized speech or behavior are generally obvious, as they often represent a dramatic change from a person's normal behavior. However, differentiating the various causes of psychosis can be difficult. In order to qualify for a diagnosis of schizophrenia,

TABLE 7-3	
EXAMPLES OF DISORGANIZED THINKING AND SPEECH	
Circumstantialities	Extremely detailed, lengthy discourse about a subject
Clang association	Repetition of words or phrases that are similar in sound, for example, red, bed, fed, led
Concrete thinking	Lack of abstraction in thinking; inability to understand metaphors and analogies
Echolalia	Parrot-like repetition of another individual's words
Flight of ideas	The topic of conversation changes repeatedly and rapidly, often after just a word or phrase
Loose association	Absence of the normal connectedness of thought, ideas, and topics
Pressured speech	Speaking quickly, almost as if the words are being forced
Word salad	String of words that is not connected in any way

two or more of the signs of psychosis must be present for at least 1 month, and at least one of those symptoms must be delusions, hallucinations, or disorganized speech. More importantly to occupational therapy practitioners, there must be a significant level of dysfunction in work, self-care, and/or interpersonal relations since the onset of the disturbance.

The symptoms of schizophrenia vary from one individual to another; however, this disease primarily affects thought and perception. Auditory hallucinations are common and often interfere with the individual's ability to attend to what is going on around him or her. Affect tends to be either flat or inappropriate to the situation, with an individual laughing or smiling when nothing funny has been said. Frequently an individual who is experiencing hallucinations will be observed muttering to him- or herself. Body awareness and sense of self are impaired, and the individual has difficulty accomplishing activities where the hands are not visible, such as tying an apron behind the back, combing hair without standing in front of a mirror, or even washing the back of the body in the shower. In addition, individuals with this disorder have difficulty establishing the appropriate distance to stand or sit from others and establishing and maintaining eye contact.

Schizophrenia occurs in three phases: (1) prodromal, (2) active, and (3) residual. In the prodromal phase, initial changes in behavior may be subtle and occur at a young age. At some point, however, these changes in behavior and thinking become so disruptive that they can no longer be ignored. Changes in cognition lead to the inability to recognize patterns in situations and environments, which affects the ability to transfer learning from one environment to another. This transfer is known as *generalization.* The ability to distinguish and focus on relevant stimuli may be diminished, and familiar cues may go unrecognized. Information processing becomes slowed, affecting functioning in school or at work.

Avolition affects the desire to complete normal activities. Over time, the person becomes less able to perform basic ADLs, including sleeping, bathing, and eating, and starts to avoid social interaction. Intentional social isolation eventually evolves into limited engagement in the community. Affective flattening may occur and includes unchanging facial expression, poor eye contact, and lack of vocal inflection.

In the active phase, symptoms associated with the prodromal phase become more severe, and the person may need to be hospitalized. Social or environmental changes, such as going away to college, alcohol or drug use, or experiencing a significant loss, may trigger this phase. Speech and behavior may become grossly disorganized, and the intensity and/or frequency of positive symptoms increase.

As the individual enters the residual phase, psychotic symptoms abate; however, they may not disappear entirely. Typically the individual continues to have difficulty with energy, motivation, concentration, sequencing of complex movements, perception, and proprioception, all of which interfere with occupational performance. Once these symptoms are stabilized, the individual is able to focus on returning to activities and occupations that he or she associates with quality of life.

Relapses may occur at any time during treatment and recovery. Two of the major factors associated with relapse are noncompliance with medication and increased levels of stress, which may exacerbate the disorder. The term *exacerbation* refers to an increase in the severity of a disease or its signs and symptoms. Combining medication with psychosocial treatment has been shown to lower the frequency and severity of recurrent relapses.

In the past, the progression of schizophrenia has been viewed as progressive deterioration over time; however, the current view of this disease is that it is quite complex and that the experience of one individual with this disorder is different from the next. Treatment with medication has been found to contribute to an improvement in the ability to function in everyday life; however, no medication has been found to cure the disease. Treatment approaches for this disorder will be discussed in more detail in the next chapter.

Major Depressive Disorder

According to the APA (2013), depressive disorders are characterized by feelings of sadness, irritability, and emptiness. With these disorders, the primary change is in mood rather than thought or perception, accompanied by somatic and cognitive changes that significantly affect the individual's capacity to function. The clinical diagnosis of depression disorder is complex and involves aspects of the lifespan and culture. It is associated with significant impairment in the performance of occupations; to be diagnosed, the person must demonstrate a decrease from his or her previous level of function for at least 2 weeks. Loss of interest in activities that were previously pleasurable is usually present, and the individual withdraws from social interaction. There is a diminished ability to think, concentrate, and make decisions. Appetite may be significantly increased or decreased, and fatigue and loss of energy affect performance of nearly every ADL. Feelings of worthlessness or excessive guilt may be present, along with recurrent thoughts of death and perhaps even suicide. Low self-esteem and feelings of hopelessness are common. The depressed individual demonstrates psychomotor agitation or retardation, which can be observed in his or her behavior. For example, a person with psychomotor agitation may be observed pacing, wringing the hands, or fidgeting constantly while seated. An individual with psychomotor retardation will think, move, and speak slowly. Finally, sleep disturbance is a hallmark of depression, with the individual experiencing a need for excessive sleep (hypersomnia) or a disruption in sleep (insomnia). Insomnia may take the form of difficulty falling asleep, middle-of-the-night awakening (waking up in the middle of the night, then having difficulty returning to sleep), or early morning awakening (waking up early and being unable to return to sleep at all).

The etiology of depression appears to be caused by the interrelation of biological, genetic, and psychosocial factors. Adverse childhood experiences such as trauma and stressful life experiences as an adult (i.e., divorce, loss of employment, diagnosis with a chronic or debilitating medical condition) are recognized as precipitants. The diagnosis of depression may run in families and is associated with a lack of social supports and coping skills (APA, 2013).

The course of a major depressive disorder is variable. Recovery typically begins within 3 months, and many individuals who have only been depressed for several months may experience a full recovery. Major depressive disorder recurrent (more than one depressive episode) is viewed as a progressive recurrent illness, with each episode becoming more severe and lasting longer in duration. With each recurrence, there is increased risk of work impairment and psychosocial limitations. The risk of recurrence becomes progressively lower over time, but is higher for individuals whose first episode of depression was severe or who experienced the episode at a younger age. Major depressive disorder frequently co-occurs with substance-related disorders, panic disorder, and personality disorders, as well as medical conditions such as Parkinson's disease, cancer, diabetes, heart disease, and stroke.

Bipolar Disorder

Bipolar disorders are distinguished from depressive disorders by the occurrence of manic or hypomanic (less than manic) episodes in addition to a depressive episode. A *manic episode* is a period where the individual experiences *euphoria*—an abnormally elevated mood, characterized by feelings of well-being. The person frequently reports feeling "on top of the world." This euphoria is accompanied by *expansive mood.* An expansive mood generally includes an exaggerated sense of self-importance and self-esteem (*grandiosity*) and lack of restraint in expressing one's feelings. For example, an individual who is experiencing a manic episode may have no difficulty in contacting the president of a large corporation to demand appointment to the position of vice president, as he believes that all "of the people" with whom he works are "inept" and that his "superior intelligence" dictates that he should be in a position of authority, even though he is a new graduate and has only been employed by this company for 2 weeks. Manic episodes are also associated with increased irritability and anger when the individual is unable to get what he or she wants, beliefs are challenged, and/or ambitions are thwarted. Demonstration of *lability of mood*—sudden alterations between euphoria and irritability—is commonly observed during a manic episode.

In addition to mood changes, other symptoms demonstrated by an individual who is experiencing a manic episode include impulsivity, distractibility, decreased need for sleep, pressured speech, racing thoughts, flight of ideas, increase in goal-directed activity (although the person seldom completes the goals), psychomotor agitation, inattention to details, and excessive involvement in pleasurable activities that have a high potential for negative consequences (i.e., gambling, substance use, barhopping, "hooking up"). Wearing clothing, makeup, accessories, and jewelry in bright colors and "outlandish" combinations are commonly seen during a manic episode.

The etiology of bipolar disorder is similar to that of depression and appears to be caused by the interrelation of biological, genetic, and psychosocial factors. The disturbance is severe enough to cause significant impairment in occupational performance and interpersonal relationships. Recurrence may occur within months or years. Later episodes of illness occur more frequently than earlier episodes, and increased frequency in episodes is experienced in those individuals who experienced onset at a younger age. Bipolar disorders frequently co-occur with substance use disorders and anxiety disorders.

Generalized Anxiety Disorder

Generalized anxiety disorder is characterized by excessive worry or concern about events or activities that interferes with an individual's focus on the tasks at hand. The concern may be about everyday activities or routine events, but it must be out of proportion to the actual impact of the event. In addition, it must occur for the majority of days for at least 6 months. The individual with this disorder is unable to control the worry. Symptoms of anxiety include autonomic hyperactivity, increased muscle tension, irritability, difficulty sleeping, restlessness, and cognitive vigilance. Motor tension can be observed as shakiness and restlessness, and the individual will usually report frequent headaches. Changes in the autonomic system are evidenced by shortness of breath, palpitations, excessive sweating, and gastrointestinal complaints such as constipation or diarrhea. Cognitive vigilance is observed in the individual as increased irritability and a tendency to startle easily.

The cause of generalized anxiety is not known, but it is assumed that biological, psychological, and environmental factors affect its development. Many individuals diagnosed with this disorder state that they have experienced anxiety all of their lives. The symptom of excessive worrying takes time and energy, which interferes with virtually every aspect of the person's life. Research has shown that the earlier an individual is diagnosed with this disorder, the more disabling it is (APA, 2013). Generalized anxiety disorder frequently co-occurs with panic disorder and substance use disorder. Panic disorder is diagnosed by recurrent, unexpected *panic attacks*. "A panic attack is an abrupt surge of intense fear or intense discomfort that reaches a peak within minutes, and during which time four or more of a list of 13 physical and cognitive symptoms occur" (APA, 2013, p. 209). Table 7-4 lists the symptoms associated with a panic attack.

Substance Use Disorders

In the DSM-5, the term *substance* is used to describe alcohol, caffeine, cannabis, hallucinogens, inhalants, opioids, sedatives, hypnotics and anxiolytics, stimulants, and tobacco. Substance-related disorders involve the use and abuse of alcohol and illicit dugs. No matter what the substance, the constant and most significant symptom defining a substance use disorder is that the individual continues to use it despite the fact that it has created problems in everyday life. For example, the person may use larger amounts of the substance or take it over a longer period than was intended. The individual may find that he or she is unsuccessful in cutting back on the amount used or in quitting use of it altogether. The individual with a substance use disorder has an intense desire for the substance, which is defined as *craving*, and will continue to use it despite experiencing recurrent social and personal problems associated with its effects. Furthermore, the person may spend the majority of his or her time obtaining and using the substance at the expense of engaging in occupations associated with important life roles at work, school, or home. Additional time is spent recovering from the use of the substance. The individual may withdraw from hobbies that were previously found to be pleasurable, as well as family functions. He or she may even engage in substance use in situations where it is physically dangerous, such as driving a car. Finally, substance use continues despite the fact that the individual with substance use disorder understands he or she may have physical and/or psychological problems as a result.

Substance-related disorders are characterized by tolerance, withdrawal, and relapse. It is important to understand these terms in order to be aware of the potential impact that these conditions may have on a client. **Substance use** refers to when a person ingests, smokes, sniffs, or injects a mind-altering substance. **Tolerance** is defined as the need to increase the amount of drug used in order to experience its full effects, and it occurs as the body accommodates to the substance. **Withdrawal** refers to the physiological and emotional effects that can accompany reduced use of the substance. Withdrawal symptoms and their intensity vary depending on the substance. Some examples of physical symptoms include sweating, tachycardia, heart palpitations, muscle tension, tremor, nausea, vomiting, and diarrhea. Emotional symptoms may include depression, poor concentration, anxiety, restlessness, irritability, and insomnia. When a person experiences both substance tolerance and withdrawal, he or she is said to be addicted to the substance. **Relapse** occurs when an individual resumes use of a substance after a period of abstinence.

Substance use disorders range in severity from mild to severe. "Individuals ages 18-24 have relatively high prevalence rates for use of virtually every substance. Intoxication is usually the initial substance-related disorder and often begins in the teens" (APA, 2013, p. 487). Prognosis depends on environmental factors (i.e., cultural factors, attitude toward substance use, and availability of the substance) and genetics, as substance use disorders tend to run in families. Abuse and dependence are more common in men than women, and abuse is higher among people who are unemployed (Sadock, Sadock, & Ruiz, 2014). Disruption in meaningful activities and roles across the lifespan can result from these disorders.

	TABLE 7-4

PHYSICAL AND COGNITIVE SYMPTOMS OF PANIC ATTACK

Physical Symptoms	• Heart palpitations • Sweating • Trembling or shaking • Shortness of breath • Chest pain or discomfort • Nausea or abdominal distress • Feeling dizzy, faint, or lightheaded • Numbness or tingling in the hands and/or feet • Chills or heat sensations • Feeling unable to swallow; a sensation of choking
Cognitive Symptoms	• Derealization (feelings of unreality) and/or depersonalization (being detached from oneself) • Fear of losing control of oneself • Fear of dying

Personality Disorders

The term ***personality*** refers to the combination of psychological characteristics or traits that create an individual's distinctive character. These characteristics form a complex pattern that remains constant across different social and personal situations and is largely outside the person's awareness. An individual's personality affects how he or she perceives, thinks, and feels about him- or herself, others, and the world in general.

Personality traits influence the consistency of emotional responses, as well as their intensity and appropriateness to the situation. An individual diagnosed with a personality disorder demonstrates traits that differ substantially from the norm. These traits are maladaptive and can lead to functional impairment and emotional distress. Impulse control, mood regulation, and judgment are three areas in which this dysfunction may be observed. Table 7-5 contains a list of personality disorders along with a definition of each.

Personality disorders become apparent during adolescence and early adulthood, when they begin to cause significant impairment in the development of and ability to effectively function in life roles and perform significant tasks associated with those stages in human development. Research shows that personality disorders likely have a genetic component, as they tend to run in families. Biological factors such as hormones and overactivity in parts of the brain have also been associated with the disorder. Finally, an individual at risk for developing a personality disorder due to these genetic and biological factors will be especially vulnerable to the impact of environmental influences that occur during childhood. Checkpoint 7-3 helps students to compare the symptoms associated with mental health disorders and identify any commonalities among them.

PART 3: EVALUATION OF OCCUPATIONAL FUNCTION

The focus of occupational intervention in mental health is on the performance of occupations that the clients need and want to accomplish. Therefore, evaluation and assessment must center on function. By understanding how client factors, performance skills, and performance patterns are interrelated and influenced by contexts and environments, practitioners can better evaluate performance-related concerns. Treatment plans are then created to support and/or develop functional performance, depending on the client's needs.

According to Brown (2012), the origin of a referral for occupational therapy services varies depending on the treatment setting. Psychiatrists usually are responsible for referrals to occupational therapy in inpatient and hospital-based outpatient settings. Often, occupational therapy is a "blanket referral" in those settings, meaning that any client admitted to the unit or outpatient program is automatically referred for occupational therapy evaluation. In

TABLE 7-5	
PERSONALITY DISORDERS	
Paranoid	This disorder is characterized by a pervasive distrust of other people. The individual finds it particularly difficult to engage in close relationships. He or she is extremely guarded and suspicious, and is constantly on the lookout for clues or suggestions to confirm his or her fears and distrust of others.
Schizoid	The person with this disorder is detached and aloof, and engages in introspection and fantasy. He or she has no desire for social or sexual relationships, and is therefore indifferent to others as well as social norms and conventions.
Schizotypal	This disorder is characterized by odd appearance, behavior, thinking, and speech. A person with schizotypal disorder often fears social interaction and sees other people as ill-intentioned and potentially harmful.
Antisocial	The person with this disorder disregards social rules and obligations and displays a lack of concern for the feelings of others. He or she acts impulsively, lacks guilt, and fails to learn from experience.
Borderline	The person with this disorder is said to lack a sense of self, and consequently experiences feelings of emptiness. He or she fears abandonment. There is a pattern of becoming involved in intense, unstable relationships. The person demonstrates emotional instability, outbursts of anger, and aggressive, impulsive behavior. Suicidal threats and acts of self-harm are common.
Histrionic	People with histrionic personality disorder lack a sense of self-worth, and consequently depend on the attention and approval of others. They crave excitement and act on impulse or suggestion. These individuals generally take great care of their physical appearance and behave in a manner that is overly charming or inappropriately seductive. They are especially sensitive to criticism and rejection and react badly to loss or failure.
Narcissistic	The person has a grandiose sense of self-importance and a need to be admired. He or she lacks empathy and readily exploits others to achieve his or her goals.
Avoidant	The person diagnosed with this disorder believes that he or she is socially inept, unappealing, or inferior and lives in fear of being embarrassed, criticized, or rejected. The individual usually avoids meeting people unless he or she is certain of being liked.
Dependent	The person with this personality disorder lacks self-confidence and has an excessive need to be taken care of. He or she looks for help to make everyday decisions. He or she greatly fears abandonment and may go to considerable lengths to secure and maintain relationships.
Obsessive-Compulsive	The person with this disorder is characterized by excessive preoccupation with details, rules, lists, order, organization, or schedules. His or her perfectionism is so extreme that it may prevent a task from being completed.

CHECKPOINT 7-3. ANALYZE
Compare the symptoms listed for each of the mental health disorders described in this chapter. What symptoms do the disorders have in common?

community-based settings, referrals may come from a variety of mental health professionals (i.e., psychologist, social worker, case manager, nurse) and agencies, such as the court system, foster care system, and vocational services. In some settings, such as a psychiatric clubhouse, the client may be a self-referral.

A referral may be for consultation only, or come with the expectation that the client will be evaluated and receive occupational therapy services. According to the Occupational Therapy Practice Framework (AOTA, 2014),

> The evaluation consists of the occupational profile and analysis of occupational performance. The occupational profile includes information about the client and the client's needs, problems, and concerns about performance in areas of occupation. The analysis of occupational performance focuses on collecting and interpreting information using assessment tools designed to observe, measure, and inquire about factors that support or hinder occupational performance. (p. S13)

Occupational therapists working in mental health may evaluate clients as part of a team approach to treatment. For example, the information needed for the occupational profile may be obtained from a variety of individuals, with each member of the treatment team contributing information that pertains to his or her areas of expertise. Although the information gathered may be interesting to all members of the treatment team, only the occupational therapy practitioners will use it in the design of an individualized intervention plan that is uniquely focused on the use of occupations. A list of potential questions to guide the occupational therapy practitioner through the interview process and the development of the occupational profile is found in Table 7-6.

The analysis of occupational performance entails collecting and interpreting information that identifies supports/strengths and barriers/challenges to occupational engagement and performance. Once this information is gathered, it is shared with the client. Later, this list of strengths and challenges is prioritized in order to design the treatment plan. It cannot be emphasized enough that only clients can identify the occupations that give meaning to their lives. By seeking and using their input, practitioners help foster the client's involvement and increase their motivation for treatment. Without effective assessment, it is difficult to create a reliable baseline upon which change can be measured. Without client buy-in, it is impossible to reliably determine whether a poor outcome was due to ineffective treatment, lack of motivation, or a combination of both factors. Checkpoint 7-4 helps students identify how the symptoms of mental illness affect the performance of occupations.

A frame of reference is defined as "a collection of ideas or theories that provide a coherent conceptual foundation for practice" (Creek, 2003, p. 53). It provides a theoretical foundation or base for evaluation and treatment, and is used to determine how the occupational therapy practitioner addresses a client's strengths and challenges during evaluation and treatment planning. On the other hand, a practice model provides specific guidelines for putting theory into practice. Using clinical reasoning, occupational therapists select a frame of reference or practice model based on how effectively it addresses potential and identified problems. Table 7-7 outlines some of the models and theories commonly used to treat individuals diagnosed with the mental health disorders discussed earlier in this chapter.

The occupational therapy practitioner synthesizes information from the occupational profile in order to decide which specific occupations and contexts need to be addressed. A combination of evaluation methods is used by the occupational therapist and occupational therapy assistant during the evaluation process. Table 7-8 provides a list of these methods, along with examples of each. The decision as to which portion of the evaluation may be completed by the occupational therapist is described in the document Standards of Practice, written by the AOTA.

The Standards of Practice for Occupational Therapy (AOTA, 2005) describe the role of the occupational therapist and the occupational therapy assistant in the provision of occupational therapy services. An occupational therapist initiates and directs the screening and evaluation process, analyzes and interprets the data, and documents the results in accordance with federal and state law, regulatory and payer requirements, and AOTA documents. An occupational therapy assistant contributes to the evaluation process by administering delegated portions of standardized assessments (after demonstrating competency) and by providing verbal and written reports of observations of client performance to the occupational therapist in accordance with federal and state laws, other regulatory and payer requirements, and AOTA documents. The occupational therapist documents evaluation results; however, the occupational therapy assistant may contribute to this documentation.

Occupational therapy practice acts differ from state to state, and practice guidelines may supersede AOTA official documents. Occupational therapy practitioners should therefore review practice guidelines in their state to understand their respective responsibilities in the occupational therapy evaluation process. In addition, it is important

TABLE 7-6
CONTENT FOR THE OCCUPATIONAL PROFILE

- Why is the client seeking service?
- Does the client have any concerns about participation in occupations or daily life activities?
- What is the client's occupational history?
- In what occupations does the client feel most successful?
- What aspects of the environment or contexts are currently supporting participation?
- Can the client identify any existing or potential barriers to success in desired occupations or daily life occupations?
- What are the client's values and interests?
- What are the client's daily life roles?
- What are the client's patterns of engagement in occupations, and have they changed over time? If so, why?

CHECKPOINT 7-4. EVALUATE
Review the list of occupations that are found in the Occupational Therapy Practice Framework. How might the symptoms of mental illness affect the performance of ADLs? Refer back to Table 7-2 as you consider this question.

TABLE 7-7
FRAMES OF REFERENCE AND PRACTICE MODELS

Psychodynamic Frame of Reference	Explains how mental processes (i.e., perceptions, thoughts, and feelings) influence an individual's selection of, participation in, and satisfaction with occupation. Mental processes may be conscious and unconscious.
Cognitive Behavior Model	Used when the goal is to broaden a client's knowledge about his or her cognitive function and beliefs and how they mediate and influence his or her behavior. Focuses on skill building to improve the ability to problem solve and change behavior.
Model of Human Occupation	Utilizes a system's perspective to describe the nature of human occupation as it develops across the lifespan. It emphasizes the interaction between the person, the task, and the environment.
Sensory Motor Model	Addresses behavior and performance problems related to central nervous system dysfunction in sensory processing. Requires that therapeutic activities and occupations be selected based on their ability to potentially produce an integrated, organized response within the central nervous system.

TABLE 7-8
EVALUATION METHODS
REVIEW OF MEDICAL RECORDS
OBSERVATION
Checklists • Comprehensive Occupational Therapy Evaluation (COTE) • The Neuropsychiatric Institute Interest Checklist (NPI) • Activity Interest Checklist • The Role Checklist • Instrumental Activities of Daily Living Scale
Interviews • Occupational Performance History Interview (OPHI) • Model of Human Occupation Screening Test (MOHOST) • Occupational Circumstances Assessment Interview and Rating Scale (OCAIRS)
Questionnaires • Occupational Questionnaire • Adolescent/Adult Sensory Profile • Canadian Occupational Performance Measure (COPM) • Occupational Self-Assessment (OSA) • Community Integration Questionnaire
Assessments • Bay Area Functional Performance Evaluation (BAFPE) • Milwaukee Evaluation of Daily Skills (MEDL) • The Kohlman Evaluation of Living Skills (KELS) • Lowenstein Occupational Therapy Cognitive Assessment

to note that the involvement of the occupational therapy assistant in the evaluation process is limited when using assessments such as the Sensory Integration Praxis Tests or the Assessment of Motor and Process Skills, which require specialized training that is only available only to occupational therapists.

SUMMARY

This chapter explored the achievement of life roles and occupational identity in the mid-lifespan and discussed the influence of environment, contexts, and client factors on their development. Mental health disorders that are typically diagnosed during this period were described, along with their potential impact on occupational performance. The evaluation process was detailed, including frames of reference, evaluation methods, and the role of the occupational therapy assistant in this process.

PART 4: APPLICATIONS

Five case studies follow, each of which is described in a different Spotlight (Spotlights 7-1 through 7-5). In each case, the individual is at a different stage of the mid-lifespan spectrum. Please note that these Spotlights will also be referenced in the following chapter. Although occupational therapists provide treatment related to personal strengths and deficits in areas of occupation, a diagnosis based on

SPOTLIGHT 7-1. SARAH

The client is a 25-year-old, White, married, employed female who presented to the emergency room of Backus Hospital with a chief complaint of suicidal thoughts. She reported that she experienced periods of depression in the past from which she recovered; however, recently she has begun to experience thoughts of suicide. The client acknowledged a plan in which she would take an overdose of "any medication" that is available to her because "nobody cares" about her. The psychiatrist noted that the client has been experiencing generalized anxiety with mild panic attacks. There is no history of alcohol or drug abuse, visual or auditory hallucinations, confusion, or thought disorder. Prior to marriage, the client had an active social life with her girlfriends.

The client presented as slightly disheveled with soiled clothing and uncombed hair. Affect was sad, and the client appeared to have difficulty gathering her thoughts before responding to interview questions. She reported that her employer has informed her that she is welcome to take whatever time she needs to "get back to her old self" and that her job is waiting for her when she recovers.

The client was oriented to date, month, and year. She described a feeling of dread in the morning, interrupted sleep at night, poor appetite, and lack of interest to "do anything."

DSM-5 Diagnoses: Major Depressive Disorder, Recurrent, Severe; Generalized Anxiety Disorder, Severe; Panic Disorder, Mild (APA, 2013)

SPOTLIGHT 7-2. LUWILLOW

The client is a 34-year-old African American woman with five children ranging in age from 5 to 18. All children are currently enrolled in school. She was referred for evaluation to the community mental health center by the Department of Children and Family Services (DCF), who mandated that she be seen for evaluation. The client reports that her husband has a history of alcohol abuse, and that DCF became involved with the family when the children mentioned in school that their father had driven drunk while they were in the car. The client reports that she has been the victim of domestic violence "for years" and plans to walk away from her 19-year marriage. She hopes to relocate to another state in order to be closer to her parents, as she does not feel she can raise her children alone. The client did not complete high school or receive her General Educational Development Certificate of High School Equivalency. She has been employed for the past 5 years as a companion to a blind, elderly woman ("She couldn't see my bruises—it worked out fine.") The client reluctantly reported that she experiences "bad dreams" every night, is easily startled, and has had "physical reactions" to most things. "Sometimes I feel like I am having a heart attack. It comes out of nowhere." The client expressed a desire to work on her "issues" with her minister instead of the clinic, as she is uncomfortable speaking with a therapist.

DSM-5 Diagnosis: Post-Traumatic Stress Disorder (APA, 2013).

symptoms and their impact on functioning is usually required when seeking reimbursement for services across all treatment settings. Thus, the diagnoses from the DSM-5 (APA, 2013) have been included in each case study.

After reading each Spotlight, answer the following questions:

1. a. What are the client's strengths?
   b. What are the identified problems?
   c. What are the developmental expectations and life roles typically associated with an individual at that age?
   d. What outcomes are desired by the client? How do they relate to occupational performance?

2. a. What symptoms are typically associated with the diagnoses given to the client?
   b. Which of those symptoms is the client experiencing

3. What additional information would you like to know to better understand the client and complete the occupational profile?

REFERENCES

American Occupational Therapy Association. (2005). Standards of practice for occupational therapy. *American Journal of Occupational Therapy, 59,* 663-665. doi:10.5014/ajot.59.6.663

SPOTLIGHT 7-3. CODY

The client is a 45-year-old, unemployed, White male who resides in a homeless shelter. He was referred by his case manager at the homeless shelter to the partial hospitalization program at Backus Hospital for psychiatric evaluation. The client is single and the father of four grown children. He receives Supplemental Security Income, and his oldest son is the payee. The son provides the client with a $25 to $50 per week allowance for incidental expenses.

The client was released yesterday from the local jail after being arrested for disorderly conduct in the park. According to other individuals from the shelter, he had consumed "four or five" 40-oz containers of beer and "a pint or more" of vodka. The client has no memory of the drinking episode or his behavior. He presents as a thin individual, with hand tremors and poor eye contact. He reported that he received his first drink at the age of 3 from his grandmother, who thought it would be funny to see him drunk. Over the years, he has stopped and started drinking at different points in his life. His longest period of sobriety was for 5 years during his marriage. Most recently, he began drinking again because he was feeling depressed after his girlfriend broke up with him. "I don't blame her. I don't have a job, I'm homeless and my family doesn't want me. I wish I had a normal life." The client was encouraged to seek treatment by his son with the hope that he can find sobriety.

DSM-5 Diagnosis: Alcohol Use Disorder; Severe (APA, 2013)

SPOTLIGHT 7-4. SANTIAGO

The client is a 57-year-old Hispanic male who carries a long-term diagnosis of chronic schizophrenia. He has had two brief hospitalizations for erratic behavior and agitation within the past month. The client was accompanied by the police to the emergency room after neighbors reported that he was walking up and down the street screaming that his brain hurt. The client reports that he was first seen by a psychologist in grade school when his foster parents became concerned with his behavior. He recalls his first hospitalization occurring in his 20s. He has had multiple hospitalizations since then, five of which occurred during the last 10 years at a former state hospital with lengths of stay exceeding 6 months each time. The client currently acknowledges auditory hallucinations in the form of voices, although he cannot describe what the voices are saying. He also describes visions of different colors and "thinking pain." The client admitted that he abused alcohol and smoked marijuana daily in his 20s and 30s; however, he has not used alcohol or marijuana in over 20 years. The client graduated from high school and attended a community college for two semesters to study the visual arts before dropping out. He is currently unemployed, lives alone in a supported apartment, and receives Social Security Disability Insurance. His typical day is described as watching television and smoking three to four packs of cigarettes. Over the years he has worked "under the table" doing construction and landscaping. His last job was 10 years ago in supported employment as a landscaper and janitor with a local mental health agency. The client has five older siblings who live in other states with whom he communicates regularly by phone. He has never married and has no children. He reports that he is "sick and tired" of coming to the hospital and just wants "to be well." He is a thin man who presents with disheveled hair, mismatched clothing, and flat affect.

DSM-5 Diagnoses: Schizophrenia, Multiple Episodes, Severe; Alcohol Use Disorder in sustained remission and Cannabis Use Disorder in sustained remission (APA, 2013)

American Occupational Therapy Association. (2010). Standards of practice for occupational therapy. *American Journal of Occupational Therapy, 64*, 106-111/

American Occupational Therapy Association. (2014). Occupational therapy framework: Domain and process. (3rd ed.). *American Journal of Occupational Therapy, 68*(Supplement 1), S1-S51.

American Psychiatric Association. (2013). *Diagnostic and statistical manual of mental disorders* (5th ed.). Washington, DC: Author.

Boyt Schell, B. A., Gillen, G., & Scaffa, M. (2014). Glossary. In B. A. Boyt Schell, G. Gillen, & M. Scaffa (Eds.), *Willard and Spackman's occupational therapy* (12th ed., pp. 1229–1243). Philadelphia, PA: Lippincott Williams & Wilkins.

Brown, C. (2012). *Occupational therapy practice guidelines for adults with serious mental illness*. Bethesda, MD: American Occupational Therapy Association, Inc.

Brown, C., & Stoffel, V. (2011). *Occupational therapy in mental health*. Philadelphia, PA: F. A. Davis

Cambridge Dictionary Online (2014). Retrieved from http://dictionary.cambridge.org/us/dictionary/american-english/community.

Craig, G. C., & Baucum, D (2002). *Human development*. (9th ed.). Saddle River, NJ: Prentice Hall.

Creek, J. (2003). *Occupational therapy defined as a complex intervention*. Southwark, London: College of Occupational Therapists.

SPOTLIGHT 7-5. SHOSHANA

The client is a 26-year-old female, who was accompanied by her mother to the emergency room. Her mother reported that the client had not slept for 3 days. Last evening she was found baking cakes, redecorating her bedroom, rearranging the furniture in the living room, and running through the lawn sprinkler (naked) during the middle of the night. This morning her mother discovered that her daughter had charged over $1,000 on her credit card to purchase baking pans, knives, and an oven. When questioned about these purchases, her daughter stated that she was practicing to be a contestant on the show Top Chef. The mother reported that her daughter had been treated on an outpatient basis for depression 6 months ago, and that she had responded well to treatment. "When she started to get active and involved in everything I thought she was just feeling better—but this behavior is crazy! It reminds me of my husband's sister."

While her mother spoke, the client moved continually around the room, spinning, dancing, and humming. At one point she took the paper off the exam table and began to wrap herself in it. When the psychiatrist asked her to sit down, the client yelled, "You are interrupting the creative process!" and threw the paper at him. A few seconds later she abruptly stopped moving, smiled seductively at him, and asked the psychiatrist if he wanted to examine her ("I can do a strip dance for you.")

The client denied any substance abuse. Questions about family history revealed that the client's aunt had been diagnosed with bipolar disorder in her mid-20s.

DSM-5 Diagnosis: Bipolar I, Severe (APA, 2013).

Dempster, E., Viana, J., Pidsley, R., & Mill, J. (2013). Epigenetic studies of schizophrenia: Progress, predicaments, and promises for the future. *Schizophrenia Bulletin, 39*(1), 11-16. doi:10.1093/schbul/sbs139.

Drapalski, A. L., Medoff, D., Unick, G. J., Velligan, D. I., Dixon, L. B., & Bellack, A. S. (2012). Assessing recovery of people with mental illness. *Psychiatric Services 63*(1), 48-53.

Havighurst, R. J. (1972). *Developmental tasks and education* (3rd ed.). New York: D. McKay Co.

Humphry, R. (2009). Occupation and development: A contextual perspective. In E. B. Crepeau, E. S. Cohn, & B. A. B. Schell, (Eds.). *Willard and Spackman's occupational therapy* (pp. 22-32), Philadelphia, PA: Lippincott Williams and Wilkins.

Kaluger, G., & Kaluger, M. (1974). *Human development: The span of life.* St. Louis, MS: Mosby.

Kielhofner, G. (1995). *A model of occupation: Theory and application.* Baltimore, MD: Lippincott Williams and Wilkins.

Papalia, D., Olds, S. W., & Feldman, R. D. (2002). *Human development.* (10th ed.) New York, NY: McGraw-Hill.

Prasad, K. M., Talkowski, M. E., Chowdari, K. V., McClain, L., & Yolken, R. H. (2010). Candidate genes and their interactions with other genetic/environmental risk factors in the etiology of schizophrenia. *Brain Research Bulletin, 83*(3-4), 86-92.

Sadock, B., Sadock, V., & Ruiz, P. (2014). *Kaplan and Sadock's synopsis of psychiatry: Behavioral sciences/clinical psychiatry.* (11th ed.). Philadelphia, PA: Lippincott Williams and Wilkins.

Thompson A. D., Nelson B., Yuen H. P., Lin A., Amminger G. P., McGorry P. D.,...Yung A. R. (2014). Sexual trauma increases the risk of developing psychosis in an ultra high-risk "prodromal" population. *Schizophrenia Bulletin, 40*(3), 697-706.

Useem, J., & Useem, R. (1963). Men in the middle of the third culture. *Human Organizations, 22*(3), 168-179.

8

Intervention Strategies
Combining Performance and Skills

Christine A. Manville, EdD, OTR/L

KEY TERMS

- Ambivalence
- Direct Services
- Illness Management and Recovery (IMR) Group
- Indirect Services
- Intervention Plan

- Just Right Challenge
- Long-Term Goal
- Motivation
- Motivational Interviewing (MI)
- Occupational Therapy Group

- Recovery
- Short-Term Goal
- Wellness Recovery Action Plan (WRAP) Training
- Wellness Tools

CHAPTER LEARNING OBJECTIVES

After completion of this chapter, students should be able to:

1. Describe the occupational therapy intervention process in a mental health treatment setting.

2. Contrast the role of the occupational therapy assistant with the occupational therapist in intervention planning.

3. Determine how the treatment setting and length of stay affect the selection of approach to intervention and anticipated treatment outcomes.

4. Create clear, concrete, and measurable treatment goals to address problems in the performance of tasks and occupations due to symptoms of mental illness.

5. Compare the use of various treatment methods to accomplish identified goals.

6. Summarize how the practice of occupational therapy complements the Recovery Movement and how occupational therapy practitioners can contribute to its success.

Manville, C.A., Keough, J. L.
Mental Health Practice for the Occupational Therapy Assistant (pp. 193-206).
© 2016 Taylor & Francis Group.

CHAPTER OUTLINE

INTRODUCTION

In the last chapter, the achievement of occupational identity in the mid-lifespan was discussed, along with the influence of the environment, contexts, and client factors on its development. Mental health disorders that are typically diagnosed during this period were described, along with their potential impact on occupational performance. An overview of the evaluation process was provided that included frames of reference and practice models, evaluation methods, and the role of the occupational therapy assistant in this process.

The next step in the occupational therapy process is treatment planning. Occupational therapists and occupational therapy assistants who work in the practice area of mental health may provide services to clients directly or indirectly. *Direct services* are interventions that are completed when in direct contact with the individual. They include meeting one-on-one with the client, as well as providing treatment in therapeutic groups. These services are implemented in a variety of settings that may include inpatient psychiatric units, residential treatment programs, outpatient programs, psychosocial clubhouses, group homes, transitional living programs, and schools, among others. *Indirect services* are provided by the occupational therapist, who operates in the role of the consultant on behalf of the individuals in the aforementioned settings. It includes consultation to national, community, and state agencies (i.e., National Alliance on Mental Illness [NAMI], Visiting Nurse Association, hospice, vocational rehabilitation); businesses (i.e., nursing homes, senior centers, postsecondary educational institutions); and individuals who deliver direct services to people who are experiencing mental illness, including their caregivers and family members. Indirect consultation may focus on outcomes such as maintaining activities of daily living (ADL) skills, enhancing development of instrumental activities of daily living (IADL) skills, improving participation in desired occupations, increasing engagement within the community, and

promoting quality of life. In this chapter, the focus will be on developing intervention plans in which the occupational therapist and occupational therapy assistant are providing direct services to individuals who are experiencing severe or persistent mental illness. Checkpoint 8-1 asks students to explain the difference between direct and indirect services, and provide examples of each in mental health practice.

PART 1: INTERVENTION PLANNING

The intervention planning process includes consideration of which skilled services will be provided by occupational therapy practitioners. It requires collaborating with the client to create treatment goals and outcomes that will facilitate his or her engagement in desired occupations. Occupational therapists combine information about the client gathered during the evaluation process with their knowledge of practice models, frames of reference, and theories of practice in order to create the written intervention plan.

The *intervention plan* directs the actions of the occupational therapist and occupational therapy assistant. It lists client goals as well as the occupational therapy approaches and types of interventions that will be used to reach identified outcomes. The occupational therapist is responsible for creating and documenting the intervention plan, although the occupational therapy assistant may contribute to the process.

Variables in the Planning Process

Many variables must be considered in the creation of the treatment plan. These include, among others, client health and well-being, existing performance skills and performance patterns, the discharge context and environment, client factors, activity demands, the environment in which the intervention will be provided, and available evidence to support the use of potential treatment methods.

CHECKPOINT 8-1. EXPLAIN

Explain the difference between direct and indirect services. Provide an example of each type of service in the practice area of mental health.

CHECKPOINT 8-2. DESCRIBE

Describe the role of the occupational therapy assistant in the goal-planning process and list the treatment variables that have been considered up to this point in the intervention plan. Provide a specific example for each variable you list.

After the client's current strengths and challenges have been evaluated in order to determine the baseline level of function and the discharge context and environment have been identified, the next step is to collaborate with the client on the creation of goals for the treatment plan. It is not always possible to obtain client input on goals, however, due to the individual's mental status. Attention, memory, thought, emotions, and higher-level cognitive skills are all potentially affected by mental illness. It becomes particularly important, then, to review the data from medical records in order to identify the client's general health and well-being, prior level of functioning, existing occupations, and any previously determined needs and goals. Family members and caretakers may be available for interview by the occupational therapy assistant or the occupational therapist in order to supplement this information. The occupational therapy assistant then helps the occupational therapist create treatment goals. Checkpoint 8-2 requires students to describe the role of the occupational therapy assistant in the goal-planning process and the treatment variables that have been addressed up to this point in the intervention plan.

The type of setting in which the individual is currently receiving services is usually indicative of the client's cognitive status, as well as the most appropriate intervention approach. For example, if the client is hospitalized on a general inpatient psychiatric unit, it can be assumed that he or she is extremely disorganized and/or unable to care for him- or herself, as these are criteria generally set by the third-party payers who authorize hospitalization. At times, the person may be at risk for harming him- or herself or others, or require medical supervision for withdrawal from alcohol or drugs. Treatment in this setting is generally short term, with an anticipated outcome of improvement in the performance skills required for the anticipated discharge environment. In the American Occupational Therapy Association (AOTA) Occupational Therapy Practice Framework (OTPF; 2013, p. S23), performance skills are defined as "observable elements of action that have an implicit functional purpose…encompassing multiple capacities (body functions and body structures) and, when combined, underlie the ability to participate in desired occupations and activities." What is clear from this definition is that these skills are needed as the foundation for successful performance in desired occupations. Impairment of client factors or performance skills typically requires the restoration or remediation of existing skills. When the symptoms of mental illness are so severe that hospitalization is required as the treatment setting, it can be anticipated that the individual's process skills, in particular, have been affected. Boyt Schell, Gillen, and Scaffa state that process skills are "observed as a person (1) selects, interacts with, and uses task tools and materials; (2) carries out individual actions and steps; and (3) modifies performance when problems are encountered" (2014, p. 1239). Descriptions of some of the client factors and process skills that may be affected by mental illness are listed in Table 8-1.

In order for a client to learn new activities and occupations, several variables must be considered. The first is the level of foundational knowledge that the individual currently possesses in regard to the how, where, when, and why the activity is performed. Next is the range and level of performance skills required for successful completion of the activity. In other words, although the client may possess knowledge, it should not be assumed that the individual has the skills needed to translate that knowledge into actual performance of the activity, or that he or she can generalize how to perform it from one setting to another. Finally, the client must be motivated to perform the activity in a variety of contexts and environments. The significance of knowledge, skills, and motivation on the learning process is discussed in more detail in Chapter 14.

Due to the client's mental status, the focus during inpatient hospitalization is usually on the individual developing self-awareness of personal symptoms of mental illness and a basic understanding of how these symptoms may affect his or her ability to interact with people and objects in the environment. As an individual's mental status improves, or when the client resides in the community while receiving occupational therapy services, the focus of treatment outcomes shifts toward enhancement of occupational performance, maintenance of health, and prevention of illness. As such, the significant learning variables to be addressed include (1) increasing knowledge related to those issues and (2) implementation and ongoing practice of skills required for occupational success. At this stage, clients are

TABLE 8-1	

EXAMPLES OF CLIENT FACTORS AND PROCESS SKILLS THAT MAY BE AFFECTED BY MENTAL ILLNESS

CLIENT FACTORS	
Attention	Sustained concentration, distractibility, and attention
Consciousness	State of alertness and awareness
Emotional	Range and regulation of emotions
Energy and drive	Appetite, energy level; impulse control; motivation
Memory	Working long-and short-term memory
Orientation	To self and others and person, place, and time
Perception	Discrimination of auditory, gustatory, olfactory, proprioceptive, tactile, vestibular, and visual input
Proprioception	Aware of body position and place
Thought	Awareness of reality; coherent and logical thought
PROCESS SKILLS	
Attends	Does not look away from what he or she is doing
Continues	Performs without interruptions; continues without pause until the action is completed
Heeds	Performs and completes the task specified by another individual
Initiates	Starts or begins a step without hesitation
Organizes	Logically positions tools and materials in an orderly fashion
Paces	Performs a consistent rate of performance throughout a task
Sequences	Performs steps in a logical order with a lack of randomness or repetition

Adapted from American Occupational Therapy Association. (2014). Occupational therapy practice framework: Domain and process. (3rd ed.). *American Journal of Occupational Therapy, 68*(Suppl. 1), pp. S1-S51.

usually able to collaborate in the goal-planning process and can identify which occupations are significant to them. However, some individuals, such as those who have permanent residence in a group home or who are residents in long-term residential treatment programs, may continue to work simultaneously on improving performance skills. Still other individuals, such as young adults in a transitional living program, may begin to explore promotion of health and wellness within the community while also working to enhance performance skills. Performance contexts and patterns become important considerations for this population, with the most important learning variable being the client's level of motivation to implement what has been learned. Table 8-2 illustrates how anticipated treatment outcomes, treatment settings, treatment focus, and variables in the learning process relate to one another.

Steps in the Planning Process

Step 1: Needs Identification

This step requires occupational therapy practitioners to review existing medical records and interview family and caregivers, as needed, to fill in any gaps that may exist in understanding the client. The occupational therapist must analyze evaluation results as they relate to the identified discharge environment. It is necessary to consider the discharge environment since the performance skills that will be needed are determined by the demands of that particular context. The discharge environment dictates which occupations the client must perform, as well as the level of support that will be available to assist the individual in that process. For example, the only expectation for an individual returning to a group home after hospitalization might be that he

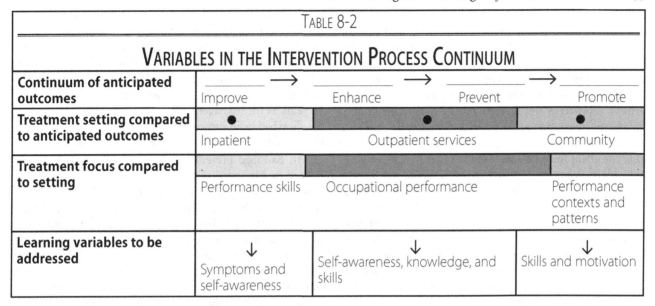

TABLE 8-2			
VARIABLES IN THE INTERVENTION PROCESS CONTINUUM			
Continuum of anticipated outcomes	Improve ⟶	Enhance ⟶	Prevent ⟶ Promote
Treatment setting compared to anticipated outcomes	● Inpatient	● Outpatient services	● Community
Treatment focus compared to setting	Performance skills	Occupational performance	Performance contexts and patterns
Learning variables to be addressed	↓ Symptoms and self-awareness	↓ Self-awareness, knowledge, and skills	↓ Skills and motivation

or she maintains good hygiene, since meal preparation and housekeeping chores are done by the staff in the home. Staff will prompt the individual to shower, if necessary, and perhaps temporarily supervise that process until the individual is able to once again accomplish this activity independently. However, a student returning to live in a dorm at college must be able to complete ADLs, concentrate in class, and effectively manage his or her time without supervision. If the client is unable to effectively perform these activities without additional support, he or she may need to consider temporarily moving back to his or her parents' home as she resumes classes or perhaps take a semester off until he or she is able to independently resume the student role.

"A person usually requires occupational therapy intervention because he is unable to meet the demands of his physical or social environments...because the demands have changed, the client has changed or he has never been able to cope adequately" (Creek & Lougher, 2008, p. 111). When the client seeks help, it is up to the occupational therapist and occupational therapy assistant to identify the gaps in self-awareness, knowledge, and/or performance skills that exist between the performance level at which the client is currently functioning (baseline) and the level at which he or she must function by discharge.

Next, the occupational therapist must analyze why these gaps exist, because this will affect the intervention approach and treatment methods selected for use. It is important to seek feedback from the client during this process as a multitude of factors may account for a problem. For example, existing performance skills may need remediation or enhancement in order for the client to reach a level of occupational competence, or perhaps entirely new skills must be learned. Maybe the individual has the necessary skills but has difficulty knowing when to utilize them. Another factor that could limit performance is when the

client is not motivated to use specific skills in a particular environment. Once existing problems have been identified and the probable reason for them determined, they are listed in the treatment plan.

Step 2: Setting Goals

The client and the occupational therapist collaborate to prioritize identified problems and to set treatment goals. In the treatment plan, both long- and short-term goals are listed. A **long-term goal** states a functional outcome (i.e., attend college, get a job). **Short-term goals** are the small steps that a client must take to achieve the long-term goal. They are sometimes referred to as *process goals*. Long-term goals are usually set by the multidisciplinary treatment team, whereas short-term goals are typically discipline specific. Take, for example, a 19-year-old client who has been diagnosed with a mental illness and who recently aged out of the foster care system. He has been placed into a group home. He has just started to receive services from the local mental health center, where he attends a treatment program for individuals with a desire to learn community living skills. After meeting with the client, the team collaborates on an interdisciplinary treatment plan. The long-term goals that have been identified by the client are to obtain a job and get his own apartment. Each team member then writes a short-term, weekly goal. The psychiatrist writes his goal about symptom management, the nurse creates a goal in which the client assumes responsibility for health management (i.e., attending program regularly and taking his medication as scheduled), the social worker's goal focuses on the client contacting his foster family in order to maintain them as a support system, and the occupational therapist writes a weekly goal in which the client will go online to locate employment opportunities in the neighborhood in which he resides. The client and the team agree to meet again in a week to discuss progress made toward these goals and to potentially set new ones. The method used by the occupational therapist to write the goal is described later in this chapter.

The definition of an ***occupational therapy goal*** is a "[m]easurable and meaningful, occupation-based, long-term or short-term aim directly related to the client's ability and need to engage in desired occupations" (AOTA, 2013, p. S35). As stated earlier, short-term goals refer to what the client must be able to do in order to achieve long-term goals. When considering goals, occupational therapy practitioners must consider whether to use a top-down or bottom-up approach to treatment. A top-down approach would require determination of which activities and tasks are associated with the client's occupations and life roles. They focus on overall performance and incorporate information from the occupational profile. In the bottom-up approach, the focus is on deficits in foundational components of function, including client factors and performance skills. The OTPF (AOTA, 2014) specifies that a top-down approach be used in the evaluation process. However, as described earlier in this chapter, the use of the top-down approach for occupational therapy treatment intervention may not always be possible in every setting, particularly if the treatment setting is a short-term, acute care psychiatric unit. Table 8-3 lists areas of occupation, tasks, and activities frequently addressed by occupational therapy practitioners who work in mental health settings.

Once the intervention goals are agreed upon with the client, more focused assessments may need to be carried out to further delineate baseline function. The more specific the measure, the easier it becomes to recognize and document change. Whether the occupational therapy assistant is able to participate in this evaluation will depend upon the tools selected and demonstrated competency by the occupational therapy assistant in the use of that particular assessment tool.

Step 3: Writing Goals

All occupational therapy goals should address functional, occupation-centered outcomes that contribute to the client's health and well-being and promote participation (AOTA, 2014). It is this focus on occupation that separates the role of the occupational therapist and the occupational therapy assistant from other professionals on the mental health treatment team, regardless of the treatment setting. Goals must be written so that they describe very clearly what the client will do. The more specifically the problem has been defined in the evaluation process, the easier it becomes to identify the treatment approach and write an appropriate, client-centered goal. Take, for example, Mr.

Santiago, who lives with his wife and children. Mr. Santiago has just been admitted to the hospital for depression. In an interview with the occupational therapist, his wife reports that her husband became depressed when he was laid off by his former employer, who closed his floral business due to health reasons. Mr. Santiago had been employed for 15 years as the manager of this shop. His wife stressed that the shop had been successful and that her husband is a well-respected business man within their community.

Mr. Santiago presents with poor hygiene. This is evidenced by his soiled clothing, unshaven beard, uncombed hair, and strong body odor. A review of the records and results from the interview with the client's wife indicates that Mr. Santiago already possesses grooming skills and is capable of independently showering and shaving. Mr. Santiago acknowledges that his problem is due a lack of energy and low motivation to get him out of bed each morning. This is often the case with an individual who is being treated for depression. The intervention approach in this case will be on restoration of grooming skills in preparation for Mr. Santiago seeking employment and resuming the role of an employee following his discharge from the hospital.

A goal is a "measurable and meaningful, occupation-based, long-term or short-term aim directly related to the client's ability and need to engage in desired occupations" (AOTA, 2013, p. S35). One format that can be used to write a goal is the RUMBA technique (Early, 2009). Table 8-4 outlines the RUMBA format and gives an example of how it is used to write a goal for Mr. Santiago.

While it is usually easy to observe whether an individual has showered or shaved, some goals will require more effort to write. Symptoms of mental illness can be difficult for students and entry-level practitioners to quantify (Early, 2009). For example, Mr. Santiago described decreased energy and low motivation. Although the assumption can be made that his energy and motivation levels will increase as his depression lessens, how are these changes measured? In this case, the occupational therapy practitioner will identify behavioral indicators that illustrate that such changes have occurred. For Mr. Santiago, a revised goal would be written as follows: "Client will shower *daily* for five *consecutive* days *without prompting* from the occupational therapy assistant." The action of taking a shower every day is used as the behavioral indicator for increased energy level, and the fact that Mr. Santiago independently takes a shower for 5 consecutive days is used as the indicator for improved motivation to perform daily hygiene. Checkpoint 8-3 requires the student to quantify two symptoms of mental illness typically associated with depression.

TABLE 8-3

EXAMPLES OF CLIENT ACTIVITIES AND SKILLS FREQUENTLY ADDRESSED BY OCCUPATIONAL THERAPY PRACTITIONERS IN MENTAL HEALTH PRACTICE

ACTIVITIES OF DAILY LIVING

Tasks	Activities

Bathing and showering	• Obtaining required supplies (washcloth, towels, soap, etc.)
	• Using soap and shampoo as directed
	• Systemically washing all body parts
	  ○ Bathing
	  ○ Showering

Hygiene and grooming	• Selecting and using appropriate grooming products as described
	  ○ Deodorant (when to use and how to apply)
	  ○ Body powder (when to use and how to apply)
	• Caring for hair
	  ○ Washing
	  ○ Combing
	  ○ Styling
	• Caring for nails
	• Caring for teeth
	  ○ Brushing
	  ○ Flossing
	  ○ Using mouthwash
	• Caring for skin
	  ○ Shaving
	  ○ Moisturizing

Dressing	• Selecting clothing appropriate for weather conditions • Selecting clothing appropriate for an occasion • Selecting an outfit (matching colors, etc.) • Sequence of dressing

INSTRUMENTAL ACTIVITIES OF DAILY LIVING

Tasks	Activities

Communication management	• Using a computer
	  ○ Searching the Internet
	  ○ Scanning for links
	  ○ Computer safety

Driving and community mobility	• Driving a car • Getting a driving permit • Learning to drive

(continued)

TABLE 8-3 (CONTINUED)	
EXAMPLES OF CLIENT ACTIVITIES AND SKILLS FREQUENTLY ADDRESSED BY OCCUPATIONAL THERAPY PRACTITIONERS IN MENTAL HEALTH PRACTICE	
INSTRUMENTAL ACTIVITIES OF DAILY LIVING	
Tasks	*Activities*

	• Taking the driving test
	• Using public transportation
	   ○ Reading the bus schedule
	   ○ Getting on and off the bus

Financial management	• Learning to budget (needs vs. wants)
	• Getting a bank account
	   ○ Selecting a bank
	   ○ Understanding the bank statement
	   ○ Using debit and credit cards responsibly

Health management and maintenance	• Exercise • Medication management • Diet and obesity

Meal preparation and clean-up	• Planning a meal
	   ○ What is a well-balanced meal?
	   ○ What is a serving size?
	• Preparing the meal
	   ○ Following a recipe
	   ○ Kitchen safety (i.e., using knives, cleaning food prep surfaces)
	   ○ Cooking techniques
	   ○ Using a microwave
	• Cleaning the kitchen
	• Storing leftovers safely
	• Selecting cleaning products

Safety and emergency maintenance	• Recognizing hazardous situations • Taking action in an emergency
EDUCATION	
Tasks	*Activities*

Formal education preparation	• Getting the diploma or GED
	   ○ Selecting a school
	   ○ Managing the academic schedule
	   ○ How to study

(continued)

TABLE 8-3 (CONTINUED)	
EXAMPLES OF CLIENT ACTIVITIES AND SKILLS FREQUENTLY ADDRESSED BY OCCUPATIONAL THERAPY PRACTITIONERS IN MENTAL HEALTH PRACTICE	

EDUCATION

Tasks	*Activities*

Formal education preparation *(continued)*	• Going to college
	  ◦ Understanding scholarships, loans, and grants
	  ◦ Accommodations
	  ◦ The registration process
	  ◦ Time management

Employment seeking and acquisition	• Locating employment opportunities • Completing an application • Preparing for an interview • Participating in the interview • Follow up after the interview
Job performance	• Understanding job requirements • Performing work procedures • Interacting with co-workers • Conflict in the workplace

VOLUNTEER EXPLORATION

Tasks	*Activities*
Volunteer exploration	• Locating volunteer opportunities • Selecting volunteer opportunities • Applying for volunteer opportunities

SOCIAL PARTICIPATION

Tasks	*Activities*
Community	• Locating community activities • Finding free activities
Peer, friend	• What is a friend? • Holding a social conversation • Establishing levels of intimacy
Family	• Parenting skills • Family roles • Negotiating conflict with parents

LEISURE

Tasks	*Activities*
Leisure exploration	• Identifying past and current leisure activities • Identifying new leisure activities

(continued)

TABLE 8-3 (CONTINUED)	
EXAMPLES OF CLIENT ACTIVITIES AND SKILLS FREQUENTLY ADDRESSED BY OCCUPATIONAL THERAPY PRACTITIONERS IN MENTAL HEALTH PRACTICE	
Tasks	*Activities*
Leisure participation	• Options for leisure participation in the community • Work, rest, and play—finding the balance • Types of leisure activities—passive vs active

TABLE 8-4	
GOAL WRITING FORMAT	
R (relevant)	The goal has meaning to the client.
U (understandable)	The goal is stated in terms of observable behavior, and does not contain jargon.
M (measurable)	The goal contains the criteria for success.
B (behavioral)	The goal describes what the client will do to achieve it.
A (achievable)	The goal is something the client can do in the specified timeframe.
"The client will shower and shave twice within the next 5 days, with no more than two prompts from the occupational therapy assistant."	

CHECKPOINT 8-3. APPLY
In an interview with the occupational therapy assistant, Mr. Santiago states that he feels worthless since he lost his job and does not believe that the situation will get better. Feelings of worthlessness are associated with low self-esteem, and the expressed statement that the situation will not improve is called *hopelessness*. Write one goal that addresses Mr. Santiago's low self-esteem and another to address feelings of hopelessness. Remember to describe the behavior that Mr. Santiago will demonstrate that indicates improvement in each area.

PART 2: INTERVENTION IMPLEMENTATION

Intervention is then provided to assist clients in reaching a state of physical, mental, and social well-being; identifying and realizing aspirations; satisfying needs; and changing or coping with the environment. (AOTA, 2013, p. S12)

During the past 10 to 15 years, there has been an increased effort to improve the quality of services provided to individuals who have been diagnosed with severe mental illness. A report written by the President's New Freedom Commission on Mental Health (2002) called for the transformation of the existing mental health system to one that provides access to high-quality treatment that is based on scientific evidence. The report stated that treatment should focus on not just managing symptoms associated with mental illness, but also on *recovery* from illness,

"helping people with mental illness…live, work, learn, and participate fully in their communities" (p. 27). The concept of recovery resonates with the definition of occupational therapy, which is stated as "the therapeutic use of everyday life activities (occupations) with individuals or groups for the purpose of enhancing or enabling participation in roles, habits, and routines in home, school, workplace, community, and other settings" (AOTA, 2014, p. S1). Both of these definitions address the importance of community participation for individuals in a variety of life roles in order to promote quality of life. This suggests that the profession of occupational therapy is a good "fit" with the Recovery Model.

Use of Activities

Once the client's goals have been identified, it is up to the occupational therapist and occupational therapy assistant to determine the best way to achieve them. The methods selected for service delivery must take into consideration

CHECKPOINT 8-4. FORMULATE

Refer back to the goal listed in Table 8-4. Work from that goal to formulate an example of activity synthesis, activity adaptation, and activity gradation, given what you know about Mr. Santiago and the symptoms of depression that were listed in Chapter 7.

the needs and wants of the client and the learning variables associated with those factors, the focus of treatment (i.e., occupations, activities, tasks, and skills), the intervention approach, types of interventions available to the client within that setting (i.e., one on one, therapeutic groups, community engagement), whether the occupational therapist or the occupational therapy assistant will provide the intervention, and the frame of reference or practice model selected to guide the intervention process. Referring back to the definition of occupational therapy, it is clear that this intervention will include the use of activities, but exactly *which* activities are selected will depend in large part on the information gathered during the evaluation, particularly client preferences. "When a person engages in activities out of personal choice and they are valued, these clusters of purposeful activities form occupations" (Hinojosa, Kramer, Royeen, & Luebben, 2003). Although preferred occupations will be different for each person, all activities selected for treatment should provide personal satisfaction to the client who engages in them. If an activity is not related to intervention goals, there is no reason to even consider using it with the client.

Before an activity is selected, it must be analyzed for activity demands. "Activity demands are the specific features of an activity that affect the meaning it may have for a client and the type and amount of effort required to engage in it" (AOTA, 2014, p. S12). Some of these demands are as follows:

- Actions and performance skills that are required
- Body functions and structures that are needed to perform the activity
- Resources required to complete the activity
- Sequencing and timing of the activity process
- Social demands
- Space required to complete the activity (and the location in which it will be performed)

The occupational therapist and occupational therapy assistant must also contemplate the variety, level, and range of skills needed to successfully complete the activity. This analysis is important to determine the "just right" challenge. If the challenge of a task is too low, boredom may occur. If it is too high, it may result in frustration for the client and decreased motivation to participate in further occupational therapy treatment. A just right challenge is an activity that is slightly above what a person is currently able to easily do. Successful completion of such a challenge

results in improved self-confidence and higher self-esteem. As the client demonstrates improved ability to accomplish one task, activity components from that task may be combined into new activities. This is termed *activity synthesis*. Another possibility is that an activity demand be modified to become more challenging (or less challenging if needed), which is called *activity adaptation*. If an activity is adapted in stages to become progressively more or less difficult, the occupational therapy practitioner is said to be using *activity grading*. Checkpoint 8-4 requires students to formulate activities that illustrate these terms.

It is always important to consider the individual's cognitive level of function when selecting treatment activities. In general, the more difficulty an individual demonstrates with organization of thoughts and attention to task, problem solving (ability to identify options), and decision making (choosing the best option), the more structure should be provided in order for him or her to complete a task successfully. The amount of structure and assistance given to the client should be decreased as performance skills and self-confidence improve.

Use of Self

Use of self is another treatment method utilized by occupational therapy practitioners and other health care professionals. Clients have identified the therapeutic relationship as critical to the outcome of occupational therapy intervention (Cole & McLean, 2003). They like to feel that they are respected and are active participants in their treatment (Horvath, 2000). "Rapport occurs when two or more people feel that they are *in sync* or *on the same wavelength* because they feel similar or relate well to each other" (Stewart, 1998, p. 282). This includes agreement on therapy goals and the methods that are used to achieve them. *Therapeutic use of self* is a term that is used to describe how an occupational therapy practitioner uses personal understanding about relationships, emotions, and experiences in an intentional way in order to communicate with the client (Taylor, 2008). Therapeutic use of self and methods to improve rapport with the client are covered in more detail in Chapters 12 and 14.

An example of the therapeutic use of self is found in an evidence-based counseling technique called *motivational interviewing* (MI). MI is a consumer-centered method for enhancing a client's motivation to change by exploring and resolving ambivalence (Rollnick & Miller, 1995). *Motivation* is the state of readiness or willingness to change. It fluctuates over time and situations and depends on context. **Ambivalence** is a state of uncertainty that individuals experience throughout most change processes. It occurs because of conflicting feelings about the process and outcomes of change. A client's resistance to change may be perceived by health care providers as a lack of motivation. In health care settings, resistance may be displayed by the client who passively listens to the occupational therapy practitioner and agrees to a goal, but without real intention or commitment. This can result in failure to achieve treatment outcomes.

MI recognizes that clients who may benefit from making changes in their lives are often at different levels of readiness to change their behavior. For example, some individuals may have thought about change but not taken any steps toward it. Others may be in the process of actively making changes. This variation is explained by a six-stage cycle that all individuals go through when making a change: (1) precontemplation, (2) contemplation, (3) preparation, (4) action, (5) maintenance and (6) relapse (Rollnick & Miller, 1995).

In MI, the therapist uses basic interaction skills to help clients think differently about their behavior and consider what might be gained through change. Many of the patients with whom occupational therapy practitioners work have conditions that can be improved or managed through a change in behavior. During the collaboration process that occurs in treatment planning, some clients are motivated to address behavioral changes to achieve such outcomes, whereas others may be less motivated to make changes in their lifestyle. Research has shown that the more a therapist ignores a client's ambivalence, the more likely the client will continue to resist change (Rollnick, Mason, & Butler, 1999). This suggests that MI may be a useful tool for occupational therapy practitioners to utilize.

In MI, the therapist provides a supportive, empathic atmosphere while selectively eliciting and strengthening the patient's own reasons for change. In order for a therapist to be successful at MI, he or she must possess four basic interaction skills. These skills include the ability to ask open-ended questions, the ability to provide affirmations, the capacity for reflective listening, and the ability to provide summary statements to the client. All four skills are used strategically. Once the ambivalent client is committed to change, the occupational therapy treatment plan can be implemented with greater probability of success.

The use of MI requires additional training, and both occupational therapists and occupational therapy assistants are eligible candidates. MI training is generally delivered in one workshop, but should be practiced under the supervision of a trained individual until competence is established.

Groups

Groups are an important therapy tool. Occupational therapy practitioners use groups to facilitate client engagement in meaningful tasks and activities that support participation in occupations and desired roles. Participation in groups can help participants develop knowledge and self-awareness, build specific skills, and explore new behaviors. The interaction among group members may increase an individual's motivation to make the behavioral changes required to effectively perform valued roles. The topics of how to design and lead an occupational therapy group are covered in detail in Chapters 13 and 14, respectively.

Two types of educational programs that have become popular in the Recovery Movement are **Illness Management and Recovery (IMR)** groups and the **Wellness Recovery Action Plan (WRAP)** system. Both of these programs may be taught by peer specialists and mental health professionals, including the occupational therapist and occupational therapy assistant. These programs are described next.

Illness Management and Recovery

The IMR program was developed to help individuals who are diagnosed with severe mental illness learn how to effectively manage their symptoms. The program may be taught one on one to individuals or to groups of participants. It promotes the use of self-management strategies and includes the following content:

- Psychoeducation about mental illness and its treatment

- Use of cognitive behavior approaches to improve medication adherence

- Development of a relapse prevention plan

- Social skills training to strengthen participation in community support systems

- Training in coping skills for self-management of persistent symptoms

Occupational therapists and occupational therapy assistants may consider leading IMR groups, as these topics are already familiar to occupational therapy practitioners who are employed in mental health settings. For example, the development and/or implementation of social skills and coping skills are frequently written into occupational therapy treatment goals, as use of these skills promotes successful engagement in a number of occupations. IMR sessions follow a standardized teaching format, so they can be led by even entry-level occupational therapy practitioners.

The program begins with exploration of the meaning of recovery to each client. Next, participants set personal recovery goals. The remaining curriculum taught in IMR has been scripted into a kit, which is available along with additional instructional materials, from the Substance Abuse and Mental Health Services Administration (SAMHSA). Organizations and individuals who are interested in establishing a new IMR program may obtain a free training manual from SAMHSA. After potential trainers have thoroughly reviewed the contents of the manual, they are encouraged to visit an existing IMR team to see how the information is put into practice. Finally, they are encouraged to hire a consultant for 1 year to make sure that they adhere to the IMR model as they launch their new program.

Wellness Recovery Action Plan System

WRAP is an intervention program developed by Mary Ellen Copeland. It is intended for use by adults with mental illness (Copeland, 1999). The program has been recognized by SAMHSA as an evidence-based practice. Participants work on identifying and understanding their personal wellness resources, which are termed **wellness tools**. Examples of wellness tools include things like taking a nap, listening to music, and calling a friend. After identifying wellness tools, participants develop an individualized plan to manage their mental illness that includes daily use of these resources. An important consideration is that the person who experiences the symptoms of mental illness must develop their personal WRAP, and not the mental health professionals with whom they work. Participants may seek assistance from others, however, if it is needed and desired. WRAP is intended to help individuals manage the symptoms of their illness. The anticipated outcomes for participants include improved quality of life, increased personal empowerment, and achievement of long-term life goals. The program is viewed as a useful way for participants to build healthy and successful lives within the community. These goals correspond with the domain of occupational therapy, which is the achievement of health, well-being, and participation in life through engagement in occupation. WRAP groups are led by trained facilitators, who may be mental health consumers as well as health care professionals. Instructional methods include individual and group exercises, lecture, and discussion. Both leaders and group members are encouraged to share personal examples that illustrate the key concepts discussed each week.

SUMMARY

This chapter outlined the occupational therapy intervention process and discussed the variables that must be considered when creating the intervention plan. The significance of the treatment setting when planning the intervention approach and anticipated treatment outcomes was emphasized. The use of meaningful activities and occupations as treatment methods was described. Several types of therapeutic techniques and programs for which occupational therapy practitioners can receive additional training were detailed. These included MI, IMR programs, and WRAP training.

PART 3: APPLICATIONS

In Chapter 7, five case studies were presented, each of which was described in a different Spotlight. In each case, the individual was at a different stage of the mid-lifespan spectrum and had been given a diagnosis from the *Diagnostic and Statistical Manual of Mental Disorders*. After reviewing these Spotlights, answer the following questions for each case:

1. In which occupations is the client currently experiencing problems? What information in the study supports your answer?

2. In what setting will the client most likely receive services? Why? Based on this setting and information described in the case, what occupational therapy treatment approach(es) will likely be selected for use with the client? Refer to Table 8-2 and the OTPF while contemplating this question.

3. Write one long-term and one short-term treatment goal for each client.

REFERENCES

American Occupational Therapy Association. (2013). Guidelines for documentation of occupational therapy. *American Journal of Occupational Therapy, 67*(Suppl.), S32-S38. doi:10.5014/ajot.2013.67S32.

America Occupational Therapy Association. (2014). Occupational therapy framework: Domain and process. (3rd ed.). *American Journal of Occupational Therapy, 68*(Supplement 1), p. S1-S51.

Boyt Schell, B. A., Gillen, G., & Scaffa, M. (2014). Glossary. In B. A. Boyt Schell, G. Gillen, & M. Scaffa (Eds.), *Willard and Spackman's occupational therapy* (12th ed., pp. 1229-1243). Philadelphia, PA: Lippincott Williams & Wilkins.

Copeland, M. E. (1999). *Winning against relapse: A workbook of action plans for recurring health and emotional problems.* Dummerston, VT: Peach Press.

Creek, J. & Lougher, L. (2008). *Occupational therapy and mental health.* Philadelphia. PA: Elsevier.

Early, M. B. (2009). *Mental health concepts and techniques for the occupational therapy assistant.* Philadelphia, PA: Lippincott, Williams & Wilkins.

Hinojosa, J. & Blount, M. L. (2009). Occupation, purposeful activities, and occupational therapy. In J. Hinojosa & M. L. Blount (Eds.), *The texture of life: Purposeful activities in context of occupation* (3rd ed., pp. 1-19). Bethesda, MD: AOTA Press.

President's New Freedom Commission on Mental Health. (2002). Achieving the promise: Transforming mental health care in America. Retrieved from http://govinfo.library.unt.edu/mentalhealthcommission/reports/FinalReport/downloads/downloads.html.

Rollnick, S. & Miller, W. R. (1995). What is motivational interviewing? *Behavioral and Cognitive Psychotherapy, 23,* 325-334.

Rollnick, S., Mason, P., and Butler, C. (1999). *Health behaviour change: A guide for practitioners.* London: Churchill Livingstone.

Trombly, C. (1993). Anticipating the future: Assessment of occupational function. *American Journal of Occupational Therapy, 47,* 253-257.

9

Occupational Environment of the Late Lifespan

Jeremy L. Keough, MSOT, OTR/L

KEY TERMS

- Antecedent-Behavior-Consequence
- Cognitive Disability Theory (CDT)
- Competency-Environment-Press
- Complexity
- Context/Environment
- Dynamic Systems Theory (DST)

- Flow
- Interdisciplinary Team
- Medical Model
- Medicare
- Model of Human Occupation (MOHO)
- Needs-Driven Dementia Compromised Behavior
- Occupation
- Occupational Performance Fit

- Parameters
- Performance Mode
- Person-Environment-Occupation (PEO) Model
- Phase Shifts
- Progressively-Lowered Threshold
- Self-Organization
- Social Model
- Theory of Retrogenesis

CHAPTER LEARNING OBJECTIVES

After completion of this chapter, students should be able to:

1. Identify the characteristics of aging through the late lifespan.

2. Recognize environmental/contextual influences that affect the provision of health care services in the late lifespan.

3. State influential legislation affecting health care services for those in the late lifespan.

4. Describe differences between medical model services and community-based services affecting the late lifespan.

5. Explain the use of occupational therapy theory and models as they apply to persons with dementia.

6. Apply the use of occupational therapy theory and models as they apply to persons with dementia.

Manville, C.A., & Keough, J. L.
Mental Health Practice for the Occupational Therapy Assistant (pp 207-227).
© 2016 Taylor & Francis Group.

CHAPTER OUTLINE

INTRODUCTION

Aging in the late lifespan encompasses many factors. These factors affect people differently over time, as well as individually due to personal differences. These factors, among many, can include social beliefs, legislative influences, and settings where services are provided.

Certainly life experiences will present differently between the ages of 60 to 70, 70 to 80, 80 to 90, and 90 to 100 years of age or over. Many people accept the late lifespan to begin about 65 years of age, to accompany retirement, whereas old age may be considered closer to the later years of the late lifespan. Although age is a sequential aspect of the late lifespan, no formal age can be attributed to specific characteristics. Certainly genetics, familial patterns of living, lifestyle choices, and the environment exert a significant influence on the aging process. The domains of the Occupational Therapy Practice Framework (OTPF) help to identify the unique events that occur in the late lifespan.

PART 1: OCCUPATIONAL ENGAGEMENT IN THE LATE LIFESPAN

Occupational Therapy Domains: Participation in Occupation

Occupation is one domain of the OTPF. As described earlier in this text, this domain includes activities of daily living (ADLs), instrumental activities of daily living (IADLs), rest, sleep, education, work, play, leisure, and social participation. Most significantly, as a person ages, work occupations can change. People may change from working as a necessity to working for enjoyment.

Additionally, as people progress through the late lifespan, they may experience the change from being an active employed member of society to a more dependent member of society. Productivity may change to appear in different forms. Leisure occupations may replace work occupations, and education pursuits may be undertaken. A person in the late lifespan may choose to learn how to play the guitar or take high school or college classes.

As the late lifespan progresses, people may experience greater limitations in engagement in IADLs and ADLs. Rest and sleep occupations can change with increased use of siestas and naps, as well as changes in sleep patterns. Social participation can also change with increased isolation from family and friends over time. The inability to drive may further isolate a person from friends and family. Greater assistance may be needed to allow a person to remain in the home. *Anhedonia* is a term used to identify when a person lacks pleasure from past pleasurable experiences. Occupational therapy assistant practitioners can help individuals identify and participate in meaningful occupations in the late lifespan. This can include new occupations as well as resumption of occupations that are important to an individual. Occupational therapy practitioners may also initiate approaches to maximize performance in ADL and IADL tasks.

Client factors are another domain of the OTPF. Values, beliefs, spirituality, body functions, and body structures are client factors specific to each person. One example of a change in client factors during the late lifespan can be identified by the perceived loss of status derived from work or other occupations. A person may perceive a loss of beauty or recognize the triviality of small problems as changes in beliefs and values occur. A person may also develop an appreciation of the "small things," develop a greater spiritual connection, and develop new meanings through self-reflection. Physical changes in body structures and body functions can lead to a change in health, illness, decreased energy, weight gain, and a change in strength (American Psychological Association [APA], n.d.; Besdine, 2013). Most significantly, a person's perception of death and even his or her own mortality can change. Occupational therapy assistant practitioners can assist clients in maintaining functional participation and engagement in life tasks as they experience changes in values, beliefs, spirituality, body functions, and body structures. Occupational therapy practitioners can assist clients by enhancing, modifying, or developing new strengths in client factors.

Changes in the domain of performance skills can also occur during the late lifespan.

Examples of performance skills include motor and praxis skills, sensory perceptual skills, emotion regulation skills, cognitive skills, communication skills, and social skills. This is not an all-encompassing list. Motor skills can become delayed or absent, and sensory perception skills can become impaired or diminished in the late lifespan (APA, n.d.; Besdine, 2013). Cognitive skills can change, such as a decline in short-term memory (recent memory), decreased problem solving, slower information processing, and loss of information (APA, n.d.; Besdine, 2013). A person may experience a better understanding of cause and effect. Social skills may resemble characteristics of the prior generation and social groups of the aged. Emotional issues can also materialize in the late lifespan to include a sense of loss, grief, resolving grief, depression, and the stress response. Occupational therapy practitioners can assist clients by enhancing, modifying, or developing new strengths in performance skills.

Performance patterns are also a domain of the OTPF. Performance patterns include habits, routines, roles, and rituals. Specific life events help to describe the varying patterns of living that can occur in the late lifespan. These events in the late lifespan can include the following:

- Retirement
- Death of a spouse
- Last child leaving the house ("empty nest syndrome")
- Birth of a grandchild
- Birth of a great-grandchild
- Inability to live alone
- Inability to drive

This is not an all-inclusive list. Each event encompasses specific habits, routines, roles, and rituals that a person in the late lifespan may experience. Unfortunately, individuals may develop deviations and rigidities in performance patterns that do not foster mental health and wellness.

Occupational therapy practitioners assist clients in refining, developing, and participating in habits, routines, roles, and rituals that support their engagement in life occupations.

Finally, the context/environment domain of the OTPF can include cultural, personal, physical, social, temporal, and virtual contexts. Examples can include differing cultural contexts for people in the late lifespan. Personal and social contexts are affected and change through the loss of personal contacts, loss of loved ones and friends, and when placement is necessary to meet an individual's medical needs. Personal and social context can be seen in a person's "freedom to speak his or her mind." Temporal context is displayed with freedom from the alarm clock, lack of need to maintain day of the week or date, and freedom from rigid schedules. Occupational therapy assistant practitioners collaborate with the occupational therapist to identify issues with the environment and context. Occupational therapy assistant practitioners provide recommendations to adapt, modify, or maintain environmental and contextual influences that affect a person's ability to participate in daily life.

The OTPF domains as applied to the late lifespan present a weaving of the multiple possible engagements in life that contrast with the middle and early lifespans. All of the domains in the OTPF contribute to occupational performance, participation, and engagement in occupations. Impairments, activity limitations, and participation restrictions all affect a person's quality of life, wellness, health, and engagement in life. Awareness of the unique experience of the late lifespan will assist occupational therapy practitioners in providing services to meet individual needs.

Mental Health, Wellness, and Mental Illness Over the Late Lifespan

Occupational engagement, mental health, and wellness have been described through the OTPF domains earlier. Mental health and wellness in the late lifespan may also be described as "active aging." The World Health Organization (n.d.) defines active aging as "The process of optimizing opportunities for health, participation, and security in order to enhance quality of life as people age." Active aging includes contributing to employment, families, peers, communities, and nations. Active aging also reflects emotional, vocational, physical, spiritual, intellectual, social, and environmental wellness. Wellness or well-being includes happiness, life satisfaction, and overall health.

At times, members of our society unknowingly or consciously prolong myths, stereotypes, and misunderstanding about aging people. The perpetuation of these untruths is called ageism. Ageism is defined as prejudice or discrimination against a particular age group, namely the elderly. Ageism is inappropriate and can have negative consequences for aging individuals when people make judgments or decisions that have no merit. This can lead to physical or emotional abuse, neglect, verbal abuse, restraint, and seclusion of the aging person. Simon Tan (2011) and the Oregon Department of Human Services (n.d.) identify common myths and stereotypes of aging. These can be found in Checkpoint 9-1.

Underestimating the potential of an aging person is a common misperception of the elderly. This corresponds with the myths that older people are not productive or

CHECKPOINT 9-1. IDENTIFY THE MYTHS ASSOCIATED WITH AGING

- The older population is all alike.
- Most elderly people have cognitive impairments.
- Forgetfulness means that dementia is starting.
- Everyone who ages gets dementia.
- Elderly people are on easy street and have no worries.
- Elderly people are set in their ways and can't change.
- Older people are not productive and are incompetent.
- The elderly are more forgetful and are slow to learn or can't learn new things.
- Most elderly people are lonely and socially isolated.
- A person becomes more religious as they age.
- Elderly people are irritable and not easy to get along with.
- Elderly people do not participate in sexual activity.
- All older persons are depressed.

Adapted from Oregon Department of Human Services. (n.d.). Myths and stereotypes of aging. Retrieved from www.oregon.gov.; Tan, S. (2011). Myths and aging. Retrieved from http://psychologytoday.com.

are incompetent. Leven and Jonsson (2002) identify this misperception when people underestimate the ability of persons with dementia. This misperception underestimates the potential for clients to improve effectively and functionally and perceives that mental deterioration is an unavoidable part of aging (Green, Ingram, & Johnson, 1993). Consequences can include rigid regulations, restricted schedules, lack of privacy, and mixed lifestyles. All of these consequences can cause problems for persons in the late lifespan. An example of this type of misperception is the belief that all elderly people will be incontinent. Incontinence is not a part of aging or dementia and is often created from the overbearing restrictions placed on persons, that is, "don't get up unless someone is with you."

Persons in the late lifespan often do need increased time to rest or sleep. Holthe, Thorsen, and Josephsson (2007) found that persons with dementia exhibited intermittent participation patterns. Additionally, persons with cognitive impairments may have deficits with initiation and sustained participation in goal-directed activities. Inactivity and not doing anything should not necessarily reflect an impairment or disability. Leven and Jonsson (2002) indicate that passing time is a relaxing and unchallenging aspect of typical occupational patterns. Also, "doing" describes engaging in occupational performance as a part of healthy everyday life. Being in "the atmosphere of doing" is additionally beneficial and rewarding for persons in the late lifespan, even if they are not the main person performing the "doing."

Gutman and Schindler (2007) recently suggested that music and drawing have been shown to activate the brain's

reward system. They suggested that cognitively stimulating activity may lead to flow, which also activates the brain's reward system. *Flow* is defined as the state when people experience deep feelings of gratification and elation in response to a highly desired activity. Deep concentration, decreased anxiety, absorption in the activity, personal satisfaction, and oneness with the activity describe a state of flow. Flow is one area from which a person may find enjoyment and pleasure in activity participation. A person in the late lifespan would certainly benefit from the continued experience with music, art, and flow. In particular, an experience of flow may lead to improved well-being, emotional health, and enhanced quality of care for persons with dementia. Occupational therapy assistant practitioners provide interventions and approaches that help clients experience flow.

Another common misperception of the elderly is that an elderly person, particularly someone with dementia, is not able to learn things. The American Psychiatric Association (2000) identifies that "[n]ew learning is impaired in people who have dementia." Basic adaptation, communication patterns, and behaviors can display some of the simplest forms of learning. These can occur throughout a person's life (Wertheimer et al., 1992). Behavior is an example where a person with dementia or cognitive impairment may react to his or her environment. Gugel (1994) identified that even though behavior appears to be random and unpredictable, it is often purposeful and predictable, as it satisfies an individual's need. A key concept is that behavior can change. Also, behavior can change to fulfill an individual's need. A person with cognitive impairments, though, does not

TABLE 9-1

LEARNING STRATEGIES OF PEOPLE DIAGNOSED WITH DEMENTIA

IMPAIRED LEARNING CAPACITY	RESIDUAL LEARNING POTENTIAL
Examples of impaired learning capacity include:	*Examples of possible intact learning potential include:*
• Recall/memorization • Effortful learning strategies • Capacity to associate ideas • Storage of information • Develop automatisms • Power of initiation • Goal orientation • Self-directed learning • New learning	• Flow • Reductionistic techniques • Participant's perception of self in the environment • Unambiguous time and space cues • Spatial orientation • Process Strategies and sequence order structures • Remaining motor memory • Procedural learning • Space retrieval techniques

Compiled from American Psychiatric Association. (2000). *Diagnostic and statistical manual of mental disorders, DSM-IV-TR.* (4th ed.). Washington, D.C.: Author.; Borell, L., Bernspång, B., Nygård, L., & Rönnberg, L. (1993). Supporting everyday activities in dementia: An international study. *International Journal of Geriatric Psychiatry, 8,* 395-400.; Gutman, S. A., & Schindler, V. P. (2007). The neurological basis of occupation. *Occupational Therapy International, 14*(2), 71-85.; Hayes, R. L., & Keller, S. M. (1999). Why won't Australian occupational therapists adopt Allen's cognitive disabilities theory? *Australian Occupational Therapy Journal, 46,* 188-192.; Holthe, T., Thorsen, K., & Josephsson, S. (2007). Occupational patterns of people with dementia in residential care: An ethnographic study. *Scandinavian Journal of Occupational Therapy, 14*(2), 96-107.; Josephsson, S., Bäckman, L., Borell, L., Nygard, L., & Bernspång, B. (1998). Effectiveness of an intervention to improve occupational performance in dementia. *Occupational Therapy Journal of Research, 15*(1), 36-49.; Leven, N. V., & Jonsson, H. (2002). Doing and being in the atmosphere of the doing: Environmental influences of occupational performance in a nursing home. *Scandinavian Journal of Occupational Therapy, 9,* 148-155.; Warchol, K. (2000). The challenge of dementia care: Focusing on remaining abilities, not deficits, creates a positive foundation for treatment. *OT Practice, 22*(5), 15-19.; Wertheimer, J., Boula, J. G., Brull, J., Gutt, A. M., Pierrehumbert, B., Rufini, J....Monagéro, J. (1992). Learning process in Dementia. *International Journal of Geriatric Psychiatry, 7,* 161-172.

typically learn the same way an elderly person without cognitive impairments would learn. New learning is impaired in persons with dementia.

Often a person with dementia or cognitive impairments is able to access residual memory to improve functional performance. This can be seen when a person with dementia displays a higher level of ability in occupationally meaningful tasks compared with activities that are new and have no meaning or purpose to the individual. In this example, simply referring to accessing residual lifelong memory and rote performance deemphasizes a person's ability to change behaviors and adapt to the environment. It is important to note, though, that as the presentations of dementia progress, a person's capacity to learn or adapt will also become more impaired. However, learning and adaptation are still possible. It is important to restate that new learning is impaired with persons with dementia.

Quite often occupational therapy education relies on typical methods of instruction, handouts, and demonstration to enable learning. Information is passed from the therapist, who is considered the expert, to the willing recipient, who is usually the client. The therapist then expects the client to instantaneously carry over the instruction or

continue learning through self-directed methods or reinforcement in further therapy sessions. Occupational therapy assistant practitioners may use recall, effortful learning strategies, association, information storage, automatisms, and initiation as methods of learning, as displayed in Table 9-1. These learning approaches attempt to access new learning, which is impaired in persons who have dementia, but may be appropriate for aging clients who present with intact cognitive functioning. Occupational therapy assistant practitioners must utilize different learning approaches with people who have dementia or cognitive impairments.

Table 9-1 also identifies learning strategies that may be successful with individuals who have dementia or cognitive impairments. Occupational therapy assistant practitioners apply learning strategies that include flow, reductionist techniques, perception of the environment, time and space cues, spatial orientation, process strategies, sequence order structures, remaining motor memory, procedural learning, and space retrieval techniques. Flow and how it can be beneficial for a person with dementia was described earlier in this chapter and will be described in Chapters 10 and 11. Reductionistic techniques and methods describe reducing the environmental demands and stress on a person to help him or her function better. This allows the person to function at his or her optimum level of ability. Time and space cues refer to how a person organizes his or her occupational performance in the context of time and space. Often, this is accompanied by procedural memory and process strategies. Procedural memory is typically less impaired. *Procedural memory* is defined as the presence of previous experiences that alter or facilitate an individual's performance (Josephsson, Bäckman, Borell, Nygard, & Bernspång, 1998). Process strategies may be used to access procedural memory to maximize functional ability. Likewise, space retrieval techniques include using approaches that access intact memories to use specific information that may enhance function. External memory cues may be an example. Spatial orientation cues refer to the physical layout and context of the lived space.

Motor memory is another aspect with residual learning capacity. Hoppes, Davis, and Thompson (2003) found that persons with dementia performed better on motor tasks in familiar environments than in unfamiliar environments. Borell, Bernspång, Nygård, and Rönnberg (1993) also identified that aspects of motor memory are preserved in persons with dementia. Motor memory refers to the ingrained, lifelong learned movement patterns that people utilize daily in their engagement in occupations. An example includes a person opening a bottle. The person may utilize a basic movement sequence learned to remove the bottle cap. Normally a person would adapt this basic movement pattern to adjust to opening a new unexperienced type of bottle cap. This new experience would then be added to the person's repertoire of movement strategies. A person with dementia or cognitive impairments may not be able to incorporate this new learning due to impairments. Occupational therapy assistant practitioners utilize the residual basic motor sequence pattern of movement and try to enhance an aspect of occupational performance that is desired.

Similar to the misperception that an elderly person is not able to learn new things is the misperception that a person with dementia or cognitive impairments is incapable of adapting to the environment. Leven and Jonsson (2002) identified that people with dementia continually adapt to disability and impairments as well as to how care is provided. A person's self-reference provides an individual a foundation from which to adapt to changes that affect him or her. The perceptions of a person with dementia are that person's reality. Examples of factors that influence a person's self-reference will be individualized and specific to the contexts of each person. Toth-Cohen (2000) identified that a person with dementia may be able to retain aspects of the cultural structure, customary perceptions, beliefs, and the home/institutional culture. These aspects can be different for people of the same culture as well as people of differing cultures. Occupational therapy assistant practitioners provide education to staff that may maximize the participation

for a client. This education can include specifics on who a client is and his or her individual intricacies.

Holthe, Thorsen, and Josephsson (2007) found that people with dementia do change their occupational patterns due to the presentation of dementia, social influences, and environmental changes. They identified that the home environment presented significant differing contexts on persons with dementia compared with institutionalized care. In particular, institutionalization appears to make individuals with dementia react as guests in the institutional setting. Clients appear to wait for permission to do things or for staff to initiate interaction. Also, the social environment is different for persons with dementia. At home, the person with dementia will experience more family social dynamics. In institutions, persons with dementia experience more of a micro-social environment with interactions among various small groups of people. The home compared with the institutional environment provides significantly different contexts affecting participants. Occupational therapy assistant practitioners may address self-determination, social interaction, and the ability of a person to find continuity in occupational patterns at home and with placement in an institution.

Finally, another misperception is that elderly persons, as well as persons with dementia, are not able to express themselves functionally. Persons with cognitive impairments can have agitation, combativeness, or behavioral exacerbations in their daily lives. Often no records are maintained as to why individuals with cognitive impairments act or behave this way in their environment. Occupational therapy assistant practitioners have to address the physical environment and the multiple contexts of the person in order to provide interventions for agitation, combativeness, and behavior exacerbations. Mahaffey (2009) suggests that feeling engaged in meaningful life roles provides a sense of control and satisfaction for a client. Occupational therapy assistant practitioners are well trained to help clients engage in meaningful life roles.

One plausible explanation for behavioral and emotional exacerbations is that an individual with cognitive impairments continues to perceive his or her surroundings and is not able to meet his or her self-perceived notion of what is deemed consistent or acceptable for him- or herself. Holthe et al. (2007) found that institutionalized persons with dementia liked activities that did not reveal their impairments or weaknesses. This could be a plausible explanation for why people do not expose their impairments early in the dementia process (Hayes & Keller, 1999). A perception of weakness, not empowerment, and long-term stress can also lead to debility and further mental health impairments (Norman, 2007). Negative emotions of elderly persons can be portrayed as frustration, loneliness, sadness, anger, guilt, stress, and fatigue (Hall & Skelton, 2012). Persons with dementia or cognitive impairments at different levels of ability can experience meaningful interactions that establish trust, rapport, expression of feelings, and acceptance of change (Greene, Ingram, & Johnson, 1993). Factors that affect a person's feelings include the cultural tendency to do certain things a particular way. "Good manners" is one example and is still important to people with cognitive impairments. Feelings of control and satisfaction would most certainly impede the development of negative emotions and behavior exacerbations. Occupational therapy assistant practitioners can educate staff on appropriate communication approaches with clients.

Unfortunately, prejudice, discrimination, and elder abuse can occur when myths and stereotypes on aging are perpetuated. Occupational therapy practitioners have a professional, ethical, and legal responsibility to report prejudice, discrimination, and elder abuse whenever it is encountered. Abuse can include physical abuse, emotional abuse, sexual abuse, exploitation, neglect, and abandonment (Waite, 2014). Guardianship and conservatorship may be necessary when a person is not able to care for or make decisions for him- or herself. Guardianship and conservatorship will necessitate consultation with case/social workers and legal counsel. Occupational therapy assistant practitioners should be aware of professional standards, state requirements, and organizational reporting guidelines if abuse is identified. Ethical and legal issues are discussed in greater detail in Appendix C.

The Centers for Disease Control and Prevention (CDC) identified that the life expectancy for 2010 in the United States was 78.7 years of age (2014). They identified the leading causes of death to be heart disease, cancer, chronic respiratory diseases, stroke, accidents, Alzheimer's disease, diabetes, nephritis, pneumonia/influenza, and intentional self-harm. Degenerative diseases of the aging also include Parkinson's disease, arthritis, cataracts, glaucoma, and hearing loss. Alzheimer's disease is the most common form of dementia and the sixth leading cause of death. Alzheimer's disease is an increasing cause of death, whereas other causes have been decreasing in significance. Occupational therapy assistant practitioners working in the late lifespan will often encounter people diagnosed with dementia, delirium, and depression.

Dementia and delirium are both classified under neurocognitive disorders (APA, 2013).

Delirium presents as a disturbance in attention, awareness, and cognition that develops over a short period and is not explained by a preexisting condition. Dementia is characterized by a chronic progressive and irreversible cognitive loss that affects the ability of a person to function optimally in daily tasks of interest. A person's cognitive, behavioral, and emotional functioning, as well as physical motor ability, are affected. At first, IADL tasks may become more impaired early in the onset of dementia. As the disorder progresses, ADL tasks often become affected. The Alzheimer's Association (2012) identifies the following seven stages of dementia:

1. Stage 1: No Impairment
2. Stage 2: Very Mild Decline
3. Stage 3: Mild Decline
4. Stage 4: Moderate Decline
5. Stage 5: Moderately Severe Decline
6. Stage 6: Severe Decline
7. Stage 7: Very Severe Decline

People often progress through the stages of dementia differently or may even skip a stage.

Persons with dementia are at increased risk for malnutrition, falls, untreated medical conditions, accidental death, wandering, increased emotional distress, and negative attitudes from community members (Alzheimer's Association, 2012).

The Alzheimer's Association (2012) estimates that 5.2 million people who are 65 years of age or older have a diagnosis of dementia. Additionally, 200,000 people who are older than 65 years of age are estimated to have dementia. Padilla (2011) shared that dementia is expected to double worldwide in the next 20 years. Greater emphasis is developing for community-based care versus dependence on the traditional medical model. Up to 70% of persons with dementia live in the community and only 3 out of every 10 people with dementia will need institutional care. Unfortunately, family members and caregivers can experience the negative consequences of dementia. They can experience stress, depression, anxiety, emotional distress, decreased quality of life, and decreased health. Often caregivers need assistance to adapt and construct roles (Keady, Woods, Hohn, & Hill, 2004). It is becoming more common for people in the community to identify a family member who is experiencing dementia. This will necessitate greater resources to meet the needs of caregivers and family members in the future.

People with dementia and cognitive impairments can enjoy themselves, be happy, and experience care from those around them to maximize their quality of life. Spotlight 9-1 lists important considerations for the occupational therapy assistant when working with a person diagnosed with cognitive impairments. These recommendations highlight specific aspects that are essential for the occupational therapy assistant to create meaningful change.

The CDC (2012) identifies that depression is not a normal part of aging; however, older adults do experience a greater risk for developing depression. The CDC reports the majority of older adults are not depressed. They identified that depression occurs in about 1% to 5% of older adults living in the community, whereas depression may develop in about 11.5% to 13.5% of older adults who require some sort of health care. A person diagnosed with depression may present with feelings of hopelessness, pessimism, guilt, worthlessness, and/or helplessness. He or she may

---

SPOTLIGHT 9-1. IMPORTANT CONSIDERATIONS FOR THE OCCUPATIONAL THERAPY ASSISTANT

- Dementia is a word, not the person! See the person, not the diagnosis of dementia.
- Focus on the presentations of dementia, not the diagnosis.
- Respect the client; treat him or her like you would treat any other person.
- A tenet of medicine is do no harm. Apply the tenet, "Don't take away anything from the client" when working with a person with dementia.
- Know the culture and passed lived experience of the person with dementia.
- Enter the reality of the person with dementia. Remember his or her perception is his or her reality.
- Every person will have differing presentations of dementia and progress differently through the disorder.
- Allow the person the ability to make choices.
- Give a client time to respond, don't interrupt. Stop talking.

---

also present with irritability, restlessness, fatigue, loss of appetite, suicidal ideation, change in sleep patterns, loss of interest in activities, and cognitive difficulties.

Although these disorders affect a person's mental health and ability to function, every person can still achieve mental health, wellness, and quality of life in the late lifespan. Identification of symptoms of mental illness may be more important to identify if a mental health concern exists. A Place for Mom (n.d.) identifies 10 symptoms of mental illness. These symptoms include the following:

1. Sad or depressed mood lasting greater than 2 weeks.

2. Social withdrawal, loss of enjoyment in previous interests.

3. Unexplained fatigue, energy loss, and sleep changes.

4. Confusion, disorientation, and problems with concentration/decision making.

5. Increase or decrease in weight or eating habits.

6. Memory loss, especially recent or short-term memory.

7. Feelings of worthlessness, helplessness, or guilt.

8. Unexplained physical complaints. (An elderly person may be more likely to report physical symptoms versus psychiatric complaints.)

9. Changes in appearance or self-care.

10. Trouble with finances or home management.

Legislation Affecting the Occupational Therapy Services

Government legislation has significantly affected the provision of health care services in the late lifespan. Legislation is often a reflection of the general public's beliefs, values, and desires for how care should be provided for populations in our society. In the United States, influential legislation affecting the late lifespan traces back as far as the 1960s through to the most recent proposed legislation. Quite often, legislation can provide a funding resource for mandates. It can also indicate the need for therapy services and identify the types of services in certain settings.

A brief listing of legislation affecting the provision of health care for individuals in the late lifespan can be found in Checkpoint 9-2. As can be seen in Checkpoint 9-2, flurries of bills were enacted in the 1960s. The economic distress of the 1970s and 1980s shifted the focus of legislative concerns elsewhere. The 1980s produced amendments to acts that affected health care by refining how services were delivered. Influential legislation and further amendments that refined health care approaches continued to be enacted in the 1990s and start of the millennium. The most recent legislation, The Patient Protection and Affordability Act, continues to affect the future of health care in the United States.

The social upheaval of the 1960s led to significant changes in the health care policy in the United States. The Community Mental Health Centers Act of 1963 (PL 8-164) provided states a financial incentive to deinstitutionalize. Up until this time, the mental health care needs of individuals were mostly met through state institutions. Individuals were reintroduced into the community where treatment could be provided in the least restrictive environment. Alternatives to institutionalization were created in the community. The themes of "treatment in the least restrictive environment" and "treatment in the community" appear common in the late lifespan for the current provision of health care in the United States (Accordino, Porter, & Morse, 2001; Werner & Tyler, 1993).

Another significant legislation in the 1960s was Title 18 of the Social Security Act, also known as *Medicare*. It was enacted in 1965 and administered by the federal government. Medicare initially was created as a health insurance plan for the elderly. It is divided into Medicare Part A and Medicare Part B Insurance. Medicare Part A covers

CHECKPOINT 9-2. IDENTIFY LEGISLATION AFFECTING THE LATE LIFESPAN				
		Legislation	*Year*	*Public Law*
1960s	1	Community Mental Health Act	1963	PL 8-164
	2	Title 18 of Social Security Act-Medicare	1965	Title 18
	3	Medicaid Act	1965	PL 89-97
	4	Older Americans Act (OAA)	1965	PL 89-73
1980s	5	Alcohol Abuse, Drug Abuse, and Mental Health Amendments	1984	HR- 5413
	6	State Mental Health Planning Act	1986	HR- 4326
	7	"Mental Health Systems Act" became the Omnibus Budget and Reconciliation Act (OBRA)	1981/1987	PL 97-35 PL 100-203
1990s	8	Britain-National Health Service and Community Care Act	1990	United Kingdom
	9	Mental Health Parity Act	1996	PL 104-204
	10	Individuals with Disabilities Act (IDEA)	1990	PL 101-476
		Americans with Disability Act (ADA)	1990	PL 101-336
2010s	11	Patient Protection and Affordability Act	2009	HR 3590
	12	The National Alzheimer's Project Act	2011	PL 111-375
	13	Amendment to the Public Health Service Act	Proposed	HR 3762

inpatient care, home health care, and initial care provided in skilled nursing facilities. Medicare Part B typically covers outpatient care and care provided in skilled nursing facilities after coverage of Part A benefits are exhausted. Medicare legislation significantly affected how fees for service health care are provided in the United States. Medicare continues to undergo amendments and revisions to coverage affecting the provision of health care for many in this country.

Along with Medicare, Medicaid (PL 89-97) was enacted in 1965 as a combined federal and state insurance program for the indigent and those not covered by Medicare (Glantz & Richmann, 1998). Werner and Tyler (1993) identified that Medicare and Medicaid in the past, however, poorly addressed psychiatric health care. Over the years, Medicaid has increasingly become a managed care plan administered by each state, in part to control costs while meeting the health care needs of participants. Tenncare in Tennessee is an example of a Medicaid managed care program.

The "Choices" program is one program offered by state Medicaid agencies that is designed to facilitate a participant's return to the community after medical care. Additionally, care can be provided to aid individuals to remain in the community. Another program provided by Tenncare is the Senior Citizen's Home Assistance Program, which again is designed to assist individuals to remain in the community. Traditional occupational therapy services may be limited or not covered under Tenncare as well as other Medicaid programs. Evidence-based practice, cost-effectiveness studies, and outcome-based studies suggest

that occupational therapy would be a beneficial service to help individuals remain in the community.

Finally, The Older Americans Act (OAA) of 1965 (PL 89-73) further expanded community-based services for the elderly (Department of Health and Human Services [DHHS], 2010). This act enabled funding for the "Meals on Wheels" program, community services employment for low-income older Americans, and elder rights protection. The OAA also created the Administration of Aging, which is part of the Department of Health and Human Services. Over the years, the OAA has undergone many revisions and amendments. A description of the OAA, which was updated in 2006, includes the following:

- Title I—Declaration of Objectives, Definitions

- Title II—Administration on Aging

- Title III—Grants for State and Community Programs on Aging

- Title IV—Activities for Health, Independence, and Longevity

- Title V—Community Service Senior Opportunities Act

- Title VI—Grants for Native Americans

- Title VII—Vulnerable Elders Rights Protection

The Administration on Aging provides a great deal of information to support the concerns of elderly persons in the community. Some agencies publish this supporting information in senior service directories or senior resource guides as a service to the community. Further information about the Administration on Aging can be found at their website: www.aoa.gov.

Health care policy legislation in the 1980s and 1990s reflected society's desire and need to control costs and address other important issues affecting Americans. The Alcohol Abuse, Drug Abuse and Mental Health Amendments of 1984 (HR-5413) and The State Mental Health Planning Act of 1986 (HR-4326) both affected the provision of community-based mental health care (Accordino et al., 2001; Kleinman, 1992). These acts provided funding for community-based mental health care through the use of grants and by enabling community mental health care providers to receive reimbursement through Medicare and Medicaid. Reimbursement sources were needed because the government had ended its financial support for community mental health care centers. Many institutions had undergone deinstitutionalization and transitioned individuals to the community. Although a large portion of costs associated with home care for individuals in the late lifespan are assumed by families, a significant portion is also covered through Medicare Part A and home health care benefits.

Perhaps the most significant legislation of the 1980s was the Mental Health Systems Act, which later became the Omnibus Budget and Reconciliation Act (OBRA) of 1981 and then 1987 (PL 97-35). OBRA mandated a comprehensive rehabilitative approach to geriatric health care through individualized care, choice, freedom, dignity, and quality of life (Keough & Huebner, 2000). OBRA encouraged intervention by occupational therapy to ensure residents in long-term care facilities maximize their level of ability and quality of life (Brown, Lohman, & Nieman, 1998). OBRA made it illegal to restrain residents in long-term care facilities for discipline, convenience, or to limit a person's mobility. Lap belts, wrist restraints, half-lap table for a wheelchair, full lap table for a wheelchair, locking a person in his or her room, and having all four side rails of a bed up are considered restraints. A physician's order will be necessary to justify the use of a restraint as medically necessary, and a time limit may be imposed on the restraint. Occupational therapy assistant practitioners may attempt restraint reduction techniques to maximize quality of life. Examples include using chair/bed alarms, environmental modifications, activity or task adaptations, chair/wheelchair/bed positioning, ability to use technology, and caregiver and client education. Finally, OBRA significantly ended the federal commitment to community health care centers (Werner & Tyler, 1993).

The 1990s saw further refinement in laws in the United States and the United Kingdom. In the United Kingdom, the National Health Service and Community Care Act of 1990 was enacted to support people to live in communities instead of institutional care (Hall & Skelton, 2012). This law is the basis for social medicine and community-based health care provided in the United Kingdom. This model of care is significantly different than the fee-for-service models of health care provided in the United States. Occupational therapy in the United States could benefit from incorporating evidence-based practice identified in countries like the United Kingdom and Scandinavia.

The 1990s in the United States saw the initial passing of the Individuals with Disabilities Act and the Americans with Disabilities Act. These acts were designed to break down barriers in the community for persons with disabilities and impairments. "Aging in Place" was created based on the concepts of these two acts. A person can become a Certified Aging in Place Specialist through the National Association of Home Builders. This certification shows that a person has a skill set to provide consultation services that may enable a person to remain living in his or her home longer. Although certification is nice to support specialization and ability to provide services, this certification is not specific to occupational therapy, and nonoccupational therapy practitioners can attain this specialization.

In the United States, the most recent and controversial legislation passed in 2009 is the Patient Protection and Affordability Act (PPACA; HR-3590). The PPACA prescribes each state to create an essential health benefit plan, which will include a "Rehabilitative and Habilitative" component (Brown, 2012). Typically, most commercial health care plans do not include options or limit options under this category. Fifty-two sections of this act were instituted by 2012. One example of this act is that children can be covered under their parents' policies until the age of 26. Starting in 2014, plans also cannot exclude participants based on preexisting conditions (Williams, 2012). The law also created the following:

- An independent Medicare advisory board to make recommendations for cost savings with Medicare.

- Community First Choice options providing attendant support for home living.

- Community Living Assistance Services and Supports, which creates a voluntary payroll deduction for a long-term care insurance program.

- Continues the Aging and Disability Resource Center (Lindberg & MacInnes, 2010).

The PPACA also has provided increased funding for services through Medicaid. The "Medicaid Money Follows the Person" (MFP) Rebalancing Demonstration Program is one example. This program provides increased funding for individuals who are institutionalized and return/transition to home with services. The Community First Choice option of the law is another example. Under this program, attendant care can be provided to aid the ability of individuals to live at home who require an institutional level of care. Additional services provided by Tenncare's Choices program to enable a person to live at home may include personal care visits, home-delivered meals, personal emergency response system, adult day care, in-home respite care, inpatient respite care, assistive technology, minor home modifications, pest control, and community-based residential alternatives.

Recently, The National Alzheimer's Project Act was passed in 2011. This act hopes to create a national plan, coordinate research, enhance outcomes, facilitate development of treatments, improve care coordination, and help with early diagnosis. This national plan to address Alzheimer's disease was created by the Department of Health and Human Services (2012). The five goals of this plan include the following:

1. Goal #1: Prevent and effectively treatment Alzheimer's disease by 2025

2. Goal #2: Enhance care quality and efficiency

3. Goal #3: Expand supports for people with Alzheimer's disease and their families

4. Goal #4: Enhance public awareness and engagement

5. Goal#5: Improve data to track progress

The national plan provides a significant change from the past when no national plan was in place to address the chronic progressive disorders of dementia-related disorders. These goals can greatly influence the role of occupational therapy in the community.

Finally, occupational therapy has also championed an amendment to the Public Health Service Act (HR-3762, 2011). This act would add occupational therapy as a behavioral and mental health profession to be included under the National Health Service Corps (HR-3762). Unfortunately, this amendment never came to fruition due to legislative gridlock. In a partial victory, the Centers for Medicare and Medicaid Services did include occupational therapy as a service that must be available in participating community mental health centers in 2013. Curtin (2008) stresses the importance of occupational therapy to continue the roles of advocates and lobbyists to help meet client needs. Occupational therapy must remain proactive and advocate for the future role that this act may enable the profession.

Since the 1960s, the United States has embarked on a fee-for-service reimbursement model of health care, which has increasingly become more managed in an effort to control costs and increase efficacy and efficiency. Third-party payers or providers typically manage and provide coverage similarly to Medicare. Unfortunately, fee-for-service reimbursement models in the United States can lead to fragmented care, less-than-ideal follow-up, and legislation that can be limiting or suppressive. The reliance on Medicare and traditional models of reimbursement has delayed the development of community-based treatment approaches for people with mental health care needs in the late lifespan.

Until recently, a diagnosis of dementia could have resulted in a denial of services. Advocacy efforts led to a reversal of this trend in Medicare at the turn of the century. Legislation provides occupational therapy the opportunity to meet individual needs in the medical model and community. In particular, occupational therapy has the opportunity to further strengthen our role in meeting individual needs in the community.

PART 2: TREATMENT SETTINGS

Occupational therapy practitioners work in a variety of settings where services may be provided over the late lifespan. Many settings are based within the medical model, whereas others are located within the community. Quite often, individuals enter a medical facility for health reasons necessitating an occupational therapy evaluation. Table 9-2 illustrates the variety of settings that may be encountered over the late lifespan. Medicare and private insurance usually provide coverage for most admissions to medical facilities. Most community-based care, however, is managed and assumed by the individual, caregiver, or family members.

The family physician or emergency room physician may be the first person to encounter a person in the late lifespan with health care needs. Admissions to a hospital can be due to medical conditions such as pneumonia, cardiac problems, or a fractured hip. Behavioral and cognitive impairments may also contribute to the need for hospital care. Injuries can occur due to forgetfulness, weakness, or decreased safety. The person may display an exacerbation of behaviors affecting function in the home due to a host of causes. Medicine mismanagement can also occur when a caregiver is not available to assist with taking medication. Holthe et al. (2007) identify that the primary priority of staff in the medical setting is the physical and medical needs of the client.

Clients can also access the medical model when living at home. A person in the late lifespan living at home can access the medical model through visiting the primary care physician, outpatient therapy, and accessing home health care services. Home health care services are usually covered by Medicare Part A benefits. A physician is also required to have a face-to-face encounter with the client prior to the start of home health care services to be reimbursed by Medicare. At this time, occupational therapy is not considered a "standalone" service by Medicare for in-home health care. This means that another qualified service must be initiated by home health care to allow occupational therapy to be provided. If home health care is not an option, outpatient therapy may be a consideration. Although outpatient therapy is an option, at times it is harder to achieve occupational therapy goals in outpatient therapy due to complex cognitive and behavioral impairments.

Occupational therapy assistants provide interventions to help a person remain in the community. This can

TABLE 9-2		
TREATMENT SETTINGS OF THE LATE LIFESPAN		
REIMBURSEMENT MODELS	MEDICALLY BASED SETTINGS	COMMUNITY BASED SETTINGS AND RESOURCES
Medicare Part A and B Medicaid Health Insurance and Private Pay	Emergency rooms	
	Geropsychiatric/specialty units	
	Acute care hospital floor	
	Inpatient rehabilitation	
	Outpatient rehabilitation	
	Skilled nursing facility/specialty units	
	Home health care	
Typically families assume financial responsibility. Insurance programs may provide some coverage but may be limited.		Home
		Group homes
		Adult day centers
		Assisted living facility
		Alzheimer's Association
		Area agency on aging
		Churches
		Friends and neighbors
		Elder abuse services
		Housekeepers
		Caregiver support groups

include educating family members and caregivers on care needs, community resources, and care assistance options in the community. Occupational therapy practitioners apply approaches to increase the independent ability to engage in life tasks, improve safety, and adapt or modify the environment. Occupational therapy assistants may also provide services to enable a person to engage and interact in the community. Occupational therapy assistant practitioners provide services to maximize overall health, well-being, and quality of life. Caregivers may also need training and education, as well as assistance, in developing their caregiver roles. These services will be identified in greater detail in Chapters 10 and 11.

Institutionalization may become necessary when a person's needs cannot be met at home. This can include admission to a geropsychiatric hospital unit or skilled nursing facility. A person may return home once stabilized, or require further care remaining at the institution. Alternative settings in the community that help meet individual needs include group homes, assisted living facilities, and adult day care centers. Although insurance programs and third-party payers cover some costs, individuals and their families usually have to make up the difference.

It is an oversimplification to assume that a person with cognitive and behavioral impairments, medical complexity, or advanced age will be institutionalized or live in a skilled nursing facility one day. Golden and Lawlor (2006) identified that most people with mild-to-moderate dementia live in the community, and almost all have a primary caregiver. Holden and Woods (1995) also identified that a majority of people with dementia in the United Kingdom live alone or with family. Padilla (2011) identified that up to 70% of people with Alzheimer's disease in the United States are cared for at home. The Alzheimer's Association (2012) identified that up to 800,000 people with dementia live alone. Half of these people don't have an identifiable caregiver. Occupational therapy assistant practitioners help to identify the most appropriate community setting to include home, assisted living facilities, group homes, specialized care homes, and respite care or day programs. Occupational therapy assistant practitioners advocate for clients and provide consultative services in collaboration with the occupational therapist.

Several themes appear to apply with the selection of a setting for persons in the late lifespan. First, is the setting cost effective and does it meet the needs of the individual

(Brown et al., 1998)? The setting of choice usually provides the least restrictive environment and the lowest level of care to meet the individual's needs. Many considerations determine the most appropriate level of care for each individual. Factors that influence the choice of setting for an individual may include the following:

- The level of cognitive or behavioral impairment
- Financial resources
- Time
- Setting availability
- Social dynamics of the family

The level of cognitive and behavioral impairments also may affect the choice of a setting. A diagnosis of dementia does not mean that a person will need to live on a locked unit one day, necessitate living in a skilled nursing facility, or require a visit to the geropsychiatric center at a hospital. Brown et al. (1998) identify that clients function best in their typical home environment. As a person progresses with dementia, symptoms and behaviors can vary, and unique behavioral manifestations can be created (Cheney, 2011). Likewise, a person's ability to adapt to familiar and unfamiliar movements and environments may decrease over time. As the dementia progresses to the advanced stages of the disorder, it can become too much for the family and caregivers to handle, thus requiring institutionalization. Occupational therapy assistant practitioners provide services to support caregivers and so the client can remain in the home environment. Services may provide solutions to alleviate problem behaviors and agitation.

Financial reimbursement for occupational therapy services can be a challenge to providing care within the medical model and community in the United States. Priebe and Fakhoury (2007) identify that socioeconomic and funding influence community practice. Quite often, private insurance plans may limit coverage for mental health benefits. Due to this lack of coverage, most people with cognitive and behavioral impairments may not be seen in the medical model until after a fall or other medical condition that causes hospitalization (Buchmueller, Cooper, Jacobson, & Zuvellers, 2007). Occupational therapy assistant practitioners make referrals to other practitioners, including social workers and case managers. They provide specific information on the client that facilitates the provision of available services to meet the client's needs.

Another consideration is the financial resources enabling a person to live at home. Quite often Social Security is used by seniors to support living in the community. Social Security may be used instead by the nursing home to finance long-term care. Another consideration is that more extended families are living together due to the economic hardships in recent years. These extended families may choose to support their family members with cognitive and behavioral impairments in the home in order to maintain the ability to keep the house as a living space for the entire family. This may be evident when the family is dependent on a person's Social Security income to maintain the home. Additionally, these families may not be able to support copayments for outpatient therapy, medications, attendants, and home health care, which may be beneficial.

The context of time influences the choice of setting. Overall, people are living longer, and cognitive and behavioral impairments increase in incidence with age (Bree & Meldrum, 2005). More complex and challenging disabilities and impairments can become present as the person advances in age (Goode, Haley, Roth, & Ford, 1998). Kleinman (1992) identifies that over time, medical model sources of care may become more necessary. A person admitted to the hospital will most likely stay there a very short time. Once the client is stabilized, discharge planning has already been initiated so that the client is ready to transition to the next lower level of care. The duration of time needed for the client may reflect the choice of facility. Skilled nursing facilities and assisted living facilities can provide respite care over short or long periods. Additionally, skilled nursing facilities may have the availability to transition the individual to become a long-term client of the facility. Day care centers and in-home respite care may be chosen to provide assistance over short periods, such as hours and days, instead of weeks and months.

Availability also influences the choice of setting. Families that live in rural areas may have less availability for different types and options of settings and services. In particular, small rural communities may not have local access to choose between assisted living facilities or community services such as Meals on Wheels. Additionally, if a setting is at full capacity, there may be a waiting list. Rural areas may have to rely more on informal support services such as churches, family members, friends, and neighbors. Barriers to quality care may include insufficient time, ineffective reimbursement, limited availability to specialists, inadequate coverage of medications, and lack of interdisciplinary teams in either rural or urban areas. Bennett, Shand, and Liddle (2011) also identify that a reactive approach versus a proactive approach, staffing, and organizational structure can be barriers to quality care.

Finally, the social dynamics of the family and society may influence the choice of setting. Group homes, specialized senior homes, and home care by families in some countries are more the norm for people in the late lifespan. In the United States, a significant proportion of individuals live in the community. A greater number of community living options are emerging to include senior apartments, independent living facilities, senior living communities, assisted living facilities, dementia homes, and respite care facilities. Occupational therapy assistant practitioners can assist families to identify the most appropriate community settings available and help to maximize function in each environment.

Documentation may vary between community-based models of care compared with care provided within the medical model. Documentation in community models of care may have minimal requirements, as documentation may not be necessary for reimbursement. The medical model often does require specific information in documentation, as it is usually tied to reimbursement. An example of required documentation in home health care is the Outcome and Assessment Information Set (OASIS) evaluation. Medicare requires the OASIS evaluation to start home health services. OASIS is not a service occupational therapy assistants will be expected to perform. Additionally, certain information is required for each therapy visit, such as pain levels, basic health information, start and end time of services, and what skilled services were provided. Medicare also requires specific documentation for other services.

Medicare requires specific information in the treatment of persons with dementia in long-term care facilities. The occupational therapist will complete Form 700 for the initial evaluation of occupational therapy services and Form 701 for the reevaluation of occupational therapy services thereafter. Occupational therapists will create the long-term occupational therapy goals. The occupational therapy assistants can collaborate with the occupational therapist in development of the short-term goals.

Medicare does have specific criteria to guide in the provision of occupational therapy services in long-term care facilities. Specific criteria are highlighted here (Butler, 2013):

- Medicare does not reimburse occupational therapy services for "maintenance" care. Restorative nursing and the certified nursing assistant staff are expected to be able to provide nonskilled maintenance services. Medicare does reimburse for skilled services to develop, set up, and educate staff on a functional maintenance program (FMP) for a person with dementia.

- Medicare will reimburse for occupational therapy services to modify or adapt a documented functional maintenance program that no longer is appropriate for a person with dementia.

- Medicare Part A and Medicare Part B will cover occupational therapy services to identify a baseline level of functioning for new residents admitted to a long-term care facility with no previous history of therapy provided.

- Medicare will not cover occupational therapy services for functional maintenance program problems that are created by not being maintained or followed through by nontherapy staff.

- Long-term goals and short-term goals are always needed with Form 700 and Form 701.

- Goals can focus on the caregiver or family and what they will be expected to demonstrate to meet the needs of the individual.

- Goals should be measurable and reflect an improvement of functional status.

- In long-term care facilities, restorative nursing should not be used concurrently with skilled occupational therapy, physical therapy, and speech therapy services. Medicare will cover concurrent therapy services with restorative nursing care when the resident is receiving a low rehabilitation category of care.

PART 3: OCCUPATIONAL THERAPY PRACTICE MODELS AND THEORY

Occupational therapy provides a unique service to treating impairments, activity limitations, and participation restrictions over the late lifespan. A wide variety of practice models and theories exist to help guide occupational therapy practitioners. Three theoretical approaches are highlighted that particularly apply to the late lifespan. These theoretical models and theories include the following:

- Cognitive Disabilities Theory (CDT) by Claudia Allen

- Person-Environment-Occupation (PEO) Model

- Complexity Science and Dynamic Systems Theory (DST)

This is not an all-inclusive list. Many other approaches can also guide occupational therapy practice with individuals in the late lifespan. The authors believe that these three approaches provide distinct explanations for the variety of approaches available in occupational therapy. Checkpoint 9-3 displays additional practice models and theories that can be applied by occupational therapists to working with people in the late lifespan.

Cognitive Disability Theory

The *Cognitive Disability Therapy (CDT)* is a function-based theory that was organized by Claudia Allen, OTR/L. Instead of solely identifying impairments and disability, the CDT theory identifies what the client may be able to do with his or her remaining skills and abilities. The CDT believes that observable, measurable limitations in routine task behavior can identify information-processing capabilities of the brain. Impairments in sensorimotor processing result in decreased safety and a failure to change or adapt. Function is identified when a person is able to change or adapt as needed. The CDT is broken down into hierarchical

CHECKPOINT 9-3. COMPARISON OF MODELS AND THEORIES USED BY OCCUPATIONAL THERAPISTS	
Models and Theories	*Summary*
Model of Human Occupation	Occupation-based model that views how people participate in life occupations and achieve positive adaptations
Theory of Retrogenesis	A reverse developmental theory whereby the progression of dementia corresponds to the developmental sequence of the brain earlier in life (Warchol, Copeland, & Ebell, 2006).
Social Model	Looks at social relationships, environmental barriers, and social stressors to promote social relationships and social advocacy (Kleinman, 1992).
Occupational Science	The variety of ways people engage in the meaningful daily tasks that affect themselves, communities, and contexts around individuals.
Competency-Environmental Press Model	Enhancement of positive behavior through matching the level of ability with the environmental press (Piersol, Earland, & Herge, 2012).
Progressively-Lowered Threshold Model	Modification of environmental stressors to meet the functional capacity facilitating occupational function (Piersol et al., 2012).
Need-Driven Dementia Compromised Behavior Model	Modification of the environment to promote function by meeting individual needs (Piersol et al., 2012).
Antecedent- Behavior- Consequence Model	Identification of behavioral triggers, the behavior, and the consequence in order to modify the antecedent (trigger) or to modify the behavior (Piersol et al., 2012).

levels to identify what abilities may be present. It helps to do the following:

- Identify what ADL and IADL tasks a client is capable of completing at various levels of ability and modes of performance.
- Identify the amount and type of supervision and assistance that may be necessary for each mode of performance (Hayes & Keller, 1999).
- Assess cognition by observing function (Warchol et al., 2006).
- Remain focused on function and remaining capabilities of a person.
- Demonstrate improvements in function and safety.
- Aid the development of realistic goals and intervention plans.

Key performance levels of ability, called **performance modes**, distinguish how a client will be able to function in meaningful occupational tasks (Bieber & Keller, 2005). These six modes begin at 1.0, the lowest level of ability, and progress to 6.0, which is the highest level of ability. Table 9-3 identifies each performance mode level of the CDT and gives a rough description of the performance capability at each mode.

These performance modes can be further broken down into 26 modes of performance to define what a person is capable of performing (Warchol et al., 2006). These 26 modes proceed in 0.2 increments, such as 2.2 or 2.4. It is important to note that the ability levels between these modes of performance are not equally dispersed between modes. Additionally, a therapist can use an odd mode, such as 2.1 or 2.3, if the therapist determines through clinical judgment that the client exceeds the ability level of the lower even performance mode but does not quite display the level of ability for the even upper mode level. Occupational therapy assistant practitioners need to develop service competency with the CDT before collaborating with the occupational therapist to identify performance modes. Table 9-4 identifies key performance modes within the CDT.

Several assessment tools have been refined and developed to screen and evaluate using the CDT. The Routine Task Inventory-Expanded (RTI-2) and Allen Diagnostic Module-2 (ADM2) are assessment tools that can be used to identify a performance mode. One of the most common screening tools used by occupational therapy practitioners is the standardized Allen Cognitive Level Screen—5th Edition (ACLS-5). A practitioner may first use the ACLS-5 to identify a performance mode level and then confirm the score with the RTI or CDT assessment tools. Occupational therapy assistants can perform the ACLS-5, as it is a standardized screening tool. The occupational therapy assistant may also help or collaborate with the occupational therapist in determining the performance mode.

The ACLS was first developed in 1978 to apply to the then Allen Cognitive Disabilities Model for adults diagnosed with psychiatric disorders and adults with dementia. The ACLS-5 is a leather lacing task that can be used to

TABLE 9-3

COGNITIVE DISABILITY THEORY PERFORMANCE MODE LEVELS
PERFORMANCE MODE LEVELS

Level	Summary	Mode Level Functional Ability
1.0	Automatic actions	Protective reflexes, minimal movement, and ability to respond to strong stimuli
2.0	Postural actions	Can overcome gravity; gross body movements present
3.0	Manual actions	Handles objects and can perform repetitive actions
4.0	Goal-directed actions	Can sequence through a familiar task
5.0	Exploratory actions	Can problem solve with trial and error; independent learning possible; learning possible through exploring
6.0	Planned actions	Abstract thinking present and can plan ahead

identify global processing capabilities. The Large Allen Cognitive Level Screen, 5th Edition (LACLS-5) was also developed for the elderly. The ACLS-5 and LACLS-5 are designed to screen for global cognitive processing ability, ability to learn, and performance abilities for individuals between the 3.0 and 5.8 modes of performance. Along with a standardized process for the therapist to follow, the therapist utilizes observation of performance to identify performance modes.

Although the CDT is very useful with clients with psychiatric disorders or cognitive impairments, it presents several weaknesses. Weaknesses of the CDT include that it is not widely known and utilized by the interdisciplinary team. This can be a strength for occupational therapy, as this model allows an approach that will be profession specific. Weaknesses of the CDT also include that performance of the ACLS-5 can be affected by visual impairments or motor impairments. A person's cognitive ability can also fluctuate between performance modes due to a host of influences. Changes in performance modes are typically not significant. Norman (2007) identified some of these influences, which include environmental stressors, medication, illicit substances, interpersonal stresses, time of day, and illnesses. Another weakness is the ability to grasp or see the leather or lacing can be impaired. The ACLS-5 can also yield inaccurate scores if the client has performed the screening tool before and has learned how to complete the task. Overlearned tasks can yield inaccurate scores. The ACLS-5 does not screen for persons with cognitive scores below performance mode 3.0.

Person-Environment-Occupation Model

The ***Person-Environment-Occupation (PEO)*** model provides an explanation for the complex dynamic relationship between the person, environment, and occupation. It provides a systematic approach to identify and address occupational performance (Strong, Rigby, Steward, Law, Letts, & Cooper, 1999). *Occupational performance fit* is the result of the interaction between the person, environment, and occupation at a given time. When a person is not in harmony with one of these factors, it will affect the other parts of the system, leading to a decreased occupational performance fit. Likewise, when all factors are ideal, an optimum occupational performance fit can be achieved.

There are three main factors in the PEO model. The *person* can represent a client, a group of clients, and organizations. *Occupation* refers to a task, multiple tasks, or activities that people participate in daily. *Environment* refers to the physical, social, cultural, virtual, and temporal contexts. The interaction between these factors is considered occupational performance fit. In addition, the interaction between person/occupation, person/environment, and environment/occupation can be considered. The areas of overlap are always changing over time. Examples can be seen when support systems are provided and impairments remediated. The area of overlap between factors will increase, reflecting an occupational performance fit in harmony. Likewise, the development of impairments, activity limitations, and participation restrictions will shrink the overlapping space between factors, reflecting a less-than-ideal occupational performance fit.

An application of the PEO model can be applied to a person with cognitive impairments in the late lifespan and his or her occupational performance fit with self-feeding; the person, environment, and occupation can all be considered. First, examples of person factors may include the ability to attain food, cognitive skills needed to eat, motor ability to bring utensils to the mouth, and the person's interest in self-feeding. Examples of environment factors may include dishware available, the use of microwaves or stoves, the

TABLE 9-4

KEY PERFORMANCE MODES

PERFORMANCE MODE LEVEL	PERFORMANCE MODE	SUMMARY OF SIGNIFICANT PERFORMANCE MODES FUNCTIONAL ABILITY
1.0		Withdrawing from stimulation
	1.2	Responds positively to pleasant stimuli; nonverbal
	1.6	Spontaneous movement in bed
	1.8	Raises body through partial movement, 50% assistance transitional movements
2.0		Overcome gravity
	2.2	Ability to stand, righting reactions
	2.4	Ability to walk; unsteady gait
	2.6	Ability to walk to a highly familiar location
3.0		Tunnel vision 14" to front, able to name, grasp, and release objects
	3.2	Clumsy grasp; speaks short phrases; easily distracted
	3.4	Sustains actions 1 min.; sequences through highly familiar objects
4.0		Sequences through steps of short-term actions; decreased quality of performance
	4.4	Ability to complete a goal; can identify a problem exists but decreased efficiency and effectiveness in problem solving
	4.6	Ability to scan the environment; may be able to live at home independently with ADL tasks; may need assistance with some IADL tasks
5.0		Follows simple written directions with verbal explanations; blames others for errors; may live alone with weekly checks
	5.4	Self-directed learning; independently makes changes to increase efficiency; responds to feedback
	5.6	Can drive; can complete child care
6.0		Planned actions

environment of the dining room, and if self-feeding is conducted with friends or alone. Finally, examples of occupation factors may include the food choice for the meal, the time needed to eat, and waiting for staff to bring the food and set up the meal. These are only a few of the possible descriptions that can be possible within each factor.

Quite often, though, deficits to a particular factor will result in a less-than-ideal occupational performance fit. Cognitive impairments, motor impairments, and visual impairments may affect the person factor. The person may not want to eat the meal provided or forget about his or her need to eat. The environment may be limited by a loud, distractible room that may not resemble a dining room. Additionally, occupation may be limited when the person is not given the opportunity to choose between meal options that may not otherwise be typical for the person. By identifying the factors in the PEO model leading to a less-than-ideal occupational performance fit, the occupational therapy practitioner can adapt, modify, and remediate the factors to maximize the available occupational performance fit.

Complexity Science and Dynamic Systems Theory

Dynamic Systems Theory (DST) principles provide an approach for analyzing and influencing nonadaptive occupational performance patterns. The DST is defined as systems that change over time and are characterized by complexity, randomness, and nonlinearity (Gray, Kennedy, & Zemke, 1996; p. 301). The focus of the dynamic system in occupational therapy is the emerging pattern(s) of human engagement in occupation(s). The individual or client is seen as an active participant rather than a passive recipient of perceptual information regarding his or her experience of the occupation(s). DST describes how order, patterns, and reason can be found in complex, random, and nonlinear organizations.

An individual provides an example of a complex, random, and nonlinear organization. Individuals unconsciously search out patterns of stability and make decisions daily regarding his or her personal engagement in occupations. These decisions act as control and order parameters that aid in creating patterns and organization over time. Four key concepts underlie the DST. These four concepts include complexity, self-organization, phase shifts, and parameters.

Complexity describes the multiple possible variations in a system, also referred to as degrees of freedom. Complexity also identifies that a system increases in complexity over time. Complexity is further created through a nonlinear cause and effect whereby the sum is not equal to the parts of the system, such as the motor development in a person. The developmental sequence of motor development, a hierarchal model, describes how one level of motor ability enables the formation of the next sequential level of motor ability. This is not the only method whereby movement develops, however. Motor development also occurs from nonlinear methods that do not reflect a cause-and-effect relationship. Additionally, complex behavioral patterns and influences from the context differ between people depending on their perceptions. Complexity can be very involved.

The second concept is self-organization. *Self-organization* refers to the ability of complex systems to form patterns over time. Patterns may evolve and develop at differing levels for a person. The numerous possible variations in a system allow for countless patterns to develop. Patterns form over the context of time and are irreversible after their formation. Within a person, this historical pattern of formation provides a self-referential context that can affect the person's present and future engagement in occupational performance.

Phase shifts reflect the small changes in a system that can create greater effects over time. An example of this phenomenon is the "butterfly effect" whereby a butterfly beating its wings in one part of the world influences the formation of a tornado in another part of the world. Even the smallest changes can have a significant effect on the system at a particular time. Changes occur in a system when the system is in disequilibrium and self-organization of new patterns is enabled to develop. These slight changes can be maximized in therapy by using slight variations as change agents during the occupational therapy process.

Finally, *parameters* include both control and order parameters. Control parameters are variables that may lead changes in a system over time, whereas order parameters are variables that have an unchanging influence on the system over time. An example of a control parameter is an aging driver's reaction time because it governs important aspects of his or her driving behavior. An example of an order parameter is the same aging driver's unchanging intention to drive safely. Occupational therapy interventions may be considered an example of a control parameter in a system where new emerging occupational patterns are developed.

The DST suggests that a person with cognitive impairments in the late lifespan may still be able to perceive chaos, disorganization, and order. The DST also suggests that a person with cognitive impairments tries to organize this information and perception to form patterns. A person's experiences over time provide a pattern of self-reference that individualizes that person and anchors him or her in interpreting information. Utilizing information concerning who a person is may aid the therapist in helping the client interpret information and make order in his or her life (Wheatley, 1992). Knowledge about what is meaningful to a client gives the therapist a way to use these meanings as order parameters (Kelso, 1995). These order parameters can be used to help the client adapt to the changing control parameters of aging and cognitive impairments. This can also explain why a person with cognitive impairments may perform poorly with changes in the environment. Since our self-reference is tied to the contexts we live in, a change in environment takes away an important order parameter that can result in compromises in occupational performance.

SUMMARY

As the population ages, more people are susceptible to developing cognitive and behavioral impairments. This means that more extended families will experience the need to provide for their aging family members throughout the late lifespan. It is a fact that people with cognitive impairments in the late lifespan can have an increased quality of life, live safely, and function at the highest level of ability with therapeutic intervention. This dispels that notion that a person with cognitive impairments, such as dementia, can't benefit from occupational therapy services. Medicare acknowledged this at the turn of the century, in 2001. Medicare sided with evidence-based practice by ending their discriminatory practices of denying services for therapy just because there was a diagnosis of dementia. Occupational therapy has the potential to support clients and their families to remain home living in their communities.

The occupational therapy process, therapeutic use of self, and "occupation" are hallmarks of occupational therapy utilized over the late lifespan (Harrison, 2005; Mahaffey, 2009). The use of occupation as a means as well as an end goal remains specific to occupational therapy. Occupations provide a unique approach to create positive change through the professional approach of occupational therapy (Brown, 2009). Kleinman (1992) has also suggested

---

SPOTLIGHT 9-2. HALLMARKS OF OCCUPATIONAL THERAPY APPLIED IN THE LATE LIFESPAN

OCCUPATIONAL THERAPY PROCESS:

OCCUPATION

THERAPEUTIC USE OF SELF

ACTIVITY ANALYSIS

DEVELOPMENTAL PERSPECTIVE

FUNCTIONAL OUTCOMES

Question: What do you think is another hallmark used by occupational therapy when providing services in the late lifespan? Be prepared to justify your choice to the class.)

Compiled from American Occupational Therapy Association. (2014). Occupational therapy practice framework: Domain and process. (3rd ed.). *American Journal of Occupational Therapy, 68*(Suppl. 1), S1-S48. doi: 10.5014/ajot2014.682006.

---

that activity analysis, a developmental perspective, and emphasis on functional outcomes are also specific to occupational therapy in the late lifespan. Spotlight 9-2 identifies hallmarks of occupational therapy applied in the late lifespan. They will also be described in greater depth in other sections of this book. Chapters 10 and 11 will build on the information provided in this chapter to highlight the use of occupation over the late lifespan. Additionally, these chapters will describe the unique approach by occupational therapy that may contribute to the effectiveness of occupational therapy services for persons over the late lifespan.

PART 4: APPLICATIONS

The following activities will help you identify key aspects of this chapter that were highlighted in this text. Activities can be completed individually or in a small group to enhance learning.

As a Group

1. Make a list (identify) the strengths and weaknesses of institutional care and community based care.

   a. From your list, which has more strengths and weaknesses?

   b. From your list, identify two to three weaknesses that you can think can affect or promote change as an occupational therapy assistant?

   c. What setting do you think would be the hardest to work in? Explain your response.

2. Have one student apply the standardized ACL-5 or LACL-5 screen to another student. Take turns administering the evaluation. In collaboration with your instructor, identify what ACL level was identified.

   a. Was it hard to follow the standardized instructions? Explain your answer.

   b. What was the hardest aspect of administering the ACL leather lacing screen?

   c. What was your ACL level score? _____ Is this what you expected? Give examples for when your ACL level score may change.

   d. Remember, service competency is necessary to administer standardized assessments. Do you feel you have attained service competency with administering the ACL screen? How can you develop service competency?

3. Pick an activity of daily living that you performed this morning or daily.

   a. Describe the:

   Occupation

   Environment

   Person

   b. Identify characteristics that exist between the:

   Occupation

   Environment

   Person

Individually

4. Identify one part of the Patient Protection and Affordability Act (HR-3590) to research. Find more information to share with your class (1 page, double spaced, 1" margins, APA style format, 12" font, with references).

    a. Identify suggestions on how aspects of this law can influence/affect the provision of occupational therapy positively.

    b. If possible, make suggestions for what occupational therapy could do to advocate for persons with dementia under this aspect of the law.

5. Identify one legislative act or amendment to report to the class. Write a description of what you learn (3 pages double spaced, 1" margins, APA style format, 12" font and with references).

6. Considering yourself as a dynamic complex system, identify examples using the key concepts as they apply to your life.

    a. Complexity

    b. Self-organization

    c. Phase shifts

    d. Control parameters

    e. Order parameters

7. Instructing, teaching, and enabling learning are important aspects of the occupational therapy process. Quite often, occupational therapy utilizes demonstration, memorization, recall, and self-directed learning, which may not generalize well with persons with cognitive impairments such as dementia. Give an example of how each of the following areas can be utilized in the learning process with persons with dementia.

    a. Flow

    b. Reductionist techniques

    c. Client perception of the environment

    d. Client perception of him- or herself

    e. Unambiguous time/space cues

    f. Spatial orientation

    g. Sequence order/process structures

    h. Remaining motor memory

    i. Procedural memory

REFERENCES

A Place for Mom (n.d.). 10 symptoms of mental illness in the Elderly. Author. Retrieved from www.aplaceformom.com.

Accordino, M. P., Porter, D. F., & Morse, T. (2001). De-institutionalization of persons with severe mental illness: Context and consequences. *Journal of Rehabilitation, 67*(2), 16-21.

Alzheimer's Association. (2012). Alzheimer's disease facts and figures. Author. Retrieved from www.alz.org.

American Occupational Therapy Association. (2014). Occupational therapy practice framework: Domain and process (3rd ed.). *American Journal of Occupational Therapy, 68*(Suppl. 1), S1-S48. doi: 10.5014/ajot2014.682006.

American Psychiatric Association. (2000). *Diagnostic and statistical manual of mental disorders,* DSM-IV-TR, (4th ed.). Washington, DC: Author.

American Psychiatric Association. (2013). *Diagnostic and statistical manual of mental disorders,* DSM-V (5th ed.). Washington, DC: Author.

American Psychological Association. (n.d.) Older adults' health and age-related changes. Retrieved from www.apa.org.

Bennett, S., Shand, S., & Liddle, J. (2011). Occupational therapy practice in Australia with people with dementia: A profile in need of change. *Australian Occupational Therapy Journal, 58,* 155-163.

Besdine, R. W. (2013). Changes in the body with aging. Retrieved from www.merckmanuals.com.

Bieber, D. C., & Keller, B. (2005). Falls and the client with dementia: Using the occupational profile and Allen cognitive level to direct care. *Gerontology Special Interest Section Quarterly, 28*(2), 1-4.

Borell, L., Bernspång, B., Nygård, L., & Rönnberg, L. (1993). Supporting everyday activities in dementia: An international study. *International journal of Geriatric Psychiatry, 8,* 395-400.

Bree, P., & Meldrum, J. (2005). Primary healthcare teams and dementia. *Nursing Older People, 17*(5), 20-22.

Brown, C. (2009). Pain, ageing and dementia: The crisis is looming, but are we ready?. *British Journal of Occupational Therapy, 72*(8), 371-375.

Brown, D. (2012). AOTA, state associations collaborate on health reform advocacy. *OT Practice, 17*(17), 6.

Brown, P., Lohman, H., & Nieman, M. (1998). Practice settings. In H. Lohman, R. L. Padilla, & S. B. Byers-Connon (Eds.), *Occupational therapy with elders: Strategies for the COTA* (pp. 81-88). New York: Mosby.

Butler, L. (2013). Therapeutic approaches to dementia. Cross-Country Education Presentation in Knoxville, TN. February 7, 2013.

Buchmueller, T. C., Cooper, P. F., Jacobson, M., & Zuvekas, S. H. (2007). Parity for whom? Exemptions and the extent of state mental health parity legislation. *Health Affairs, 26*(4), 483-487.

Centers for Disease Control and Prevention. (2012). Depression is not a normal part of growing older. Retrieved from www.cdc.gov/aging/mentalhealth/depression.htm.

Centers for Disease Control and Prevention. (2014). Deaths and mortality. Retrieved from www.cdc.gov.

Cheney, P. (2011). The dementia dilemma: Strategies for home care treatment. *Home & Community Health Special Interest Section Quarterly, 18*(3), 1-4.

Curtin, M. (2008). Therapists as advocates and lobbyists. *International Journal of Therapy and Rehabilitation, 15*(3), 120-121.

Department of Health and Human Services. (2010). Older Americans Act. Author. Retrieved from www.aoa.gov.

Department of Health and Human Services. (2012). National plan to address Alzheimer's disease. Author. Retrieved from http://aspe.hhs.gov.

Glantz, C. H., & Richman, N. (1998). Public policy and aging. In H. Lohman, R. L. Padilla, & S. Byers-Connan (Eds.), *Occupational therapy with elders: Strategies for the COTA* (pp. 49-59). New York: Mosby.

Golden, J., & Lawlor, B. (2006). Treatment of dementia in the community. *British Medical Journal, 333*(7580), 1184-1185.

Goode, K. T., Haley, W. E., Roth, D. L., & Ford, G. R. (1998). Predicting longitudinal change in caregiver physical and mental health: A stress process model. *Health Psychology, 17*(2), 190-198.

Gray, J. M., Kennedy, B. L., & Zemke, R. (1996). Dynamic systems theory: An overview. In R. Zemke & F. Clark (Eds.), *Occupational science: The evolving discipline* (pp. 297-308). Philadelphia, PA: F. A. Davis.

Greene, J. A., Ingram, T. A., & Johnson, W. (1993). Group psychotherapy for patients with dementia. *Southern Medical Journal, 86*(9), 1033-1035.

Gugel, R. N. (1994). Behavior approaches for managing patients with Alzheimer's disease and related disorders. *Medical Clinics of North America, 78*(4), 861-867.

Gutman, S. A., & Schindler, V. P. (2007). The neurological basis of occupation. *Occupational Therapy International, 14*(2), 71-85.

Hall, L., & Skelton, D. A. (2012). Occupational therapy for people with dementia: A review of the United Kingdom literature. *British Journal of Occupational Therapy, 75*(6), 281-288.

Harrison, D. (2005). Context of change in community mental health occupational therapy: Part one. *International Journal of Occupational Therapy and Rehabilitation, 12*(9), 396-400.

Hayes, R. L., & Keller, S. M. (1999). Why won't Australian occupational therapists adopt Allen's cognitive disabilities theory?. *Australian Occupational Therapy Journal, 46*, 188-192.

Holden, U., & Woods, R. T. (1995). *Positive approaches to dementia care.* New York: Churchill Livingstone.

Holthe, T., & Thorsen, K., & Josephsson, S. (2007). Occupational patterns of people with dementia in residential care: an ethnographic study. *Scandinavian Journal of Occupational Therapy, 14*(2), 96-107.

Hoppes, S., Davis, L. A., & Thompson, D. (2003). Environmental effects on the assessment of people with dementia: A pilot study. *American Journal of Occupational Therapy, 57*(4), 396-402.

H. R. 3762—112th Congress. (2011). To amend the public health service act to include occupational therapists as behavioral and mental health professionals for purposes of the national health service corps. Retrieved from www.govtrack.us/congress/bills/112/hr3762.

Josephsson, S., Bäckman, L., Borell, L., Nygard, L., & Bernspång, B. (1998). Effectiveness of an intervention to improve occupational performance in dementia. *Occupational Therapy Journal of Research, 15*(1), 36-49.

Keady, J., Woods, B., Hohn, S., Hill, J. (2004). Community mental health nursing and early intervention in dementia: developing practice through a single case history. *International Journal of Older People in Nursing, 13*(66), 57-67.

Kelso, J. A. (1995). *The self-organization of brain and behavior.* Cambridge, MA: The MIT Press.

Keough, J., & Huebner, R. (2000). Treating dementia: The complementing team approach of occupational therapy and psychology. *The Journal of Psychology, 134*(4), 375-391.

Kleinman, B. (1992). The challenge of providing occupational therapy in mental health. *American Journal of Occupational Therapy, 46*(6), 555-557.

Leven, N. V., & Jonsson, H. (2002). Doing and being in the atmosphere of the doing: Environmental influences on occupational performance in a nursing home. *Scandinavian Journal of Occupational Therapy, 9*, 148-155.

Lindberg, B., & MacInnes, G. (2010). Health care reform provisions affecting older adults. The Gerontological Society of America. Retrieved from www.geron.org/uploads/documents/HCRprovisions.pdf.

Mahaffey, L. (2009). Using theory and the therapeutic reasoning process to guide the occupational therapy process for older adults with mental illness. *OT Practice, 14*(5), CE1-CE8.

Norman, J. (2007). Impossible to ignore. A mental health crisis changes a community and a reporter's focus. *Nieman Reports, 52-54.*

Oregon Department of Human Services. (n.d.). Myths and stereotypes of aging. Retrieved from: http://wwworegon.gov.

Padilla, R. (2011). Effectiveness of occupational therapy services for people with Alzheimer's disease and related dementias. *American Journal of Occupational Therapy, 65*(5), 487-489.

Piersol, C. V., Earland, T. V., & Herge, E. A. (2012). Meeting the needs of caregivers and persons with dementia. *OT Practice, 17*(5), 8-12.

Priebe, S., & Fakhoury, W. (2007). De-institutionalization and re-institutionalization: Major changes in the provision of mental healthcare. *Psychiatry, 6*(8), 313-316.

Strong, S., Rigby, P, Stewart, D., Law, M., Letts, L., & Cooper, B. (1999). Application of the Person-Environment-Occupation model: A practical tool. *Canadian Journal of Occupational Therapy, 66*, 122-133.

Tan, S. (2011). Myths and aging. Retrieved from http://psychologytoday.com.

Toth-Cohen, S. (2000). Role perception of occupational therapist's providing support and education for caregivers of person's with dementia. *American Journal of Occupational Therapy, 54*(5), 505-515.

Waite, A. (2014). Elder abuse: Knowing when, why, and how to intercede. *Occupational Therapy Practice, 19*(3), 9-12.

Warchol, K. (2000). The challenge of dementia care: Focusing on remaining abilities, not deficits, creates a positive foundation for treatment. *OT Practice, 22*(5), 15-19.

Warchol, K., Copeland, C., & Ebell, C. (2006). *Dementia theory: Achieving positive outcomes for the person with dementia.* Hillsborough, NC: Dementia Care Specialists, Inc.

Wertheimer, J., Boula, J. G., Brull, J., Gutt, A. M., Pierrehumbert, B., Rufini, J.,…& Monangéro, J. (1992). Learning process in Dementia. *International Journal of Geriatric Psychiatry, 7*, 161-172.

Werner, J. L., & Tyler, M. (1993). Community-based interventions: A return to community mental health centers' origins. *Journal of Counseling & Development, 71*, 689-692.

Wheatley, M. J. (1992). *Leadership and the new science: Learning about organization from an orderly universe.* San Francisco: Berrett-Koehler Publishers.

Williams, J. (2012). Obamacare: What's already in effect. Tennessee Occupational Therapy Association. Retrieved from http://tnota.org/obamacare-whats-already-in-effect.

World Health Organization. (n.d.). What is active aging?. Retrieved from www.who.int.

Participation in Occupation in the Late Lifespan

Janice Ryan, OTD, OTR/L

KEY TERMS

- Adaptive Capacity
- Adaptive Response Model
- Brain Reward Center
- Centering
- Complex Adaptive System
- Complexity Science
- Developmental Learning

- Environmental Fit
- Fight-Flight-Freeze
- Flow
- Grounding
- Homeostasis
- Neuroplasticity
- Occupational Pattern Adaptation

- Relaxation Response
- Resilience
- Self-Organization
- Sensory Modulation
- Spiritual Context
- Therapeutic Adaptation

CHAPTER LEARNING OBJECTIVES

After completion of this chapter, students will be able to:

1. Identify adaptive responses as part of the occupational therapy process to achieve adaptive occupational participation patterns that support well aging.

2. Recognize factors from complexity science that help to explain the adaptive process.

3. Compare and contrast adaptive patterns, symptoms, behaviors, and functions that maintain healthy occupational participation patterns.

4. Demonstrate knowledge of occupational therapy evaluation tools used to identify or quantify occupational participation patterns.

5. Analyze how standardized occupational therapy evaluations are linked to theory and performed to attain client-specific information.

6. Link contextual information, client-specific factors, and occupational therapy theory to the occupational therapy process.

Manville, C.A., & Keough J. L.
Mental Health Practice for the Occupational Therapy Assistant (pp 229-257).
© 2016 Taylor & Francis Group.

CHAPTER OUTLINE

INTRODUCTION

> ...people will forget what you said, people will forget what you did, but people will never forget how you made them feel. (Maya Angelou, n.d.)

Occupational therapy practitioners encourage therapeutic adaptation during the occupational therapy process. Occupational therapy leader Lorna Jean King (1978) proposed that the adaptive response is the science that supports occupational therapy practice. Schkade and Schultz (1992) also introduced occupational adaptation as a frame of reference for practice, research, and student practitioner development. Occupational adaptation occurs continuously throughout a person's life.

Events that require personal, environmental, or occupational context adaptations are common during the late lifespan. Such events include life changes that require intrapersonal (within oneself), interpersonal (interaction with other people), and naturalistic learning. These learning types occur through seeing, understanding, and influencing natural system patterns that occur in oneself, environment, or occupational context. Retirement, personal illness, and the death of a spouse are late life events that encourage the development of new occupational patterns.

Coping with change is a form of intrapersonal learning that is required for successfully dealing with every life transition associated with aging, including accepting one's own personal mortality. Healthy occupational participation patterns support this intrapersonal learning process. They help aging adults control stress through positive forms of coping. Participating in activities and occupations that are personally rewarding and that support new learning are known to positively influence mental health and cognition during the aging years (Carver, 2006; Eoyang, 2012; Gray, 2004; Gutman & Schindler, 2007). This chapter focuses on the identification of contextual influences, client factors, and evaluation tools that can be used to assist clients in well aging or community mental health programs. It includes a discussion of the Person-Environment-Occupation (PEO) Model, the Cognitive Disability Model, and the Adaptive Response Model, all of which offer frameworks for treatment approaches.

Current knowledge of complex adaptive systems and complexity science affirms the belief that occupational pattern adaptation is at the core of all occupational therapy practice (Yerxa, 1967; Zemke & Clark, 1996). Complexity science offers a way to practice, teach, and research the occupational therapy process. Importantly, complexity science is leading to new ways to recognize and measure the patterned changes of occupational pattern adaptation displayed by clients during occupational therapy (Champagne, 2008; Eoyang & Holladay, 2013; Ryan & Griswold, 2011).

Complexity science models and tools (Eoyang, 1997) already inform the actions of businesses and organizations, and have been used to develop leadership (Quade & Holladay, 2010) and self-awareness (Tytel & Holladay, 2011) in the general population. Models and tools from complexity science can assist practitioners to understand the core occupational therapy process that is required to promote health and wellness during aging years. This process is commonly referred to as *occupational pattern adaptation*.

A model developed from complexity science principles of the adaptive action cycle (Human Systems Dynamic Institute, n.d.) has been modified for use in occupational therapy. The **Adaptive Response Model** can be used as a teaching aid to support occupational therapy assistant students to analyze, synthesize, and comprehend the assessment of occupational participation patterns in aging adults. This includes assessment of cognitive control, affective state, and the complex neuro-occupational dynamics of developmental learning.

In order to facilitate occupational pattern adaptation, occupational therapy practitioners must be able to identify

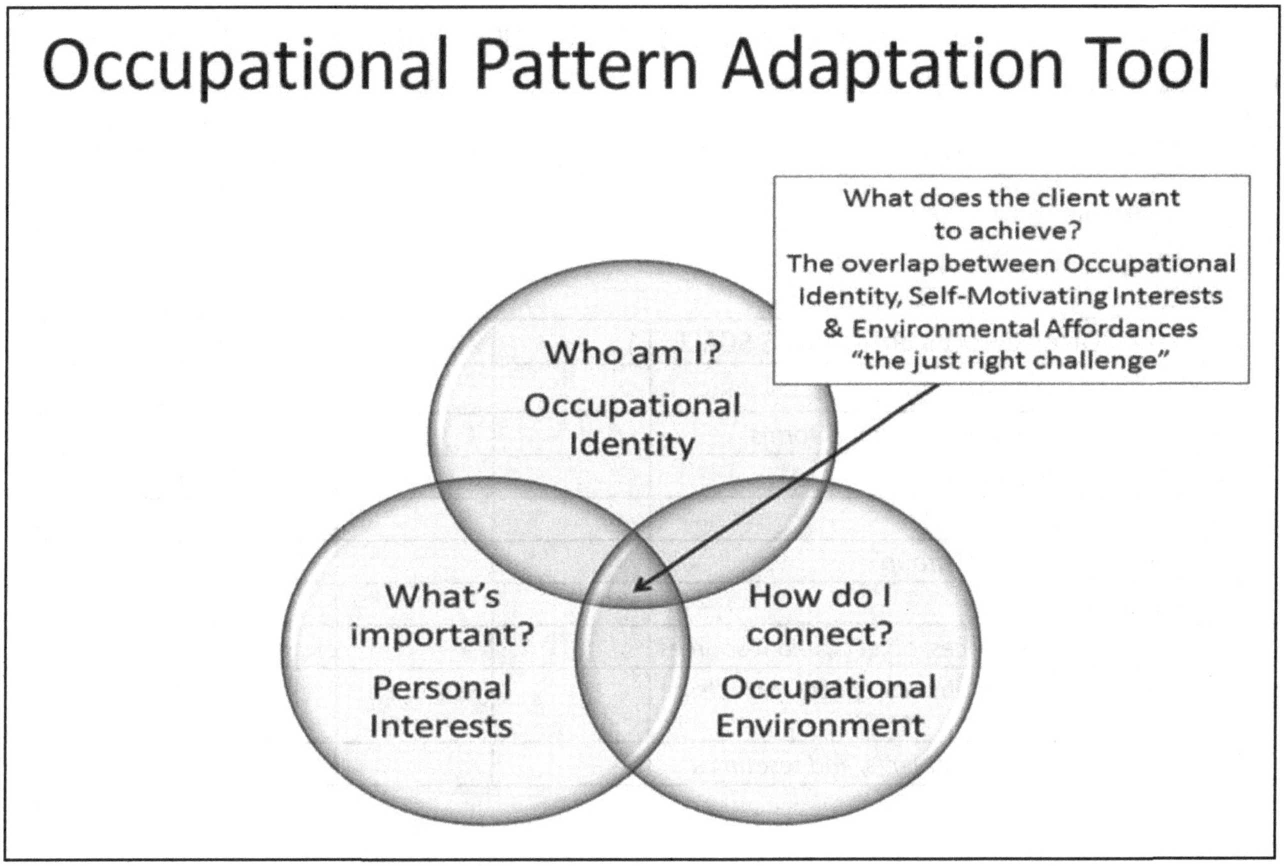

Occupational Pattern Adaptation Tool

What does the client want to achieve?
The overlap between Occupational Identity, Self-Motivating Interests & Environmental Affordances "the just right challenge"

Who am I?
Occupational Identity

What's important?
Personal Interests

How do I connect?
Occupational Environment

Figure 10-1. The occupational pattern adaptation tool. (Reprinted with permission from Ryan, J. (2013). Treating the brain as an adaptive system in clients with dementia: Facilitating the neurobiology of action system processes. Poster at the 2013 American Occupational Therapy Association Annual Conference, San Diego, CA.)

SPOTLIGHT 10-1. COLLECTING DATA FOR STEVE'S OCCUPATIONAL PROFILE

- The Occupational Therapy Practice Framework: Domain and Process was published by AOTA in 2002. It provides a way to organize assessment of mental and cognitive health in aging clients.

- Steve's occupational profile demonstrates how data may be collected using other standardized assessments that answer the three questions critical to understanding how client self-motivation develops through occupational pattern adaptation.

- Data on Steve's occupational patterns of daily living and personal interests were gathered by using subtests from the Model of Human Occupation (Kielhofner, 2002).

Steve's Occupational Profile:
Steve is a 58-year-old man receiving outpatient mental health services due to a dual diagnosis of depression and alcoholism lasting 2 years. Until he was laid off approximately 3 years ago, Steve worked in middle management at a carpet manufacturing company. After 1 year of unsuccessful interviews and job searching, Steve shared that he "just lost hope" of being hired. The stresses of financial worries began taking its toll on

(continued)

and quantify complex adaptive system patterns. Figure 10-1 illustrates the occupational participation adaptation tool. The *occupational participation adaptation tool* shows the relationship between client information commonly gathered during occupational therapy assessment and what the client wants to achieve.

Spotlight 10-1 presents the occupational profile of Steve that is used to illustrate concepts in this chapter. By understanding how the occupational profile connects to client-centered practice, occupational therapy assistants can be prepared to facilitate developmental learning in aging clients.

The occupational pattern adaptation tool offers a way to turn concept into practice in an era that values holistic and client-centered approaches. It requires the user to visualize the inter-relationships between the occupational profile and

---

SPOTLIGHT 10-1. COLLECTING DATA FOR STEVE'S OCCUPATIONAL PROFILE (CONTINUED)

his marriage. His wife works at a department store for only slightly above minimum wage. They have two grown children.

Over time, Steve became more depressed and apathetic, and developed a pattern of drinking heavily. He recently agreed to seek mental health services when his wife threatened divorce. Steve and his wife Lisa both contributed information during the initial occupational therapy assessment process.

Steve's Occupational Patterns of Daily Living

OCCUPATIONAL BEHAVIOR SETTINGS SCALE	1	2	3	4
Home-life occupational forms			X	
Major productive role occupational forms		X		
Leisure occupational forms		X		
Home-life social group	X			
Major productive social group	X			
Leisure social group	X			
Home-life physical spaces, objects, and resources			X	
Major productive role physical spaces, objects, and resources		X		
Leisure physical spaces, objects, and resources		X		

Key:

4 = Exceptionally competent occupational functioning

3 = Appropriate satisfactory occupational functioning

2 = Some occupational dysfunction

1 = Extremely occupationally dysfunctional

Model of Human Occupation
Occupational Performance History Interview-II Occupational Behavior Settings Scale
Client Name: *Steve Block*

Date:
Steve's Personal Interests:
Model of Human Occupation
OPHI-II Interest Checklist
Client Name: *Steve Block*

Date:

(continued)

SPOTLIGHT 10-1. COLLECTING DATA FOR STEVE'S OCCUPATIONAL PROFILE (CONTINUED)

ACTIVITY	WHAT HAS BEEN YOUR LEVEL OF INTEREST						DO YOU CURRENTLY PARTICIPATE IN THIS ACTIVITY?		WOULD YOU LIKE TO PURSUE THIS IN THE FUTURE?	
	IN THE PAST TEN YEARS			IN THE PAST YEAR						
	STRONG	SOME	NO	STRONG	SOME	NO	YES	NO	YES	NO
Gardening/yard work	X					X	X		X	
Sewing/needlework										
Playing cards										
Foreign languages										
Church activities	X					X		X	X	
Radio										
Walking										
Car repair										
Writing										
Dancing										
Golf										
Football										
Listening to popular music										
Puzzles										
Holiday activities										
Pets/livestock										
Movies										
Listening to classical music										
Speeches/lectures										
Swimming										
Bowling	X					X		X	X	
Visiting										

(continued)

SPOTLIGHT 10-1. COLLECTING DATA FOR STEVE'S OCCUPATIONAL PROFILE (CONTINUED)

ACTIVITY	WHAT HAS BEEN YOUR LEVEL OF INTEREST						DO YOU CURRENTLY PARTICIPATE IN THIS ACTIVITY?		WOULD YOU LIKE TO PURSUE THIS IN THE FUTURE?	
	IN THE PAST TEN YEARS			IN THE PAST YEAR						
	STRONG	SOME	NO	STRONG	SOME	NO	YES	NO	YES	NO
Mending										
Checkers/chess										
Barbecues										
Reading										
Traveling										
Parties										
Wrestling										
House cleaning										
Model building										
Television		X			X		X			X
Concerts										
Pottery										
Camping										
Laundry/ironing										
Politics										
Table games										
Home decorating										
Clubs/lodge										
Singing										
Scouting										
Clothes										
Handicrafts										
Hairstyling										
Cycling										
Attending plays										
Bird watching										

(continued)

SPOTLIGHT 10-1. COLLECTING DATA FOR STEVE'S OCCUPATIONAL PROFILE (CONTINUED)

| ACTIVITY | WHAT HAS BEEN YOUR LEVEL OF INTEREST | | | | | | DO YOU CURRENTLY PARTICIPATE IN THIS ACTIVITY? | | WOULD YOU LIKE TO PURSUE THIS IN THE FUTURE? | |
| | IN THE PAST TEN YEARS | | | IN THE PAST YEAR | | | | | | |
	STRONG	SOME	NO	STRONG	SOME	NO	YES	NO	YES	NO
Dating										
Auto racing										
Home repairs										
Exercise		X				X		X	X	
Hunting										
Woodworking										
Pool										
Driving										
Child care										
Tennis										
Cooking/baking										
Basketball										
History										
Collecting										
Fishing										
Science										
Leatherwork										
Shopping										
Photography										
Painting/drawing										

the client-centered questions that are included with this tool and use them to facilitate therapeutic adaptation in aging occupational therapy clients like Steve. Three questions from the occupational profile overlap with questions from the occupational pattern adaptation tool. The intersection between these three questions reveals the answer to the core source of a client's self-motivation. This information can then be used to facilitate occupational pattern adaptation in aging clients.

A practitioner can help a client be successful at achieving treatment goals if those goals capture the client's self-motivation. This can be achieved by understanding the client's occupational identity, including what the client does to feel connected to his or her environment and his or her personal interests.

Mental and cognitive interventions with aging adults are more effective when occupational therapy practitioners recognize and use the occupational profile as a conceptual model of each client's occupational pattern-forming system. The key to achieving sustainable improvements in mental and cognitive function is for the occupational therapy practitioner to understand the sources of client self-motivation. Practitioners can use occupational patterns to determine the "just right" cognitive and mental health challenge for their client by tying this information together with data from standardized assessments. The Occupational Therapy

Practice Framework refers to a client's self-motivated occupational patterns as his or her spiritual context. Assessing, understanding, and using an aging client's spiritual context to facilitate occupational pattern adaptation are sometimes called the art of occupational therapy.

PART 1: OCCUPATIONAL PARTICIPATION PATTERNS IN AGING CLIENTS

Developmental Learning: Occupational Participation During the Aging Years

The Philosophy of Occupational Therapy (Meyer, 1922/1977) and other professional writings refer to human adaptation as an intuitive part of the occupational therapy process (Yerxa, 1967). Occupational therapy practitioners commonly view themselves as holistic practitioners who treat the whole person. A person is an example of a complex adaptive system. Occupational therapy for aging clients should be approached from a holistic perspective. Schkade and Schultz (1992) proposed that occupational adaptation provides a perspective to promote the development of holistic practice.

There is increasing evidence that adaptive capacity is a critical component of well aging. People constantly adapt through learning that occurs over time, otherwise referred to as *developmental learning*. Though the term **complex adaptive system** was not used, Schkade and Schultz (1992) were among the first to propose that occupation and adaptation evolve as a single system. An increasing number of neuroscientists and psychologists are studying complex adaptive systems that support this assumption (Carver, 2006; Freeman, 1995, 2000; Gray, 2004). Psychologists propose that the social approach-and-avoidance system that exists within every human brain shapes affect or mood, cognitive control, adaptive responses, and all adaptive actions. This includes occupational engagements that help an aging client cope with stress.

In their model of occupational adaptation, Schkade and Schultz (1992) made two assumptions that correlate with occupational therapy applications of complexity science principles. These two assumptions are as follows:

1. Occupation provides the means by which human beings adapt to changing needs and conditions, and the desire to participate in occupation is the intrinsic motivational force leading to adaptation.

2. Occupational adaptation is a normative process that is most pronounced in periods of transition, both large and small. The greater the adaptive transitional needs, the greater the importance of the occupational adaptation process, and the greater the likelihood that the process will be disrupted (Schkade & Shultz, pp. 829-830).

Schultz and Schkade (1997) were recognizing an unconscious cognitive process of experiential or developmental learning that continues throughout the lifespan. Current learning theories are finding a place in today's health care practice (Braungart, Braungart, & Gramet, 2011). Figure 10-2 illustrates the Human Systems Occupational Therapy Adaptive Response Model. The Human Systems Occupational Therapy Adaptive Response Model provides a way to visualize this learning, which is also called naturalistic learning by Harvard psychologist Howard Gardner (Gardner, 1999).

The Adaptive Response Model is useful as a means to teach occupational therapy assistant students how to recognize naturalistic learning in clients. Holistic, client-centered care of aging adults requires a practitioner to visualize how clients can still learn through adaptation as a "complex relationship among person, environment, and participation in occupations" (Law, 2002, p. 640). **Naturalistic learning** occurs through seeing (or sensing), understanding, and influencing the patterns of living things. It can be used by practitioners for clinical reasoning and can also be used by clients of any age to learn from their just right challenge.

Spotlight 10-2 refers to Steve's case study to use the Adaptive Response Model. The Adaptive Response Model facilitates Steve's developmental learning during the assessment. It also highlights the process of clinical reasoning. The art of holistic, client-centered practice is clarified by understanding Steve's occupational profile as natural patterns that can support future learning. The Adaptive Response Model provides valuable clinical insights to identify and understand Steve's occupational patterns.

Complexity science is the study of dynamic "systems that change with time," such as human beings (Gray, Kennedy, & Zemke, 1996, p. 301). Adaptive responses can develop into new adaptive actions within the time it takes in a therapy session to shift a motor or cognitive control pattern. The future of mental health occupational therapy with aging populations was enhanced when neuroscientists discovered that all adaptive actions are supported by the integration of cognitive control and emotion (Freeman, 1995, 2000; Gray, 2004). The new paradigm understanding of cognitive control explains why a single positive shift in self-perception can change the cognitive and mental health of aging individuals. It also explains why information from the occupational profile is useful for knowing how to facilitate self-motivation in any client.

Occupational therapy acknowledges that the environment and context have a major influence on occupational patterns (Dunn, Brown, & McGuigan, 1994). Lorna Jean King (1978) identified two types of adaptation that are at the core of occupational therapy practice. She proposed the

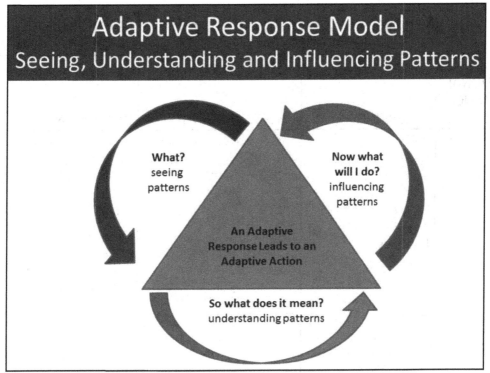

Figure 10-2. The Human Systems Occupational Therapy (HSOT) Adaptive Response Model. (Reprinted with permission from Ryan, J. (2013). Treating the brain as an adaptive system in clients with dementia: Facilitating the neurobiology of action system processes. Poster at the 2013 American Occupational Therapy Association Annual Conference, San Diego, CA.)

SPOTLIGHT 10-2. FACILITATING STEVE'S DEVELOPMENTAL LEARNING DURING ASSESSMENT

- Steve's occupational profile helps to focus practitioner observations on the occupational patterns critical to development of client self-motivation.

- By focusing attention in the core areas of occupational history, occupational patterns of daily living, and occupational interests, answers begin to emerge to the client question, "What do I want to achieve?"

- By understanding how clients come to answer this question, occupational therapy assistants can become increasingly skillful at facilitating this client discovery.

STEVE'S OCCUPATIONAL PERFORMANCE PATTERNS	OBSERVING	UNDERSTANDING	INFLUENCING
Occupational History "Who am I?"	**Past:** middle manager at a carpet manufacturing company **Now:** unemployed for 2 years	**Past:** Self-Perceptions were that his life was on track and successful. Positive affect supported self-motivation **Now:** Negative self-perceptions and depression are blocking self-motivation to take adaptive actions.	His therapist begins to teach him about developmental learning and how his occupational history, current mood and self-motivation are all interrelated parts of a complex adaptive system. Steve begins to see that his mood challenges need to be addressed in occupational therapy in order to reach his "What do I want to achieve?" goals.

(continued)

SPOTLIGHT 10-2. FACILITATING STEVE'S DEVELOPMENTAL LEARNING DURING ASSESSMENT (CONTINUED)			
STEVE'S OCCUPATIONAL PERFORMANCE PATTERNS	**OBSERVING**	**UNDERSTANDING**	**INFLUENCING**
Patterns of Daily Living *"How do I connect?"*	**Roles:** Steve sees his role as a provider for his family as the most important way he connects with the world. **Routines:** Steve is bored and unmotivated by his daily routines. **Habits:** Steve's drinking has become a habit that temporarily reduces feelings of anxiety.	Through developmental learning Steve begins to become aware of how mood is negatively influenced when a person feels disconnected from their primary life roles, occupational context and environments. He also learns that his drinking habit has been used to reduce feelings of anxiety associated with this disconnection.	His therapist begins to teach Steve how he can receive emotional self-regulation benefits from adding healthy leisure and social activities to his routine. Steve decides he wants to focus his energy in occupational therapy on activities that will improve his mood and feelings of productivity.
Personal Interests Values and Needs *"What's important?"*	**Past:** gardening, church, bowling, television, exercise **Now:** television	Steve begins to recognize the core value he places on feeling productive for his family. He understands that, if he is to achieve his goals, he must pay attention to the personal feelings generated by his occupational patterns and life environments. He decides it is important for him to return to some of the environments that felt good to him in the past.	Steve decides that he will participate in an early morning exercise group, very similar to the routine he followed for years before work. His therapist suggests and Steve agrees that isometric exercises should be included for their emotional self-regulation benefits. He also decides he wants to participate in a computer skills class that might prepare him for his job search and for re-entering the workforce. His therapist encourages this, reminding him that exploratory computer-based learning also provides emotional self-regulation benefits.

process labels of developmental learning and therapeutic adaptation. **Developmental learning** might be defined as the natural process of learning from patterns of experience that involve ongoing adaptive responses. **Therapeutic adaptation** may be defined as an adaptive response facilitated by a practitioner in treatment to promote the natural process of developmental learning. Developmental learning and therapeutic adaptation are utilized in the well population, as well as those with impairments, activity limitations, or disabilities. Checkpoint 10-1 helps identify the similarities and differences between developmental learning and therapeutic adaptation.

Person-environment-occupation fitness (or pattern harmony) is at least temporarily lost following an illness, injury, or significant life transition (Jackson, Carlson, Mandel, Zemke, & Clark, 1998). Occupational therapy clients commonly lose this state of coherence between their own natural patterns and their current environment. Occupational therapy clients need occupational pattern changes for a couple of reasons. First, they have not yet or do not have the

CHECKPOINT 10-1. UNDERSTAND

Summarize the similarities and differences between developmental learning and therapeutic adaptation. Give an example of a behavior that demonstrates each concept.

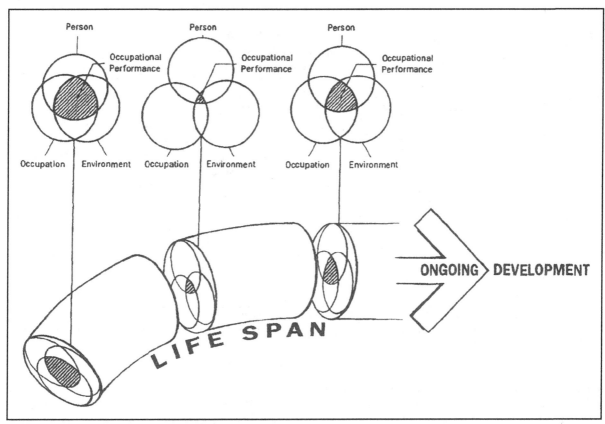

Figure 10-3. The PEO Model of Occupational Performance across the Lifespan. (Reprinted with permission from Rigby, P., & Letts, L. (2003). Environment and occupational performance: Theoretical considerations. In L. Letts, P. Rigby, & D. Stewart (Eds.). *Using environments to enable occupational performance* (pp. 17-32). Thorofare, NJ: SLACK Incorporated.)

capacity to positively adapt to recent life changes. Second, they are experiencing maladaptive patterns of thought, feeling, or self-perception due to unrecognized needs for environmental or occupational pattern adaptation.

The PEO Model and variations of person-environment-occupation (PEO) fitness over the lifespan are illustrated in Figure 10-3. Occupational performance tends to become more stable during the young adult years due to more personal control of the environment and occupational contexts. During aging years, occupational performance becomes less predictable as positive visions of future occupational performance tend to be reduced. During the late aging years PEO fitness is less stable. Adaptive capacity can also be lost when a client does not have a healthy spiritual context.

Internal environment adaptation is a way to understand developmental learning. Categorized into the learning patterns identified by Gardner (1999), developmental learning includes intrapersonal, interpersonal, and naturalistic learning patterns. This includes learning about the self,

others, and natural processes such as occupational patterns through observance and experience. Figure 10-4 illustrates an occupational pattern-forming system. It shows how personal identity develops through two-way occupational exchanges with the environment.

The Occupational Pattern-Forming System Model (Messbauer & Ryan, 2014) illustrates how occupational patterns naturally develop through occupational exchanges with the external environment. *Occupational pattern adaptation* is developmental learning that occurs during PEO exchanges. Developmental learning occurs across the lifespan, but not all responses, choices, and actions are adaptive. Nonadaptive coping strategies, such as reduced participation in healthy occupations in favor of isolation or addictions, may result in clients needing occupational therapy.

The "outcomes of good fit are adaptive behavior and positive affect" (Rigby & Letts, 2003, p. 25). When the demands of an environment lack fitness with a person's capacities or occupational identity, the person is likely to

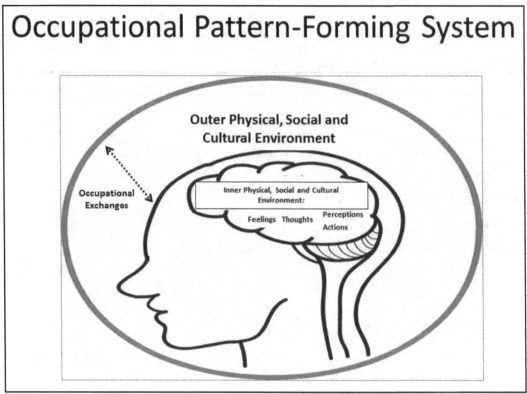

Figure 10-4. The Natural Occupational Pattern-Forming System. Model. (Reprinted with permission from Ryan, J. (2013). Treating the brain as an adaptive system in clients with dementia: Facilitating the neurobiology of action system processes. Poster at the 2013 American Occupational Therapy Association Annual Conference, San Diego, CA.)

develop stress, tension, negative affect, and eventually maladaptive behavior. When the requirements and opportunities of an environment are too predictable or uninteresting, a person commonly develops boredom and may develop a lack of attention to environment.

Through a complexity science lens, reduced occupational participation tends to occur when healthy occupational pattern flexibility and complexity are lost. This commonly happens during stressful and traumatic transitions and events. Brain scan research has shown that social pain produces activation patterns in the brain similar to those created when a person experiences a physical threat (Eisenberg, Lieberman, & Williams, 2003). Both physical and social discomfort can lead to avoidance of occupational participation over time.

The positive occupational pattern adaptation that occurs during new experiential learning is compromised if the brain is also putting energy into making sense of negative stress. In this way, occupational performance and patterns of participation may be negatively affected while adjusting to unwelcome changes. It can also lead to nonadaptive coping patterns that compromise well aging. Sometimes nonadaptive coping patterns are carried over from mental health challenges during earlier years. Other times nonadaptive coping patterns seem to emerge during stressful transitions related to aging.

The cumulative influences of prolonged stress can take their toll during the aging years. This makes understanding stress-related conditions an important aspect of occupational therapy client care. The Social Readjustment Rating Scale (Holmes & Rahe, 1967) can be used to increase a client's self-awareness in order to move forward toward an adaptive response and past feelings of guilt, grief, or loss. Stress is an unconscious cognitive process experienced as an affective state. Occupational therapy assistants must know how to see (sense), understand, and influence the patterned effects of negative mood on occupational participation and performance.

The Social Readjustment Rating Scale (Holmes & Rahe, 1967) suggests that change requires (1) effort to adapt and (2) an effort to regain stability. Although some people are better able to cope with stress than others, the total score can be considered an approximation of the level of cumulative stress. A total of 150 or less suggests low stress and low probability of developing stress-related conditions. If the total is 300 or more, a person is estimated to have an 80% chance of developing a stress-related condition. This includes a variety of physical conditions, cognitive challenges, and maladaptive behaviors. Checkpoint 10-2 helps with understanding of the Social Readjustment Rating Scale.

CHECKPOINT 10-2. APPLY

Go online and search for information on the Social Readjustment Rating Scale. Administer it to yourself. What does your score mean?

SPOTLIGHT 10-3. STEVE'S TOTAL STRESS RATING

- The Social Readjustment Rating Scale is a cumulative inventory of common stressful events described with a value that represents a life-changing unit.

- Since stress is cumulative, values are multiplied by the number of times the life event has happened during the last 12 months.

- Thomas Holmes and Richard Rahe (1967) created this rating scale as a standardized measurement to reflect the impact of a wide variety of stressors.

- Steve's Social Readjustment Rating Scale reflects the stressors that were part of his life during the 12-month period after he lost his job.

Steve's Cumulative Stress in Life Changing Units

Life Event	Value
Death of Spouse	100
Divorce	73
Marital separation	65
Jail term	63
Death of close family member	63
Personal injury or illness	53
Marriage	50
Fired at work	47
Marital reconciliation	45
Retirement	45
Change in health of family member	44
Pregnancy	40
Sex difficulties	39
Gain of new family member	39
Business readjustment	39
Change in financial state	38

Death of close friend	37
Change to a different line of work	36
Change in number of arguments with spouse	35
Home Mortgage over $100,000*	31
Foreclosure or mortgage or loan	30
Change in responsibilities at work	29
Son or daughter leaving home	29
Trouble with in-laws	29
Outstanding personal achievement	28
Spouse begins or stops work	26
Begin or end school	26
Change in living conditions	25
Revision of personal habits	24
Trouble with boss	23
Change in work hours or conditions	20
Change in residence	20
Change in schools	20
Change in recreation	19
Change in church activities	19
Change in social activities	18
Mortgage or loan of less than $100,000*	17
Change in sleeping habits	16
Change in number of family get-togethers	15
Change in eating habits	15
Single person living alone	**
Other- describe	**

Total: 441

* the mortgage figure was updated from the original figure of $10,000 to reflect inflation.

** Estimate the impact on yourself

Spotlight 10-3 identifies Steve's total stress rating. The Social Readjustment Rating Scale was used to identify the cumulative health care influences of unaddressed negative stress.

Elisabeth Kubler-Ross was a psychiatrist who pioneered research, conceptual modeling, and practice strategies in the area of death and dying. The Kubler-Ross Model of the Five Stages of Grief has strongly influenced the way the United States serves the terminally ill and their families (Kubler-Ross, 1969). Hospice and palliative care services use this model to understand common behavioral patterns of terminally ill clients—the same stages that are identified in people who are grieving the loss of a loved one or who are recovering from stressors that generate a variety of negative emotions, such as depression, anxiety, and fear. The five stages of the Kubler-Ross Model are as follows:

1. *Denial:* A temporary defense during which a person believes the diagnosis must be a mistake. The

Kubler-Ross Model refers to this as the "I feel fine" or "This can't be happening, not to me" stage. Denial can be characterized by an unconscious or even conscious refusal to accept the reality of the situation.

2. *Anger:* An attachment of feelings such as rage or envy at one's self or others. This stage may involve blaming self or others for the disease and is described as the "Why me? It's not fair!" stage. Anger is often directed at close family members and can cause difficulty for the caregiver.

3. *Bargaining:* Involves a hope that the person can delay his or her death. This stage can be characterized by the words, "I'll do anything for a few more years." It involves an acceptance of the situation but a need to negotiate for a postponement of death.

4. *Depression:* Characterized by sadness accompanied by increased understanding of the certainty of death. This stage is a precursor to acceptance that involves strong emotions such as fear, sadness, and regret. A sense of hopelessness associated with this stage has been identified as a feeling that, "I'm so sad, why bother with anything?"

5. *Acceptance:* A coming to terms with the client's or his or her loved one's death. Sometimes the person who is dying actually enters this stage before his or her loved ones. It is characterized by feeling, "It's going to be okay" or "I can't fight it, I may as well prepare for it."

Spotlight 10-4 shows an application of the Kubler-Ross Model to Steve's case study. The Observing-Understanding-Influencing cycle is an application of the Adaptive Response Model that was introduced in Figure 10-2. This demonstrates how the proposed stages of grief and loss can be associated with a wide variety of stressful life transitions. In Steve's case, he experienced his late-life job loss as a catastrophic event leading to further life meaning challenges. The patterns of behavior associated with grief contributed to depression, alcohol addiction, and eventually the fear of losing his marriage to divorce. In Steve's case, personal interests he associated with getting reconnected to a career and a positive occupational identity were selected as initial adaptive actions to be supported in treatment.

Personal Fitness With Environment: A Key to Well Aging

Occupational performance challenges are recognized as a source of social stress and identity confusion (Christiansen, 1991, 1999; Hasselkus, 2002). Increasingly, social psychologists (Ogden, Minton, & Pain, 2006) focus on the therapeutic power of positive emotions to change lives and client behavior. Social and emotional wellness strategies are being applied to the general population and are called positive psychology or the psychology of success (Dweck, 2006).

Self-perceptions of *environmental fit* are believed to occur through a survival-based system in the brain and body that self-regulates affect and action. Since it has served this evolutionary role, it is also called the approach-and-avoidance system (Carver, 2006). This is the occupational pattern-forming system previously pictured in Figure 10-4. Occupational patterns tend to be shaped through attraction to pleasant feelings such as flow (Csikszentmihalyi, Abuhamdeh, & Nakamura, 2005) and avoidance of negative emotions associated with unpleasant stress. The occupational pattern adaptation tool helps to organize and understand collective results from standardized and unstandardized assessments. Occupational therapy assistants can then visualize ways to facilitate the positive feelings that come from improving PEO fitness in treatment as well as in home programs.

Survival requires the body's physiology to be maintained within a certain homeostatic or system stability range. Hunger, thirst, fear, and pain are feelings that serve as an internal trigger for a physiological corrective response. Thoughts, feelings, and self-perceptions also act as internal cues that inform a person about his or her current emotional fit within social and cultural environments. Magnetic resonance imaging (MRI) studies show that the prefrontal cortex of the brain, which is responsible for cognitive control, is negatively influenced by social interactions in which one feels physically or socially isolated and/or victimized (Eisenberg, Lieberman, & Williams, 2003). The central nervous system acts continually to monitor the human interior and exterior environments of everyday life. Visceral muscles and heart rate levels are two examples of internal body systems that serve to detect body state change and restore physical system *homeostasis.* This rebalancing occurs within an internal adaptive system. Emotion and cognitive control are integrated by triggering self-regulatory adjustments such as heart rate, hormone secretion, and breathing (Ogden, Minton, & Pain, 2006).

Recent advances in brain technology, such as neurological imaging, have allowed scientists to view brain function during occupational participation (Nattkemper, 2004). This includes functional MRI, positron emission tomography, and electroencephalographs (Bankman & Morcovescu, 2002). This research has demonstrated the benefits of engagement in meaningful and purposeful occupations to reduce the stress of anxiety or boredom.

The reduction of stress and stress-related diseases can slow cognitive decline. The capacity to adapt to change in positive ways during aging is called resilience. *Resilience* is the adaptive capacity that supports healthy adjustments to the inevitable internal and external system stressors common during aging years. It is the combined patterns of adapting to change and regaining a feeling of stability.

Stress responses tend to block the emotional integration required for cognitive control of an adaptive response. Table 10-1 lists emotional self-regulation challenges that interfere

SPOTLIGHT 10-4. STEVE OVERCOMING THE PATTERNS OF GRIEF AND LOSS

- Patterns of recovery from grief and loss naturally follow the course of developmental learning, but usually happen over a long period and with no cognitive awareness.

- After Steve is taught about his own capacity for developmental learning in occupational therapy, he begins to recognize its pattern.

- In other words, Steve's occupational therapy assistant has facilitated Steve's capacity to observe, understand, and influence his own behavior patterns.

- This leads to those self-motivating "ah-ha" moments that accompany developmental learning.

Steve Overcoming the Patterns of Grief and Loss

PATTERNS LEADING TO STEVE'S ACCEPTANCE	OBSERVING	UNDERSTANDING	INFLUENCING
Denial	Steve did not accept his progressive problems with drinking at first. It required cumulative stress to move him past the denial stage.		
Anger		When Steve became aware of his cumulative stress, he still didn't have the understanding required to get help. Anger is a natural reaction to the fear and anxiety Steve was feeling. Anger began to compromise his marriage.	
Bargaining			Steve finally decided he would influence the situation after his wife threatened divorce. At this point, Steve bargained with his wife and she agreed to accompany him to seek mental health services.
Depression	Steve's occupational history shows that he entered a depressed emotional state after 1 year of unsuccessful job searching. He said, "I just lost hope."	Steve did not understand the interconnected relationship between his mood, self-motivation, and his inability to take adaptive action until learning about this in occupational therapy.	Steve's newly learned capacity to use developmental learning to increase coping and self-motivation during the occupational therapy assessment began to influence behavior through a series of adaptive responses.

(continued)

SPOTLIGHT 10-4. STEVE OVERCOMING THE PATTERNS OF GRIEF AND LOSS (CONTINUED)

Acceptance	Observing the outcomes of initial adaptive responses added to self-motivated choices and adaptive actions.	As stressors were reduced, Steve's adaptive capacity increased.	Steve began to unconsciously recognize and repeat patterns of developmental learning and adaptive actions.

with healthy developmental learning. This table demonstrates how physical conditions and negative thoughts, feelings, self-perceptions, and environmental conditions result in compensatory actions in the form of negative patterns of coping behavior. A high level of **adaptive capacity** allows for cognitive system flexibility so that stressors can be endured more calmly and recovered from more quickly.

Currently, research differentiates the emotionally self-regulating benefits of meaningful and purposeful occupations during aging into three categories. The first category includes activities and occupations that are interpreted in the brain as rewarding. The second category includes activities and occupations that produce the relaxation response for stress reduction. Finally, the third category includes novel activities and occupations that create new neuronal connections in the brain called **neuroplasticity** (Doidge, 2007; Gutman & Schindler, 2007; Jacobs, 2001). All three of these emotionally self-regulating processes are promoted in aging clients through occupations that self-regulate affect and action. Table 10-2 illustrates the emotional self-regulation activity checklist. The emotional self-regulation activity checklist demonstrates a way to informally identify which rewarding and relaxing activities center or ground a person's arousal level for coping with life stress. The positive feelings and homeostatic adjustments associated with emotional self-regulation of stress are supportive of well aging. Checkpoint 10-3 helps identify occupational patterns using the Emotional Self-Regulation Activity Checklist.

Spirituality also can affect healthy occupational participation during aging years. The American Occupational Therapy Association (AOTA) defined the **spiritual context** as "the fundamental orientation of a person's life; that which inspires and motivates that individual" (2008, p. 609). The spiritual context might be thought of as a vehicle by which human participation is self-motivated by intrinsic components of the activity. These include activities that promote a sense of reward, a relaxation response, developmental learning, or a purpose with infinite social or cultural meaning (Carse, 1986). Figure 10-5 illustrates the spiritual context. It displays the transformative homeostatic balance achieved during the meaning-making process where emotional integration and cognitive control support an adaptive response. This is represented as Meaning Making on a PEO Landscape Diagram and represents the concept of

the spiritual context from the AOTA occupational therapy practice framework (AOTA, 2008).

Aging clients tend to experience a greater sense of health and wellness through meaningful and purposeful occupational participation patterns. Primary roles such as husband, wife, parent, or teacher may have infinite social and cultural meanings. These roles and routines act as self-motivators for occupational participation and provide a source of healthy social identity complexity (Roccas & Brewer, 2002). Self-motivating spiritual roles, routines, or rituals are often a boost to occupational participation for this same reason.

Healthy spiritual and religious practices that promote positive emotions such as love and altruism have been shown to promote neuroplasticity in the brain (Post, 2007). Although reward and relaxation responses are categorized separately for occupational therapy practice purposes, they are really complementary processes within a shared system. When a positive mood shift occurs during a developmental learning opportunity, its self-motivating influence makes an adaptive response possible (Jackson, 1996; Scheufele, 2000; Siegel, 2012).

Personal Fitness With Occupational Contexts: Maintaining Occupational Participation During the Aging Years

The occupational therapy terms of centering and grounding may be thought of as two ways to describe a cognitively self-organizing experience through a complexity science lens. They distinguish between transformative shifts in a client's spiritual context. **Centering** activities promote self-motivation by producing a feeling of personal reward and positive anticipation. **Grounding** activities promote self-motivation by facilitating the relaxation response and a sense of calm anticipation. Neuroscientists and psychologists believe this may assist neurons to secrete neuromodulators that support an unconscious adaptive response through the approach-and-avoidance system in the brain (Carver, 2006; Freeman, 1995).

Although the approach-and-avoidance system works as an interconnected whole, occupational therapy activities

TABLE 10-1

EMOTIONAL SELF-REGULATION CHALLENGES

PHYSICAL CONDITIONS	THOUGHTS	FEELINGS	SELF-PERCEPTIONS	COMPENSATORY ACTIONS	ENVIRONMENTAL CONDITIONS
Pain/ headache/ stomach problems	Reduced attention	Anger	Meaningless Life/Unsatisfying Lifestyle	Loss of Self-Control	Disconnected from meaningful physical, social, and cultural roles
Muscle tension	Negative thoughts about others	Fear/ anxiousness	Purposeless Life/unfulfilling roles or non-fulfilling role expectations	Social isolation	Disconnected from purposeful physical, social, and cultural routines or rituals
Stress/ increase sweating	Forgetfulness	Depression	Vulnerability/environmental conditions block development of positive self-perceptions, choices, and actions	Drink/use drugs	Disconnected from Physical, Social & Cultural Opportunities to Take Adaptive Actions for Feeling Better
Sleep disorders	Rumination	Loneliness	Loss of sense of occupational competence/setting goals, organizing time, working toward goals	Remove self from challenging/problem contexts	Disconnected from physical, social, and cultural opportunities to experience and interpret personal goals/ areas of interest
High blood pressure/ heart palpitations	Confusion	Overwhelmed	Loss of sense of personal effectiveness/not meeting personal performance standards	Yell/scream/cry	Disconnected from anticipating a positive life plan that includes making personal choices
Fatigue/ numbness/ apathy	Trouble solving problems	Emptiness	Loss of sense of having and needing an occupational identity	Overeat/not eat	Disconnected from anticipating and experiencing daily life comforts, pleasures, and enjoyments
Anxiety/ shakiness/ hyperactivity	Poor concentration	Boredom	Loss of sense that personal values and interests can be participated in/developed	Physical violence toward self or others	Disconnected from prior habits of meaning/feelings of personal, social, and cultural stability
Irritability	Negative thoughts about self	Moodiness	Loss of sense that personal thoughts and feelings can be changed for greater satisfaction	Sleep more	Disconnected from desired feelings of love/social bonding and support

TABLE 10-2

THE EMOTIONAL SELF-REGULATION CHECKLIST

CENTERING ⟶		⟵ GROUNDING
(INCREASING PLEASURE-REDUCING BOREDOM)		(INCREASING COMFORT-REDUCING ANXIETY)
Positive interpersonal relationships		Progressive relaxation
Positive self-talk		Deep breathing
Joyful religious, social, and cultural rituals/relational prayer		Meditation, mindfulness and contemplative prayer
Fast upbeat music/songs		Slow rhythmic musical/instrumentals
Laughter/singing joyously/choir		Humming/ singing quietly and rhythmically
Dancing, aerobics, energizing yoga poses		Isometric exercises, relaxing yoga poses
Power walking/group walking		Leisure walking/calm settings
Novel/interesting multi-sensory environments		Familiar/predictable multi-sensory environments
Visualizing loved ones/successful and joyful social exchanges		Visualizing pleasant scenery and natural/open environments
Teamwork	INTEGRATION OF EMOTION AND COGNITIVE CONTROL	Working in a quiet space
Social community service		Task-oriented community service
Reminiscing together		Cleaning and polishing
Work with novelty and surprise		Predictable/planned work
Creative expression		Home and yard work
Reading romance or mystery novels		Reading educational and self-affirming books
Working collaboratively on a project		Winning a competition/marking jobs off a list
Collaborative computer-based learning		Exploratory computer-based learning
Virtual games: X-Box		Virtual games: Wii (Nintendo)
Writing poetry or narratives		Journaling about feelings to let go
Swimming		Hot shower/bath
Meaningful relationship hugs		Comforting hugs
Caring for meaningful people or pets		Caring for meaningful objects or spaces
Enjoying an ocean breeze or warm sun		Wrapping in a heavy blanket
Face-paced social events		Alone time
Bright/rhythmic light patterns		Slow swinging or rocking
Drinking coffee/energizing herbal tea		Drinking water, relaxing herbal teas
Tasty or complex food		Chewy or crunchy food

Reprinted with permission from Ryan, J. (2013). Treating the brain as an adaptive system in clients with dementia: Facilitating the neurobiology of action system processes. Poster at the 2013 American Occupational Therapy Association Annual Conference, San Diego, CA.

CHECKPOINT 10-3. ANALYZE

Using the Emotional Self-Regulation Activity Checklist found in Table 10-2, identify the activities that are a part of your own occupational patterns.

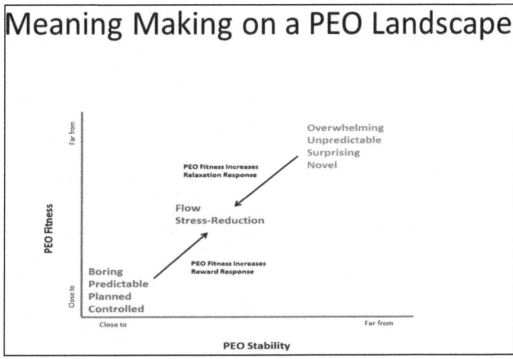

Figure 10-5. The spiritual context: Meaning Making on a PEO Landscape Diagram. (Reprinted with permission from Ryan, J. (2013). Treating the brain as an adaptive system in clients with dementia: Facilitating the neurobiology of action system processes. Poster at the 2013 American Occupational Therapy Association Annual Conference, San Diego, CA.)

influence the system in two complementary ways. Activities that are primarily self-motivating may be thought of as having a centering influence as they activate reward centers in the brain. These activities can also be identified by their ability to support feelings of social connectedness, positive emotion, and/or social identity. These activities tend to have a positive social purpose because they promote interpersonal bonding, empathy, collaborative processes, and community building (Champagne, Ryan, Saccamondo, & Lazzarini, 2007; Freeman, 1995).

Activities that are primarily self-motivating may be thought of as having a grounding influence as they promote the relaxation response in the brain. Herbert Benson, MD identified the relaxation response and has since proven its powerful stress-reducing benefits during mindfulness and meditation (Benson, 1975/2000; Gutman & Schindler, 2007). Occupational therapy commonly refers to the challenging patterns of reactive stress as the *fight-flight-freeze* response. It influences the shaping of occupational patterns in many clients receiving sensory integration treatment at any age (Dunn, 2009; Frick & Young, 2009).

Although the fight-flight-freeze response was vital for self-preservation in the wild, its current neurobiological influence shapes the boundaries of what the public often thinks of as a personal comfort zone. Extreme examples of these sensory defensive behaviors are associated with people who have developmental challenges, such as symptoms associated with autism spectrum disorders. Although these

responses are commonly more subtle in the general population, the neurobiological surge associated with a physical or social threat creates the unhealthy effects of cumulative stress. The extreme reaction to traumatic events, such as symptoms associated with posttraumatic stress disorder (van der Kolk, McFarlane, & Weisaeth, 1996), develops through the same approach-and-avoidance system as the fight-flight-freeze response.

Rewarding and relaxing feelings act as behavioral attractors that shape a person's personality and occupational patterns through the approach-and-avoidance system (Carver, 2006). This is a process called system *self-organization*. The process of self-organization follows a set of interaction rules to establish ordered patterns across space and time. Developmental learning of motor patterns in babies (Howle, 2002), cognitive control patterns in small children (Siegel, 1999), and occupational patterns through the lifespan (Champagne et al., 2004, 2005) are examples of self-organizing human systems.

Self-organization of the approach-and-avoidance system into a state of cognitive control may be thought of as an adaptive response at the transformative center of the Meaning Making on a PEO Landscape Diagram. Feelings of connectedness with the occupation and environment become a behavioral attractor for habit formation. Feelings of stress and fear create boundaries that shape a person's comfort zone through approach-and-avoidance patterns of occupational participation. Habits that create meaning for

SPOTLIGHT 10-5. STEVE'S EMOTIONAL SELF-REGULATION CHECKLIST

Integration of Emotion and Cognitive Control

Progressive Relaxation
Deep Breathing
Meditation, Mindfulness and Contemplative Prayer
Slow Rhythmic Music/ Instrumentals
Humming/ Singing Quietly & Rhythmically
Isometric Exercises/ Relaxing Yoga Poses
Leisure Walking/ Calm Settings
Familiar/ Predictable Multi-Sensory Environments
Visualizing Pleasant Scenery & Natural/ Open Environments
Working in a Quiet Space
Task-Oriented Community Service
Cleaning & Polishing
Predictable/ Planned Work
Home & Yard Work
Reading Educational & Self-Affirming Books
Winning a Competition/ Marking Jobs off a List
Exploratory Computer-based Learning
Virtual Games: Wii
Journaling about Feelings to Let Go
Hot Shower/ Bath
Comforting Hugs
Caring for Meaningful Objects or Spaces
Wrapping in a Heavy Blanket
Alone-Time
Slow Swinging or Rocking
Drinking Water, Relaxing Herbal Teas
Chewy or Crunchy Food

an individual reinforce engagement in experiences for positive feelings. Sometimes these positive feelings are sensory pleasures such as the scent of a garden. Other times they are emotional experiences such as the feeling of social bonding. They can also be the subtle but real pleasure of a meaning-making experience such as playing an instrument. This has been called the feeling of *flow* (Csikszentmihalyi, 1997).

Research has shown that the neurological system is stimulated and a sense of well-being is promoted during flow experiences. The mesocorticolimbic system is a reward pathway in the brain that connects the **brain reward centers** deep in the limbic system with the frontal lobe (Gutman & Schindler, 2007). It plays a key role in the self-motivating experience of flow during meaningful and purposeful occupations. Researched activities commonly associated with flow include "music, drawing, meditation, reading, arts and crafts, and home repairs" (Gutman & Schindler, p. 71).

Aging clients with challenges related to Parkinson's disease, dementia, depression, and aphasia have demonstrated functional benefits attributed to the stimulation of alternative pathways that occurs during music. Studies with artists have shown that these positive influences are also associated with creative drawing and other activities that tend to naturally produce the feeling of flow. **Flow** describes a state associated with meaningful and purposeful activity characterized by the following:

- Complete absorption in the activity and diminished awareness of the external environment

- A sense of oneness with the activity

- Total immersion in the present moment and a lost sense of time

- Lost fear or anxiety—everyday worries fade as people become increasingly engrossed in the activity

- Immense feelings of personal satisfaction—the activity is rewarding in itself (Gutman & Schindler, 2007, p. 75)

Flow activities include creative expression, occupations in the workplace, education, music, gaming, sports, religion, and spirituality (Csikszentmihalyi, 1997; Keller & Bless, 2008; Peifer, 2012). The mesocorticolimbic system is activated during the pleasant feelings that accompany flow, along with subtle shifts in emotional self-regulation. These shifts are associated with changes in affect and mood, and are considered likely contributors to the development of identity, attachment, personality development, and expression.

Spotlight 10-5 illustrates the Emotional Self-Regulation Activity Checklist. It uses Steve's case study to demonstrate how this checklist can be used to identify centering or grounding activities. These activities may be used to facilitate the reward or relaxation response.

The mesocorticolimbic system also seems to contribute to development of new occupational participation patterns by "motivating people to repeat pleasurable activities that promote survival and avoid activities that cause harm" (Skuse, Morris, & Lawrence, 2003). This is developmental learning, and begins with an adaptive response. Three examples of developmental learning in childhood are the development of occupational performance skills associated with motor, cognitive, and social competence. Three examples of developmental learning in aging adults include the following:

1. Emergent coping strategies that follow life transitions

2. New learning that occurs when a lifelong learner moves out of his or her comfort zone

3. Transformative shifts in emotional self-regulation from regular meditation or yoga

The understanding of flow has contributed to the development of positive psychology principles that are being used by the general population to improve mood, affect, attention, and self-motivation (Csikszentmihalyi, 1997). It is easy during times of stress to lose motivation to be involved with leisure or social interests. The sciences of physical medicine and stress reduction have proven the well-aging benefits of participating in rewarding and relaxing activities during aging years (Blood & Zatorre, 2001) to overcome or prevent these self-defeating feelings. The *relaxation response* is triggered as an interdependent emotional shift away from reliance on a reactive approach-and-avoidance system.

PART 2: ASSESSING OCCUPATIONAL PATTERNS IN AGING CLIENTS

Three occupational therapy practice models are presented to guide occupational therapy practitioners to meet the needs of aging clients. They are the PEO Model, Cognitive Disability Theory, and complexity science models. The PEO Model and Cognitive Disability Theory led to the development of standardized assessments. The PEO Model contributed to development of the Canadian Occupational Performance Measure (COPM) (Law, Baptiste, Carswell, McColl, Polatajko, & Pollock, 2005). The Cognitive Disability Model led to development of Claudia Allen's Cognitive Levels (Allen, 1985; Pollard & Olin, 2005). These standardized assessments help identify and link phenomena to the evaluation and treatment process in occupational therapy.

Complexity science principles and methods apply to the third set of practice tools and models. These principles and methods are currently used worldwide in related disciplines to respond to what has been called a human systems dynamics paradigm shift (Eoyang, 2012; Eoyang & Holladay, 2013). Occupational scientists and practice leaders (Royeen, 1997, 2002; Yerxa, 1967; Zemke & Clark, 1996) have challenged the profession to develop ways to apply complexity science in occupational therapy. Rather than offering a standardized assessment, Human Systems Occupational Therapy (HSOT) tools and models are currently being used to teach, explain, and increase the measurability of the central practice technique of facilitating occupational pattern adaptation in occupational therapy.

Assessing Occupational Participation and Performance Using the Person-Environment-Occupation Model

A group of Canadian occupational therapists introduced the PEO Model that identifies goodness-of-fit in the occupational performance system. The occupational performance system is made up of three parts: the person, environment, and occupation (Law, Cooper, Strong, Stewart, Rigby, & Letts, 1996). Goodness-of-fit between these three parts is considered a key influence on the development of occupational patterns. Self-directed occupational choices develop into habits, routines, and roles throughout the lifespan because they "meet intrinsic needs for self-maintenance,

expression and fulfillment" (Letts, Rigby, & Stewart, 2003, p. 27). As people age, environmental fit requires adaptive responses to life transitions to maximize goodness-of-fit.

The COPM was developed to identify occupational therapy clinical observations and clinical analysis of environmental fit over the lifespan, especially during times of transition and aging. Figure 10-6 displays an occupational therapy practitioner administering the standardized COPM. The COPM assesses individual occupational performance patterns that are influenced by the PEO system. It is designed to identify occupational performance issues by asking clients to rate by importance what they want to, are expected to, or need to do in a regular day. Clients are interviewed about the general areas of self-care, productivity, and leisure. A client's level of satisfaction is also considered.

By recognizing leisure activities as equal to self-care and productivity, the COPM is compatible with holistic quality-of-life goals that include rewarding and relaxing leisure activities as well as lifelong learning. The PEO Model and the COPM are client centered due to their interest in client satisfaction. This means that the COPM recognizes that the internal environment of thoughts, feelings, self-perceptions, and actions largely shape a person's occupational patterns on an unconscious level.

The PEO Model and the COPM can be used to help practitioners suggest adaptations to occupational context and the environment that can increase a client's performance or satisfaction. After intervention, a reassessment is beneficial so that new performance and satisfaction scores can document intervention outcomes. Examples of COPM assessment and reassessment outcomes are provided from Steve's occupational therapy intervention in Spotlight 10-6.

Assessing Cognitive Pattern Complexity and Flexibility Using the Cognitive Disability Model

Claudia Allen began developing the Cognitive Disability Model in the 1960s (Allen & Blue, 1998). The Cognitive Disability Model is foundational knowledge for much of today's cognitive occupational therapy practice. Years of practice informed Allen on the cognitive performance patterns she repeatedly observed in treatment. From her experiences, she developed a behavioral level of cognitive performance. The books *Understanding Cognitive Performance Modes* (Allen, Earhart, & Blue, 1995) and the second edition of *Allen's Cognitive Levels* (Pollard & Olin, 2005) describe the cognitive performance levels that can be applied in multiple types of settings and facilities worldwide.

The Allen's Cognitive Levels (ACL) rating is commonly assessed using the leather lacing screening tool as well as an assortment of standardized activities. Assessments have been developed using a variety of craft activities such as woodworking, placemats, and bookmarks. After selecting

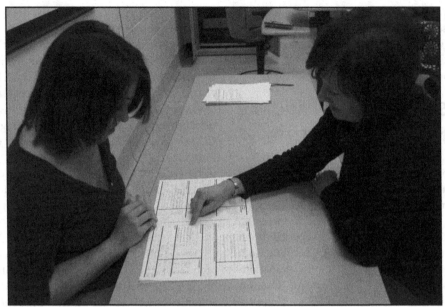

Figure 10-6. An occupational therapy practitioner administering the COPM.

SPOTLIGHT 10-6. STEVE'S CANADIAN OCCUPATIONAL PERFORMANCE MEASURE

STEP 1:
IDENTIFICATION OF OCCUPATIONAL PERFORMANCE ISSUES

STEP 2:
RATING
IMPORTANCE

To identify occupational performance problems, concerns and issues, interview the client, asking about daily activities in self-care, productivity and leisure. Ask clients to identify daily activities which they want to do, need to do or are expected to do by encouraging them to think about a typical day. Then ask the client to identify which of these activities are difficult for them to do now to their satisfaction. Record these activity problems in Steps 1A, 1B, or 1C.

Using the scoring card provided, ask the client to rate, on a scale of 1 to 10, the importance of each activity. Place the ratings in the corresponding boxes in Steps 1A, 1B, 1C.

STEP 1A: Self-care   IMPORTANCE

Personal Care
(e.g., dressing, bathing,
feeding, hygiene)

Functional Mobility
(e.g., transfers,
indoor, outdoor)

Community Management
(e.g., transportation,
shopping, finances)

STEP 1B: Productivity

Paid/Unpaid Work   Finding a job   10
(e.g., finding/keeping   preparing resume   9
a job, volunteering)   arranging interviews   9

Household Management   dealing with problems/   10
(e.g., cleaning,   conflicts
laundry, cooking)

Play/School
(e.g., play skills,
homework)

(continued)

SPOTLIGHT 10-6. STEVE'S CANADIAN OCCUPATIONAL PERFORMANCE MEASURE (CONTINUED)

STEP 1C: Leisure

Quiet Recreation (e.g., hobbies, crafts, reading)
gardening — IMPORTANCE: 4

Active Recreation (e.g., sports, outings, travel)
attending church services — 8

Socialization (e.g., visiting, phone calls, parties, correspondence)
talking on the phone — 6

STEPS 3 & 4: SCORING - INITIAL ASSESSMENT and REASSESSMENT

Initial Assessment:			Reassessment:	
OCCUPATIONAL PERFORMANCE PROBLEMS	PERFORMANCE 1	SATISFACTION 1	PERFORMANCE 2	SATISFACTION 2
1. Finding a job	1	1	5	6
2. dealing with conflicts	2	3	5	5
3. preparing resume	8	7	9	10
4. arranging interviews	7	6	8	7
5. attending church	3	7	9	8

SCORING:

Total Score = Total performance or satisfaction scores ÷ # of problems

	PERFORMANCE SCORE 1	SATISFACTION SCORE 1	PERFORMANCE SCORE 2	SATISFACTION SCORE 2
	21 / 5	24 / 5	36 / 5	36 / 5
	= 4.2	= 4.8	= 7.2	= 7.2

CHANGE IN PERFORMANCE = Performance Score 2 7.2 – Performance Score 1 4.2 = 3.0

CHANGE IN SATISFACTION = Satisfaction Score 2 7.2 – Satisfaction Score 1 4.8 = 2.4

---

the craft that is most self-motivating for a client, the Allen Diagnostic Rating Scale is used. The Allen Diagnostic Rating Scale is used to observe and rate client's cognitive performance patterns as the client completes simple, moderate, and complex stitch designs. There is both a standard and a large leather lacing screening tool for clients with vision loss or severely challenged manual dexterity. Figure 10-7 displays an occupational therapy practitioner administering the standardized leather lacing screening.

ACL and diagnostic modules are divided into six developmentally arranged categories, with level 6 representing the highest cognitive complexity. An individual may be able to live independently at home or in the community with an ACL level of 4.6 or above. This is important, as health and wellness interventions in the community most often will be applied at or above this cognitive level. Clients with cognitive challenges may progressively lose their cognitive performance, receive lower ACL level ratings, and require greater levels of assistance for safety and activities of daily living. The following is a brief description of each of the cognitive levels within the cognitive disabilities model:

- **Level 6:** An important ACL level, level 6 criteria is the functional application of a high level of abstract thought. In the words of Allen, this rises above survival-based behaviors and allows a person to "understand divergent opinions leading to continual searching for truth, analyzing facts, and questioning accuracy of others" (Pollard & Olin, 2005, p. 13). Allen describes learning at this level as exploratory but with internalized rather than manual trial-and-error processing.

  ○ At ACL level 6, people can observe, understand, and respond adaptively to symbolic or abstract cues that are not directly related to their personal experience. ACL level 6 recognizes imagination and a high level of conceptual ability as key components of cognitive complexity. Rather than learning through imitation, people at ACL level

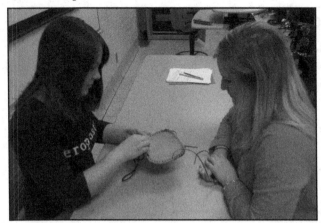

Figure 10-7. Occupational therapy assistant students practicing the ACL leather lacing screen.

6 flexibly shift between deductive and inductive reasoning for creative problem solving and novel idea generation. Allen describes ACL level 6 as a state of cognitive control that supports high-level social behavior, achieving shared goals through compromise rather than force or manipulation.

- **Level 5:** ACL level 5 is the highest level of survival-motivated behavior by which a person attends to personally relevant cues for self-directed developmental learning. An important difference between ACL level 6 and level 5 is a lack of capacity to imagine the thoughts of others for empathic understanding and high-level social system influence. Developmental learning occurs at ACL level 5 on the scale of sensory motor performance with observable, manual trial-and-error problem solving. "Spontaneous motor actions are exploratory, with an effort to imitate the novel actions of others. One's purpose is to achieve self-control through the experience of inductive reasoning" (Pollard & Olin, 2005, p. 15). An example of Steve's rating on the ACL leather lacing screening is provided in Spotlight 10-7.

- **Level 4:** At ACL level 4, practitioners often need to model familiar multistep activities in order for a client to mirror exact actions. An important difference between ACL level 5 and level 4 is an increased level of dependence on external environmental cues to feel connected to the spatial and temporal context of familiar occupations. The increasing distortion of time and space during the progression of dementia contributes to difficulties with sequencing and transitioning between the steps of familiar multistep goals. Familiar multiple-step tasks include things such as activities of daily living. The capacity to live safely at home alone is commonly gone in ACL Level 4; however, a person may be able to live at home alone at ACL level 4.6 or higher. Confusion increases while attempting to navigate the environment.

- **Level 3:** At ACL level 3, practitioners often need to provide separate cues for each step of familiar multistep occupations. Again, familiar multistep occupations can include activities of daily living, for example. An important difference between ACL level 4 and level 3 is a greater need to self-activate "attention through the experience of touching" (Pollard & Olin, 2005) objects and surfaces within the physical environment. This means the use of familiar rather than novel tools is increasingly important for sustaining manual actions such as grooming or leisure activities. A narrowed temporal context limits client performance to completion of one step at a time.

- **Level 2:** At ACL level 2, practitioners usually need to provide direct physical assistance for even one step of a familiar, goal-directed activity. An important difference between ACL level 3 and level 2 is a greater focus on use of attention and proprioceptive cues to increase personal comfort and reduce fight-flight-freeze responses. Self-generated adaptive responses are usually automatic motor and postural actions.

- **Level 1:** At ACL level 1, practitioners are usually limited to activities that focus on facilitating a positive mood or affect. Practitioners also provide cognitive support of client consciousness during meaningful relationships, family visits, and spiritual preparation for end of life. An important difference between ACL level 2 and level 1 is a greater focus on sustaining arousal level rather than attempting even automatic motor and postural actions.

Observing and Understanding Human System Patterns Using Human Systems Occupational Therapy Practice Tools and Models

The HSOT occupational pattern adaptation tool helps guide assessment with standardized and nonstandardized assessments, incorporates a client's occupational history and activities of daily living, and identifies personal interests to focus client-centered interventions. The COPM, the ACL, and subtests from the *Model of Human Occupation* (Kielhofner, 2002) were used in the example of Steve's case study. This same information can be gathered from a variety of other standardized assessments such as the Activity Card Sort (Baum & Edwards, 2008).

The occupational pattern adaptation tool can be used to guide assessment in any practice area. It promotes positive client change through self-awareness, client-centered goal development, and adaptive responses. For example, occupational pattern adaptation is required when a client needs to develop new daily living routines after experiencing a stroke. In mental health settings, changing nonadaptive

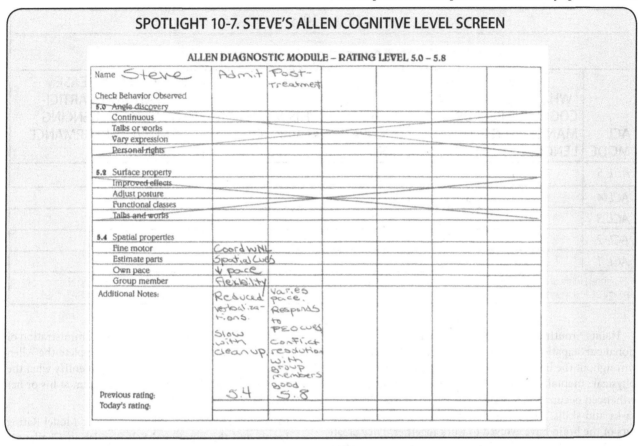

thoughts, feelings, and self-perceptions are typically the first step toward taking adaptive action.

The Adaptive Response Model is useful to the occupational therapy assistant when identifying assessment results in collaboration with the occupational therapist. The Adaptive Response Model supports the client and therapist to observe, understand, and influence occupational patterns. Clinical problem solving is enhanced when a practitioner makes safety or home program recommendations using the Adaptive Response Model.

The Emotional Self-Regulation Checklist and the Meaning Making on a PEO Landscape Diagram are useful in identifying and teaching clients how to use healthy coping mechanisms. An occupational therapy assistant is shown in Figure 10-8 administering the Emotional Self-Regulation Checklist. This model can be used when explaining how a client benefits from centering or grounding activities during stressful transitions. Both models are also helpful for explaining the quality-of-life benefits of activities that fit a client's spiritual context.

SUMMARY

An individual's adaptive capacity or resilience is a strong contributor to healthy aging and overcoming emotional or

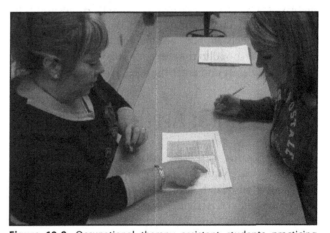

Figure 10-8. Occupational therapy assistant students practicing administration of the Emotional Self-Regulation Checklist.

physical challenges. Often, the treatment of two clients with similar impairments and disabilities may lead to very different outcomes due to their differences in individual adaptive capacity (Champagne et al., 2007; Christiansen, 1991). Occupational therapy practitioners can facilitate the just right challenge for clients throughout the lifespan by applying the science of complex adaptive systems to occupational therapy services. Understanding the dynamic system relationship between person, environment, and occupation is a key to the art and science of occupational therapy.

TABLE 10-3			
FOR APPLICATION QUESTION 3			
ACL MODE	"WHAT ARE COMMON COGNITIVE PERFORMANCE PATTERN CHALLENGES?"	"WHAT DOES THIS MEAN FOR OCCUPATIONAL PARTICIPATION?"	"HOW CAN I INCREASE OCCUPATIONAL PARTICIPATION BY INFLUENCING COGNITIVE PERFORMANCE PATTERNS?"
ACL 5			
ACL 4			
ACL 3			
ACL 2			
ACL 1			

Reprinted with permission from Ryan, J. (2013). Treating the brain as an adaptive system in clients with dementia: Facilitating the neurobiology of action system processes. Poster at the 2013 American Occupational Therapy Association Annual Conference, San Diego, CA.

Habits, routines, and roles are spontaneous occupational participation patterns that serve important functions throughout the lifespan. They develop as a way to conserve physical, mental, and emotional energy. It also leads to enhanced occupational performance during well-practiced tasks and skills. The relaxation response and reward centers of the brain have evolved to work together. They create a positive and supportive influence on cognitive control, adaptive responses, and individual actions. Applications of the PEO Model, the Cognitive Disability Model, and HSOT tools and models support occupational therapy practitioners as they respond to the current human systems dynamics paradigm shift and enter the age of complexity.

PART 3: APPLICATIONS

The following activities will help you identify key aspects of this chapter that were highlighted in this text. These questions also highlight the chapter objectives at the start of the chapter. Activities are suggested to be completed individually or in a small group to enhance learning.

1. With a partner, take turns role-playing a client and a therapist during the administration of the COPM. The student role-playing the therapist will be responsible for administering the COPM to the client. Follow steps 1 through 3 of the COPM on the COPM initial assessment form. List the client's five most important occupational performance problems, a performance score, and a satisfaction score. Don't forget to record additional notes and background information in the appropriate place on the form.

2. View the "Administering the ACL" video. Individually or in groups, divide into pairs to take turns role-playing a client and therapist during the administration of the ACL leather lacing screening. Complete the Allen Diagnostic Model Rating Levels, and identify what the client (student) should be able to perform at his or her level of cognitive ability.

3. In groups, refer to the Allen Diagnostic Model Rating Levels and the Emotional Self-Regulation Challenges Activities Checklist found in Table 10-2. After analyzing differences between cognitive performance modes, groups will present their ideas for improving client safety at each ACL mode. Fill in Table 10-3 with ideas for improving client safety at each ACL mode level. Each group should consider ways to adapt the therapeutic relationship, the occupational context, and the physical environment.

4. Refer to the Allen Diagnostic Model Rating Levels and the Emotional Self-Regulation Challenges Activities Checklist found in Table 10-2. Fill in Table 10-4 with ideas for increasing a client's occupational participation at each ACL mode. After analyzing the differences between cognitive performance modes, groups will present their ideas. Each group should consider ways to adapt the therapeutic relationship, the occupational context, and the physical environment.

5. In groups, answer the centering and grounding discussion questions found in Table 10-5. This will help synthesize understanding of material and build empathy for therapeutic relationships when treating aging adults.

6. In groups, refer to the Meaning Making on a PEO Landscape Diagram. Discuss how using the Emotional Self-Regulation Checklist might make it easier to identify coping mechanisms to help aging clients experiencing dramatic life transitions. List your results.

	TABLE 10-4		
	FOR APPLICATION QUESTION 4		
ACL MODE	**"WHAT ARE COMMON COGNITIVE PERFORMANCE PATTERN CHALLENGES?"**	**"WHAT DOES THIS MEAN FOR OCCUPATIONAL PARTICIPATION?"**	**"HOW CAN I INCREASE OCCUPATIONAL PARTICIPATION BY INFLUENCING COGNITIVE PERFORMANCE PATTERNS?"**
ACL 5			
ACL 4			
ACL 3			
ACL 2			
ACL 1			

Reprinted with permission from Ryan, J. (2013). Treating the brain as an adaptive system in clients with dementia: Facilitating the neurobiology of action system processes. Poster at the 2013 American Occupational Therapy Association Annual Conference, San Diego, CA.

TABLE 10-5
FOR APPLICATION QUESTION 5
CENTERING AND GROUNDING DISCUSSION QUESTIONS

1. After self-administration of the Emotional Self-Regulation Checklist students will be asked to discuss which occupational patterns they use to regulate their own emotional state.

2. Do they see any patterns in their own lives in which they participate in these centering or grounding activities? Examples: time of day, occupational context, social or physical environment.

3. Do they seem to use more centering or more grounding occupational patterns in their current life?

4. After reviewing these patterns, are there any that they would consider support feelings of flow? That support feelings of self-motivation? That they would consider part of their spiritual context?

5. Have they ever used any of these activities or recommended them in treatment?

6. Which would they consider a coping strategy and therefore an example of their own intrapersonal learning? Has anyone experienced a life transition that seemed to naturally increase any of these occupational patterns?

7. Now relate these occupational patterns to others. This could be family members, friends, and acquaintances. If students have had clinical experience, they can relate these occupational patterns to observations of clients.

8. Finally, after this exercise in intrapersonal, interpersonal, and naturalistic learning, discuss the benefits and uses of centering or grounding occupational patterns when treating aging client populations. Examples: people with dementia, depression, or addictions

Reprinted with permission from Ryan, J. (2013). Treating the brain as an adaptive system in clients with dementia: Facilitating the neurobiology of action system processes. Poster at the 2013 American Occupational Therapy Association Annual Conference, San Diego, CA.

REFERENCES

Allen, C. K. (1985). *Occupational therapy for psychiatric diseases: Measurement and management of cognitive disabilities*. Boston, MA: Little & Brown.

Allen, C. K., & Blue, T. (1998). Cognitive disabilities model: How to make clinical judgments. In N. Katz (Ed.), *Cognition and occupation in rehabilitation: Cognitive models for intervention in occupational therapy* (pp. 225-280). Bethesda, MD: American Occupational Therapy Association.

Allen, C. K., Earhart, C. A., & Blue, T. (1995). *Understanding cognitive performance modes*. Ormond Beach, FL: Allen Conferences.

American Occupational Therapy Association. (2008). Occupational therapy practice framework: Domain and process (2nd ed.). *American Journal of Occupational Therapy, 62, 625–683.*

Angelou, M. (n.d.). In *Brainy Quote*. Retrieved from www.BrainyQuote.com.

Bankman, I. N., & Morcovescu, S. (Eds.). (2002). *Handbook of medical imaging: Processing and analysis.* Orlando, FL: Academic Press.

Baum, C. M., & Edwards, D. (2008). *Activity card sort* (2nd ed.). Bethesda, MD: American Occupational Therapy Association.

Benson, H. (1975/ 2000). *The relaxation response.* New York, NY: HarperCollins Publishers.

Blood, A. J., & Zatorre, R. J. (2001). Intensely pleasurable responses to music correlate with activity in brain regions implicated in reward and emotion. *Proceedings of the National Academy of Sciences, 98,* 11818-11823. (Electronic version)

Braungart, M. M., Braungart, R. G., & Gramet, P. (2011). Applying learning theories to healthcare practice. In Bastabel S., Gramet, P., Jacobs, K., Sopczyk, D. L. (Eds.), *Health professional as editor.* (pp. 51-89). Sudbury, MA: Jones & Bartlett Learning.

Carse, J. P. (1986). *Finite and infinite games: A vision of life as play and possibility.* New York, NY: Free Press.

Carver, C. S. (2006). Approach, avoidance, and the self-regulation of affect and action. *Motivational Emotion, 30,* 105-110.

Champagne, T. (2008). *Sensory modulation & environment: Essential elements of occupation* (3rd ed.). Southampton, MA: Champagne Conferences & Consultation.

Champagne, T., Ryan, J., Saccamondo, H. & Lazzarini, I. (2007). A nonlinear dynamics approach to exploring the spiritual dimensions of occupation. *Emergence: Complexity & Organization, 9*(4), 29-43.

Christiansen, C. (1991). Performance deficits as sources of stress: Coping theory and occupational therapy. In C. Christiansen & C. Baum (Eds.). *Occupational therapy: Overcoming human performance deficits.* Thorofare, NJ: SLACK.

Christiansen, C. (1999). Defining lives: Occupation as identity: An essay on competence, coherence, and the creation of meaning. *American Journal of Occupational Therapy, 53,* 547-558.

Csikszentmihalyi, M. (1997). *Finding flow: The psychology of engagement with everyday life.* New York, NY: Basic Books.

Csikszentmihalyi, M., Abuhamdeh, S., & Nakamura, J. (2005). Flow. In A. Elliot, *Handbook of competence and motivation* (pp. 598-698). New York, NY: The Guilford Press.

Doidge, N. (2007). *The brain that changes itself.* New York, NY: Viking Press.

Dunn, W. (2009). *Living sensationally: Understanding your senses.* Philadelphia, PA: Jessica Kingsley.

Dunn, W., Brown, C., & McGuigan, A. (1994). The ecology of human performance: A framework for considering the effect of context. *American Journal of Occupational Therapy, 48*(7), 595-607.

Dweck, C. S. (2006). *Mindset: The new psychology of success: How we can learn to fulfill our potential.* New York, NY: Ballantine Books.

Eisenberg, N. I., Lieberman, M. D., & Williams, K. D. (2003). Does rejection hurt? An MRI study of social exclusion. *Science, 302,* 290-292.

Eoyang, G. H. (2012). *The human systems dynamics paradigm shift.* Unpublished manuscript.

Eoyang, G. H., & Holladay, R. J. (2013). *Adaptive action: Leveraging uncertainty in your organization.* Stanford, CA: Stanford University Press.

Freeman, W. (1995). *Societies of brains: A study in the neuroscience of love and hate.* Hillsdale, NJ: Lawrence Erlbaum Associates Publishers.

Freeman, W. (2000). *How brains make up their minds.* New York, NY: Columbia University Press.

Frick, S. M., & Young, S. R. (2009). *Listening with the whole body: Clinical concepts and treatment guidelines for therapeutic listening.* Madison, WI: Vital Links.

Gardner, H. (1999). *The disciplined mind: Beyond facts and standardized tests.* New York, NY: Simon and Schuster.

Gray, J. M., Kennedy, B. L., & Zemke, R. (1996). Dynamic systems theory: An overview. In R. Zemke & F. Clark (Eds.). *Occupational science: The evolving discipline.* Philadelphia, PA: F. A. Davis.

Gray, J. R. (2004). Integration of emotion and cognitive control. *American Psychological Society, 13*(2), 46-48.

Gutman, S. A., & Schindler, V. P. (2007). The neurological basis of occupation. *Occupational Therapy International, 14*(2), 71-85.

Hasselkus, B. R. (2002). *The meaning of everyday occupation.* Thorofare, NJ: SLACK.

Holmes, T. H., & Rahe, R. H. (1967). The social readjustment rating scale. *Journal of Psychosomatic Research, 11*(2), 213-21.

Howle, J. M. (2002). *Neuro-developmental treatment approach: Theoretical foundations and principles of clinical practice.* Laguna Beach, CA: North American Neuro-Developmental Treatment Association.

Human Systems Dynamics Institute. (n.d.a.). Adaptive action. Retrieved from http://wiki.hsdinstitute.org/adaptive_action.

Human Systems Dynamics Institute. (n.d.b.). Radical inquiry. Retrieved from http://wiki.hsdinstitute.org/radical_inquiry.

Human Systems Dynamics Institute. (n.d.c.). CDE. Retrieved from http://wiki.hsdinstitute.org/cde.

Human Systems Dynamics Institute. (n.d.d.). Landscape Diagram. Retrieved from http://wiki.hsdinstitute.org/landscape_diagram.

Jackson, S. A. (1996). Toward a conceptual understanding of the flow experience in elite athletes. *Research Quarterly for Exercise and Sport, 67,* 76-90.

Jackson, J., Carlson, M., Mandel, D., Zemke, R., & Clark, F. (1998). Occupation in lifestyle redesign: The well-elderly study occupational therapy program. *American Journal of Occupational Therapy, 52,* 330.

Jacobs, G. D. (2001). The physiology of mind-body interactions: The stress response and the relaxation response. *Journal of Alternative and Complementary Medicine, 7,* S83-S92.

Keller, J., & Bless, H. (2008). Flow and regulatory compatibility: An experimental approach to a flow model of intrinsic motivation. *Personality and Social Psychology Bulletin, 34,* 196-209.

Kielhofner, G. (2002). *Model of human occupation: Theory and application* (3rd ed.). Philadelphia, PA: Lippincott Williams & Wilkins.

King, L. J. (1978). Toward a science of adaptive responses: 1978 Eleanor Clarke Slagle Lecture. *American Journal of Occupational Therapy, 32*(7), 429-437.

Kubler-Ross, E. (1969). *On death and dying.* New York, NY: Routledge.

Law, M. (2002). Participation in the occupations of everyday life: 2002 Distinguished Scholar Lecture. *American Journal of Occupational Therapy, 56,* 640-649.

Law, M., Baptiste, S., Carswell, A., McColl, M. A., Polatajko, H., & Pollock, N. (2005). *Canadian Occupational Performance Measure* (4th ed.). Ottawa, Ontario: Canadian Association of Occupational Therapists.

Law, M., Cooper, B., Strong, S., Stewart, D., Rigby, P., & Letts, L. (1996). The Person-Environment-Occupation Model: A transactive approach to occupational performance. *Canadian Journal of Occupational Therapy, 63*(1), 9-23.

Lazzarini, I. (2004). Neuro-occupation: The nonlinear dynamics of intention, meaning and perception. *British Journal of Occupational Therapy, 67*(8), 342-352.

Lazzarini, I. (2005). A nonlinear approach to cognition: A web of ability and disability. In N. Katz (Ed.). *Cognition & occupation across the lifespan* (pp. 211-233). Bethesda, MD: American Occupational Therapy Association.

Letts, L., Rigby, P., & Stewart, D. (2003). *Using environments to enable occupational performance.* Thorofare, NJ: SLACK.

Meyer, A. (1922/1977). The philosophy of occupational therapy. *American Journal of Occupational Therapy, 31,* 639-642.

Nattkemper, T. W. (2004). Multivariate image analysis in biomedicine. *Journal of Biomedical Informatics, 37,* 380-391.

Ogden, P., Minton, K., & Pain, C. (2006). *Trauma and the body: A sensorimotor approach to psychotherapy.* New York, NY: W. W. Norton.

Peifer, C. (2012). Psycophysiological correlates of flow-experience. In S. Engeser (Ed.). *Advances in flow research* (pp. 139-164). New York, NY: Springer.

Pollard, D., & Olin, D. W. (2005). Allen's cognitive levels: Meeting the challenges of client focused services (2nd ed.). Monona, WI: SELECT One Rehab – Publication and Distribution.

Post, S. (2007). *Altruism and health perspectives from empirical research.* New York, NY: Oxford University Press.

Quade, K., & Holladay, R. (2010). *Dynamical leadership: Building adaptive capacity for uncertain times.* Apache Junction, AZ: Gold Canyon Press.

Rigby, P., & Letts, L. (2003). Environment and occupational performance: Theoretical considerations. In L. Letts, P. Rigby, & D. Stewart (Eds.). *Using environments to enable occupational performance* (pp. 17-32). Thorofare, NJ: SLACK.

Roccas, S., & Brewer, M. B. (2002). Social identity complexity. *Personality and social psychology review, 6*(2), 88-106.

Royeen, C. (Ed.). (1997). *Neuroscience & occupation: Links to practice.* Bethesda, MD: American Occupational Therapy Association.

Royeen, C. (2002). Occupation reconsidered. *Occupational Therapy International, 9*(2), 112-121.

Ryan, J. (2013). Treating the brain as an adaptive system in clients with dementia: Facilitating the neurobiology of action system processes. Poster at the 2013 American Occupational Therapy Association Annual Conference, San Diego, CA.

Ryan, J., & Griswold, D. (2011). The neuro-occupational potential of multi-sensory environments in cognitive treatment. Presentation at the 2011 Tennessee Occupational Therapy Association Annual Conference, Nashville, TN.

Scheufele, P. M. (2000). Effects of progressive relaxation and classical music on measurements of attention, relaxation, and stress response. *Journal of Behavioral Medicine, 23,* 207-228.

Schkade, J., & Schultz, S. (1992). Occupational adaptation: Toward a holistic approach for contemporary practice: Part 1. *American Journal of Occupational Therapy, 46*(9), 829-837.

Schultz, S., & Schkade, J. (1997). Adaptation. In C. Christiansen & C. Baum (Eds.). *Occupational therapy: Enabling health and well-being* (2nd ed.). Thorofare, NJ: SLACK.

Siegel, D. J. (1999). *The developing mind: How relationships and the brain interact to shape who we are.* New York, NY: The Guilford Press.

Siegel, D. J. (2010). *The mindful therapist: A clinician's guide to mindsight and neural integration.* New York, NY: W. W. Norton.

Siegel, D. J. (2012). *Pocket guide to interpersonal neurobiology: An integrative handbook of the mind.* New York, NY: W. W. Norton.

Skuse, D., Morris, J., & Lawrence, K. (2003). The amygdala and development of the social brain. *Annals of the New York Academy of Science, 10008,* 91-101.

Tytel, M., & Holladay, R. (2011). *Simple rules: A radical inquiry into self.* Circle Pines, MN: Lagumo.

van der Kolk, B. A., McFarlane, A. C., & Weisaeth, L. (Eds.). (1996). *Traumatic stress: The effects of overwhelming experience on mind, body and society.* New York, NY: The Guilford Press.

Yerxa, E. J. (1967). Authentic occupational therapy. *American Journal of Occupational Therapy, 21,* 1, 1-9.

Zemke, R., & Clark, F. (1996). *Occupational science: The evolving discipline.* Philadelphia, PA: F. A. Davis.

11

Improving Occupational Performance During the Late Lifespan

Janice Ryan, OTD, OTR/L

KEY TERMS

- Action Systems
- Emotional Resiliency
- Emotion-Focused Coping Cues
- Emotion-Focused Coping Resources
- Explicit Memories
- Fight-Flight-Freeze
- Generative Group Engagements
- Identity Cues
- Implicit Memories

- Mindful State of Consciousness
- Modeling
- Multisensory Cues
- Multisensory Environments
- Neuroadaptation
- Occupational Contexts
- Palliative
- Play Therapy
- Positive Approach
- Praxis

- Priming
- Problem-Focused Coping Cues
- Problem-Focused Coping Resources
- Self-Actualization
- Self-Organized Learning System
- Spatial Navigation
- Therapeutic Cues
- Therapeutic Exchange

CHAPTER LEARNING OBJECTIVES

After completion of this chapter, students will be able to:

1. Recognize common adaptive responses that occur over the late lifespan through developmental learning.

2. Describe self-actualizing occupational performance patterns that form at Allen Cognitive Levels Level 6.

3. Identify pattern rigidities that can affect health, well-being, and participation in life during engagement in occupations.

4. Apply four simple rules to target the adaptive response during occupational therapy.

5. Summarize how to create an adaptive response during occupational therapy using the therapeutic exchange, therapeutic environment, and occupational context.

6. Select traditional, holistic, and client-centered occupational therapy interventions that achieve occupational therapy outcomes that meet the needs of the client.

Manville, C.A., & Keough, J. L.
Mental Health Practice for the Occupational Therapy Assistant (pp 259-284).
© 2016 Taylor & Francis Group.

CHAPTER OUTLINE

INTRODUCTION

Feelings of worth can flourish only in an atmosphere where individual differences are appreciated, mistakes are tolerated, communication is open, and rules are flexible—the kind of atmosphere that is found in a nurturing family. (Virginia Satir, n.d.)

Occupational performance is a dynamic and complex adaptive system that every occupational therapy assistant targets in practice. It is "shaped by the transaction that occurs among the person, environment, and occupation in which the person engages" (Law, Cooper, Strong, Stewart, Rigby, & Letts, 1996). Occupational therapy assistants can create an adaptive response in treatment by focusing on the therapeutic exchange, therapeutic environment, or occupational context. Therapists can target the adaptive response in psychosocial treatment by applying four simple rules that are described throughout this chapter. Traditional, holistic, and client-centered occupational therapy interventions all serve a purpose to meet the needs of clients.

Community and population-based settings are common in contemporary psychosocial occupational therapy treatment during the late lifespan. The principles of self-organized learning systems can be used to target the adaptive response during treatment in these settings (Braungart, Braungart, & Gramet, 2011; Coombs & Smith, 1998). Real-world settings provide a complex system of variables in which a person's motivations, coping resources, and personal abilities can be facilitated. These elements combine to shape new behavioral patterns through the process of developmental learning.

As stated earlier, occupational therapy has targeted the adaptive response as a way to generate positive behavior pattern changes from the inception of the profession (Meyer, 1922/1977). Technology, adapted environments, and new research on coping processes have broadened clinical reasoning and practice possibilities for psychosocial occupational therapy. Treatment strategies recognize the importance of targeting client behavioral change as a complex adaptive system made up of interconnected parts. Occupational therapy assistants can develop strong clinical problem-solving skills by applying the knowledge that a human system is made up of the person, environment, and occupational context.

The adaptive response in this chapter is identified as a way for occupational therapy practitioners to clearly understand how to provide client-centered treatment. Emphasis is placed on patterns of treatment to address the mood, motivation, and cognitive challenges that may block a client's capacity for an adaptive response. Students can learn how to analyze adaptive response patterns and predict treatment outcomes within the scope of the Occupational Therapy Practice Framework (American Occupational Therapy Association [AOTA], 2014). This chapter focuses on emphasizing the following approaches in the late lifespan:

- Mind–body approaches that include exercise and the expressive and creative arts.

- Positive coping processes and the cues that can prompt their use, including the use of identity cues for clients with dementia.

- Programs that focus on therapeutic environments.

- Programs that focus directly on functional performance.

- Capacity with treatment tools and an understanding of the role of personal identity, environment, and occupation in setting a client's emotions.

- Mindfulness practice tools such as meditation, visualization, stress-relief activities, and the Adaptive Response Model (Eoyang, 2008; Ryan, 2013; Siegel, 2010).

- Sensorimotor approaches and positive psychology used to enhance treatment outcomes through the application of emotional self-regulation (Champagne, 2008; Champagne, Ryan, Saccamondo, & Lazzarini, 2007; Fosha, Siegel, & Solomon, 2009; Snow & Bunn, 2003).

PART 1: ADAPTIVE RESPONSES DURING OCCUPATIONAL THERAPY SERVICES OVER THE LATE LIFESPAN

Developmental Learning and Adaptive Responses Over the Late Lifespan

Neuroadaptation, self-organizing learning systems, and praxis influence developmental learning and adaptive responses over the late lifespan. The complexity science of *neuroadaptation* explains why a good fit between person, environment, and occupational patterns is a key contributor to healthy aging (Schaffer & Gage, 2004). Neuroadaptation may be thought of as a brain–mind–body system. It is involved in the adaptive response required for coping with stress, setting and achieving goals, and ongoing developmental learning. Psychosocial neuroadaptation supports unconscious action-oriented coping resources such as "optimism, mastery, self-esteem, and social support" (Taylor & Stanton, 2007). Neuroadaptation has an influence on retrieval of memories and development of new thoughts, ideas, and goals (Schaffer & Gage, 2004). The anticipatory energy generated by having a positive outlook, ongoing relationships, and future goals contribute to healthy aging.

The educational concept of a *self-organized learning system* can easily be adapted for occupational therapy. It naturally creates the flow of client-centered therapy (Eoyang & Holladay, 2013). This is because it is composed of or includes the following:

- A positive and encouraging therapist
- Self-motivating therapeutic activities
- A well-designed environment
- An active exploratory learning approach
- Cues to trigger the adaptive response cycle

A model of the adaptive response cycle can be found by returning to Figure 10-2 in Chapter 10. Following the same three-step cycle but focusing on clinical action, the *praxis,* or action planning, for a client-centered treatment session flows naturally into the SOAP note documentation format. Figure 11-1 demonstrates the way adaptive responses and actions between client and therapist can be documented in a Subjective Assessment Objective Plan (SOAP) note format. Opportunities to use this model to develop SOAP note documentation and student capacities for client-centered practice are embedded in this chapter's Spotlights and Application questions.

A self-organized learning system sets the conditions for developmental learning, regardless of whether a person is ready to learn something new about his or her environment, develop a new plan of action, or put an existing plan into action. Self-organized learning systems allow clients to learn through self-motivated learning, exploration, or even a sense of playful discovery. Four simple rules are applied throughout this chapter for creating a plan of action to treat clients by targeting the adaptive response. These four simple rules are as follows:

1. Rule #1: Use positive coping cues.
2. Rule #2: Target performance as a self-organized learning system.
3. Rule #3: Use self-motivating activities.
4. Rule #4: Offer only achievable challenges.

Adaptive responses and actions are unconscious responses that develop as action systems in the brain. *Action systems* are brain networks with a neurobiological and human evolutionary purpose (Ogden, Minton, & Pain, 2006). Sensorimotor, emotional, and cognitive responses are shaped by these self-organizing action systems. Some action systems activate the response to threat. Other action systems "stimulate us to form close attachment relationships, explore, play, participate in social relationships, regulate energy (through eating, sleeping, etc.), reproduce, and care for others" (Ogden, Minton, & Pain, 2006, p. 108). Eight different action systems and descriptions of each can be seen in Checkpoint 11-1. The blending of action system networks begins with an adaptive response and influences all unconscious action-oriented behaviors. Action systems are a strong influence on the psychomotor and affective aspects of experiential learning.

Adaptive responses are involved in neuroplasticity or brain rewiring. Neuroscientists propose that three internal states or conditions must be present at the same time for brain rewiring to occur (Sara, 2000). Psychologists tend to agree that motivation, ability, and a personally relevant cue must be present for developmental learning to occur (Fogg, 2009; Unsworth, Spillers, & Brewer, 2011). In treatment, these are called *therapeutic cues* and can serve as self-motivators. Specific types of therapeutic cues will be discussed later in the chapter.

Natural cues can be part of the environment, the occupation, or the therapeutic exchange. Positive environmental cues that naturally generate a neuroadaptive system response include the sight of appealing food when a person is hungry, a nice hotel when traveling late, or the

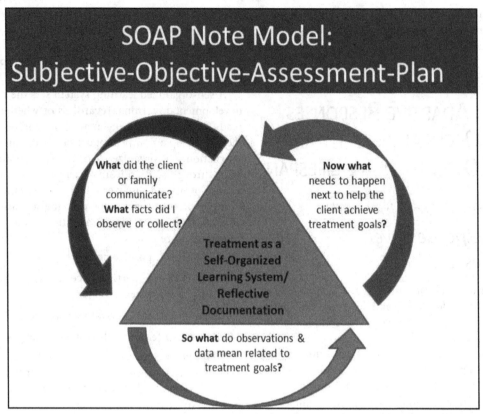

Figure 11-1. The Human Systems Occupational Therapy (HSOT) SOAP note model. (Reprinted with permission from Ryan, J. (2013). Treating the brain as an adaptive system in clients with dementia: Facilitating the neurobiology of action system processes. Poster at the 2013 American Occupational Therapy Association Annual Conference, San Diego, CA.)

CHECKPOINT 11-1. DESCRIBE THE EIGHT ACTION SYSTEMS	
Eight Action Systems	
Defense	Activated whenever danger is sensed and leads to fight- flight-freeze behaviors.
Energy regulation	Regulation of defense behaviors by the energy regulation system, self-regulates for adaptive actions and responses.
Attachment	Blocked by the defense system when feelings of insecurity are strong. Linked to sociability for bonding when feelings of safety and security are strong.
Sociability	Supportive of unified community behaviors, establishment of "common good" philosophies and collaborative behavior patterns.
Exploration	Linked to the attachment system because a sense of safety and security is required for exploratory learning.
Caregiving	Modulates adaptive actions and responses related to care and protection of offspring.
Play	Linked to the attachment system because a sense of safety and security is required for playful emotions and behaviors.
Sexuality	Linked to all the other action systems to optimize inter-generational benefits of pair bonding and reproduction.
Reprinted with permission from Ryan, J. (2013). Treating the brain as an adaptive system in clients with dementia: Facilitating the neurobiology of action system processes. Poster at the 2013 American Occupational Therapy Association Annual Conference, San Diego, CA.	

CHECKPOINT 11-2. UNDERSTAND
Identify a personal example of a positive environmental cue and a negative environmental cue. What behaviors do these cues prompt for you?

mood-enhancing experience of a beautiful sunset. Negative environmental cues that naturally generate a neuroadaptive system response include the smell of something burning, a fire alarm, or a red traffic light.

Positive environmental cues promote behaviors such as risk taking and willingness for change. In contrast, the unconscious meanings of negative environmental cues activate avoidance behaviors associated with anxiety, agitation, or fear. *Fight-flight-freeze* behavior patterns may be thought of as hard-wired reactions to negative environmental cues. Checkpoint 11-2 asks you to identify a positive environmental cue and a negative environmental cue.

In practice, fight-flight-freeze behaviors may appear as obvious survival-based reactions. Examples of fight-flight-freeze behaviors can include physical outbursts, refusals to participate, or extreme difficulty with making decisions. These behaviors tend to be more common in clients functioning at a low Allen Cognitive Level (ACL) of ability. It is beneficial to remember that there are more subtle demonstrations of these stress response patterns in less cognitively or psychosocially challenged clients. Avoid triggering subtle reactive stress responses when working with any clients, family members, or fellow workers. Subtle reactive stress responses may appear as a tendency to become:

- Anxious, angry, or agitated
- Depressed, withdrawn, or disengaged
- Disoriented or confused

Emotional resiliency may be thought of as a key component of healthy mental and cognitive aging. It includes the emotional capacity to adapt to change, even to a stressful loss. This response occurs quickly enough to rebound before the physical effects of stress take a permanent toll on health and function. Occupational therapy assistants often enter the life of a client after one or more challenging losses. Practitioners are challenged to address activities of daily living (ADL) goals that require client self-motivation and willingness to change in order to be accomplished. Targeting a client's neuroadaptive capacity to regain self-motivation and openness to change is a key contributor to the achievement of any treatment goals.

Research that applies new brain technologies has shown that neuroplasticity or neuroadaptive brain rewiring can occur throughout the lifespan (Doidge, 2007). This means the neurological pathways developed in the early lifespan can be influenced in ways that allow aging clients to meet new environmental demands. An example of this is demonstrated each time a client learns to don a shirt with the use of one arm following a stroke. A more subtle example

occurs over time as clients adapt to age-related changes in eyesight, hearing, and physical capacities.

Neuroadaptation is considered an important part of well aging (Roccas & Brewer, 2002). It is required for the reshaping of well-practiced brain networks to develop new motor plans after a stroke, for example. Neuroadaptation is also required for new life routines after retirement or new roles after the loss of a loved one. Occupational therapy assistants are working in a variety of community-based settings that can support healthier aging. Well-aging practice settings that will be discussed include aging in place programs and holistic wellness centers.

Occupational therapy treatment goals usually include some kind of patterns that are in need of change. Treatment goals may address nonadaptive motor, process, or interaction skill patterns developed secondary to disease, as well as injury or aging. Other times, treatment is designed to address nonadaptive performance patterns from the past, such as habits, routines, or roles that are no longer adaptive or helpful for the client.

Occupational therapy assistants often treat clients with functional limitations, such as those following a hip replacement, or obvious physical challenges, such as those that accompany a diagnosis of stroke. Often, these clients have secondary challenges that further compromise treatment outcomes, such as depression or poor motivation. An example of the way an occupational therapy assistant considers primary and secondary challenges was provided in Chapter 10, in the case study of Steve. Steve developed depression, substance abuse, and loss of motivation after being laid off from his job. Steve's primary social role change and secondary emotional challenges were considered by the occupational therapy practitioner during activity selection, treatment planning, and selection of outcomes.

Spotlight 11-1 provides another clinical spotlight about Steve. It identifies the long-term goals of the intervention plan and illustrates how the occupational therapy assistant targets the adaptive response as documented in her SOAP note. Steve has already regained stability following changes that occurred in his social, emotional, and occupational patterns due to his early life challenges. He has now retired and has been in good health until recently, when he fell down a flight of steps in his home. In this scenario, treatment is being provided through an aging in place program. His occupational therapy assistant is targeting developmental learning in Steve's use of adaptive equipment for functional independence, adjustment to an adapted home environment, and the loss of previous life roles.

SPOTLIGHT 11-1. STEVE

The Treatment Plan

Teresa reviewed the occupational therapy evaluation and treatment plan completed by the occupational therapist prior to her first therapy session with Steve. Steve's long-term goals included:

1. Client will independently perform activities of daily living 3 out of 4 days.

2. Client will identify and independently perform an activity from three valued life roles.

3. Client will identify and independently perform a daily stress management routine 3 out of 4 days.

Targeting Adaptive Responses in Treatment Week One

Teresa, Steve's occupational therapy assistant, is working with Steve to help him cope with the stresses that accompany life role changes. These stresses have resulted from a severe fall resulting in a fractured right hip and wrist. Steve has returned home and has already been provided with recommendations for environmental and occupational context adaptations by the acute care occupational therapist. Steve's wife is concerned because Steve resists using equipment that had been recommended for safety, mobility, and energy conservation. He forgets to use his walker, refuses to use his long-handled reacher, and is becoming increasingly passive in his day-to-day activities.

Teresa knows that she needs to cue Steve's neuroadaptive responses. This will require her to learn some important information. Teresa initiated treatment using activities designed to cue Steve's self-awareness for coping with change and developing self-motivation. These activities were primarily used to enhance Steve's self-awareness of his limitations, values, and neuroadaptive capacities. These activities were also used to increase Teresa's capacity to provide client-centered treatment. Teresa collaborated with the occupational therapist to create short-term goals. The following are the short-term goals identified in the "Plan" section of Steve's first SOAP note.

Short-Term Goals

1. Client will identify current barriers to activities of daily living independence.

2. Client will select three valued roles after completing the occupational pattern adaptation tool and a role checklist.

3. Client will identify three stress management activity interests after completing the Emotional Self-Regulation Checklist.

Documenting Adaptive Responses in Treatment Week Two

Subjective	"I miss the yard work I used to do."
Objective	Client completed Mindful Attention-Awareness Scale. Created Mindful Awareness Journal. Independently used walker to ambulate on uneven surface 30 ft. to retrieve bird seed from garden shed. Used long-handled reacher two times while setting up bird-watching area in yard.
Assessment	Client showed increased self-motivation and independence using adapted equipment in valued life role as yard maintainer. Appears interested in using expressive media and natural settings to improve self-awareness and regulate emotions. Appears to have interest and capacity to add hobbyist role with multistep woodworking project.
Plan	Discuss journal entries as self-motivated. Set new ADL independence goals. Begin woodwork project building a birdhouse.

Steve's occupational performance goals reflect actions that might be used to regain ACL 6 ability. ACL 6 may be thought of as a well-aging state of cognitive ability. As stated in Chapter 10, ACLs descend based on a client's cognitive and occupational performance patterns. Factors such as postsurgery pain and use of pain medications can temporarily compromise a client's ability to cope with change. Steve's clinical spotlight shows how the occupational therapy assistant utilized the long-term goals as a starting point for targeting adaptive responses in treatment.

Carl Rogers (1951, p. 487) gave the name *self-actualization* to describe an advanced state of social and emotional wellness that can be achieved during the late lifespan. He said, "The organism has one basic tendency and striving—to actualize, maintain, and enhance the experiencing organism" throughout the lifespan. A well-aging client can continue to sustain or regain person-environment-occupation (PEO) fit following a variety of life transitions by continuing to respond adaptively.

Individuals continue to learn from experience throughout their entire lifespan using the neuroadaptive process. Carl Rogers recognized that self-actualization can only occur naturally when a person has the capacity to use independent, creative thought (Rogers, 1959). Within the context of occupational therapy, therapeutic cues of various types can be used to promote the neuroadaptive process of self-actualization.

Self-actualizing occupational performance patterns include concepts such as quality of life; self-actualization; and physical, mental, and spiritual health. Holistic wellness centers have become popular for people during the late lifespan. Many of these programs are designed to serve clients within a specific sociocultural, ethnic, or religious group and to address physical, mental, and spiritual health. Others use complementary therapy approaches such as mind, body, and energy work (Davis, 2004). Populations and complementary approaches are described next.

- Population-based programs are usually designed to serve a specific ethnic or religious group, and are created to provide therapeutic cues with a unifying community theme. Therapeutic activities may include exercise, dance/movement, music, art, drama, poetry, and play therapy. These may be familiar to most members of the population being served. Movement activities often use music from a specific culture, whereas art activities incorporate symbols and activities with sociocultural meaning for that population. Increasing numbers of online creative communities and resources provide culturally specific music, activities, and art for nonspecialized treatment programs (TIPETILC, n.d.).

- Complementary therapy approaches are also gaining in popularity. This is partly due to increased research evidence of the health benefits of therapeutic exchanges, environments, and occupations. These reduce stress and enhance coping resources. Yoga, tai chi, and Pilates are examples of mind–body work programs that improve physical performance such as balance and reducing falls. Two examples of energy work are therapeutic touch (Davis, 2004) and the use

of a mindful, present-centered focus during treatment (Siegel, 2010).

Quality of life is associated with the harmonious striving for health in body, mind, and spirit. The increase in popularity of holistic wellness programs for adults during the late lifespan is due to their ability to address physical, mental, and spiritual health areas. The neuroscience and psychology of positive experience now supports an increased focus on mental and spiritual wellness as it relates to healthy aging. Research on coping processes following stress and trauma have also increased understanding of the importance of continued developmental learning for emotional self-regulation and resiliency during the aging years.

Two categories of coping behaviors are approach and avoidance. Table 11-1 illustrates behavior patterns associated with positive approach and avoidance and negative approach and avoidance behaviors. Positive approach and avoidance behaviors are adaptive actions and responses. Negative approach and avoidance behaviors may be thought of as habitual patterns that tend to block adaptive actions and response. Negative approach and avoidance behaviors may be thought of as subtle forms of fight-flight-freeze responses.

Nonfunctional Developmental Learning and Adaptive Responses

Occupational therapy assistants work in a variety of community-based settings that target adaptation in the late lifespan due to a loss of ability, new environmental challenges, and stressful roles. Practice approaches that target the emotional self-regulation and social challenges experienced by caregivers of people with dementia is an emerging area of practice for occupational therapy. Practice approaches are currently being used with clients who have developed psychosocial and cognitive rigidities due to dementia. Residential dementia care programs are a common practice setting.

Enjoying "life, and contributing to the social and economic fabric of a community" remains a core motivator for most aging clients (Townsend, 1997, p. 1810). Caregivers of people with severe challenges, such as dementia, have been identified as a population that commonly experiences stress-related challenges and reduced quality of life. Spotlight 11-2 presents Steve and the interaction with his caregivers. The occupational therapy assistant helps Steve's wife sustain her own adaptive capacity for self-actualization after he develops ACL Level 4-3 dementia. Spotlight 11-2 focuses only on treatment plan goals that might be written for Steve's caregiver-wife Lisa.

Occupational therapy assistants can provide dementia care providers support for their adaptive capacity through

TABLE 11-1

NATURAL AND THERAPEUTIC APPROACH AND AVOIDANCE COPING

	APPROACH COPING	AVOIDANCE COPING
Positive	**Allowing engagement** with cues in one's environment, occupational context or interpersonal exchanges that promote **healthy** energy regulation, attachments, sociability, exploration, caregiving, playfulness or sexuality. This is a neuroadaptive coping response that can be promoted in therapy.	Setting boundaries that **prevent engagement** with cues in one's environment, occupational context or interpersonal exchanges that promote **unhealthy** energy regulation, attachments, sociability, exploration, caregiving, playfulness or sexuality. This is a neuroadaptive coping response that can be promoted in therapy.
Negative	**Habituated patterns of engagement** with cues in one's environment, occupational context or interpersonal exchanges that promote **unhealthy** energy regulation (**fight or flight** behaviors) that block attachments, sociability, exploration, caregiving, playfulness or sexuality. This is a non-adaptive coping response that is avoided in therapy.	**Habituated patterns of disengagement** with cues in one's environment, occupational context or interpersonal exchanges that block development of the **healthy** energy regulation (**freeze** behaviors) required for attachments, sociability, exploration, caregiving, playfulness or sexuality. This is a non-adaptive coping response that is avoided in therapy.

Reprinted with permission from Ryan, J. (2013). Treating the brain as an adaptive system in clients with dementia: Facilitating the neurobiology of action system processes. Poster at the 2013 American Occupational Therapy Association Annual Conference, San Diego, CA.

SPOTLIGHT 11-2. STEVE

The Treatment Plan

Steve's functional ability has declined to ACL Level 4.3, and occupational therapy services have been resumed. Teresa is again serving as Steve's occupational therapy assistant. The occupational therapist has written three long-term goals that address Steve's therapeutic needs. This case study scenario will focus on the long-term goals written for Steve's primary caregiver, his wife Lisa.

Teresa reviewed the treatment plan written by his occupational therapist prior to her first therapy session. The treatment plan specifically addresses the stress-based behaviors that often accompany the dementia caregiver role. The long-term goals for occupational therapy address Lisa's needs to be able to continue to strive for self-actualization while carrying out her caregiver role. The long-term goals include:

1. Client's caregiver will independently perform caregiver role without reporting negative approach or avoidance coping behaviors 3 out of 4 days.

2. Client's caregiver will identify and independently perform an activity from three valued life roles besides caregiver.

3. Client's caregiver will identify and independently perform a daily stress management routine 3 out of 4 days.

Targeting Adaptive Responses in Treatment Week One

Steve's occupational therapy assistant is now addressing the treatment goals. Lisa has experienced increased stress from the life role changes that have resulted from Steve's severe fall. Steve and Lisa have expressed the desire for Steve to be able to live at home as long as possible. Lisa, however, has begun to show physical indicators of a high level of stress, including high blood pressure, depression, and a constant feeling of fatigue.

Teresa knows that she needs to learn some important information in order to cue Steve's neuroadaptive responses. Teresa initiated treatment using activities designed to cue Lisa's self-awareness for coping with change, reducing depression, and increasing her coping resources. These activities were primarily used to enhance Lisa's self-awareness for the use of more positive approach and avoidance coping patterns. The

(continued)

SPOTLIGHT 11-2. STEVE (CONTINUED)

activities were also used to increase Teresa's capacity to provide client-centered treatment for Lisa as well as Steve. The following are the short-term goals identified in the "Plan" section of the first SOAP note entry that address Lisa's needs.

Short-Term Goals:

1. Client's caregiver will identify her current negative approach and avoidance coping behaviors.

2. Client's caregiver will select three valued roles to perform besides caregiver after completing the occupational pattern adaptation tool and a role checklist.

3. Client's caregiver will identify three positive coping behavior interests after completing the Emotional Self-Regulation Checklist.

Documenting Adaptive Responses in Treatment Week Two

Subjective	"I called three friends this week."
Objective	Client's caregiver completed Mindful Attention-Awareness Scale. Created Mindful Awareness Journal. Independently arranged dementia respite services for Monday and Wednesday mornings weekly. Was self-motivated to call three friends and to set a lunch date during first day of respite services.
Assessment	Client's caregiver showed improved positive approach coping for independent problem solving by pursuing valued life role of friend. Appears interested in using expressive media and religious participant role to further develop positive approach coping. Appeared less depressed and more engaged in learning new strategies for dementia caregiver role.
Plan	Client's caregiver—Discuss journal entries as self-motivated. Set new coping goal to promote religious participant role. Begin practicing the positive dementia caregiver approach, play therapy, and generative engagement dynamics with client and caregiver.

emotional self-regulation. Such activities may include the following:

- Activities and occupations that produce the feeling of flow. Flow is a natural characteristic of self-motivating activities. These may be thought of as activities that generate a neuroadaptive reward or the relaxation response (Metz & Robnett, 2011).

- Activities and occupations that promote use of the left hemisphere. In general, these activities promote a feeling of mental stimulation as well as a sense of achievement. They include activities that use logical problem solving such as calculations and analysis, symbol and code games, word finding and crosswords, categorization and sequencing puzzles such as card games, and solving/reading mystery stories (Gutman & Schindler, 2007).

- Activities and occupations that promote self-actualization by promoting mindfulness, attention, and enjoyment. By beginning with activities that are already meaningful, the client will be able to develop new life roles. He or she can include activities that

encourage lifelong learning, living in appreciation of the present, a trust in intuitive feelings regarding environmental fit, creative thinking, and placing value in living a fulfilling life (Rogers, 1961).

Cognitive ability during the aging years is influenced by both the explicit and the implicit memory systems. ***Explicit memories*** are conscious ones that can be verbalized (Harrison, Son, Kim, & Whall, 2012). They are holistic memories that can be remembered as a unified experience. Explicit memories include the event, its time of day, where it happened, objects, and people who were present. They are developed through multisystem adaptive responses and integrative processes.

Explicit memories tend to be lost during the progression of dementia. This may be related to their dependence on a brain area called the *hippocampus*. The hippocampus is an important memory storage system that tends to be vulnerable to the influences of stress (Miller & O'Callaghan, 2005). Explicit memories include memorized knowledge and autobiographical details about one's life history.

The implicit memory system works quite differently. **Implicit memories** are stored as step-by-step procedures in the brain that can often be performed without conscious thought (Harrison et al., 2012; Machado et al, 2009). These memories may be thought of as filling in the "background" rather than the "foreground" of occupational performance. For example, one of the cognitive capacities assessed by the ACL is a client's implicit memory of the procedural process of lacing.

A second form of implicit memory is the association between a feeling or emotion and a life experience. These are stored within the limbic system and are more resilient during the progression of dementia. Implicit memories may be thought of as neuroadaptive responses that may have been shaped during very early developmental learning. Early family attachment patterns are one example of this type of memory. A person with dementia may feel positive emotions while sitting in the kitchen with family members even though he or she may have forgotten the names of family members due to the implicit memory of earlier life experiences.

Implicit memories allow a person with dementia to remember general information about life events after the details have been forgotten. For example, a person with dementia may have lost explicit memory of the day, time, and year he or she was married, but enjoy reminiscing about the events of the day in general. Sometimes environmental cues reactivate more details about these memories. Examples include hearing a song that was played on the person's wedding day, walking into a church, and seeing a wedding picture.

Spotlight 11-3 again highlights the case study of Steve. It portrays how the occupational therapy assistant can apply the same simple rules to target adaptive responses in a long-term care environment. In this scenario, Steve's performance ability has declined to the ACL 3.2. Steve is now living in a long-term care facility. A person at ACL 3.2 requires more consistent use of therapeutic cues and exchanges, as well as a just-right environmental fit to meet treatment goals.

PART 2: ADAPTIVE RESPONSES DURING OCCUPATIONAL THERAPY AS A SELF-ORGANIZED LEARNING SYSTEM

Positive Coping Cues

There are two types of positive coping cues. One is positive emotion-focused coping cues, and the other is positive problem-focused coping cues. Both are important environmental or therapeutic cues that support a client's capacity to achieve therapeutic adaptation. Positive **emotion-focused coping cues** may be used by occupational therapy assistants to activate the emotional self-regulation action system required for client self-motivation. Positive emotion-focused coping cues may be part of the environment, occupation, or therapeutic exchange. Developmental learning of new occupational performance patterns will flow more naturally when the therapist is able to facilitate a positive shift in emotional self-regulation. Emotion-focused coping cues may be used in treatment to enhance participation while not competing with the therapeutic goals. Some examples of emotion-focused coping cues that are useful with clients who have dementia include the following:

- Playing a client's favorite song to bring back implicit memories of earlier dancing years can trigger self-motivation to participate in an exercise dance group.

- Offering a therapeutic activity stored as a positive implicit memory. Examples can include a woodworking project for a handyman or folding children's clothes for a mother. A positive implicit memory can trigger self-motivation to participate in the activity group. Other memories and a greater willingness to engage in other functional activities develop by participating in the conversation and reminiscence that accompanies a favorite activity.

- Creating a familiar social dynamic. Eating breakfast at a family-style table can trigger self-motivation to participate and more mindful participation in a morning news and orientation group.

Positive emotion-focused coping cues generate a **palliative** adaptive response within the context of dementia care and treatment when mood improves without directly changing the physical condition of the client (Taylor & Stanton, 2007). However, since one adaptive response tends to set the conditions for another, an increase in self-motivation may lead to increased attention and memory retrieval. Linking together strands of interrelated adaptive responses can help a client make significant functional gains.

Self-motivation is the underlying adaptive response required to increase focused attention for new learning when treating clients with the cognitive capacity to benefit from activities that go beyond a palliative approach. Therapeutic activities that might be used with clients within the boundaries of their current ability to achieve functional goals may require a more mindful state of consciousness. These activities can be embedded in treatment or a home program and can include the following:

- Expressive and creative arts

- Meditation or contemplative prayer

- Journaling or therapeutic dialogue

- Visualization and imagery

SPOTLIGHT 11-3. STEVE

The Treatment Plan

Steve's functional ability has continued to decline to ACL Level 3.2. He is now living in a skilled care environment. Greg is Steve's occupational therapy assistant. The occupational therapist has written the long-term goals to address Steve's client-centered needs. Greg also recognized the importance of establishing a self-organized developmental learning environment for Steve. This involved teaching and coaching Steve's new caregivers and activity or life enrichment coordinators. Greg realized the importance of preparing for his first session. Any client at ACL Level 3.2 may exhibit negative coping behaviors. Preparation for the first therapy session included learning about:

- Positive coping cues that have been useful for Steve in the past.
- Implicit memory and core identity cues that might be beneficial to embed in Steve's environment, occupational contexts, and daily interpersonal exchanges.
- Life role activities that are likely to be self-motivating for Steve's weekly routine.
- Steve's current ACL level in order to teach and coach Steve's activity or life enrichment coordinators how to offer only achievable challenges.

Greg reviewed the data in Steve's chart that provides the same types of information as the occupational pattern adaptation tool and role checklist. Greg planned the first therapy session with a focus on creating a therapeutic exchange that offered cues to communicate an interest in knowing. This therapeutic exchange displayed:

- Who is Steve?
- How can Steve connect with his physical, social, and cultural environment at his new home?
- What is important to Steve?

Greg also reviewed the treatment plan written by Steve's occupational therapist. Steve's long-term goals included:

1. Client will don shirt with moderate assist except buttons 3 out of 4 days.
2. Client will demonstrate self-motivation to participate in two out of three activity groups provided daily for 1 week.
3. Client will demonstrate no negative coping behaviors when participating in a 15-minute bird watching group three out of four times.

Documenting Adaptive Responses in Treatment Week One

Steve's occupational therapy assistant is working to help him cope with the stresses that accompanied the move into a long-term care setting. These stresses accompanied the dramatic changes in life environment, occupational context, and interpersonal exchanges. Greg knows that the neuroadaptive response of positive coping with stress can be blocked by a poor environmental fit. Greg considered the importance of bonding with Steve during his first therapy sessions. Greg knew that he can expect greater positive coping capacities due to this empathic bonding. Steve's SOAP note after his first week of treatment is as follows.

Subjective	"Get out of my room!"
Objective	Resident refused to interact with therapist in his room. Forcefully requested therapist to leave his room six times during first 5 minutes of session. Hit at therapist with palm of hand one time during first 5 minutes of session. Following identity cue of resident's favorite song, increased eye contact and reduced agitation. Following identity cue of therapist sitting in front and at eye level with resident to sand a bird house, increased communication with therapist. Following multisensory integration cues of actively feeling and holding birdhouse, resident independently rubbed with sandpaper 10 seconds.

(continued)

SPOTLIGHT 11-3. STEVE (CONTINUED)

Assessment	Resident progressed from negative approach to positive approach coping behaviors in one session. Appears to have interest and capacity to participate in woodworking group. Appears to remember bird house identity cue for previously enjoyed life role of yard mainter.
Plan	Carry out session during woodworking group. Introduce to yard environment to assess reaction. Continue to increase neuroadaptive coping response for donning shirt with moderate assist.

Documenting Adaptive Responses in Treatment Week Two

Steve's progress in one-on-one treatment sessions during the week was likely to have a carry-over effect during the second week of therapy. Greg had saved introduction of therapeutic group experiences until the second week of therapy. Greg knew that there are more potential stresses in group activities. Steve's SOAP note after his second week of treatment is as follows.

Subjective	"Who are you?"
Objective	Resident demonstrated calm speech but focused only on identity cue of favorite music during first 5 minutes of session. After multisensory cues of therapist humming along with music, resident used eye contact and tolerated therapist rubbing hands. Resident smiled when lotion was rubbed on hands. Resident was pushed (in wheelchair) to woodworking group with no refusals or indications of distress. Watched other group members for 10 minutes before therapist put wooden birdhouse on table at midline. Resident self-motivated to pick up sandpaper. Sanded with three prompts for 5 minutes. When provided with screwdriver and partially screwed-in nail as an implicit memory cue, resident used screwdriver independently for 20 minutes. Used eye–hand coordination appropriate for use of screwdriver. Therapist propelled resident in wheelchair to yard environment. Resident smiled when taken past vegetable garden area.
Assessment	Resident showed increased positive approach coping for interacting with therapist, tolerating handling of hands by therapist. Resident showed decreased negative approach coping with no fight-flight-fear reactions during session. Resident showed self-motivation and independence for one-step woodworking project. Showed positive responses to implicit memory cues related to two previous life roles, including woodwork hobbyist and yard maintainer.
Plan	Submit request for resident to be included in woodworking, bird watching, and gardening groups. Teach and coach life enrichment coordinator in use of client-centered identity cues to facilitate performance. Use implicit memory and multisensory cues as needed to facilitate shirt donning with moderate assist.

Documenting Adaptive Responses in Treatment Week Three

Greg recognizes that Steve's progress in establishing better environmental fit in his new long-term care community is likely to have continued to reduce his negative approach and avoidance behaviors. During week three, Greg will turn group activities over to his life enrichment coordinator and will turn his focus directly on the functional goal of donning his shirt with moderate assistance. The following is Steve's SOAP note after his third week of treatment.

(continued)

SPOTLIGHT 11-3. STEVE (CONTINUED)

Subjective	"I can't."
Objective	Resident demonstrated calm speech but refused initially when provided with verbal request and shirt for donning. After multisensory cues of therapist humming resident's favorite song without the music, resident used eye contact and tolerated therapist rubbing shirt sleeve on hands and arms. Resident tolerated therapist placing first sleeve over hand and independently pulled shirt up to shoulder following verbal assist and modeling.
Objective	Therapist brought shirt around back to second arm. Resident put second hand through sleeve after priming three times. Therapist pulled shirt to shoulder for donning shirt with max assist.
Assessment	Resident dons shirt with max assist with therapist in homelike environment, a therapeutic occupational context, and exchanges.
Plan	Repeat shirt donning to facilitate moderate assistance except buttons. Teach and coach resident caregivers cues used to facilitate shirt donning with maximal assist. Initiate caregiver record keeping of daily independence level in resident donning of shirt.

Emotion-focused coping resources are the underlying emotional self-regulation strategies that can be used to support healthy coping behavior. Rather than activities, these are patterns of thought that support and promote coping, self-motivation, attention, adaptive action, and learning. Therapists can teach clients about the benefits of emotion-focused coping resources and coach them while they develop their self-regulation strategies. They are also part of the *mindful state of consciousness* that consists of good self-awareness and the positive sense of being in control of one's own PEO fitness decisions. Emotion-focused coping resources can include the following:

- Reframing negative thoughts
- The flow of positive thinking
- Mindfulness

Positive *problem-focused coping cues* can be used by occupational therapy assistants to trigger context-specific neuroadaptive responses. Positive problem-focused coping cues support a client's capacity to take intentional adaptive actions designed to change life problems. For clients with the cognitive capacity, these adaptive actions are the ones required to improve self-awareness and increase the client's sense of being in control of his or her own PEO fitness decisions. Examples of problem-focused coping cues for clients with a high level of cognitive capacity include the following:

- Computer-based or reading materials to promote self-education
- Job search skills practice
- Leisure skills interest questionnaires

Problem-focused coping cues can also be used in a palliative manner for clients with dementia. Retrieval of implicit memories will flow more naturally when a therapist understands how to facilitate a positive shift in adaptive actions. As stated earlier, problem-focused coping is specific to the occupational context. Problem-focused coping cues can be used in treatment to target an adaptive response in clients without the internal coping or adaptive capacity to improve their own PEO fitness. Examples include the following:

- Teaching dementia caregivers to follow a set of simple rules to improve the client's capacity to function more independently in his or her new assisted living community.
- Recommending the family of a client with dementia remove throw rugs from their home to prevent falls.
- Arranging the tools a client with dementia needs for tooth brushing by placing them in the client's visual space in the correct sequence for use.

Problem-focused coping resources are the environmental resources that support healthy coping behavior. These are commonly the social, cultural, and economic resources a person has that support coping rather than activities, emotional, or cognitive states. Examples of problem-focused coping resources that allow a person to positively change his or her PEO fitness include the following:

- Strong family attachments
- Financial security
- Meaningful community relationships
- Purposeful life roles, routines, and habits

Positive coping cues may be embedded in therapeutic environments to serve the needs of clients with severe cognitive and psychosocial challenges. Coping cues may also need to be embedded in therapeutic environments for

Self-Identifying Preferences

Name: ____________________ **Date:** ____________

Self-identifying preferences: social, spiritual and sensory preferences that may help to connect the individual to meaningful experiences from their past.

Favorite Rituals:

____ weekly religious rituals, LIST: ____________

____ daily religious rituals, LIST: ____________

____ holiday rituals, LIST: ____________

____ other rituals, LIST routines that feel central to life meaning: ____________

Favorite Service Projects:

____ teaching Sunday School or school (circle)

____ religious service projects, LIST: ____________

____ community service projects, LIST: ____________

____ other service projects, LIST: ____________

Favorite Social Events:

____ family parties, LIST: ____________

____ small gatherings with friends (showers, etc.), LIST: ____________

____ large social gatherings, LIST: ____________

Favorite Relationships:

____ being with young people, LIST: ____________

____ being with people your own age, LIST: ____________

____ being with family, LIST: ____________

____ talking about family from childhood, LIST: ____________

____ writing letters, cards, LIST: ____________

____ photos and albums, LIST: ____________

____ being with animals, LIST: ____________

____ other relationships, LIST: ____________

Favorite Routines:

____ self-care (lotion, manicure, pedicure, etc.), LIST: ____________

____ family-care (coupon clipping, shopping, etc.), LIST: ____________

____ physical exercise, LIST: ____________

____ home-care (table setting, sweeping, dusting , etc.), LIST: ____________

____ nature-care, (yards, birds, etc.) LIST: ____________

____ food preparation, LIST: ____________

____ laundry sorting and folding, LIST: ____________

____ clothing care (sewing, sock sort, shining shoes, etc.), LIST: ____________

Favorite Hobbies:

____ flower arranging	____ stuffed animals
____ wood crafts	____ reading
____ games and cards	____ puzzles
____ yarn crafts	____ paper crafts
____ sports participation	____ sports appreciation
____ music participation	____ music appreciation
____ art projects	____ art appreciation

List others (be specific): ____________

Favorite Jobs:

____ pipe construction	____ money management, coin sort
____ office work	____ garage jobs

List others (be specific): ____________

Life Fulfillment Preferences: (Which lifestyle moto best captures the identity of your loved one?)

____ Life fulfillment comes from growing in truth and wisdom.

____ Life fulfillment is all about the relationships we develop along the way.

____ Life is what you make it through the experiences you have along the way.

____ Other? ____________

Meaningful Sensory Experiences or Strategies:

Color(s): ____________

Music (describe genre, speed, mood, etc.): ____________

Sleep routine (bed clothes, position, mattress, pillow, etc.): ____________

Relaxation positions (chairs, etc.): ____________

Favorite environments (calming, busy, etc.): ____________

Calming environments or habits: ____________

Lighting: ____________

Aromas: ____________

Fidgets: ____________

Ways to "wake up": ____________

In three sentences or less, describe individual's personal identity:

Important habits or routines:

Important "dislikes" to avoid:

Figure 11-2. Lifespan identity and implicit memory questionnaire. (Reprinted with permission from Ryan, J. (2009). *A social-spiritual model of dynamic memory care.* Self-published training manual.)

clients with extreme challenges in internal coping or adaptive capacities. Therapeutic environments, occupations, and exchanges are all often required to be addressed in treatment for clients dealing with the overwhelming stress of living with dementia.

Two therapeutic environments in which the neuroadaptive response may be facilitated for clients with dementia are the positive implicit memory and multisensory environment. Ways to target occupational performance by using implicit memory cues as a self-organized learning system will be provided. Examples include self-organized learning systems that have three types of embedded implicit memory cues. These include the therapeutic environment, occupational context, and therapeutic exchange.

Target Performance as a Self-Organized Learning System

Occupational performance can be enhanced in treatment by targeting the adaptive response as a self-organized learning system. Emotion-focused coping cues in the form of positive implicit memories can be embedded into the therapeutic environment, occupational context, or therapeutic exchange. Positive implicit memories can be reactivated by therapists as identity cues that support capacity for a client at any stage of dementia. This enables the client to feel more connected to his or her physical, social, and cultural environment.

Coping cues that make a positive difference in occupational performance for people with dementia are commonly associated with their youth identity. Steve's case study in Spotlight 11-3 reflects coping cues that are associated with his youth identity. This is due to the belief that memories tend to be lost in the reverse order in which they were developed (Rogers & Lasprilla, 2006). Another viewpoint is that many of the memories developed during youth create emotional self-regulation action system networks that have been used repeatedly throughout the client's entire lifespan (Ogden, Minton, & Pain, 2006).

Activity questionnaires that focus therapist attention on early life history and interests are beneficial for planning therapeutic activities. This is due to the reality that people with dementia tend to remember earlier life memories longer during the progression of cognitive decline. Figure 11-2 provides an example of the questionnaire used by Steve's occupational therapy assistant to collect data on

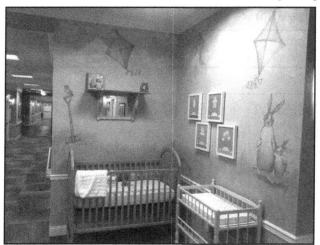

Figure 11-3. Identity cues in the environment. (Reprinted with permission from Morning Pointe of Lexington East, Lexington, KY. Independent Healthcare Properties & Morning Pointe Assisted Living [www.morningpointe.com].)

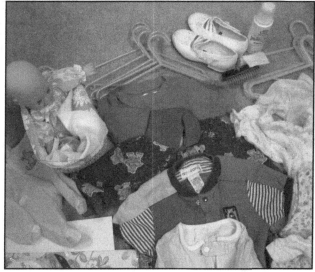

Figure 11-4. Identity cues in the occupational context. (Reprinted with permission. Photo taken by Janice Ryan, OTD, OTR/L, Program Developer/Consultant. Human Systems Occupational Therapy.)

lifelong history and interests from multiple generations of his family.

Figure 11-3 is a photo of an implicit memory environment that matches a client's core life identity. These have been embedded into the therapeutic environment of a memory care space with a primary emotion-focused coping purpose. Occupational therapy assistants can use a memory care space such as this to carry out group activities with residents who are mothers and grandmothers. These implicit memory cues are of a specific type called core *identity cues*. Pleasurable daily routines built around baby care themes can be used by occupational therapy assistants to support a rich therapeutic activity program in a positive *implicit memory environment*.

People with dementia perform better in environments containing familiar objects (Hoppes, Davis, & Thompson, 2003) that act as implicit memory or identity cues. Many of these benefits begin with improved emotional self-regulation that sets the conditions for improved performance. The primary and secondary benefits of improved emotional self-regulation and performance commonly flow into advantages for the whole community. A process is provided that changes challenging resident behavior patterns. Examples of changing challenging resident behavior patterns can include the following:

- Diverting attention from worrying or pacing
- Reducing fight-flight-freeze behaviors of many kinds
- Enhancing self-awareness for self-motivated occupational participation
- Enhancing self-in-environment connectedness to reduce physical wandering, elopement, and stress-based disengagement

Occupational performance can also be enhanced by embedding implicit memory cues into the occupational context. The AOTA lists seven *occupational contexts* to include the cultural, physical, social, personal, spiritual, temporal, and virtual contexts (AOTA, 2014). Examples of ways implicit memory cues have been shown to promote occupational performance include the following:

- Focusing attention on repetitive sensorimotor patterns and activities that reduce anxiety and promote the relaxation response.
- Focusing attention on personally enjoyable activities that reduce depression and promote the reward response.
- Enhancing a client's capacity to complete occupational patterns independently once modeled or primed by the therapist. *Modeling* is the therapeutic process of demonstrating the occupational pattern before asking the client to demonstrate it independently. *Priming* is the therapeutic process of physically assisting the occupational pattern once or twice before asking the client to demonstrate it independently.
- Retrieving implicit memory of the next step of a familiar sequenced activity.

Positive implicit memory or identity cues embedded in the occupational context can further enhance occupational performance. Positive implicit memory cues are evident in the memory care space pictured in Figure 11-3. Figure 11-4 shows familiar baby care supplies that can be used in activities to promote occupational performance. Some of the core identity cues of motherhood have been embedded in the therapeutic activity through object symbols. Checkpoint 11-3 asks students to identify examples of positive and negative environmental cues.

CHECKPOINT 11-3. APPLY

List as many therapeutic activities as you can think of that could be designed for a group of mothers with dementia using core identity cues associated with motherhood.

SPOTLIGHT 11-4. STEVE

The Treatment Plan

Greg remains Steve's occupational therapy assistant and he has lived in his new long-term care environment for just over 3 weeks. Steve has developed self-motivation to participate in bird watching, woodworking, and gardening groups when he receives a visual cue (passes by a group that happens to be occurring) or physical assistance (is led to the group by a caregiver). Greg is informed at a team meeting that caregivers have attempted to use verbal cues to prompt Steve to attend his favorite groups independently. They report that Steve tends to wander the halls unless he arrives by chance and sees the group occurring. Greg is also told that Steve is distracted whenever he passes by windows, forgetting about the group.

Greg considers the spatial navigation required of Steve to walk from his apartment to each group. After reviewing Steve's self-identifying preferences form, Greg recognizes Steve's pattern for preference for the outdoors. Greg decides to use multisensory cues to coach Steve to independently find the bird watching and gardening activity area. As always, Greg reviews the treatment plan written by Steve's occupational therapist. Greg decides that the long-term goal of donning a shirt can easily be embedded into this daily routine. Steve's long-term goals remain the same as in Spotlight 11-3.

Long-Term Goals

1. Client will don shirt with moderate assist except buttons 3 out of 4 days.

2. Client will demonstrate self-motivation to participate in two out of three activity groups provided daily for 1 week.

3. Client will demonstrate no negative coping behaviors when participating in a 15-minute bird watching group three of four times.

Documenting Adaptive Responses in Treatment Week Three

The following is Steve's SOAP note after his third week of treatment.

Subjective	"This feels good."
Objective	Resident followed three-part visual-spatial cues for way finding to outside activity area with minimal assistance in 5 minutes. Independently followed verbal prompt to get bucket of seed from garage. Followed verbal prompt and visual cue to take seed bucket to courtyard door. Donned oversized work shirt with minimal assist for first sleeve, maximal assist for positioning and donning second sleeve.
Assessment	Resident progressed in spatial navigation of new environment. Was self-motivated and more independent in donning shirt when activity is embedded in the meaningful routine of attending bird watching group. Appears to be adjusting well to new environment.
Plan	Repeat therapeutic activity next session. Coach morning caregivers in routine. Schedule for morning activities of daily living (ADLs) to address long-term goal 1.

Spotlight 11-4 describes how Steve's occupational therapy assistant used implicit memory cues to help create an environment. This environment enabled Steve to navigate his new long-term care community, develop new daily routines, and reduce the risk for falls. Emotion-focused coping cues were used to increase self-in-environment awareness and attention for the ultimate goal of improving functional performance. ***Spatial navigation*** within

TABLE 11-2
THE POSITIVE APPROACH

• Come from the front	• Offer your hand
• Go slowly	• Use the person's preferred name
• Get to the side	• Wait for a response before you start talking or doing
• Get low—sit down.	

Reprinted with permission from Ryan, J. (2013). Treating the brain as an adaptive system in clients with dementia: Facilitating the neurobiology of action system processes. Poster at the 2013 American Occupational Therapy Association Annual Conference, San Diego, CA.

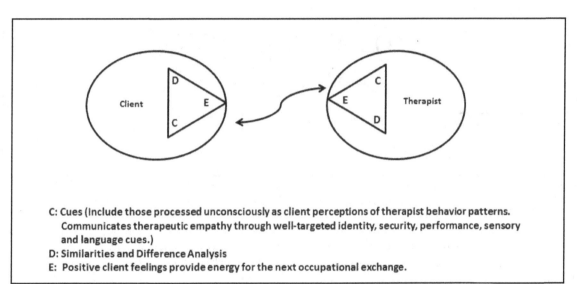

C: Cues (Include those processed unconsciously as client perceptions of therapist behavior patterns. Communicates therapeutic empathy through well-targeted identity, security, performance, sensory and language cues.)

D: Similarities and Difference Analysis

E: Positive client feelings provide energy for the next occupational exchange.

Figure 11-5. Play therapy for people with dementia. (Reprinted with permission from Ryan, J. (2013). Treating the brain as an adaptive system in clients with dementia: Facilitating the neurobiology of action system processes. Poster at the 2013 American Occupational Therapy Association Annual Conference, San Diego, CA.)

long-term care environments has been shown to improve with the use of well-placed identity cues (Harrrison et al., 2012; Kessels, Doormaal, & Janzen, 2011; Vezina, Robichaud, Voyer, & Pelletier, 2011). These forms of identity cues are also considered likely to reduce falls, as people may feel more secure when they understand their environment (Bieber & Keller, 2005).

Finally, occupational performance may be enhanced by embedding implicit memory or identity cues into the therapeutic exchange. Embedding implicit memory into the therapeutic exchange follows the principles of positive psychology (Dweck, 2007; Prehn & Fredens, 2011) and human systems dynamics (Eoyang & Holladay, 2013). Positive implicit memory or identity cues embedded in therapeutic exchanges may support occupational performance. It provides a sense of safety for the client to use a positive approach pattern rather than avoidance patterns. Three examples are provided for the use of positive implicit or identity cues embedded in the therapeutic exchange:

1. The positive approach (Snow & Bunn 2003)

2. Play therapy for people with dementia (Ryan, 2013)

3. Generative group engagements (Human Systems Dynamics Institute, n.d.c.)

Positive approach patterns were identified by Snow and Bunn as a way to approach and interact with clients with dementia that signal they are safe, secure, and respected. This approach has been used extensively to teach caregivers how to interact more successfully with people who have dementia. Table 11-2 describes the seven steps of the positive approach.

Play therapy for people with dementia combines the comforting support of empathic therapeutic exchanges with the clinical skill of facilitating the neuroadaptive response (Ryan, 2013). Figure 11-5 illustrates a Human Systems Occupational Therapy (HSOT) Practice Model for this ***therapeutic exchange*** supporting a client's need for the following:

- Empathic understanding of fight-flight-freeze behaviors

- External assistance for regulating emotions

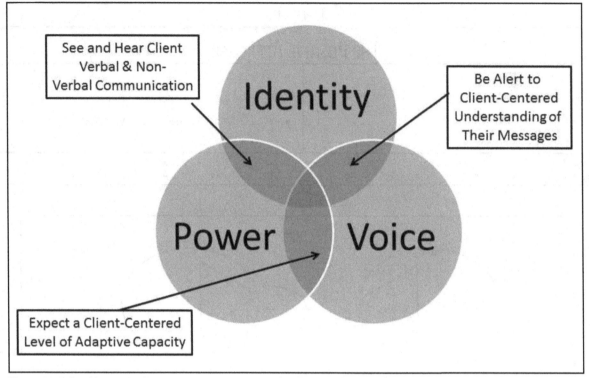

Figure 11-6. Coaching generative group activities. (Reprinted with permission from Ryan, J. (2014). The nonlinear neurodynamics of play therapy for people with dementia. Presentation at the 2014 Society for Chaos Theory in Psychology in Life Sciences Annual Conference, Milwaukee, WI.)

- Therapeutic facilitation of an adaptive response

The feelings of security and safety experienced by clients with dementia during play therapy are believed to activate the play action system. It has also been theorized that a more self-regulated state tends to increase a client's capacity to respond to a broader range of therapeutic cues (Roccas & Brewer, 2002). Occupational therapy services that incorporate this approach prepare the client's nervous system for developmental learning within the scope of his or her current adaptive capacity.

Generative group engagements use the Human Systems Dynamics Institute (n.d.) Model found in Figure 11-6 in order to promote more positive or generative therapeutic group exchanges. This approach is believed to promote feelings of security and safety within group activities. The feelings of security and safety seem to support the client's capacity to use his or her exploratory action system for developmental learning and sociability. During the progression of dementia, clients can re-experience the most positive dynamics of their interpersonal life experience through the feelings of generative engagements.

The Human Systems Dynamics Model of Generative Engagement created by Holladay and Nations (Human Systems Dynamics Institute, n.d.) has been adapted for use by occupational therapy practitioners. These same principles can be taught to memory care givers using The Simple Rules of Relationship-Based Memory Care (Ryan,

2009). Refer to Table 11-3 for the application of the Simple Rules Model (Human Systems Dynamics Institute, n.d.). This approach can be used to teach long-term care community caregivers how to use daily exchanges with community members. It promotes daily exchanges that naturally provide the just-right performance, security, identity, and language cues to promote emotion-focused coping in residents with dementia while maintaining their safety in a long-term care environment.

Multisensory environments (Messbauer, 2010; Messbauer & Ryan, 2013) provide a therapeutic environment that is filled with emotion-focused coping cues for clients who do not have the capacity to self-regulate their emotions. Personally meaningful music, visual, movement, touch, and pressure sensations are all promoters of self and self-in-environment awareness (Messbauer, 2010). ***Multisensory integration cues*** may be thought of as foundational for coping with physical changes (Botta et al., 2011). Examples of the problem-focused coping achievements that can emerge after self-regulatory emotions are modulated by the multisensory environment include the following:

- Improved eye-contact
- More neuroadaptive visual scanning of environment
- Increased attention to eye–hand tasks
- Enhanced communication

TABLE 11-3
RELATIONSHIP-BASED MEMORY CARE LIST OF SIMPLE RULES (AN APPLICATION OF THE HSD SIMPLE RULES MODEL [HUMAN SYSTEMS DYNAMICS INSTITUTE, N.D.])

• Consider safety first	• Learn to speak nonverbally
• Watch for changes in health and wellness	• Use the power of first impressions
• Report all changes to nursing staff	• Use simple language
• Use personal meanings	• Stay observant to respond quickly to change
• Encourage current abilities	• Be in a joyful relationship

Reprinted with permission from Ryan, J. (2009). *A social-spiritual model of dynamic memory care.* Self-published training manual.

- More complex occupational participation patterns

- More complex occupational performance patterns

Spotlight 11-5 shows how Steve's occupational therapy assistant used the multisensory environment to enhance the outcomes of Steve's treatment. Steve's therapist used the therapeutic environment as a preparatory activity for functional goals, since all treatment goals must be functional and measurable. Steve's SOAP note demonstrates how treatment within a multisensory environment can be documented.

The timing and synchronization of a variety of multisensory inputs have been shown to influence the brain circuitry. They increase a person's ability to perceive natural cues from his or her environment (American Friends of Tel Aviv University, 2013; Schmitz, De Rosa, & Anderson, 2009). This is believed to occur by reducing the distractions of cognitive "noise" that prevent clear perceptions of the external environment (Collier, McPherson, Ellis-Hill, Staal, & Bucks, 2010). The first neuroadaptive responses observed in clients receiving treatment within a multisensory environment are commonly consistent with a reduced stress response.

Problem-focused coping, self-motivation, decision making, and performance may all be enhanced by first matching the client's internal emotional state and then appropriately shifting multisensory integration cue intensity (Messbauer, 2010). An adaptive response is always the goal, just as with implicit memory environments. Treatment in multisensory environments can also be used to decrease frequency of the fight-flight-freeze response, enhance positive self-regulated emotions, improve sleep patterns, and decrease challenging behaviors. Figures 11-7 and 11-8 illustrate multisensory environments that might be used in occupational therapy. The American Association of Multi-Sensory Environments (AAMSE, n.d.) is the regulating board designed to ensure quality control of treatment within multisensory environments. Occupational therapy assistants with special training can learn to perform multisensory environment treatment (www.aamse.us/) for clients with severe cognitive and psychosocial challenges.

Self-Motivating Activities

Self-motivating activities are believed to naturally increase emotion and problem-focused coping due to the feeling of flow. The natural benefits of self-motivating activities for reducing stress are well accepted in occupational therapy and are believed to provide meaning and purpose. Self-motivating activities benefit people with dementia in four specific ways. These include the following:

- Self-motivating activities tend to be familiar. Familiar activities facilitate implicit memories or unconscious knowledge of the use of familiar tools. This may increase the speed and accuracy of tool use.

- Self-motivating activities tend to be activities with which a person has had prior success. Motor skills are performed with greater skill and accuracy when they match prior occupational performance successes.

- Self-motivating activities tend to be ones that are simple enough for independence. Processing abilities such as attention are enhanced by using motor patterns that are simple enough for independence.

- Self-motivating activities tend to be ones that provide natural identity cues. Identity cues are valuable for priming more mindful consciousness and memory throughout the progression of dementia.

Activity-focused treatment (Hellen, 1998) is included in every occupational therapy program that addresses quality of life. All activity-focused treatment is designed to provide holistic benefits to body, mind, and spirit. The qualities of

SPOTLIGHT 11-5. STEVE

The Treatment Plan

Since emotional self-regulation tends to be chaotic and dependent on day-to-day stresses in people with dementia, Greg decides during the fourth week of treatment to address Steve's goals in the community's multisensory environment. Greg knows that multisensory integration cues can influence Steve's deep approach-avoidance system for more successful goal attainment. Greg also knows that all documentation must clearly reflect gains toward achieving functional long-term goals rather than goals related to the multisensory environment. Steve's long-term goals remain the same.

Long-Term Goals

1. Client will don shirt with moderate assist except buttons 3 out of 4 days.

2. Client will demonstrate self-motivation to participate in two out of three activity groups provided daily for 1 week.

3. Client will demonstrate no negative coping behaviors when participating in a 15-minute bird watching group three out of four times.

Documenting Adaptive Responses in Treatment Week Four

Steve's occupational therapy assistant has made great progress in helping Steve achieve his long-term goals. However, Steve's activities of daily living performance patterns remain unpredictable and tend to be related to environmental factors from day to day. Steve is more comfortable with some caregivers due to personal identity preferences and tends to perform better when they are working. Since he tends to be sensitive to occupational context, Steve's performance is even compromised when his caregiver is hurried and stressed. Steve's sensitivity to loss of good environmental fit tends to provide daily challenges that tend to dysregulate performance, attention, and behavior.

During week 4, Greg decides to treat Steve in the multisensory environment. He anticipates that an enhanced sensory environment might support Steve's emotional self-regulation and his adaptive capacity for achieving long-term goal 1. The following is Steve's SOAP note after his week 4 treatment conducted in the multisensory environment.

Subjective	Caregiver said, "I've never seen him so calm at dinner."
Objective	Resident entered therapeutic environment independently but demonstrated no coordinated eye–hand use, no eye contact with therapist, and no generative communication. Used eyes and hands together for preparatory activity, clapping and playing tambourine for 15 minutes after therapist modeling. After independent participation in preparatory activity with music, visual stimulation, and rhythmic movement for 20 minutes used activity-related verbalizations and eye contact with therapist for remainder of session. After preparatory activities, resident donned oversized work shirt independently except for buttons before completing a simple three-step woodworking project.
Assessment	Resident progressed from nongenerative activity and social engagement with therapist to generative engagement and independent participation in donning oversized shirt in one session. Responded well to use of therapeutic environment to prepare for functional goals.
Plan	Repeat use of preparatory activity. Follow with donning of own shirt to continue to work toward long-term goal 1.

self-motivating activities are believed to benefit people with dementia because they provide a sense of the following:

- A clear progress goal
- Receiving clear sensory feedback
- Positive anticipation

Achievable Challenges

All occupational therapy programs for clients with dementia are designed to offer achievable challenges that will not frustrate the client. Three popular programs used

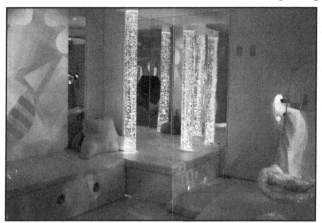

Figure 11-7. Multisensory Environments, picture one. (Reprinted with permission. Photo taken by Linda Messbauer, OTR/L, Sensational Environments.)

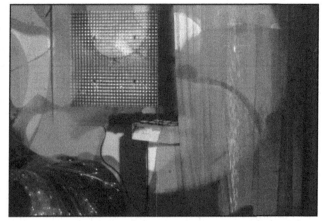

Figure 11-8. Multisensory environments, picture two. (Reprinted with permission. Photo taken by Linda Messbauer, OTR/L, Sensational Environments.)

by occupational therapists will be introduced. These three programs provide structure that reduces the likelihood that untrained caregivers will frustrate themselves and the person with dementia. These include the following:

- Tailored activity program
- Montessori-based activities
- Forget-me-not approach

TAP provides a home-based occupational therapy program designed to reduce the challenges of keeping people with dementia at home. It focuses on training families to provide activities that are within a client's capabilities and customized to his or her interests and history. TAP uses activities that are personalized to match an individual's sensorimotor, physical, and cognitive abilities.

Negative behavior patterns addressed by TAP include resistance to activities of daily living, aggressive vocalizations, and physically aggressive behaviors. These defense action system behaviors tend to reduce quality of life and safety for people with dementia and their families. It is believed that reduction of caregiver burden will allow people with dementia to stay at home longer and reduce the stress-based challenges of caregivers (Ballard, Lowery, Powell, O'Brien, & James, 2000). Though representing a freeze rather than a fight or flight reaction, "even passive behaviors (withdrawal, apathy) are sources of frustration and sadness to families" (Colling, 2004; Gitlin et al., 2009).

Another popular dementia care treatment approach (use) the Montessori-based activities for persons with dementia (Camp, 1999). It targets very simple, sequenced, one-step activities that were commonly developed during early sensory motor experience. This approach presents each activity at a level that is compatible with the person's ability. Activities include the use of simple sensory, form, object, and picture matching. They also ask for size discrimination and ordering of objects by size. They commonly involve very early one-step sensorimotor activities

such as scooping, pouring, squeezing, and caring for one's personal environment.

The forget-me-not approach (Warchol, Copeland, & Ebell, 2002) is designed primarily for use in the integrated development of long-term care activity programs. Table 11-4 demonstrates two ways that ACLs have been adapted so that they can be taught to the daily caregivers of people with dementia. An adapted version of the Functional Assessment Staging of Alzheimer's Disease (FAST) is used by the creators of the forget-me-not approach and is taught by Dementia Care Specialists. Gemstone States is a practical adaptation of the ACL for teaching caregivers and is used in trainings provided by the creators of the positive approach (Reisberg, 1988; Snow & Bunn, 2003). Both are useful for monitoring the shifts that occur in people with dementia related to neuroadaptive and behaviorally adaptive responses that occur during occupational therapy treatment.

SUMMARY

The importance of meaningful and purposeful activities and occupational engagements during the aging years has been emphasized with research on consciousness as "the feeling of what happens" (Damasio, 1999). Therapeutic environments, occupational context, and therapeutic exchanges with occupational therapy practitioners can be used as powerful tools for promoting an adaptive response. Spotlight 11-6 describes the epilogue for Steve to help understand the outcomes of occupational therapy services.

Occupational therapy assistants can become skillful at promoting self-actualization in well-aging clients and aging clients with high cognitive capacity. Likewise, occupational therapy assistant practitioners can also have a positive impact on clients in the late lifespan with cognitive challenges or lower cognitive capacity. Examples include the

		TABLE 11-4	
		TARGETING ADAPTIVE CAPACITIES	
STAGE	**FAST**	**FUNCTIONAL CHALLENGES**	**TARGETING ADAPTIVE CAPACITIES**
Early Dementia (Diamond)	3-4	Compromised function in less familiar occupational contexts: meeting job demands, finding way when traveling and increasingly when driving in community, increased difficulty planning and structuring days.	Benefits from PEO cues for adaptation to new environments when traveling or finding way in community. Remains independent on familiar multi-step activities and finding way in familiar environments.
Early-Moderate Dementia (Emerald)	5	Compromised function in planning and structuring less familiar multi-step activities: selecting appropriate clothes, cooking, cleaning, paying bills and finding way to unfamiliar rooms and locations when walking.	Benefits from PEO cues for selection of rewarding and relaxing activities to increase comfort for way finding, for planning and structuring less familiar multi-step activities. Remains independent on highly familiar multi-step activities and finding way to familiar rooms and locations when walking.
Moderate Dementia (Amber)	6	Compromised independence in familiar multistep activities including basic ADL's such as dressing, bathing and toileting. Increased difficulty finding way to familiar rooms and locations when walking.	Benefits from PEO cues for selection of rewarding and relaxing activities to increase comfort for basic ADL's and way finding. Remains independent on highly familiar one-step activities, using hands to pick up objects and initiate but not sequence multistep activities.
Severe Dementia (Ruby)	7	Compromised speech and ambulation. Requires maximal assistance for all ADL's. Capacity to perform familiar leisure activities limited to ones with gross body movements such as clapping, catching or hitting a balloon.	Benefits from relaxing or rewarding multisensory environments to promote coping with physical changes, self-awareness, speech, assistance in familiar leisure activities and one-step ADL's. Remains able to visibly respond with a smile to favorite music, voice, and familiar, smiling people.
Severe/ End Stage (pearl)	8	Compromised postural and head control for sitting up. Capacity to use non-verbal communication is limited to sounds such as grunts, single words or subtle shifts in facial expressions.	Responds to relaxing or rewarding multisensory environments with subtle expressions of comfort such as breathing rate changes and very subtle interpersonal exchanges such as blinking or turning head to track familiar, smiling people.

Adapted from Snow, T. & Bunn, M. (2003). *Accepting the challenge: Providing the best care for people with dementia.* [DVD]. Eastern North Carolina: Alzheimer's Association.; Reisberg, B. (1988). Functional assessment staging (FAST). *Psychopharmacology Bulletin, 24,* 653-659.

reduction of external controls such as restraints, seclusion, and psychopharmaceuticals, as well as improved quality of life, wellness, and ability to remain in the community. Research applying complexity science and brain technology has affected occupational therapy services in the late lifespan. This includes a new understanding of the therapeutic benefits of enriched environments, meaningful occupations, and joyful relationships in the treatment of both well-aging and impaired clients.

PART 3: APPLICATIONS

The following activities will help you identify key aspects of this chapter that were highlighted in this text. In particular, these questions also highlight the chapter objectives at the start of the chapter. Activities are suggested to be completed individually or in a small group to enhance learning.

SPOTLIGHT 11-6. EPILOGUE FOR STEVE

Steve has adapted well to the previously unfamiliar environment of his long-term care community. He adapted quickly enough to achieve all three of the long-term goals from his treatment plan. Steve achieved these three goals partly due to his occupational therapy assistant's knowledge of the skillful use of a variety of therapeutic approaches.

Greg, his occupational therapy assistant, knew that the use of a multisensory environment in treatment would be an effective strategy for promoting emotional self-regulation. He knew that an emotionally self-regulated state is essential for the development of positive coping strategies. Greg also knew that reactivation of Steve's meaning-making process is a natural way to promote positive coping.

Steve achieved his three long-term goals at a time when new residents commonly lose function following a move to an unfamiliar environment. Greg knew that independence and occupational performance often decrease when a person with dementia leaves the familiar home environment so he adapted Steve's new home with meaningful identity cues. By understanding how to target Steve's meaning-making system, Greg supported his adaptive capacity and therefore assisted him to sustain a higher level of function during this time of transition.

Along with direct treatment, Steve benefited from the use of identity cues that helped him to connect to his new physical, social, and cultural environment. His independence was enhanced by Greg's active approach to coaching his new caregivers. Through this indirect service approach, Steve benefited from the community knowledge of who he is, what is important to him, what he is capable of, and how to motivate him.

Steve developed positive rather than negative coping behaviors after the move to his new home. He quickly developed a meaningful daily and weekly routine that activated his meaning-making process. Steve bonded with Greg and others because he felt safe and respected in his new home. Steve's functional independence and occupational performance were enhanced by Greg's direct, indirect, and preparatory occupational therapy services.

---

1. Individually, re-read Steve's case study in Spotlight 11-1. Apply the SOAP Note Model provided in Figure 11-1 to write a SOAP note for a therapy session with Steve. Be prepared to share with the class.

2. Re-read Spotlight 11-2. Use the Activity Analysis Form. Complete an activity analysis on one of the emotional self-regulation activities you are considering recommending for Lisa. Share this with the class.

3. Using the *Lifespan History and Interest Questionnaire* in Figure 11-2 to plan a treatment session for Steve. Be prepared to share ideas with the class.

4. Divide into pairs of two for role-play. Refer to the positive approach in Table 11-2. Both pair members will take a turn teaching and demonstrating the positive approach while the other member plays a client with dementia.

5. Review the Play Therapy Model in Figure 11-5. There are 5 categories of cues you will use to improve occupational performance, followed by a list of cues you will use to understand how they overlap and fit together. After you finish, you will have 3 cues in each column. The answer key follows at the end of this section. Label your paper to categorize these into the following columns:

a. Emotion-focused coping cues: used to promote a positive feeling or reduce stress

b. Problem-focused coping cues: used to solve performance problems

c. Implicit memory cues: used to promote an unconscious memory from the past

d. Identity cues: used to remind a person about their life story

e. Multisensory integration cues: used to promote function through self-in-context awareness

- Teaching a dementia caregiver to lay the client's clothes out in the morning to promote independent dressing

- A long-term care environment that feels comfortable and home-like

- A menorah when working with a Jewish client or a cross when working with a Christian client

- Using the vestibular and proprioceptive input of a favorite rocking chair to help an agitated client relax

- A favorite song that lifts a client out of boredom and into self-motivated occupational engagement

- Giving a client a Leisure Skills Interest Questionnaire to help them develop new life goals

- An environment with personal sociocultural meaning such as a nursery for a mother

- Using the sight and smell of a favorite food to help a client feel hungry

- The use of gardening activities to bring back the sequenced pattern of planting a seed

- A smile from the therapist

- The use of therapeutic touch to bring back the memory of being held lovingly

- The use of a family picture to help a client remember their wedding day

- Using the weight and feel of a heavy blanket to help a client sleep

- Pointing to a client's flaccid arm to teach them to put their sleeve on that arm first

- The use of a family meal to bring back the memory of happy family attachments

6. After completing Application Question 5, have a class discussion on the following topics: How does each category of cues provide client energy for an adaptive response? How can each be embedded into a therapeutic exchange, environment, and occupation?

7. Divide into groups of four to six students. Take turns leading a dementia care staff training group. Refer to the seven simple rules of relationship-based memory care in Figure 11-6. Use these simple rules to teach the staff (your group members) how to carry out a generative group engagement. Provide several examples of what each student did well, along with one or two recommendations for improvement as a group after each student has lead the group.

8. Read an article on reimbursable occupational therapy services. Be prepared to answer the following questions in class:

- Why is it important when using treatment approaches that focus on an adaptive response to always document how the adaptive response contributes to a functional goal?

- Why is it important when treating within a therapeutic environment to focus your SOAP note on the measurable changes you observe during treatment that contribute to your functional goals?

Answer Key for Question 5

a. Emotion-focused coping cues are used to promote a positive feeling or reduce stress.

- A smile from the therapist

- A long-term care environment that feels comfortable and home-like

- A favorite song that lifts a client out of boredom and into self-motivated occupational engagement

b. Problem-focused coping cues are used to solve performance problems.

- Pointing to a client's flaccid arm to teach them to put their sleeve on that arm first

- Giving a client a Leisure Skills Interest Questionnaire to help them develop new life goals

- Teaching a dementia caregiver to lay the client's clothes out in the morning to promote independent dressing

c. Implicit memory cues are used to promote an unconscious memory from the past.

- The use of therapeutic touch to bring back the memory of being held lovingly

- The use of gardening activities to bring back the sequenced pattern of planting a seed

- The use of a family meal to bring back the memory of happy family attachments

d. Identity cues are used to remind a person about their life story.

- An environment with personal sociocultural meaning such as a nursery for a mother

- A menorah when working with a Jewish client or a cross when working with a Christian client

- The use of a family picture to help a client remember their wedding day

e. Multisensory integration cues are used to promote function through self-in-context awareness.

- Using the sight and smell of a favorite food to help a client feel hungry

- Using the vestibular and proprioceptive input of a favorite rocking chair to help an agitated client relax

- Using the weight and feel of a heavy blanket to help a client sleep

REFERENCES

American Association of Multi-Sensory Environments. (n.d.). Retrieved from www.aamse.us/.

American Occupational Therapy Association. (2014). Occupational therapy practice framework: Domain and process (3rd ed.). *American Journal of Occupational Therapy, 68*(Suppl. 1), S1-S48. doi: 10.5014/ajot2014.682006.

American Friends of Tel Aviv University. (2013). "Bursts of brain activity may protect against Alzheimer's disease." *Medical News Today.* Retrieved from www.medicalnewstoday.com/releases/259370.php.

Ballard, C., Lowery, K., Powell, I., O'Brien, J, & James, I. (2000). Impact of behavioral and psychological symptoms of dementia on caregivers. *International Psychogeriatrics, 12*(S-1), 93-105.

Bieber, D. C. & Keller, B. (2005). Falls and the client with dementia: Using the occupational profile and Allen Cognitive Level to direct care. *American Occupational Therapy Association Gerontology: Special Interest Section Quarterly, 28*(2), 1-4.

Braungart, M. M., Braungart, R. G., & Gramet, P. (2011). Applying learning theories to healthcare practice. In: Bastabel S., Gramet, P., Jacobs, K., Sopczyk, D. L. (Eds.), *Health professional as editor.* (pp. 51-89). Sudbury, MA: Jones & Bartlett Learning.

Botta, F., Santangelo, V., Raffone, A., Sanabria, D., Lupianez, J., & Belardinelli, M. O. (2011). Multisensory integration affects visuospatial working memory. *Journal of Experimental Psychology: Human Perception and Performance, 37*(4), 1099-1109.

Camp, C. J. (Ed.) (1999). *Montessori-based activities for persons with dementia (Vol. I).* Beachwood, OH: Myers Research Institute.

Champagne, T. (2008). *Sensory modulation & environment: Essential elements of occupation* (3rd ed.). Southampton, MA: Champagne Conferences & Consultation.

Champagne, T., Ryan, J., Saccamondo, H., & Lazzarini, I. (2007). A nonlinear dynamics approach to exploring the spiritual dimensions of occupation. *Emergence: Complexity & Organization, 9*(4), 29-43.

Collier, L. McPherson, K., Ellis-Hill, C., Staal, J., & Bucks, R. (2010). Multisensory stimulation to improve functional performance in moderate to severe dementia-interim results. *American Journal of Alzheimer's Disease & Other Dementias, 25,* 698-703.

Colling, K. B. (2004). Caregiver interventions for passive behaviors in dementia: Links to the NDB model. *Aging & Mental Health, 8,* 117-125,

Coombs, S. J., & Smith, I. D. (1998). Designing a self-organized conversational learning environment. *Educational Technology, 38*(3), 17-28.

Damasio, A. (1999). *The feeling of what happens: Body, emotion and the making of consciousness.* New York, NY: Harcourt Brace Jovanovich.

Davis, C. M. (2004). *Complementary therapies in rehabilitation: Evidence for efficacy in therapy, prevention, and wellness.* Thorofare, NJ: SLACK, Inc.

Doidge, N. (2007). *The brain that changes itself.* New York, NY: Viking Press.

Dweck, C. S. (2007). *Mindset: The new psychology of success: How we can learn to fulfill or potential.* New York, NY: Ballantine Books.

Eoyang, G. H. (2008). *Human Systems Dynamics Professional: Certification Training.* (Available during training from Human Systems Dynamics Institute, 50 East Golden Lake Road, Circle Pines, MN, 55014).

Eoyang, G. H., & Holladay, R. J. (2013). *Adaptive action: Leveraging uncertainty in your organization.* Stanford, CA: Stanford University Press.

Fogg, B. J. (2009). A behavior model for persuasive design. Persuasive [Online]. ISBN 978-1-60558-376-1/09/04.

Fosha, D., Siegel, D. J. & Solomon, M. F. (Eds.) (2009). *The healing power of emotion: Affective neuroscience, development & clinical practice.* New York, NY: W. W. Norton.

Gitlin, L. N., Winter, L., Earland, T. V., Herge, E. A., Chernett, N. L., Piersol, C. V., & Burke, J. P. (2009). The Tailored Activity Program to reduce behavioral symptoms in individuals with dementia: Feasibility, acceptability, and replication potential. *The Gerontologist, 49*(3), 428-439.

Gutman, S. A., & Schindler, V. P. (2007). The neurological basis of occupation. *Occupational Therapy International, 14*(2), 71-85.

Harrison, B. E., Son, G., Kim, J., & Whall, A. L. (2012). Preserved implicit memory in dementia: A potential model for care. *American Journal of Alzheimer's Disease & Other Dementias, 22*(4), 286-293.

Hellen, C. R. (1998). *Alzheimer's disease: Activity-focused care* (2nd ed.). Boston, MA: Butterworth/ Heinemann.

Hoppes, S., Davis, L. A., & Thompson, D. (2003). Environmental effects on the assessment of people with dementia: A pilot study. *American Journal of Occupational Therapy, 57*(4), 396-402.

Human Systems Dynamics Institute. (n.d.a). Adaptive action. Retrieved from http://wiki.hsdinstitute.org/adaptive_action.

Human Systems Dynamics Institute. (n.d.b). CDE. Retrieved from http://wiki.hsdinstitute.org/cde.

Human Systems Dynamics Institute. (n.d.c). Generative engagement. Retrieved from http://wiki.hsdinstitute.org/generative_engagement.

Human Systems Dynamics Institute. (n.d.d). Same and different. Retrieved from http://wiki.hsdinstitute.org/same_and_different.

Human Systems Dynamics Institute. (n.d.e). Simple rules. Retrieved from http://wiki.hsdinstitute.org/simple_rules.

Kessels, R. P. C., van Doormaal, A., & Janzen, G. (2011). Landmark recognition in Alzheimer's dementia: Spared implicit memory for objects relevant for navigation. *PLoS ONE 6*(4), e18611.doi: 10.1371/journal.pone.0018611.

Law, M., Cooper, B., Strong, S., Stewart, D., Rigby, P., & Letts, L. (1996). The Person-Environment-Occupation Model: A transactive approach to occupational performance. *Canadian Journal of Occupational Therapy, 63*(1), 9-23.

Machado, S., Cunha, M., Minc, D., Portella, C. E., Velasques, B., Basile, L. F., Cagy, M., Piedade, R., & Ribeiro, P. (2009). *Alzheimer's Disease and Implicit Memory, 67*(2A), 334-342.

Messbauer, L. (2010). *The art and science of multi-sensory environments.* Available during training from the American Association of Multi-Sensory Environments, Chattanooga, TN: Orange Grove Center.

Messbauer, L., & Ryan, J. (2013). Applications of multi-sensory environments in treatment of adult clients with functionally significant brain system challenges. Poster at the 2013 American Occupational Therapy Association Annual Conference, San Diego, CA.

Metz, A. E., & Robnett, R. (2011). Engaging in mentally challenging occupations promotes cognitive health throughout life. *Gerontology Special Interest Section Quarterly.* Bethesda, MD: American Occupational Therapy Association.

Meyer, A. (1922/ 1977). The philosophy of occupational therapy. *American Journal of Occupational Therapy, 31,* 639-642.

Miller, D. B., & O'Callaghan, J. P. (2005). Aging, stress and the hippocampus. *Ageing Research Review, 4*(2), 123-140.

Ogden, P., Minton, K., & Pain, C. (2006). *Trauma and the body: A sensorimotor approach to psychotherapy.* New York, NY: W. W. Norton.

Prehn, A., & Fredens, K. (2011). *Play your brain: Adopt a musical mindset and change your life and career.* Tarrytown, NY: Marshall Cavendish International.

Reisberg, B. (1988). Functional assessment staging (FAST). *Psychopharmacology Bulletin, 24,* 653-659.

Roccas, S., & Brewer, M. B. (2002). Social identity complexity. *Personality and Social Psychology Review, 6*(2), 88-106.

Rogers, C. (1951). *Client-centered therapy: Its current practice, implications and theory.* London: Constable.

Rogers, C. (1959). A theory of therapy, personality and interpersonal relationships as developed in the client-centered framework. In S. Koch (Ed.), *Psychology: A Study of a Science. Vol. 3: Formulations of the Person and the Social Context.* New York, NY: McGraw Hill.

Rogers, C. (1961). *On Becoming a Person: A Therapist's View of Psychotherapy.* London: Constable..

Rogers, H., & Lasprilla, J. C. (2006). Retrogenesis theory in Alzheimer's disease: Evidence and clinical implications. *Anales de Psicologia, 22*(2), 260-266.

Ryan, J. (2009). *A social-spiritual model of dynamic memory care.* Self-published training manual.

Ryan, J. (2013). Treating the brain as an adaptive system in clients with dementia: Facilitating the neurobiology of action system processes. Poster at the 2013 American Occupational Therapy Association Annual Conference, San Diego, CA.

Ryan, J. (2014). The nonlinear neurodynamics of play therapy for people with dementia. Presentation at the 2014 Society for Chaos Theory in Psychology in Life Sciences Annual Conference, Milwaukee, WI.

Sara, S. J. (2000). Retrieval and reconsolidation: Toward a neurobiology of remembering. *Learning and Memory, 7,* 73-84.

Satir, V. (n.d.) In Brainy Quote. Retrieved from www.BrainyQuote.com

Schaffer, D. V., & Gage, F. H. (2004). Neurogenesis and neuroadaptation. *NeuroMolecular Medicine, 4*(5), 1-9.

Schmitz, T. W., De Rosa, E., & Anderson, A. K. (2009). Opposing influences of affective state valence on visual cortical encoding. *The Journal of Neuroscience, 29*(22), 7199-7207.

Siegel, D. J. (2010). *The mindful therapist: A clinician's guide to mindsight and neural integration.* New York, NY: W. W. Norton.

Snow, T., & Bunn, M. (2003). *Accepting the challenge: Providing the best care for people with dementia.* [DVD]. Eastern North Carolina: Alzheimer's Association.

Taylor, S. E., & Stanton, A. L. (2007). Coping resources, coping processes, and mental health. *Annual Review Clinical Psychology, 3,* 377-401.

Townsend, E. (1997). *Enabling occupation: An occupational therapy perspective.* Ottawa, ON: Canadian Association of Occupational Therapists.

Trauma-informed Practices and Expressive Arts Therapy Institute & Learning Center. (n.d.). Retrieved from www.trauma-informed-practice.com.

Unsworth, N., Spillers, G. J., & Brewer, G. A. (2011, June). Dynamics of context-dependent recall: An examination of internal and external context change. *Journal of Memory and Language, 66.* Retrieved from www.elsevier.com.

Vezina, A., Robichaud, L., Voyer, P., & Pelletier, D. (2011). Identity cues and dementia in nursing home intervention. *PMC Canada, 40*(1), 5-14.

Warchol, K., Copeland, C., & Ebell, C. (2002). *The "Forget-Me-Not" Activity Planning Book.* Chesterfield, MO: Dementia Care Specialists.

Therapeutic Rapport
Applications of the Intentional Relationship Model

Renee R. Taylor, PhD and Su Ren Wong, BOccThy, OTR/L

KEY TERMS

- Client-Centered
- Clinical Reasoning
- Collaborative Approach
- Contemporary Era
- Desired Occupation
- Era of Inner Mechanism

- Intentional Relationship Model (IRM)
- Interactive Reasoning
- Interpersonal Characteristics
- Interpersonal Dynamics
- Interpersonal Event
- Interpersonal Reasoning

- Interpersonal Skill Base
- Mode Shift
- Narrative Approach
- Nontherapeutic Response
- Occupational Era
- Therapeutic Modes
- Therapeutic Use of Self

CHAPTER LEARNING OBJECTIVES

After completion of this chapter, students should be able to:

1. Identify historical applications of therapeutic use of self in occupational therapy.

2. Recognize the Intentional Relationship Model in occupational therapy.

3. State the elements of the Intentional Relationship Model as they apply to occupational therapy.

4. Describe interpersonal characteristics all persons have that will influence the therapeutic relationship.

5. Explain therapeutic modes in relating to the client and possible nontherapeutic responses.

6. Apply aspects of the Intentional Relationship Model in enhancing therapeutic use of self with clients.

Manville, C.A., & Keough, J. L.
Mental Health Practice for the Occupational Therapy Assistant (pp 285-305).
© 2016 Taylor & Francis Group.

CHAPTER OUTLINE

OCCUPATIONAL PROFILE

Janice is a 38-year-old single mother with two young children. She has not been able to sustain long-term paid employment for the last 6 years because of neck and low back pain. The impairments to her neck and back happened from a car accident 8 years ago. There were no significant injuries found during the initial medical examination; however, the pain persisted and over time it became unbearable. Eventually, Janice was diagnosed with nerve compression in the neck and lower back due to the formation of scar tissue. Her physician recommended surgery to release the compression. Following surgery, however, the pain remained. Janice continued to have difficulty carrying out her usual daily activities.

Janice was a successful accounting assistant prior to the injury, holding the same job for over 12 years. She took pride in her work and in her own words "could almost be labeled a workaholic." Janice was "efficient" and "meticulous" with her job and also with her housework. Janice was married to a husband who was unable to find consistent employment. This caused a strain on their relationship. Her husband left her 4 years after the automobile accident, and they have been separated ever since. Janice does not know where he is, and she cares for their children on her own. Although she receives some financial assistance from the state to care for her children, Janice occasionally has to borrow money from her family and friends to "make do" until the end of the month.

Janice is able to complete her own self-care tasks independently; however, she requires increased time due to her chronic pain. She uses most of her energy to take care of her children. Janice is moderately depressed. She has become socially isolated and feels that her pain and low energy levels prevent her from participating in social and leisure activities. The only thing that keeps Janice from feeling entirely hopeless is her relationship with her children. Her children are her main source of encouragement and support.

Janice was referred to various therapies, including occupational therapy, to address pain management. Janice did not follow up consistently with her appointments due to financial and time constraints. The medical records from her pain management therapy include terms such as *noncompliant* and *stubborn* to describe Janice. Occupational therapy is one of the therapies in which Janice has continued to participate.

INTRODUCTION

In occupational therapy, therapeutic success is often measured by the client's ability to engage in meaningful occupations. To reach the occupational goals, the therapist needs to develop an effective working relationship with the client. A growing number of studies indicate that the client–therapist relationship is a key determinant of treatment success in occupational therapy (Ayres-Rosa & Hasselkus, 1996; Cole & McLean, 2003). ***Therapeutic use of self*** is a term that is used to describe how an occupational therapy practitioner uses personal understanding about relationships, emotions, and experiences in an intentional way in order to communicate with the client (Taylor, 2008). The therapist uses an internal, reflective reasoning process in

SPOTLIGHT 12-1. STRESSFUL INTERACTIONS AND NEGATIVE CONSEQUENCES

Janice's family doctor, the referring physician, has decided to refer Janice to occupational therapy due to the concern that she was too dependent on medications. Previously, various health care practitioners had perceived their interactions with Janice as stressful and described her as noncompliant and stubborn. Both Janice and her previous therapists found their relationship difficult, and Janice missed many therapy sessions. Missed therapy sessions might have been prevented if practitioners were more knowledgeable about how to manage challenging behaviors like those in Janice's situation. Additional efforts and approaches may have aided in restoring the relationship between Janice and her therapist.

order to develop a client-centered, dynamic partnership with the client (Taylor, 2008). Therapeutic use of self is used interchangeably with the term *use of self*.

Practitioners may not realize the importance of understanding the psychology of human interaction until they experience a stressful relationship with a client. A nationwide study found that more than 80% of occupational therapists believe that therapeutic use of self was the most important determinant of successful therapy outcomes (Taylor, Lee, & Kielhofner, 2011; Taylor, Lee, Kielhofner, & Ketkar, 2009). Less than half of the therapists, however, felt that they were adequately trained in therapeutic use of self while attending school (Taylor, Lee, Kielhofner, & Ketkar, 2009). The occupational therapy training curriculum is often prioritized with academic information to ensure that practitioners graduate with a certain level of technical competence. Unfortunately, the development of therapeutic use of self has not been intentionally included into many programs. Instead, therapeutic use of self is assumed to develop along the way. As a result, health care practitioners may underestimate the skill required to achieve open communication with clients and often are unintentional in developing therapeutic rapport with clients.

If occupational therapy practitioners are intentional about relationships, they will reflect on the experience and consider how their communication might be improved in the future. It is fairly easy and sometimes more comfortable for the therapist, however, to dismiss the experience or label the client as pathological, confused, or eccentric in some way. Stressful interactions with clients can lead to negative consequences, not only for clients but also for the health care practitioner. Spotlight 12-1 describes an example of negative consequences. This could include client withdrawal from therapy or the initiation of complaints against the practitioner. In other cases, the practitioner may decide to terminate therapy prematurely. The therapist could refer the client elsewhere due to noncompliance, communication failures, or some other behavioral issue (Taylor et al., 2009).

The therapeutic use of self by the therapist is more complex than the task of building rapport with a client. This chapter begins by reviewing the literature on the use of self within the profession of occupational therapy. Next, the central concepts of the **Intentional Relationship Model** (IRM) are defined. The IRM is a conceptual practice model that explains the reasoning process and communication skills that comprise the use of self in occupational therapy. Finally, appropriate and inappropriate communication styles, known as therapeutic and nontherapeutic modes, are identified and explained using a case study for examples. This chapter provides a basic overview of the IRM.

PART 1: HISTORICAL OVERVIEW

A therapist's use of self has been identified as an important topic throughout the history of occupational therapy. The term *therapeutic use of self*, also known as *use of self*, was first described in the 1950s as an important consideration in effective occupational therapy (Frank, 1958). Use of self is said to be therapeutic when it facilitates the achievement of desired therapeutic goals (Devereaux, 1984). There have been various definitions of therapeutic use of self since the 1980s (Cara & MacRae, 1998; Denton, 1987; Hagedorn, 1995; Mosey, 1981; Schwartzberg, 1993). The Occupational Therapy Practice Framework describes therapeutic use of self as a "practitioner's planned use of his or her personality, insights, perceptions and judgments as part of the therapeutic process" (American Occupational Therapy Association, 2008, p. 653).

Strategies for effective communication within the therapeutic relationship have changed over time just as theories of practice have changed. Kielhofner (2009) identified three distinct eras in occupational therapy. Each era provides a unique perspective and emphasis on the role of the client–therapist relationship in the occupational therapy process. The three distinct eras in occupational therapy are as follows:

1. Early Occupation Era (before the 1920s)

2. Era of Inner Mechanisms (mid-20th century)

3. Contemporary Era (later part of the 20th century)

Early Occupational Era

The first era, referred to as the **Occupational Era**, reflects the values that were held by the founders of occupational therapy (Kielhofner, 2009). The earliest relevant descriptions of therapeutic use of self emerged within Europe in the late 1700s during the time of moral treatment (Bing, 1981; Bockoven, 1971). Moral treatment emphasized the development of a sense of competence and independence through engagement in everyday activities such as arts and crafts, sports, and other pursuits. When occupational therapy became more developed as a profession in the early 1900s, advocates for moral treatment recommended that therapy should be rooted in a deep understanding of the patient's personality, preferences, and interests (Bing, 1981). Interpersonal values of *consideration* and *kindness* were considered central to therapy. In this era, the purpose of the therapeutic relationship was to encourage clients to engage in occupations. The role of the therapist in creating the therapeutic relationship was to serve as an expert, model, and guide in order to persuade the client to engage in occupations.

Era of Inner Mechanisms

In the mid-20th century, a client's underlying impairment became the focus of occupational therapy treatment (Kielhofner, 2009). As the profession aligned itself with the biomedical field, the role of occupational therapy changed to that of understanding and treating pathologies of the body and mind. This was known as the **Era of Inner Mechanisms.** By the 1970s, however, some therapists believed that occupation had lost its place as the key dynamic in occupational therapy (Kielhofner & Burke, 1977; Schwartz, 2003; Shannon, 1977; Yerxa, 1967).

Occupational therapy was mainly practiced in mental health institutions during this era. In occupational therapy settings, it was common to expect that the client would express his or her unconscious motives and desires within the therapeutic relationship. One focus of therapy was to help the client become more aware of underlying motives and desires. This was believed to be at the core of pathological feelings and behaviors. The client–therapist relationship was viewed as the central mechanism for change. Understanding this relationship was largely based on principles influenced by the psychoanalytic perspective. This meant that the relationship was viewed as a way to understand a client's unconscious motives, desires, and behaviors toward others and occupations.

Contemporary Era (Return to Occupation)

The profession of occupational therapy realigned itself back to the centrality of occupation during the latter part of the 20th century. This era was labeled by Kielhofner (2009) as the **Contemporary Era** or the *Return to Occupation*. In the Contemporary Era, the emphasis on the therapeutic relationship was set aside in favor of a renewed emphasis on occupational engagement. Occupational engagement is viewed as the true mechanism for client change and positive outcomes in the occupational therapy process (Kielhofner & Burke, 1977; Schwartz, 2003; Shannon, 1977; Yerxa, 1967). Similar to the Early Occupational Era, the role of the therapeutic relationship in the Contemporary Era reverted back to the one-dimensional focus of facilitating the client's engagement in occupation.

Three central themes have been used to describe the client–therapist relationship in the Contemporary Era:

1. Collaborative and client-centered approaches

2. Caring and empathy

3. Clinical reasoning and narrative approaches

The first theme places an emphasis on the terms *collaborative* and *client-centered* (Duncan, 2011; Mosey, 1970; Parker, 2006; Townsend, 2003). A **collaborative approach** involves readjusting power imbalances between the therapist and client. It also involves increasing client control in decision making and problem solving. **Client-centered** practice focuses on the client's perspective, as well as recognition of the client's strengths, goals, and priorities. To use a collaborative, client-centered approach, the therapist needs to develop self-awareness of his or her own worldviews, values, and biases. The therapist is then able to exercise self-control and refrain from imposing his or her own personal beliefs, goals, and perception of the world on the client. The therapist does use his or her own life experiences to understand the client's perspective and to guide clinical reasoning used in the treatment process. For example, if a practitioner has a similar cultural background that values independence with a client, the therapist can understand the client's frustration when dressing requires assistance. The practitioner may then suggest the use of dressing aids to modify the task before suggesting physical assistance. If the therapist comes from a different cultural background that does not value independence, a different approach may be utilized. The lack of awareness of cultural norms between the therapist and client may lead the therapist to collaborate with the client and the family differently. The therapist may approach the family to pursue availability to help the client on a regular basis with tasks that require physical assistance.

The second theme of the Contemporary Era has been characterized by an emphasis on the qualities of *caring and empathy* within the therapeutic relationship. This can be summarized as an emphasis on the emotional exchange between the client and therapist. It includes activities that reflect the client's goals and promotes growth in the client (Baum, 1980; Devereaux, 1984; Gilfoyle, 1980; King, 1980; Peloquin, 1989a, 1989b, 1990, 1993, 1995, 2002, 2003; Yerxa, 1980).

The first quality, *caring,* is recognized as a much-needed value (Baum, 1980; Devereaux, 1980; Gilfoyle; 1980; King, 1980; Yerxa, 1980). Devereaux identified supporting skills that were found to be important in developing a caring relationship. These skills include restoring personal control

---

SPOTLIGHT 12-2. CONTEMPORARY ERA: QUALITY OF CARING

Janice's occupational therapist, Sarah, was considered caring as she had taken the effort to intimately know Janice. She connected with Janice at an emotional level rather than distancing herself from Janice's emotional pain. Sarah communicated effectively at times, which included the judicious use of touch and humor as necessary. Sarah also did not withhold information from Janice that was considered critical in allowing her to make informed decisions. Instead of focusing on Janice's impairments, Sarah showed that she cared for Janice by pointing out her strengths and capabilities in order to instill hope. This showed that Sarah believed in Janice's innate potential. Sarah understood that to be truly caring, she could not treat Janice as a passive and dependent client. Sarah used activity to restore Janice's personal control and to strengthen her will. Sarah was also caring by mindfully adapting the environmental demands according to Janice's needs rather than choosing therapeutic activities that were convenient for herself as a practitioner.

---

through activity, communicating effectively, believing in the innate potential of the individual, using touch to connect, and using humor. Spotlight 12-2 illustrates how Sarah showed the quality of caring in the case example of Janice.

The second quality, *empathy,* is the foundation for effective therapeutic use of self. Dr. Suzanne Peloquin (1989b, 1990, 1993, 1995) wrote about empathy extensively. She described empathy as a communication of partnership that involves entering the client's experience and connecting with the feelings of the client. Dr. Peloquin emphasized the role of art, literature, imagination, and self-reflection in the development of empathy in occupational therapy practitioners. She stressed, for example, the use of both fictional and nonfictional stories to illustrate the importance of empathy and negative consequences of neglectful attitudes. Candid stories by clients were used to show how practitioners' impersonal, aloof attitudes and abrasive, insensitive comments led clients to feel discouraged and hopeless (Peloquin, 1993). Dr. Peloquin expressed the belief that exposing clinicians to such stories can be a powerful motivator in the development of caring and empathy (Peloquin, 1990, 1993, 1995).

The final theme in the Contemporary Era is the use of **clinical reasoning** and *narrative approaches* that utilize the client–therapist relationship as a focal point (Clark, 1993; Fleming, 1991a, 1991b; Jonsson, Josephsson, & Kielhofner, 2001; Lyons & Crepeau, 2001; Mattingly, 1994; Mattingly & Fleming, 1994; Schell, 2003; Schwartz, 2003; Schwartzberg, 2002). Clinical reasoning emphasizes how therapists think and reflect about the occupational therapy process.

Clinical reasoning involves thinking about the client–therapist relationship as a component of the occupational therapy process. It includes making sense of assessment findings and developing a treatment plan (Mattingly & Fleming, 1994). Therapists often do much of their clinical reasoning during therapy sessions while they are interacting with the client. This is also known as **interactive reasoning** (Mattingly & Fleming, 1994). For example, a therapist may engage in interactive reasoning when wanting to gain information about a client's experience of an illness. The client may describe the challenges and lessons learned. Other clients may describe the frustration and anger about having an illness. Individual experiences can be diverse. The therapist is able to develop a more intimate understanding of the client's experience through this interaction rather than being apart from the client's experience. Interactive reasoning is referred to as an "underground practice" in occupational therapy, as relatively little is known about the mechanisms that underlie it (Fleming, 1991b, p. 1010).

Narrative approaches, on the other hand, focus on how the client conceptualizes and summarizes key events in his or her life (Kielhofner, 2004). Narrative approaches seek to organize and make sense of information. Clients are encouraged to present information about themselves through storytelling, poetry, and metaphor. Thinking in story form allows both the client and therapist to discover the meaning of impairment according to the client's unique perspective. Therapeutic approaches are then focused toward reconstructing a more hopeful narrative in order to reshape the client's life story. Spotlight 12-3 describes how Sarah helped Janice reframe her life story.

The Need for a Conceptual Practice Model

Occupational therapy literature has contributed to our understanding of the important elements of an effective therapeutic relationship. Unfortunately, most of the literature does not directly explain the specific reasoning and communication skills that are necessary for an effective therapeutic relationship. Until recently, two particular challenges have hampered the integration of contemporary interpersonal approaches into a coherent model of the therapeutic relationship. First, there was a lack of clarity and consensus regarding the exact definition, use, and relevance of the term *therapeutic use of self* in occupational therapy. Second, there was insufficient understanding about how the therapeutic relationship relates to the central focus of occupation. These observations led to the development of the conceptual practice model entitled the IRM (Taylor, 2008). This model was developed in an attempt to clarify

SPOTLIGHT 12-3. JANICE REFRAMING HER LIFE STORY

Janice presented a bleak picture of her experiences and impairments during the first few encounters with Sarah. Janice recounted how her husband deserted her, leaving her by herself to deal with financial and medical problems. She was frustrated and unable to care for her children due to uncontrolled pain. She also had nightmares of her children being taken away from her. Sarah tried to point out her strengths and the control she was regaining over her pain throughout the next few sessions. One day Janice came in smiling and told Sarah that her family had given her money that would help cover expenses over the next month. Sarah took the opportunity to modify Janice's narrative of her impairment. Sarah gave Janice time to talk about her family and also asked her about other instances when she experienced care and concern from others. Janice eventually was able to mention how she learned the importance of forgiveness and not harboring bitterness toward her husband. By giving Janice an opportunity to reframe her experience, Sarah helped Janice see that she could have a more hopeful life story.

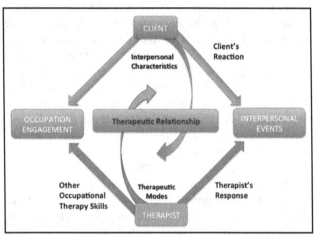

Figure 12-1. The Intentional Relationship Model. (Adapted from Taylor, R. R. (2008). *The Intentional Relationship: Occupational therapy and use of self*. Philadelphia: F.A. Davis.)

and provide more detailed guidance on how to develop and utilize therapeutic use of self in occupational therapy.

Therapeutic use of self involves a highly personal and individualized decision-making process. The process is driven by subjective and emotional reactions to clients and the use of intuition for some occupational therapy practitioners. Other practitioners perceive the process as largely rational and grounded in the application of a specific set of interpersonal guidelines. Therapeutic use of self is, in large part, the development of a knowledge base and interpersonal skills that can be applied to common interpersonal events in everyday practice. Therapeutic use of self is an occupational therapy skill that is constantly being developed, reinforced, monitored, and refined.

The IRM explains therapeutic use of self and its relationship with occupational engagement. Additionally, the model provides a means of mapping, interpreting, and responding to the unique or everyday interpersonal events. The model provides educators, supervisors, students, and practitioners a common vocabulary to describe and discuss the interpersonal phenomena that affect everyday practice.

PART 2: THE INTENTIONAL RELATIONSHIP MODEL

The IRM is an empirically based model that has been undergoing development over the past 8 years. In part, its concepts were based on practitioner responses to a large-scale nationwide survey concerning their knowledge, attitudes, and interpersonal behaviors related to the use of self (Taylor et al., 2009). The model is intended to complement, rather than replace, any single conceptual practice model. It explains the client–therapist relationship, which is an important aspect of occupational therapy not addressed extensively by other conceptual practice models. The IRM uniquely explains how the interpersonal relationship between the client and therapist influence both occupational engagement and therapeutic outcomes. Other conceptual practice models only address therapeutic concepts and strategies that are directly aimed at facilitating occupational engagement. Elements of this model provide an explanation of how they interact to optimize a successful client–therapist relationship in occupational therapy.

Elements of the Intentional Relationship Model

The IRM views the therapeutic relationship as being composed of four central elements:

1. Client and his or her interpersonal characteristics
2. Interpersonal events that occur during therapy
3. Therapist and his or her use of modes
4. Desired occupation

Figure 12-1 illustrates a diagram summarizing the IRM. The IRM explains the requirements for a functional client–therapist relationship. It incorporates guidelines for responding to common interpersonal events that frequently occur in therapy. Aspects of each element within the IRM are described in the next section.

The Client and Interpersonal Characteristics

The client is one central component of the IRM and is considered the focal point. It is the therapist's responsibility to develop a positive relationship with the client and to respond appropriately when interpersonal events occur. In order to develop this relationship and respond appropriately to the client, a therapist must work to understand the client from an interpersonal perspective. This involves getting to know a client's interpersonal characteristics. The IRM defines 12 categories of *interpersonal characteristics*. The 12 categories are presented in Checkpoint 12-1.

Fundamental to the IRM is the ability to read and understand a client's interpersonal characteristics accurately. It is important for the occupational therapy practitioner to do this as early as possible in the treatment relationship. The practitioner also needs to continually verify the accuracy of observations and perceptions regarding client behaviors. Understanding a client's interpersonal characteristics and preferences enables the therapist to adjust his or her therapeutic personality (or interpersonal mode use) accordingly. The therapist is then able to increase the potential to develop positive rapport and open communication.

Interpersonal Events That Occur During Therapy

An *interpersonal event* is defined as a naturally occurring communication, reaction, process, task, or general circumstance that occurs during therapy. It has the potential to weaken or strengthen the therapeutic relationship (Taylor, 2008). During therapy, interpersonal events may include the following kinds of circumstances:

- Client reluctance or resistance (e.g., a client refuses or feels unable to participate in an activity).

- Therapist behavior (e.g., the therapist asks a question that the client perceives as intrusive or emotionally difficult to face).

- Client display of strong emotions in therapy (e.g., an elderly client begins crying during transfer training or a child client runs up to the therapist and hugs her in the midst of a sensory motor activity).

- A difficult circumstance of therapy (e.g., a client is embarrassed due to losing bladder control, or becomes frustrated or fearful in the midst of an activity).

- An argument or conflict between the client and therapist (e.g., the client is offended by a comment made by the therapist).

- Differences concerning the aim of therapy (e.g., a client insists on a goal that the therapist believes is not attainable, or the therapist recommends a goal that the client rejects).

- Client requests that test the boundaries or limits of the therapeutic relationship (e.g., the client invites the therapist to attend her wedding or asks for her address).

These are only a few examples of the many possible interpersonal events that can occur in the course of occupational therapy.

When an interpersonal event occurs during therapy, the client interprets the event depending on his or her unique set of interpersonal characteristics. Remember interpersonal characteristics were displayed in Checkpoint 12-1. The interpersonal event may have a significant impact on the client on one occasion, whereas another time it can have minimal effect on the client. It is important that the practitioner be aware of an event when it occurs and respond appropriately.

According to the IRM, interpersonal events will happen in every therapeutic relationship. They can be perceived as a threat or an opportunity in the therapeutic process. It is essential that the therapist approach these interpersonal events intentionally, rather than ignore or minimize them. Approaching an event intentionally means using one's interpersonal reasoning skills first to decide if and when the issue should be addressed openly. Then the therapist should choose the appropriate mode or aspect of his or her therapeutic personality to best communicate with the client when working through the interpersonal event. Spotlight 12-4 describes an example of an interpersonal event during one of Janice's therapy sessions.

Interpersonal events are part of the constant give and take between the client and therapist during the occupational therapy process. Interpersonal events are different from other events in that they have the potential to trigger an emotional response, either at the time they occur or later upon reflection. If these events are ignored or responded to inappropriately, it can affect both the therapeutic relationship and the client's occupational engagement. Alternatively, these events can provide the client with opportunities for positive learning and solidify the therapeutic relationship. One of the primary responsibilities of the occupational therapy practitioner is to respond to these inevitable events in a way that leads to the strengthening of the therapeutic relationship.

The Therapist and His or Her Use of Modes

This is the third central element in the IRM. Within the IRM, the therapist is entirely responsible for making every reasonable effort to establish open and trusting communication with the client. Specifically, the therapist is responsible for bringing three main interpersonal capacities into the relationship:

1. Interpersonal skill base

CHECKPOINT 12-1. DEFINE INTERPERSONAL CHARACTERISTICS

	Interpersonal Characteristics	Description
1	Communication style	• Includes a client's tone of voice, pacing, and amount of speech or other form of communication. • A client may either have an acceptable or problematic method of communication. Examples of problematic communication include being too talkative, refusing to speak, and using a commanding tone of voice.
2	Capacity for trust	• Includes a client's level of comfort and confidence in the therapist and the therapy process. • A client shows trust by being open and comfortable about his or her thoughts, opinions, and feelings. A client who has difficulty with trust may appear skeptical of the therapist and reluctant to participate in the therapy process.
3	Need for control	• Describes a client's desire to control how needs are met during the therapy session. • Signs of a problematic need for control include clients who try to gain control of situations through aggressive or passive methods. Examples include manipulation, dominance, or criticism.
4	Capacity to assert needs	• Describes a client's ability to ask for help. The client expresses what he or she desires during therapy freely and in a manner that the therapist finds acceptable and respectful. • Clients who have difficulty in this area are observed to range from being reluctant to overly demanding in requesting help. Clients who have difficulty asserting their needs may appear excessively dependent or helpless during therapy.
5	Response to change and challenge	• Reflects a client's reaction to change or challenges during the therapy process. • It is common for clients to struggle initially with an impairment and the therapy process; however, they usually adapt to this new challenge. Clients who continue to resist change or challenge may become anxious, reluctant, easily irritated, or angry with the therapist.
6	Affect	• Refers to the client's observable expression of emotion. • A client with an unremarkable affect will show an appropriate intensity and type of emotional reaction according to the situation at hand. Problematic affect may include both overly and blunted emotional expressions and observable mood swings.
7	Predisposition to giving feedback	• Describes a client's ability to voluntarily tell the therapist what is working and going well in therapy or what is not working. • Examples of a problematic approach include using excessively negative expressions such as complaining, excessively positive expressions such as a complimenting manner, and only giving feedback at the end of a session or treatment process.

(continued)

	Interpersonal Characteristics	Description
		CHECKPOINT 12-1. DEFINE INTERPERSONAL CHARACTERISTICS (CONTINUED)
8	Capacity to receive feedback	• Reflects the client's ability to accept both positive and negative feedback from the therapist about his or her behavior or performance. • An acceptable response to any feedback is to accept it objectively, understand the meaning behind it, and make adjustments if necessary. Difficulty accepting feedback is characterized by a client ignoring and showing negative emotions such as displaying anger or anxiety.
9	Response to human diversity	• Describes a client's ability to work with and accept a therapist who might differ in an important way such as age, gender, race, ethnicity, religion, or sexual orientation. • A client who does not have a problem with diversity will not raise it as an issue or act out in some way. A client who does have difficulty with diversity will remark, question, or act out around an issue in some way.
10	Orientation toward relating	• Describes the client's degree of preference for an emotionally open connection versus a more professional or business-like relationship with the therapist.
11	Preference for touch	• Is a client's degree of tolerance or preference for touch. • Some clients may reject touch entirely because of personal preference, sensory, or pain-related issues. Others may tolerate it only with necessary treatments. Clients may also seek out or appear comforted by attempts at caring forms of touch by the therapist.
12	Capacity for reciprocity	• Describes a client's ability to consider the therapist as a person beyond the professional. • A client may be spontaneous with expressing compliments, gratitude, and other forms of appreciation toward the therapist. Clients without a desire for reciprocity will not show many of these behaviors.

Adapted from Taylor, R. R. (2008). *The intentional relationship model: Occupational therapy and use of self.* Philadelphia, PA: F. A. Davis.

2. Intentional use of therapeutic modes

3. Capacity for interpersonal reasoning

Every therapist needs to develop a "toolbox" of communication skills and professional behaviors collectively known as an *interpersonal skill base*. Although occupational therapy education provides therapists with a basic set of communication skills, no therapist is expected to be an expert in communication when first starting entry-level practice. New occupational therapy assistant practitioners need to develop their service competency with communication as soon as possible. It is the therapist's responsibility to engage in ongoing reflection concerning less-than-ideal situations and successes in relationships in order to add to the communication skills toolbox.

A *therapeutic mode* is a specific way of relating to a client. It includes verbal communication and nonverbal communication and behaviors. Therapeutic modes are communication styles that are part of a therapist's personality. They are used at a particular moment by the therapist to be most helpful to the client during therapy. *Interpersonal reasoning* is an internal process during which the occupational therapy practitioner selects the most appropriate mode for interacting with a client at a particular time. It is a complex task. First, it includes anticipating and being ready for an interpersonal event. Then it includes adjusting or changing modes according to the client's needs and personality. The IRM identifies six therapeutic modes, which will be explained later in this chapter. The six therapeutic modes are as follows:

1. Advocating

2. Collaborating

3. Empathizing

SPOTLIGHT 12-4. JANICE—AN INTERPERSONAL EVENT

One of Janice's goals was to be able to sit for 30 minutes to complete various tasks. Sarah, the occupational therapy practitioner, was addressing this goal during a therapy session by introducing Janice to various backrests she could use to sit comfortably in her chair. Suddenly, Janice started sobbing. Sarah was puzzled. Janice did not look particularly upset when she came into the session today. Sarah was sensitive and identified that this was an interpersonal event. Sarah decided to stop talking about backrests. Sarah asked Janice gently how she felt and gave her space to talk about what caused her to feel emotional. Janice could not talk immediately, and Sarah sat there quietly, supplying tissues to Janice. After a few minutes, Janice said that she had not gone to visit her mother in a long time. She explained that her mother loves to cook elaborate dinner meals and everyone would sit at the dinner table for hours. Janice reported that she went back to visit her mother for the first time in a long time as she thought she had been feeling better with therapy. Janice said that she had to stand multiple times during the course of dinner, which is one of the strategies that Sarah taught her to control her pain. Unexpectedly, Janice's mother became offended. Janice's mother perceived that she was being rude and distracted when she stood. As Sarah listened to Janice speak, Sarah realized the emotional pain that Janice was going through by not being able to sit for a long period. Sarah listened to her and sought to understand her experience. Sarah verbalized how important it was for Janice's mother to be part of her life. Sarah also responded by affirming how being able to sit was not just about sitting, but also about being able to spend time with her mother and family. Janice understood what Sarah was saying; however, she still was not very hopeful that she would be able to join family dinners again. Sarah asked Janice if she would like to continue the session by exploring how she could talk to her mother about her pain, and Janice agreed. Sarah felt it was an important interpersonal moment even though they did not have time to explore the use of backrests that session. Janice did feel more empowered about communicating about her pain.

4. Encouraging

5. Instructing

6. Problem solving

The Desired Occupation

The **desired occupation** is the task or activity that the therapist and the client have selected to address in therapy. Occupational therapy is unique in that the ultimate goal of therapy is the client's occupational engagement. The main purpose of occupational therapy is not only for clients to feel well, but also to enhance their quality of life. Desired occupations may include a wide range of tasks and activities. They can include activities of daily living, instrumental activities of daily living, rest and sleep, education, work, play, leisure, and social participation. Achievement of occupational engagement depends upon the therapist's ability to use strategies and skills from occupational therapy models that meet the client's needs. At the same time, the therapist maintains an effective relationship with the client. Intentional use of therapeutic modes will aid in maintaining an effective therapeutic relationship with the client during the occupational therapy process.

Therapeutic Modes and Nontherapeutic Responses

A **therapeutic mode** is a style of relating to a client. As mentioned earlier, the IRM identifies six therapeutic modes. A brief definition of each mode is provided in Checkpoint 12-2. Therapists naturally use therapeutic modes that are consistent with their fundamental personality characteristics. For example, a therapist who tends to be more of a listener than a talker and believes in the importance of understanding another person's perspective before making a suggestion would likely use empathizing as a primary therapeutic mode in therapy. Likewise, someone who is a natural teacher or leader might have a tendency to draw upon the instructing and problem-solving modes more often.

Therapists are also different in terms of their range and flexibility of modes when relating to clients. Some practitioners relate to clients with just one or two primary modes. Other practitioners may easily use multiple therapeutic modes depending on the characteristics of the client, the situation, or interpersonal event. One of the goals in using the IRM is to become increasingly more comfortable using any of the six modes flexibly and interchangeably (Taylor, 2008). A therapeutic mode (or set of modes) defines a therapist's general interpersonal style when interacting with a client. Therapists who are able to utilize all six modes flexibly and comfortably, and match those modes to the client and the situation, are described as having a multimodal interpersonal style.

According to the IRM, a therapist's choice and application of a particular therapeutic mode or set of modes should depend mostly on the interpersonal characteristics of the client. Certain interpersonal events in therapy frequently may call for a mode shift. A **mode shift** is a conscious

CHECKPOINT 12-2. UNDERSTAND THE SIX THERAPEUTIC MODES	
Mode	*Definition*
Advocating	Advocating describes when therapists stand up for a client's rights and ensure resources are accessible. The therapist may need to serve in different roles such as mediator, negotiator, or enforcer with external persons and organizations.
Collaborating	Collaborating emphasizes a partnership with the client to ensure that the client plays an active role in the therapeutic process. This mode provides the client with choice, freedom, and autonomy as much as possible.
Empathizing	Empathizing is when the therapist seeks to understand the client's thoughts, feelings, and behaviors. This approach focuses on ensuring that the client feels trusted and understood rather than just focusing on the client's therapy goals.
Encouraging	Encouraging describes when the therapist takes on the role of a cheerleader or motivator to instill hope and confidence in a client. This mode is used to motivate a client through positive reinforcement with an attitude of positivity and playfulness.
Instructing	Instructing is when the therapist takes on the role of teaching through clear explanations of the plan, sequence, and events of therapy. This mode gives consistent objective feedback about performance. It may also involve setting boundaries on client demands.
Problem solving	Problem solving describes when the therapist acts as a facilitator. The therapist systematically works through issues using logical thinking, outlining choices, and utilizing strategic questions. The therapist provides opportunities to ensure that the client knows the pros and cons of available choices and opportunities.

Adapted from Taylor, R. R. (2008). *The intentional relationship model: Occupational therapy and use of self.* Philadelphia, PA: F. A. Davis.

change in the therapist's approach of relating to a client. Mode shifts are frequently required in response to interpersonal events in therapy. For example, if a client perceives a therapist's attempt at problem solving is insensitive or off the mark, a therapist would be wise to switch from the problem-solving mode to an empathizing mode. This would allow the therapist to get a better understanding of the client's reaction and the root of the dilemma. Spotlight 12-5 describes a mode shift during an interpersonal event between Janice and Sarah.

Interpersonal reasoning is important to determine if a mode shift is required and then to identify which alternative mode would be best. Sometimes, an interpersonal event is seen as insignificant by both the therapist and client. This would be an example of when a mode shift would not be needed. Sometimes, the therapist is already in the right mode and a shift is not required. Other times, the situation has changed or certain client characteristics have become more important at a particular moment, necessitating a mode shift. After changing modes, it is important to get feedback from the client about whether the mode is suitable. Examples of seeking feedback include the following:

- Checking in and asking how the client feels about the situation.

- Inquiring if the client feels supported by the therapist.

- Asking if there is anything that is still bothering the client that he or she would like to talk about.

Mode shifts may occur many times during a therapy session, or not at all. To be highly adaptive, it is recommended that occupational therapy practitioners learn to use all six therapeutic modes to increase ease and comfort in applying the best approach.

Nontherapeutic Responses

A therapist's words or behavior can be said to be therapeutic if a client feels connected, supported, and understood. A therapist's response can be defined as ***nontherapeutic*** when it results in a negative emotional response from the client. There are many reasons and circumstances as to why a therapist would choose a nontherapeutic response. Therapists are human. It is common for any person to feel hurt or upset when trying to help someone and that person does not behave or respond in the way that is expected. At times, people have stressful or hectic days, act impulsively, and feel physically or mentally unwell. There are also times when a therapist may be preoccupied by daily life situations and personal problems. Therapists may unconsciously

---

SPOTLIGHT 12-5. THERAPEUTIC MODE SHIFTS

Therapeutic modes and *mode shifts* are evident in the interpersonal event presented in Spotlight 12-2. Sarah used an instructing mode when she initially introduced different backrests to Janice. Sarah taught Janice how to use the different backrests, explaining and demonstrating the pros and cons of each backrest. Sarah felt a mode shift was necessary when Janice started sobbing during her emotional interpersonal event. Sarah was initially puzzled about why Janice was sobbing. Sarah reasoned within herself that the empathizing mode was the most effective method to let Janice know that she was present with her in her struggle. The empathizing mode was effective, as Janice felt understood by Sarah.

Janice still felt helpless that her mother did not understand her though. Sarah intentionally wanted to help Janice be more empowered in her communication with her mother. Sarah used interpersonal reasoning and decided that there was a need for another mode shift. She decided to use the collaborating mode when she asked Janice if she wanted to focus on something different. Janice did want to change the direction of the therapy session. She wanted to change the focus of the session to communicating effectively about her pain with her mother. Sarah used the rest of the therapy session to consciously give Janice the lead during brainstorming. Sarah constantly asked her opinion and asked Janice how she felt about each option.

---

ignore a client when the client expects or needs their direct attention. A response cannot automatically be defined as nontherapeutic or therapeutic. That being said, some responses carry a higher possibility of being nontherapeutic. Table 12-1 shows a list of possible nontherapeutic responses that may be encountered.

When communicating with therapeutic modes or using a mode shift, the IRM emphasizes that the mode should be applied in pure form. That means the therapist should not blend the modes together. This may create confusion by sending mixed signals. Blending of modes increases the chance of creating a form of nontherapeutic response. Spotlight 12-6 describes possible nontherapeutic responses that Sarah could have used in response to an interpersonal event.

Interpersonal Dynamics

Engaging a client in therapy requires the understanding that the client exists within a wider social system. This involves understanding the client's role and relevant interpersonal dynamics that may affect participation in occupation and affect how the client reacts to the therapist. Questions help the occupational therapy practitioner understand how the client's social context facilitates or impedes occupational engagement. Questions that the occupational therapy practitioner may consider include the following:

- Who are the individuals that comprise the system, and what is their relationship to the client (e.g., parents, friends, extended family members, or other clients)?
- Who are the most engaged members of the system? Who are the most disengaged?

- Who are the most prominent or influential members? How do they exert their power? How effective are they at influencing the client?
- What does the client appear to expect or need from others in the system?
- What do others appear to expect or need from the client?
- Is communication within the system shared, open, and direct, or are there certain alliances and indirect routes of communication?
- What are the positive dynamics that support the client's best interests?
- What negative dynamics exist?
- How are disagreements or conflicts of interest managed?

Distinguishing Between Positive and Negative Dynamics of a System

A *dynamic* defines the distinctive pattern, emotional tone, and interpersonal events that comprise the interaction between individuals. Every dynamic serves a purpose even if it is not a productive or positive dynamic. A dynamic involving competition for parental approval may be observed between clients and their siblings, for example. In this case, the dynamic increases the likelihood that at least one of the siblings will receive approval from a usually critical parent. A dynamic may also become repetitive and subconscious over time.

Dynamics can be positive or negative. *Positive dynamics* work in such a way as to benefit and produce positive feelings for both persons in the relationship. Examples

TABLE 12-1

UNDERSTAND POTENTIALLY NONTHERAPEUTIC RESPONSES

RESPONSE	DESCRIPTION
Parental response	A *parental response* describes a response often used with children or younger clients that is meant to be caring but may come across as being overprotective. It may appear as if the therapist thinks that the client is incapable. *Example:* "I'm so sorry about your fall. You should really take care of yourself."
Defensive response	A *defensive response* is a response that usually clarifies and explains the therapist's rationale or gives feedback to the client. It may be perceived by the client that the therapist is trying to justify himself or herself, or give excuses for decisions, intentions, or positions. It also depends on the tone of voice and words that are chosen. *Example:* "I was only trying to help you."
Minimizing/exaggerating responses	A *minimizing response* downplays the importance of what a client says. It is often used when a therapist does not want the client to focus too much on certain preoccupations; however, it may come across as being insensitive. *Example:* "C'mon, it doesn't seem that bad!" An *exaggerating response* is the opposite of a minimizing response. A therapist adds more to what a client says. It may be used when the therapist tries to bring a client out of denial to the existing problem. The client, however, may not be ready to face the problem yet. *Example:* A client says, "I feel sad sometimes" and the therapist responds, "So, tell me more about your depression."
Responses that compare	*Responses that compare* describe when a therapist compares the client's progress or situation to another client in an attempt to motivate the person. This may encourage the client, but also may potentially be discouraging. It could be discouraging if the client has a lot of self-doubt present or if the client is unable to be receptive. *Example:* This may occur when the client is too tired, unwilling, or angry about the situation.
Premature responses	A *premature response* describes when a therapist is too eager to help or gives excessive compliments. This can occur when the therapist wants to motivate a client. This response may be perceived as nontherapeutic if the client feels the therapist is not sincere, overly positive, or unrealistic. *Example:* The occupational therapy practitioner states, "You've done an excellent job. Now we can move on to the next task" before the client even finishes the task.
Cliché responses	Although a therapist may be trying to encourage a client, the therapist can respond with a *cliché response*. Cliché responses are overused statements. They can be thought of as insincere or minimizing by the client. Example: "Every cloud has a silver lining."

Adapted from Taylor, R. R. (2008). *The intentional relationship model: Occupational therapy and use of self.* Philadelphia, PA: F. A. Davis.

of positive dynamics include *trusting* and *collaborative dynamics*. Trusting and collaborative dynamics are characterized by vulnerability and teamwork. This can be evident when a client and caregiver work to achieve a desired outcome. Most relationships with clients will be characterized by dynamics that are productive when a therapist is self-disciplined and does not treat therapeutic relationships as a way to fulfill personal needs. Spotlight 12-7 presents an example of a trusting dynamic in the case example of Janice.

SPOTLIGHT 12-6. SARAH AND POSSIBLE NONTHERAPEUTIC RESPONSES

Referring back to the situation in Spotlight 12-4, there were times when Sarah could have reacted in nontherapeutic ways. Examples include:

- When Janice was sharing her experience at dinner with her mother, Sarah could have responded, "I know how you feel." This could have been perceived as a cliché response. This response could have been nontherapeutic if Janice felt that Sarah was giving her a response for the sake of a response and not really empathizing with her.

- When Janice was sharing her experience, Sarah could have also interceded too early to talk about communication solutions. Being too quick to return to the specific intervention strategy before Janice felt accepted and understood could have been perceived as a premature response.

- Sarah could have also responded excessively by being too eager to help or have a tone in her voice that showed she was not being respectful. This could have been perceived as a patronizing response. Examples of a patronizing response include: "How can a mother do or say something like that?" or "If I was your mother, I would never say such a thing to my child!" Sarah may have just been trying to help Janice feel understood by responding this way. Unfortunately, Janice could also have perceived this as being disrespectful toward someone who Janice still respects deeply. Such a response may backfire. Janice could become upset and less connected with Sarah, resulting in the response not being beneficial.

SPOTLIGHT 12-7. JANICE AND A TRUSTING DYNAMIC

A trusting dynamic of mutual trust is observed most of the time between Janice and Sarah. For example, when Janice feels confident about Sarah's ability to teach her how to manage her housework better because of their mutual trust. Janice displayed her trust in Sarah by her earnest attempts to learn the strategies being taught. A sign of trust was also expressed when Janice asks for feedback. This showed that she was confident in Sarah's judgment, skills, and strategies. Sarah also had faith in Janice and a belief that Janice wanted to learn. Sarah returned this trust by showing a genuine interest in teaching. Evidence of the enhanced connectivity in the trusting dynamic was displayed when Sarah showed happiness or pleasure at Janice's accomplishments.

It is possible to be invited or drawn into a negative dynamic with a client even when the therapist is trying to sustain a positive dynamic. This is particularly likely when a client is accustomed to using maladaptive patterns of relating to others. It is critical to be able to recognize the difference between positive and negative dynamics for this reason.

Negative dynamics are similar to positive dynamics in that they benefit at least one individual within the system. Negative dynamics, however, are usually inefficient and involve negative feelings or outcomes for at least one member of the group. An example of a negative dynamic is when teenage clients struggle to identify themselves as individuals and don't take responsibility for the consequences of their actions. A teenager using this dynamic continues to ask parents for advice but only to protest and explain why the guidance offered is unhelpful or does not work. The same negative pattern could occur between the teenage client and the therapist. This is commonly referred to as a *help-seeking and help-rejecting dynamic.* Parents and teenagers end up feeling frustrated and unsatisfied as a result. Examples of negative dynamics that have the potential to

affect the process or outcomes of therapy are presented in Table 12-2. Although Table 12-2 provides examples of particular systems in which these dynamics are most common, any of these dynamics may occur within a relationship.

In long-term relationships, positive and negative dynamics may emerge. At times, the lines are blurred and it becomes unclear whether a dynamic is ultimately positive or negative. Sometimes, negative dynamics become so familiar that they are assumed to be positive due to their familiarity. Persons in the dynamic may not be aware that anything is wrong even though the dynamic may be hurtful or uncomfortable. An example of this type of situation is often found in an abusive relationship where there is a dominance and submission dynamic. Often, victims of abuse will not want to end the abusive relationship even though they know it is not healthy. It is also possible that dynamics that were once thought to be positive may become negative over time (and vice versa). The nature and combination of potential dynamics that can occur within a given social system are endless. Spotlight 12-8 describes a negative dynamic that Janice was involved in with her ex-husband. In this case example, Janice's husband was no

TABLE 12-2

DYNAMICS THAT AFFECT THE OCCUPATIONAL THERAPY PROCESS

DYNAMIC	DESCRIPTION
Help-seeking/help-rejecting	The *help-seeking/help-rejecting* dynamic describes when a person develops a pattern of asking for help or advice and then counteracts any help by explaining why it would not work. Possible outcomes include negative emotions and increased passivity by the help seeker. This dynamic is often seen in relationships between parents and children. If it is a long-standing pattern, it can occur in the therapeutic relationship as well.
Competitive	The *competitive* dynamic describes when an individual competes to obtain something that he or she perceives to be important and in short supply. Conflict arises between the competitors, as well as feelings of decreased self-esteem in the loser if this becomes a long-standing pattern. Examples include competition between siblings for parental attention and approval. It also can occur between clients in group therapy for resources.
Enabling negative behavior	The *enabling negative behavior* dynamic describes when a person gives consent or supports the negative behavior of another individual by enabling it. Passivity and lack of opposition for the behavior are actions that permit this dynamic. As a result, the negative behavior becomes more entrenched. This often is observed in close relationships where people are afraid of disappointing the other individual. This can also make the individual angry, or lose the relationship altogether.
Dominance/submission	The *dominance/submission* dynamic is created when there is a clear power difference between certain individuals who are constantly oppressed by others. People in power continue to oppress others to compensate for a perceived lack of control and feelings of insecurity in other aspects of their lives. Individuals who assume a submissive role do so for various reasons. Examples include perceiving that the relationship is still advantageous and easier for them in some way despite being mistreated, as well as low self-esteem. This could lead to learned helplessness, a pattern of aggression, passivity, or even abuse. These dynamics most likely occur in caregiving or couple relationships where one person is vulnerable. Abusive or abused individuals should be referred to mental health services.
Enmeshment	An *enmeshment* dynamic occurs when individuals become overly intimate, protective, and loyal to each other. There is a lack of individuality that reflects in similar behaviors and values. It can appear as being overly dependent on each other in decision making. An example is a caregiving relationship where the caregiver is too involved in the client's care. Health care professionals can find individuals secretive and controlling, which can hamper development of a therapeutic relationship. Enmeshment dynamics are most often observed in families and couples.
Disengagement	A *disengagement* dynamic is the opposite of the enmeshment dynamic. This relationship is characterized by minimal sharing of individuals or information. People in this relationship view themselves as being independent of others in values and behaviors. Individuals in this dynamic may feel isolated and disappointed in other people's lack of presence and investment. This can be caused by a lack of communication and connection between members. Caregivers may be uninvolved and unaware of a client's need for care as an example. This may result in physical or medical neglect. Similar to enmeshed relationships, disengaged relationships are most often observed in families and couples.
	(continued)

TABLE 12-2 (CONTINUED)	
DYNAMICS THAT AFFECT THE OCCUPATIONAL THERAPY PROCESS	
DYNAMIC	**DESCRIPTION**
Approach/avoidance	The *approach/avoidance* dynamic describes individuals who expect a relationship to meet their unfulfilled needs. This relationship begins with intense closeness followed by avoidance of the other person. Individuals may avoid the relationship for various reasons. The relationship is centered on an intense and unrealistic expectation to be admired or accepted. As a result, contradictory feelings about the relationship may arise, such as fear of rejection, abandonment, or feelings of suffocation by the relationship. This is often seen in couples' relationships where one partner repeatedly approaches with unrealistic expectations and the other partner repeatedly finds ways to withdraw. The outcome is a relationship that fluctuates between extreme closeness and openness to feelings of rejection and abandonment. This dynamic may occur in a therapeutic relationship where clients who seem extremely open in one session appear distant or do not show up for the subsequent session.
Idealizing/devaluing	An *idealizing* dynamic occurs when an individual admires another person in an unrealistically positive light without acknowledging the person's negative characteristics. A *devaluing* dynamic is the opposite in which the negative characteristics are exaggerated. Some people tend to have very distinctive positive or negative perceptions of people. Although it may seem flattering to be highly valued by another individual, eventually the dynamic becomes uncomfortable or infuriating. The compliments and special treatment suddenly turn to rejection and accusations. This dynamic is often observed in therapeutic relationships where the client has unrealistic expectations of the therapeutic outcomes. At the same time, the client does not want to actively participate or accept the less-than-ideal outcome.
Reluctance/reassurance	The *reluctance/reassurance* dynamic occurs when individuals are consistently self-doubting and anxious about their ability to engage in occupations. Others automatically respond through reassurance and promise of rewards. The individual may become dependent on such responses if this dynamic occurs repetitively and predictably. It can also result in slow or limited progress in therapy.
Demonstrative/ voyeuristic	The *demonstrative/voyeuristic* dynamic occurs when individuals exaggerate or dramatize their difficulties and emotions. They often demonstrate their need to be recognized and validated for their hardship. The demonstrative and voyeuristic dynamic is created when others continue to encourage this behavior or find it humorous or amusing. Voyeurism may further reinforce the demonstrative behavior. Voyeurism is neither a helpful nor ethical way of relating, especially in a therapeutic relationship.
Helpless/rescuing	The *helpless/rescuing* dynamic describes when individuals continue to appear needful and receive assistance when it is no longer necessary. This behavior is often due to a need to be loved, attended to, or cared for by others. For some individuals, any effort to help them will be futile as their needs are too strong. Other individuals consistently enable the helpless behavior by assisting without being aware that it is not necessary. This results in learned helplessness and dependency in one individual and frustration in the helper. This dynamic can be seen as a norm in some cultural contexts and may not be problematic. This is most often observed in parents of disabled children who feel guilty or responsible for the child's impairments. The parents, however, are usually unaware of the consequences of enabling the child's helpless behavior.

(continued)

TABLE 12-2 (CONTINUED)

DYNAMICS THAT AFFECT THE OCCUPATIONAL THERAPY PROCESS

DYNAMIC	DESCRIPTION
Chaotic/organizing	A *chaotic/organizing* dynamic is created when individuals who are disorganized, undisciplined, or lack self-control are reciprocated by another person who constantly compensates for that behavior. Examples include providing practical supports such as reminders or scheduling the other person's appointments. Emotional supports such as reassurance may also be provided so that the person can function. Although the organizing person may be emotionally and physically drained, the individual still continues to provide support. The other person is reinforced to continue with the chaotic behavior. This dynamic is often observed in relationships where one person has an impairment or disability such as attention deficit hyperactivity disorder.
Manipulating/conceding	A *manipulating/conceding* dynamic describes a pattern of using manipulative methods to get what a person wants or needs. These individuals have a deep understanding of what others need or want and use it to their advantage. The conceding individual is supporting the dynamic when the individual gives in to demands due to feelings of obligation or guilt. This perpetuating cycle leaves the conceding person feeling upset, angry, and unable to set limits for the manipulator. This dynamic may often be observed in parents or teachers who are unsure about disciplinary approaches and often feel guilty about setting limits consistently. It can also be observed in therapeutic relationships if a therapist is not clear about boundaries.
Scapegoating	The *scapegoating* dynamic occurs when a group of individuals conspire to influence, criticize, shame, or control another individual. Groups may choose to act in this manner if they feel the "scapegoat" is threatening or a misfit in the system. This often occurs when people are looking for someone to blame. The most powerless and vulnerable individual is usually selected as the scapegoat. This dynamic is most likely to occur within families or groups. It can also occur when a therapist forms an unhealthy alliance with one group of clients against another, or with one partner of a couple against the other.

Adapted from Taylor, R. R. (2008). *The intentional relationship model: Occupational therapy and use of self.* Philadelphia, PA: F. A. Davis.

SPOTLIGHT 12-8. JANICE AND NEGATIVE DYNAMICS

Negative dynamics were evident as Janice began to open up about her past relationship with her husband. Janice's husband was an alcoholic and was not able to hold down a job for long. Janice took on the role of being the main breadwinner for her family and supported them financially. She gave her husband money when he asked for it even though she was upset and angry inside. She grumbled but always allowed him to drink. Janice was enabling his negative behavior, as she was supporting his habits. At the same time, he was abusive when he was drinking. She was often the victim as she tried to protect her children during these moments. She gave in to her husband's threats of hurting their children by offering herself to be beaten. This was evidence of the dominance/submission dynamic in their relationship. She did not want to tell anyone about the abuse and refused help when people were concerned. Janice always downplayed her situation as not being as bad as it seemed.

longer present in her life and there was no need to manage that dynamic anymore. There could be lingering effects, however, of that dynamic on her relationship with others.

Managing Maladaptive Dynamics in a System

Every therapist will encounter negative dynamics in his or her practice of occupational therapy at some time. Understanding dynamics will enable the therapist to:

- Understand the implications of dynamics and their impact on the client and therapy process.
- Anticipate the effects of dynamics on the therapeutic relationship.
- Remain an objective observer of dynamics.
- Make an intentional decision about whether or not to manage the dynamics.

Negative dynamics are very difficult to change. They involve negative feelings for the client or other members of the relationship. Even though the client knows that it is causing hurt or pain for someone or everyone in the system, the client and other members of the system are likely to continue acting the same way. It is important to begin with empathy, knowing that systems are naturally hard to change. In order to understand a client's negative dynamics, a therapist should try to understand that:

- It is usually not one person's problem but the problem of multiple people in the system that in some way contributes to a negative dynamic.
- There is always a purpose in sustaining a negative dynamic. What needs does the negative dynamic serve for the client and other members of the system? What might the members of the system lose if they stop acting the way they do?
- What is the history behind a negative group dynamic? Did it start a long time ago or recently? Are there patterns of this dynamic that trace back to similar dynamics in childhood? How does their history put them at risk to develop and continue this dynamic?

The next step is to decide whether to remain an objective observer of the maladaptive dynamics or try to manage and remove them. In order to decide what to do, therapists should ask the following questions:

- Is the dynamic interfering with the course of therapy?
- Does the client think that this dynamic is negatively affecting his or her quality of life?
- Is the client or other group members using a similar negative dynamic within their relationship with you? If so, how will this affect the therapeutic outcomes?

Use of Modes to Improve Relationship Dynamics

Therapeutic modes are not only employed by the therapist with a client, but can also be a useful way of improving a client's dynamics with other people. The importance of mode purity and flexibility may be taught in order to ensure that negative dynamics are replaced with new positive dynamics. Suggestions that the therapist can utilize to improve a client's dynamics with other people include:

- Define the six modes using lay terminology, and discuss how they can be used in everyday interactions.
- Identify through observation the mode or modes that seem to be most comfortable to the client.
- Identify the strengths of the client's preferred modes.
- Discuss common cautions of preferred modes and encourage the client to brainstorm about the times when these modes did not work well.
- Identify the mode or modes that may need to be developed for more positive dynamics in the client's relationship.
- Weigh the pros and cons of introducing a new mode or modes into the relationship.
- Identify the likely short-term, negative but brief side effects, as well as long-term, positive dynamic changes of introducing a new mode or modes to a relationship.

The epilogue in Spotlight 12-9 describes what happened to Janice after participating in occupational therapy. Exposing clients to the concept of modes is highly challenging. It requires a tremendous amount of empathy and trust within the relationship so that the client does not feel judged or criticized for his or her current efforts in relationships. There also needs to be evidence that the client is capable of learning to use new modes.

SUMMARY

Therapeutic use of self is a fundamental aspect of occupational therapy practice. It has significant implications in terms of the process and ultimate outcomes of therapy. Initiating and maintaining a relationship that supports occupational engagement is a complex and dynamic process. Therapists must be intentional in order to be effective and responsive to a client's developing interpersonal needs during therapy. This chapter reviewed the occupational therapy literature on therapeutic use of self. It also described a conceptual practice model that addresses the need for communication skills training in occupational therapy. The

> ### SPOTLIGHT 12-9. EPILOGUE OF JANICE
>
> Janice attended 16 sessions of occupational therapy within a 6-month time period. Each session was 45 minutes long. Sarah, her occupational therapist, spent the first session assessing her participation in activities of daily living and discussing the goals of therapy. Janice was most concerned about her ability to complete her housework and take care of her children. Janice learned strategies to stay in control of her pain utilizing a combination of medical and therapeutic techniques. Therapeutic techniques included learning to pace her activities with frequent breaks and modification of household activities. She also learned to incorporate cognitive and bodily relaxation techniques in association with her daily activities. Janice felt that simply planning her time was the most important strategy. It helped her accomplish things that were important to her with less emotional stress. Toward the last few sessions, Janice felt more confident to explore work options. Janice found that she enjoyed interacting with people and decided that she did not want go back to being an assistant accountant.
>
> Janice started working a part-time position 4 hours per day as a beauty consultant with a major beauty label. This job allowed her to use her lifestyle management strategies, as she could manage her time independently. She became increasingly more aware of the state of her body and made realistic goals to accomplish each week. Janice worked out a way to actively engage her children in helping with the housework so she did not have to do everything herself. She also found that she was able to deal with her pain with less medication by employing alternative coping strategies. Janice prioritized more time with her children to fulfill her role as mother, which gives her the most meaning in life. Janice began to feel more confident and calm concerning her future. She started a relationship with a man who she says she is happy with and he treats her well. Janice continued to desire to be dependent on herself and still works to be independent from others. Although Janice continues to struggle with the helpless/rescuing dynamic, she chooses to allow her new partner to support her partially.

IRM, a conceptual practice model, was explained to guide clinical reasoning and communication in this important area of practice. This model provides practical skills necessary to create trust and effective communication during the occupational therapy process through the use of therapeutic modes. The IRM model provides new concepts and concrete, usable clinical skills that are necessary to foster and improve relationships in occupational therapy practice.

PART 3: APPLICATIONS

The following activities will help you analyze and apply key aspects of the IRM within this chapter. Activities can be completed individually or in a small group to enhance learning.

1. Think of an encounter with a friend or relative that involved a fair degree of conflict or tension. For example, you and your friend may have had different opinions or viewpoints about an important issue that you both cared about.

   a. Considering the six therapeutic modes, describe your approach to communication with your friend. What modes did you attempt to use?

   b. Were they successful or not? Why?

   c. Were there modes you wished you had used but did not?

   d. Would your approach to communication been considered therapeutic or nontherapeutic if your friend had been a client?

2. Identify a group that you participated in last week. Reflect on your behavior and communication style when you are communicating within the group. Common group situations in which students may find themselves include classroom situations, volunteer leadership roles, social groups, athletic teams, therapy, and self-improvement groups that you may have attended.

   a. Considering the six IRM modes, what was your predominant mode or modes of communication within that group?

3. As a group or individually, reflect on a situation that you found remarkable.

   a. Describe the interpersonal dynamics involved in IRM terms.

   b. What positive communications and dynamics occurred, if any?

   c. Did any maladaptive dynamics occur? If so, label and describe them in IRM terms.

4. Reflect on a recent conversation when someone was resistant to your suggestion or upset with you. Thinking about the six therapeutic modes, answer the following questions:

a. Describe the event that occurred.

b. Describe how you initially communicated with your friend before your friend became resistant or upset.

c. Was a mode shift necessary? If so, how did your communication change afterward?

5. Think about another situation when you were in a vulnerable condition and asked for help from another person. Answer the following questions:

a. What are some of the interpersonal characteristics that were evident in this situation?

b. Did the person respond in a way that showed consideration for your interpersonal characteristics? Give some examples.

c. Was there any part of the person's response that was not therapeutic or helpful to you? If so, identify some examples.

REFERENCES

American Occupational Therapy Association. (2008). Occupational therapy practice framework: Domain and process (2nd ed.). *American Journal of Occupational Therapy, 62*(6), 625-683.

Ayres-Rosa, S. A., & Hasselkus, B. R. (1996). Connecting with patients: The personal experience of professional helping. *Occupational Therapy Journal of Research, 16*(4), 245-260.

Baum, C. M. (1980). Occupational therapists put care in the health system. *American Journal of Occupational Therapy, 34*(8), 505-516.

Bing, R. K. (1981). Occupational therapy revisited: A paraphrastic journey. 1981 Eleanor Clark Slagle lecture. *American Journal of Occupational Therapy, 35*(8), 499-518.

Bockoven, J. S. (1971). Occupational therapy—a historical perspective: Legacy of moral treatment—1800's to 1910. *American Journal of Occupational Therapy, 25*(5), 223-225.

Cara, E., & MacRae, A. (1998). *Psychosocial occupational therapy: An evolving practice* (3rd ed.). Clifton Park, NY: Delmar Cengage Learning.

Clark, F. (1993). Occupation embedded in a real life: Interweaving occupational science and occupational therapy. 1993 Eleanor Clarke Slagle lecture. *American Journal of Occupational Therapy, 47*(12), 1067-1078.

Cole, M. B., & McLean, V. (2003). Therapeutic relationships re-defined. *Occupational Therapy in Mental Health, 19*(2), 33-56.

Denton, P. L. (1987). *Psychiatric occupational therapy: A workbook of practical skills.* Boston, MA: Little, Brown.

Devereaux, E. B. (1984). Occupational therapy's challenge: The caring relationship. *American Journal of Occupational Therapy, 38*(12), 791-798.

Duncan, E. A. (Ed.). (2011). *Foundations for practice in occupational therapy* (5th ed.). Edinburgh, UK: Elsevier.

Fleming, M. H. (1991a). Clinical reasoning in medicine compared with clinical reasoning in occupational therapy. *American Journal of Occupational Therapy, 45*(11), 988-996.

Fleming, M. H. (1991b). The therapist with the three-track mind. *American Journal of Occupational Therapy, 45*(11), 1007-1014.

Frank, J. D. (1958). Therapeutic use of self. *American Journal of Occupational Therapy, 8*(4), 215-225.

Gilfoyle, E. M. (1980). Caring: A philosophy for practice. *American Journal of Occupational Therapy, 34*(8), 517-521.

Hagedorn, R. (1995). *Occupational therapy: Perspectives and processes.* New York, NY: Churchill Livingstone.

Jonsson, H., Josephsson, S., & Kielhofner, G. (2001). Narratives and experience in an occupational transition: A longitudinal study of the retirement process. *American Journal of Occupational Therapy, 55*(4), 424-432.

Kielhofner, G. (2004). *Conceptual foundations of occupational therapy* (3rd ed.). Philadelphia, PA: F. A. Davis.

Kielhofner, G. (2009). *Conceptual foundations of occupational therapy practice* (4th ed.). Philadelphia, PA: F.A. Davis.

Kielhofner, G., & Burke, J. P. (1977). Occupational therapy after 60 years: An account of changing identity and knowledge. *American Journal of Occupational Therapy, 31*(10), 675-689.

King, L. J. (1980). Creative caring. *American Journal of Occupational Therapy, 34*(8), 522-528.

Lyons, K. D., & Crepeau, E. B. (2001). The clinical reasoning of an occupational therapy assistant. *American Journal of Occupational Therapy, 55*(5), 577-581.

Mattingly, C. (1994). The narrative nature of clinical reasoning. In C. Mattingly and M. H. Fleming (Eds.), *Clinical reasoning: Forms of inquiry in a therapeutic practice* (pp. 239-269). Philadelphia, PA: F. A. Davis.

Mattingly, C., & Fleming, M. H. (1994). Interactive reasoning: Collaborating with the person. In C. Mattingly and M. H. Fleming (Eds.), *Clinical reasoning: Forms of inquiry in a therapeutic practice* (pp. 178-196). Philadelphia, PA: F. A. Davis.

Mosey, A. C. (1970). *Three frames of reference for mental health.* Thorofare, NJ: Slack, Inc.

Mosey, A. C. (1981). *Occupational therapy: Configuration of a profession.* New York, NY: Raven Press.

Parker, D. M. (2006). Implementing client-centered practice. In T. Sumsion (Ed.), *Client-centered practice in occupational therapy: A guide to implementation* (2nd ed., pp. 55-73). Edinburgh: Churchill Livingstone.

Peloquin, S. M. (1989a). Moral treatment: Contexts considered. *American Journal of Occupational Therapy, 43*(8), 537-544.

Peloquin, S. M. (1989b). Sustaining the art of practice in occupational therapy. *American Journal of Occupational Therapy, 43*(4), 219-226.

Peloquin, S. M. (1990). The patient-therapist relationship in occupational therapy: Understanding visions and images. *American Journal of Occupational Therapy, 44*(1), 13-21.

Peloquin, S. M. (1993). The depersonalization of patients: A profile gleaned from narratives. *American Journal of Occupational Therapy, 47*(9), 830-837.

Peloquin, S. M. (1995). The fullness of empathy: Reflections and illustrations. *American Journal of Occupational Therapy, 49*(1), 24-31.

Peloquin, S. M. (2002). Reclaiming the vision of reaching for heart as well as hands. *American Journal of Occupational Therapy, 56*(5), 517-526.

Peloquin, S. M. (2003). The therapeutic relationship: Manifestations and challenges in occupational therapy. In E. B. Crepeau, E. S. Cohn, & B. A. Boyt Schell (Eds.), *Willard and Spackman's occupational therapy* (10th ed., pp. 157-184). Philadelphia, PA: Lippincott Williams & Wilkins.

Schell, B.A. (2003). Clinical reasoning: The basis of practice. In E. B. Crepeau, E. S. Cohn, & B. A. Boyt Schell (Eds.), *Willard and Spackman's occupational therapy* (10th ed., pp. 131-152). Philadelphia, PA: Lippincott Williams & Wilkins.

Schwartz, K. B. (2003). The history of occupational therapy. In E. B. Crepeau, E. S. Cohn, & B. A. Boyt Schell (Eds.), *Willard and Spackman's occupational therapy* (10th ed., pp. 5-13). Philadelphia, PA: Lippincott Williams & Wilkins.

Schwartzberg, S. L. (1993). Therapeutic use of self. In H. L. Hopkins, & H. D. Smith (Eds.), *Willard and Spackman's occupational therapy* (8th ed., pp. 269-274). Philadelphia, PA: Lippincott.

Schwartzberg, S. L. (2002). *Interactive reasoning in the process of occupational therapy.* Upper Saddle River, NJ: Pearson Education.

Shannon, P. D. (1977). The derailment of occupational therapy. *American Journal of Occupational Therapy, 31*(4), 229-234.

Taylor, R. R., Lee, S. W., Kielhofner, G. W., & Ketkar, M. (2009). Therapeutic use of self: A nationwide survey of practitioners' experience and attitudes. *American Journal of Occupational Therapy, 63*(2), 198-207.

Taylor, R. R., Lee, S. W., & Kielhofner, G. (2011). Practitioners' use of interpersonal modes within the therapeutic relationship: Results from a nation-wide study. *Occupational Therapy Journal of Research, 31*(1), 6-14.

Townsend, E. (2003). Reflections on power and justice in enabling occupation. *Canadian Journal of Occupational Therapy, 70*(2), 74-87.

Yerxa, E. J. (1967). Authentic occupational therapy: Eleanor Clark Slagle lecture. *American Journal of Occupational Therapy, 21, 1-9.*

Yerxa, E. J. (1980). Occupational therapy's role in creating a future climate of caring. *American Journal of Occupational Therapy, 34*(8), 529-679.

SUGGESTED READING

Taylor, R. R. (2008). *The intentional relationship model: Occupational therapy and use of self.* Philadelphia, PA: F. A. Davis.

13

Use of Therapeutic Groups in Occupational Therapy Treatment

Christine A. Manville, EdD, OTR/L

KEY TERMS

- Activity Analysis
- Activity Demands
- Activity Group
- Activity Synthesis
- Adaptation
- Behavioral Group
- Closed Group
- Cognitive
- Communication Patterns
- Didactic Teaching
- Directive Group
- Expressive Group
- Group
- Group Climate
- Group Cohesion
- Group Content
- Group Duration
- Group Frequency
- Group Gradation
- Group Interaction Skills
- Group Protocol
- Group Reality Testing
- Group Size
- Group Treatment
- Open Group
- Peer Learning
- Personal Space
- Psychodynamic Group
- Psychoeducational
- Revolving Membership
- Ringelmann Effect
- Role
- Routines
- Schedules
- Self-Help Group
- Sensory Integration
- Sensory Integration Group
- Sensory Modulation
- Support Group
- Systems Theory
- Task Group

CHAPTER LEARNING OBJECTIVES

After completion of this chapter, students will be able to:

1. Define the term *group*.

2. Summarize the benefits of using group treatment.

3. Analyze the impact of the basic elements used to frame a group on its overall effectiveness.

4. Determine the impact of those elements on the level of participation among group members.

5. Differentiate between a variety of groups on a continuum of task and interpersonal components, and note the similarities and differences among them.

6. Create a group protocol based upon client needs.

Manville, C.A., & Keough, J. L.
Mental Health Practice for the Occupational Therapy Assistant (pp 307-333).
© 2016 Taylor & Francis Group.

CHAPTER OUTLINE

INTRODUCTION

Historically, in the practice area of mental health, much of occupational therapy is carried out in activity-based groups, with the goals of developing skills and encouraging social interaction among members (Allen, 1987; Duncombe & Howe, 1985; Howe & Schwartzburg, 2001). In the group setting, the actions of doing and communicating coalesce into a powerful therapeutic tool that can be used to help clients explore and develop new or adapted roles in society (Bullock & Bannigan, 2011). The Occupational Therapy Practice Framework, 3rd ed. (American Occupational Therapy Association [AOTA], 2014) defines the term *role* as a set of behaviors expected by society and shaped by culture. In other words, a *role* is a set of expectations about the ways in which people are supposed to behave in different situations. It is through interactions with others that individuals learn significant life roles, such as "friend," "student," "employee," and "parent." Each role is structured by the expectations of others and the social and cultural systems in which it is located. Occupational therapy practitioners use groups to facilitate client engagement in meaningful tasks and activities that support participation in desired roles. Groups can help participants develop knowledge and self-awareness, build specific skills, and explore new behaviors, as well as increase the desire to make needed changes to effectively perform valued roles.

Groups are a powerful therapeutic tool, but what exactly is the role of the occupational therapy assistant in regard to group work? To answer that question, one must begin by exploring the skill set that is required of the occupational therapist and the occupational therapy assistant who work in the practice area of mental health. Understanding role delineation and supervision requirements is especially important in practice areas that have a high demand for practitioner autonomy, such as mental health, in order to ensure that both entry-level and seasoned practitioners are working within the profession's Standards of Practice and state licensure laws. Although the occupational therapist and occupational therapy assistant share a common fundamental knowledge base, their academic learning objectives differ (Accreditation Council for Occupational Therapy Education, 2013); therefore, the practice expectations for an entry-level occupational therapist and occupational therapy assistant differ as well. In all settings, the occupational therapy assistant works "under the supervision and in partnership with" occupational therapists (AOTA, 2014, p. 51). To delineate the responsibilities of each practitioner further, a document entitled "Specialized Knowledge and Skills in Mental Health Promotion, Prevention, and Intervention in Occupational Therapy Practice" (AOTA,

2010) was created to outline the knowledge, reasoning, and performance skills necessary for competent and ethical occupational therapy practice in mental health promotion, prevention, and intervention. In regard to group work specifically, it is stated that the entry-level occupational therapist is competent to design and execute group interventions, whereas the occupational therapy assistant is competent to *assist* in the design and execution of group interventions in mental health practice. In other words, an entry-level occupational therapy assistant is not expected to design or lead groups independently.

When discussing the group as a therapeutic intervention, it is important to note that the skills required to design and lead groups involve a combination of artistic and scientific abilities (Cara & MacRae, 2013). The scientific aspect refers to the framing process that incorporates the structural elements with which a group is built. Preparation for this process includes the development of a group protocol that addresses both the needs of the setting and the population with whom one works. The group protocol is a template that outlines the group and explains why it was designed, what it is used for, how it should run, and who can participate in it. Design of a group protocol requires knowledge of occupation and activity analysis, both of which are included in the curriculum taught in occupational therapist and occupational therapy assistant programs.

The artistic components are based on knowledge and include practiced application of communication techniques and group process. It requires that the occupational therapy practitioner attend simultaneously to the needs of the individual participants and the group as a whole. The effective group leader is constantly observing and analyzing interpersonal dynamics, while skillfully implementing the communication techniques required at that particular moment to effectively move the group forward. These skills cannot be learned by reading a book or taking a single college course. The art of successful group leadership requires a combination of the *knowledge* of group dynamics with *ongoing practice* in the implementation of group skills *under the supervision of a trained group leader.*

Part 1: What Is a Group?

Participation in groups is a fundamental part of life, beginning at birth. Our quality of life depends to a large degree on our ability to effectively function within the groups to which we belong, whether it is our family, the neighborhood, or the larger community (Baumeister & Leary, 1995). Socialization starts within the family unit and then continues on in play groups, classrooms, and peer groups as a child grows and learns new roles within the community setting. As adults we usually choose to participate in groups formed by individuals with common interests, such as church groups, social groups, and work groups, all of which provide us with opportunities to learn how to interact effectively with other individuals in a variety of situations. The part we elect to play in such groups may range from passive to very active. Over our lifetime, our personal identity and self-esteem are derived, in large part, from the way in which we are perceived and treated by other members in our groups. Groups are significant sites of socialization and education, and offer a setting where our relationship skills can develop and where people find companionship, help, and support. Groups make it easier for us to complete a wide variety of tasks; help us establish meaningful social bonds; encourage us to experiment with new roles; and help us create, maintain, and change our sense of self.

Disagreements are plentiful among professionals as to the correct definition of the word *group*, and many variations of the term exist. One method commonly used to define the word derives from systems theory. **Systems theory** is the interdisciplinary study of systems in science and society. It provides a theoretical framework for describing and analyzing groups of objects that work together to produce results. According to this theory, a group can be considered a system because it has identifiable parts (members), yet it is a whole entity (group), with each part interacting with and influencing the work of the other. It is therefore more than just the sum of its parts (Lewin, 1947). Thus, if one group member is nonparticipative in a session, the group as a whole can still achieve its goal. One way to visualize the group using a systems approach is to consider the example of a baseball team. There are nine individuals (members) on the field, each of whom plays a different position. Even though each individual is a skilled player, the team will not automatically win solely because these individuals are put together on the field, nor will they automatically lose just because one member is having an "off day." Rather, the goal of winning the game is achieved by members (players) *working together* as a unit.

Another way to think of a group is as a purposeful or planned coming together of members with the intention of producing change (Bruce & Borg, 2002; Hagedorn, 2000; Howe & Schwartzberg, 2001). In 1973 Mosey defined the group as "an aggregate of people who share a common purpose which can be attained only by group members interacting and working together" (p. 45). When considering both of these definitions, it is understood that not every gathering of people can be considered a group. Rather, a **group** is a collection of people who have a *shared purpose* for being together (Early, 2012).

Do occupational therapy groups differ from groups led by other health care professionals? Currently, there is no specific definition of an occupational therapy group, per se. Given the profession's core belief in the relationship between occupation and health, the assumption may be made, however, that the format of occupational therapy groups will most likely include the use of activity and emphasize occupation. In addition, they will address occupational performance skills and patterns, with the goals being to aid in adaptation; improve or enhance occupational performance and quality of life; promote role competence, client satisfaction, and health and wellness; prevent unhealthy lifestyle choices; and/or provide advocacy skills (AOTA, 2014).

Historically, occupational therapy activity groups were used primarily to treat mental illness; however, over the years the focus of groups has broadened from treatment of the mentally ill population to include client education in the "well population" as a means for illness prevention (Hildenbrand & Lamb, 2013). Occupational therapy practitioners contribute to the promotion of health and participation of people through engagement in occupation, and one of the modalities that can be used for that purpose is group work. Howe and Schwartzburg (2001) have described four factors that influence and/or justify the use of activity groups by occupational therapy practitioners for client treatment:

1. The importance of occupation to health

2. The ability to adapt group structures and goals to changing patterns of treatment

3. The importance of interpersonal relationships to wellness

4. Socioeconomic pressures that shape health care, including cost effectiveness and reimbursement.

PART 2: BENEFITS TO GROUP TREATMENT

"It is usually easier to change individuals formed into a group than to change any one of them separately" (Lewin, 1951, p. 228).

Group treatment is a planned process for creating changes in individuals, bringing them together for this purpose. In the early 20th century, physicians were using groups as a tool to help their patients with mental illness cope with their disease (Pratt, 1922). Although group treatment was initially used to increase staff efficiency, physicians soon discovered that the patients were experiencing benefits from the structure of the group itself. These benefits included the opportunity to gather support and hear information from peers who understood their problems from a personal perspective. In a later study, Lloyd and Mass (1997) had similar findings. They concluded that clients value the commonalities found with fellow group members and the opportunities to experience support, talk freely, and feel "in touch" with others.

There are other important advantages to group work as well. Some of the additional benefits of group education and treatment are as follows:

- People learn who they are by experiencing how others respond to them in groups; therefore, group treatment is often more realistic than one-on-one therapy. Feedback from fellow group members may help individuals perceive themselves more accurately and encourage them to try out new roles.

- There is a connection between problems experienced in daily life and the work world. As clients engage in group activities, they express characterlogical difficulties seen in their everyday occupations. Attention to these problems, as they emerge in the here and now, can benefit the client, since the way members behave in the context of the group is usually reflective of how they interact with others outside of the group.

- Group treatment facilitates personal growth by virtue of providing an individual with more people with whom to interact. This increases the opportunity for more feedback and different types of interactions. Participants learn about themselves by identifying with others, comparing and contrasting their experiences, values, and beliefs with fellow group members.

- *Peer learning* (learning from those one perceives as equals rather than those one perceives as authorities) feels comfortable to many people; therefore, the group supports trying out new skills and experimenting with different behaviors. Groups offer social persuasion, with the ability to change attitude and behaviors through peer pressure and social support.

- There is greater potential for skill development in activity groups, as participants can actually practice skills they wish to master, as well as learn by observation of their peers (Corey, Corey, & Corey, 2010).

- Groups provide the opportunity for reality testing. *Reality testing* is defined as "the ability to tell the difference between reality and fantasy and to share the same general ideas about reality as everyone else" (Cole, 2012, p. 22).

- Participation in groups diminishes feelings of isolation and promotes a sense of belonging.

- Activity groups permit a single occupational therapy practitioner to assess the capacities of a number of patients simultaneously, making it a time-efficient evaluation process.

- Treating people in groups means that several individuals can receive treatment at the same time; thus, group treatment is considered cost effective.

- Groups provide the occupational therapy practitioner with the opportunity for observation of members. Even though group members may be essentially nonverbal, observations can be about an individual when an activity is the primary focus of a group. By effectively communicating those observations to the treatment team, the occupational therapy practitioner plays an important role in the treatment of clients with acute psychiatric illnesses. Checkpoint 13-1 provides a list of behaviors that a leader may observe as a participant engages in an activity group. Each behavior is accompanied by a description of inappropriate and appropriate (typical) behavior, allowing the observer to better gauge the individual's function within the group.

Although there are numerous advantages to the use of group treatment, there are also limitations, given that the group must also meet the needs of every individual client. For example, on an acute care inpatient unit for individuals diagnosed with mental illness, a planned group activity may be too stimulating or require too high a degree of abstraction for the client diagnosed with schizophrenia who is currently experiencing auditory hallucinations and feelings of paranoia. Such symptoms may limit his or her ability to join in discussion and work alongside peers. Likewise, at a rehabilitation center, an individual who recently experienced a stroke may be too disoriented and confused to tolerate even minimal group interaction. Thus, the occupational therapy practitioner who is leading a group must consider the existing strengths, functional limitations, and skills of every individual in order to select appropriate group activities and promote successful group participation for all members. One particular skill that must be evaluated prior to placing a potential member into a group is the client's level of group interaction skill. A discussion on the development of group interaction skills follows.

PART 3: DEVELOPMENT OF GROUP SKILLS

How do human beings develop the ability to interact with others? An occupational therapist by the name of Anne Mosey analyzed the development of group interaction skills. She defined the term ***group interaction*** skill as:

> … the ability to be a productive member of a variety of primary groups. Through acquisition of the various group interaction subskills, the individual learns to take appropriate group membership roles, engage in decision making, communicate effectively, recognize group norms and interact in accordance with these norms, contribute to goal attainment, work toward group cohesiveness, and assist in resolving group conflict. (Mosey, 1970, p. 201)

Assessing group interaction skills informs you of a person's capabilities. In her research, Mosey identified five levels of group interaction skill, which are summarized in Checkpoint 13-2. Group interaction skills are defined as the "ability to participate in a variety of groups in a manner that is satisfying for oneself and for one's fellow group members" (Cole, 2012, p. 379). In creating these levels, Mosey suggested that people do not automatically learn interaction skills and may need help to develop them. Specifically, she claimed that such skills can be learned through task-oriented groups that are designed to use activities that help patients develop a particular level of skill. Mosey went on to say that people at different levels of group interaction skill require different levels of involvement from the group leader and varied types of interaction with other participants. Specifically, at each successive level, as social interaction becomes more important in the group, the role of the therapist becomes less directive.

Developmental groups simulate the variety of nonfamilial groups typically encountered in normal development. They are task oriented. The task in these groups does not always result in a tangible end product; at the highest level, task accomplishment is emphasized equally with meeting the needs of other group members. For best results, it is recommended that individuals be placed in a group that is functioning no more than one level above the level of group interaction skill present at the time of an individual's evaluation. Using this formula is said to facilitate growth in social skills. Information on the baseline level of group interaction skills is obtained by the occupational therapy practitioner through the client interview as well as observation of the individual in informal group situations. In order for a member to benefit from a developmental group, (1) the behavior that is interfering with development must be identified, (2) the behavior to be learned must be specified, and (3) the participant must be provided with opportunities to engage in the desired behavior. Learning of a specific group interaction skill is enhanced by feedback from fellow group members and reinforcement from the group leader. In addition, it is facilitated though availability and use of good role models.

PART 4: FRAMING THE GROUP

Groups are organized systems of interactions and relationships that are regulated by their structure. Although the definition of structure varies among researchers and professions, it appears that there are common properties used to frame any type of group. According to Schwartzburg, Howe, and Barnes (2008), group structure is created by the combination of a number of elements that includes the goals of the group, group climate, group membership, group composition, and the communication patterns between the group leader and group participants. These elements, which are described next, can be varied depending on the type and purpose of the group, as well as the needs and functional level of its members. It has been said that

CHECKPOINT 13-1. BEHAVIORAL OBSERVATIONS

(Note: The endpoints are listed for a continuum that describes inappropriate to appropriate behavior).

General Observations

Activity level	• Client is severely retarded in speech, physical reaction, and movements (hypoactive) *or* highly accelerated in speech or action (hyperactive).
	• Client speaks, reacts, and moves at a normal, appropriate rate.
Affect	• Client demonstrates continuous flat affect and/or affect inappropriate to the situation.
	• Client demonstrates facial expression that is spontaneous and appropriate to the situation.
Anxiety	• Client appears highly anxious, fidgety, and/or agitated.
	• Client appears calm, relaxed, and attentive.
Appearance	• Client's hygiene is poor and/or he or she dresses inappropriately for sex, age, or occasion and/or the clothes are unkempt.
	• Client's hygiene is adequate. He or she dresses appropriately for age, sex, or occasion, and the clothes are clean and well kept.
Bizarre behavior	• Client rocks, plays with hands, appears to be talking to self, and/or appears preoccupied with own thoughts.
	• Absence of the above.
Concept formation	• Client demonstrates an inability to understand or formulate abstract ideas. He or she only understands simple, concrete concepts.
	• The client is able to deal with both concrete and abstract concepts effectively.
Mood	• Client appears severely depressed (sad; crying; withdrawn; preoccupied with feelings) or manic (high; giggling; constant talking; pressured speech; expansive ideas).
	• Client demonstrates a positive frame of mind and appropriate responses to the situation/topic.
Reality orientation	• Client is disoriented or confused as to time, date, and place and/or he or she articulates distorted ideas or expresses delusional thinking.
	• Client is oriented to time, date, and place. He or she articulates a realistic view of him- or herself and the environment.
Self-esteem	• Client articulates an excessive amount of self-derogatory comments and/or demonstrates self-destructive behavior.
	• Client is able to identify and accept personal strengths and limitations, and expresses that he or she likes himself or herself.

Interpersonal Behavior

Amount of interaction	• Client does not interact *or* he or she talks incessantly to the point that it interferes with functioning.
	• Client demonstrates an appropriate level of interaction for group activity.
Attention from others	• Client seeks excessive attention from others and/or seeks attention, verbally and/or nonverbally, in a socially inappropriate manner.
	• Client seeks attention in a socially appropriate manner.

(continued)

CHECKPOINT 13-1. BEHAVIORAL OBSERVATIONS (CONTINUED)

(Note: The endpoints are listed for a continuum that describes inappropriate to appropriate behavior).

Interpersonal Behavior

Content of verbalizations	• Client articulates comments that are inappropriate to the situation and/or discussion topic. • Client does not articulate inappropriate comments.
Cooperation	• Client refuses to follow direction, opposes suggestions or constructive criticism, and/or refuses to participate in group. • Client willingly follows directions, accepts constructive feedback, and tries out suggestions from other group members.
Group task roles	• Client does not assume a role in selection, planning, and/or execution of the group activity. • Client assumes an active role in the selection, planning, and/or the execution of the group activity.
Independence	• Client constantly relies on others for direction, guidance, decisions, and emotional support. • Client is self-reliant in carrying out tasks.
Manner of relating	• Client relates in a guarded, suspicious manner, and/or relates negatively or with aggression, and/or dominates or overwhelms other group members, and/or relates in a condescending manner with others. • Client relates in an appropriate and spontaneous manner with others.
Responses from others	• Client's actions or speech evoke negative responses from other group members. • Client's actions or speech evoke positive responses from other group members.
Self-assertion	• Client is passive, excessively compliant, and/or unable to seek assistance when needed *or* aggressive and demanding to get own way, insisting on immediate assistance when help is needed. • Client makes wishes and desires known in an assertive, socially acceptable manner.
Sociability	• Client does not voluntarily join others in activity. He or she is withdrawn and unable to carry on a casual conversation. • Client readily and appropriately participates in group activities. He or she spontaneously carries on conversations with others.

Task Behavior

Ability to follow verbal directions	• Client is unable to follow verbal instructions (include apparent reason for the inability, such as difficulty with concentration, disorientation, anxiety, etc.). • Client is able to follow verbal directions correctly and without apparent difficulty.
Ability to follow written directions	• Client is unable to follow written instructions (include apparent reason for the problem, such as disorientation, illiteracy, etc.). • Client is able to follow written instructions correctly and without apparent difficulty.
Activity neatness	• Client performs activity in a sloppy manner. • Client performs activity in a neat, orderly manner.

(continued)

CHECKPOINT 13-1. BEHAVIORAL OBSERVATIONS (CONTINUED)

(Note: The endpoints are listed for a continuum that describes inappropriate to appropriate behavior).

Task Behavior	
Attention to detail	• Client is overly concerned with detail to the point that it interferes with his or her performance. • Client attends to detail according to the demands of the activity.
Complexity	• Client can only engage in simple, one-step activities that involve the use of few materials or tools. • Client is able to engage in activities that require the use of a variety of tools and materials and/or which require several steps for completion.
Concentration	• Client rapidly loses interest in the activity or task, and/or is highly distractible, and/or is unable to focus on just one aspect of the activity or task at a time. • Client is able to work on a given task or activity with sustained interest and attention.
Engagement	• Client does not engage in activity. • Client readily engages in activity without prompting or encouragement.
Fine motor coordination	• Small muscle movements are clumsy and/or inaccurate. • Small muscle movements are coordinated and accurate.
Frustration tolerance	• Client is easily frustrated. He or she responds to frustration with aggressive behavior and/or refuses to continue to engage in the activity or task.
Gross motor coordination	• Large muscle movements are clumsy or inaccurate. • Large muscle movements are coordinated and accurate.
New learning	• Client is unable to learn new activities *or* learns new activities very slowly. • Client learns a new activity quickly and without apparent difficulty.
Organization to task	• Client is unable to effectively organize his or her approach to the activity or task. • Client organizes a task in a logical, effective manner.
Performance standards	• Client sets unrealistically high *or* low standards for performance of an activity or task given expected, acceptable results. • Client sets standards for performance of an activity or task that are compatible with expected, acceptable results.
Problem solving	• When confronted with a problem, the client is unable to identify options or evaluate alternative courses of action in order to make a decision, and/or the client is unable to use past experience in deciding course of action, and/or the client is unable to utilize available resources appropriately. • Client identifies and solves problems that arise in the performance of an activity. He or she uses resources in an appropriate manner and is able to make use of past experiences to decide course of action.

Adapted from Fidler, G., & Fidler, J. (1963). *Occupational therapy: A communication process in psychiatry.* New York, NY: MacMillan Group.

CHECKPOINT 13-2. UNDERSTAND DEVELOPMENTAL GROUP INTERACTION SKILL LEVELS			
Level	*Description of Group*	*Expected Client Behavior*	*Activities*
Parallel group	Clients work side by side on individual projects. Consequently, little interaction is required with other individuals in the group. The role of the leader is to define the task and provide emotional support and assistance for each member as needed.	• Engages in some type of activity, but acts as if this is an individual task as opposed to a group activity *or* • Aware of others in the group, evidenced by limited verbal and nonverbal interaction with others	• Basic crafts • Imitative group exercise
Project group	This group emphasizes the completion of a short-term group task (1 to 2 hours). Members share space, tools, and supplies, which requires some level of social interaction and cooperation. The leader assumes a directive role in that she or he selects the activity and structures the tasks required for project completion. Trial and error learning is encouraged within the group.	• Occasionally engages in the group activity, moving in and out according to whim • Occasionally seeks assistance from others • Gives some assistance to others when specifically asked by leader to do so	• Craft projects requiring multiple steps
Egocentric-cooperative group	In this group the members select and implement the task over one to two sessions. Social interaction is required, and group members are expected to respond to one another's needs. The leader assumes a facilitory role as needed, making suggestions but allowing the group to choose and carry out their own plan.	• Aware of the group goal relative to task • Aware of group norms • Act as if they belong in the group • Willing to participate in activity • Meets the esteem needs of others	• Cooking group
Cooperative group	Members are encouraged to express and share thoughts and feelings while participating in a group activity. The task is not the primary focus; rather, the goal is to provide an experience in which members have the opportunity to share information and listen to one another. The leader has the role of an advisor in this group.	• Makes needs, wishes, and desires known • Participates in group activity, but concerned primarily with meeting individual needs of self and others • Tends to be most responsive to group members who are similar to him or her in some way	• Values clarification groups
Mature group	In this group, task accomplishment is balanced with need satisfaction. Members independently select, plan, and complete a group task with a specific end product. The task experience is used in order to help members learn and practice new personal roles and task roles. The function of the group takes priority over individual needs.	• Responsive to all group members • Assumes a variety of roles within the group • Shares leadership • Promotes a good balance between task accomplishment and satisfaction of the needs of group members	• Community outing

any group can be better understood by examining the basic elements upon which it is designed.

Group Content

The profession of occupational therapy is founded on the belief that engagement in meaningful activities supports health and participation in life. As such, engagement in activity is a focus of one-on-one occupational therapy intervention as well as group interventions. Occupational therapy groups in mental health settings should differ from therapy groups led by other professions in that doing, or activity, is the medium through which group members achieve their goals. Studies suggest that the use of activity in a group is more effective in promoting participation in treatment than verbal-based therapy alone (Bickes, Deloache, Spicer & Miller, 2001; Cowls & Hale, 2005; Hagedorn & Hirshhorn, 2009). Occupational therapy activity groups may utilize experiential or nonexperiential activities (Cara & MacRae, 2013; Poole, 1995). In an experiential approach, the client practices the actual activity to be learned, such as completing an employment application. In the nonexperiential approach, the client will participate in an activity that promotes development of performance skills required to enhance occupational engagement. An example of a nonexperiential activity would be role-playing how to engage in general conversation, as skills such as active listening and eye contact provide a foundation for a successful employment interview. The use of both approaches is supported by the literature. Research has shown that incorporating experiential activities reinforces the content taught in a group (Kolb, 1984; Townsend, 1996), while participation in creative activities maximizes learning potentials and forms strong memories (Hare, 1982).

According to information listed in the document "Specialized Knowledge and Skills in Mental Health Promotion, Prevention, and Intervention in Occupational Therapy Practice" (AOTA, 2010), it is expected that the entry-level occupational therapy assistant possess the skills to *assist* the occupational therapist to "[d]esign and implement individual and group interventions that support development of cognitive, sensory regulation, social, and communication skills requisite for role performance" (p. 11). This document also states that the occupational therapy assistant should possess the skills to *independently* "[d]evelop intervention sessions using activities to teach and practice new skills and when possible develop actual opportunities to engage in needed tasks such as work or school tasks" (p. 11). These statements support the role of the occupational therapy assistant, under the supervision of a licensed occupational therapist, as a leader of activity-based groups where the skills needed to perform meaningful occupations, including activities of daily living and instrumental activities of daily living, are taught to participants.

Group content is a term that describes the activities and topics incorporated into a group session (Cole, 2012; Denton, 1987). Content is used to achieve group goals; for example, collaboration on a concrete, clearly defined task encourages direct and clear communication. A group activity may be straightforward and explicit (i.e., learning how to sort laundry, practicing meal preparation), or it may be a creative exercise used to explore symbolic meaning (i.e., drawing a picture that depicts an individual's hopes and dreams). In general, the greater the complexity of the task and the more time it takes to organize the group's efforts, the less time will be available to actually engage in the activity and achieve the intended goals. The type of activity that is utilized may lend itself to large group cohesiveness or the development of small subgroups. The selection of content, however, should always be based upon (1) what participants need and are expected and able to do, (2) the level of group interaction skills, and (3) the degree to which the members are capable of cooperative effort.

Content must also take into consideration the personal context of the individual group members (i.e., age, gender, socioeconomic level, and educational level), as well as performance skills and client factors. The Occupational Therapy Framework defines **client factors** as "specific abilities, characteristics, or beliefs that reside within the client and may affect performance in areas of occupation" (AOTA, 2014, p. S7). If these skills are deficient, the leader will have to structure the activity in a way that compensates for those deficiencies. In general, the higher the level of impairment in mental functions such as attention and memory, the more structured the activity needs to be. Claudia Allen (1999) defined six cognitive levels and 52 modes of performance in her cognitive assessment tool, which allows for a detailed evaluation of client cognitive ability. She suggests grouping clients with similar cognitive levels for maximum benefit from group treatment (Penny, Mueser, & North, 1995).

It is important that the occupational therapy practitioner analyze potential activities to understand what is required of the group member and to consider how those requirements relate to individual treatment goals.

> **Activity demands** refer to the specific features of an activity that influence the type and amount of effort required to perform the activity, the social demands, sequence and timing, the required actions or skills needed to perform the activity, and the required body functions and structures used during the performance of the activity. (AOTA, 2014, p. S32)

The activity analysis should also take into consideration the specific objects and tools required and the skills required in order for members to use them effectively. Consideration of these factors is important since the less members identify with the group content and participate in the activity, the less effective the group will be. Therefore, the content should include developmentally appropriate, meaningful activities that are intended to develop performance skills and aid in adaptation. The purpose of such activities is to improve occupational performance, promote role competence, address client satisfaction, and/or enhance the quality of life of its members.

One of the biggest challenges for an entry-level occupational therapy practitioner in selecting group content is the large number of potential choices that exist. Because of this variety, and in order to save time, some practitioners rely on the use of resource books that contain handouts with preselected activities and themes for their groups. Although there is nothing inherently wrong with this method and such handouts are convenient, it should be cautioned that effective group activities should always be selected based on client need and ability, and include a focus on performance.

Group Goals

Group goals are the purpose for which the group meets. They establish a commonality that supports cohesiveness. *Group cohesiveness* is defined as the sense of solidarity the members feel toward one another and the group. It is based on a feeling of closeness and identification with other members. Cohesiveness is a critical element in any group. It serves the same purpose as trust and rapport in an effective client–therapist relationship. It ties people together with a sense of belonging and signals the health of a group. In a healthy group, individual members feel safe trying out new and unfamiliar roles because they trust that the group will not reject them if they fail. They are willing to be influenced by other members and take the risk of trying new skills and behaviors.

The clarity of goals affects cohesiveness. Without clear goals and a reason for being together, a group may flounder, fail to develop cohesiveness, and fall apart. In treatment groups, the participants need to know why they are meeting and what they can expect to accomplish. Goals with clear behavioral expectations and purpose are required to motivate individual group members to participate in groups. Therefore, if the purpose of the group is not expressly stated to participants at the beginning and the activity not understood to be relevant to group members, they may choose not to engage. Likewise, when group goals are important to a person, what other members say and feel in the group become important as well. Thus, the group becomes a powerful agent for change.

Finally, goals are important as a tool with which to assess and evaluate the success of a group. The AOTA Occupational Therapy Practice Framework (2014) defines the types of outcomes that can be used to measure group success, including improvement or enhancement in occupational performance, client satisfaction, quality of life, role competence, adaptation, health and wellness, prevention, and promoting healthy lifestyles or occupational justice. A behavioral observation form is usually filled out by the leader following each group and includes notes on all participants. Table 13-1 provides an example of a behavioral observation form that may be used. Information from the observation form is reviewed and incorporated into daily or weekly progress notes, depending on the documentation requirements of the program. Assessment and observation should focus on individual goals, as well as the purpose of the group as a whole.

Group Climate

Group climate refers to the emotional environment within the group. The climate determines whether a member feels safe and accepted by his or her peers and able to express thoughts and emotions. Group climate is influenced by context and environment. The term *context* refers to a number of interrelated conditions that "are within and surrounding the client" (AOTA, 2014, p. S42). In the Occupational Therapy Practice Framework, contexts are described as cultural, personal, temporal, and virtual. Environment, on the other hand, refers to the physical and social environments. The *physical environment* refers to the nonhuman environment—the building and the room within which the group is located and the objects found within it, such as chairs, tables, and lights. The *social environment*, on the other hand, is created by the expectations of the program in which the group is run, as well as the staff who are employed to work in that program. The social environment contributes to the "atmosphere" of the institution, which may encourage or discourage interaction between group members. Both the physical and social environments are important considerations in analysis of potential group activities. Although group leaders may have limited control over the social environment of the facility in which the group is held, there may be instances where improvements can be made in the physical environment in which the group is conducted.

Many disciplines have affirmed the important impact of environmental variables on human behavior (Bell, Green, Fisher, & Baum, 2001; Gieryn, 2000). Physical factors may create stress for group members and consequently facilitate or block effective communication within the group. The environment can, among other things, be too large or small, too hot or cold, too noisy, and/or contain too many distractions. A small group held in a large space may contribute to an atmosphere of isolation and loneliness that results in decreased communication. A room that is too warm may contribute to increased irritability and aggressive behavior among members. The same is true for noise and distractions. In general, the louder the noise, the more likely it is to produce distraction and irritation, and possibly sensory overload. In general, individuals cope with overload in a group by reducing their interaction with one

TABLE 13-1

EXAMPLE OF A BEHAVIORAL OBSERVATION FORM

Client: _____   Date: _____

Context of Observation (Check all that apply):

Group Activity: _____   Individual Activity: _____

Unstructured activity: _____   Structured Activity: _____

Interview: _____   Other (Specify): _____

1. Significant Problem ☐   **2. Moderate Problem** ☐   **3. Minor Problem** ☐   **4. No Problem** ☐

GENERAL BEHAVIOR	COMMENTS	1	2	3	4
Activity level					
Affect					
Anxiety					
Appearance					
Bizarre behavior					
Concept formation					
Mood					
Reality orientation					
Self-esteem					
Comments:					

INTERPERSONAL BEHAVIOR	COMMENTS	1	2	3	4
Amount of interaction					
Attention from others					
Content of verbaliza-tions					
Cooperation					
Group task roles					
Independence					
Manner of relating					
Responses from others					
Self-assertion					
Sociability					
Comments/group Interaction skill level:					

TASK BEHAVIOR	COMMENTS	1	2	3	4
Ability to follow verbal directions					
Ability to follow written directions					
Activity neatness					

(continued)

TABLE 13-1 (CONTINUED)					
EXAMPLE OF A BEHAVIORAL OBSERVATION FORM					
TASK BEHAVIOR	**COMMENTS**	**1**	**2**	**3**	**4**
Attention to detail					
Complexity of task					
Concentration					
Engagement					
Fine motor coordination					
Frustration tolerance					
Gross motor coordination					
Ability to process new learning					
Organization to task					
Performance standards					
Problem solving					
Comments:					

Adapted from Fidler, G., & Fidler, J. (1963). *Occupational therapy: A communication process in psychiatry.* New York, NY: MacMillan Group.

CHECKPOINT 13-3. APPLY

You have been instructed by the occupational therapist to plan a reminiscence group for six individuals who are diagnosed with Alzheimer's disease and reside in an assisted care facility. What would be the ideal environment in which to hold this group in order to obtain maximum engagement from the participants?

---

another, ignoring select aspects of the situation ("zoning" out of the discussion) and shutting down altogether (closing their eyes, falling asleep). Overcrowding a small room with a large group of people is likely to increase social interaction, but it will also magnify the potential for interpersonal conflict among group members. Too much conflict can decrease the likelihood of productive group work. On the other hand, the use of a quiet, well-lit room that is not cluttered and allows for comfortable seating in a circular arrangement where everyone can see each other generally promotes social interaction and facilitates discussion. That being said, occupational therapy practitioners may find that they are limited as to where groups can take place due to safety concerns. For example, if the group consists of members who have been diagnosed with dementia and are restricted to a locked unit, the choice of rooms in which to hold a group will be limited. In those instances, it is very important to carefully consider the elements of group composition in an effort to compensate for potential problems in the physical environment. Checkpoint 13-3 provides the reader with an opportunity to practice designing a physical environment for a specified population.

Group Composition

Another factor that affects the level of participation within a group is its **composition**. This is defined by several variables, including the differences and similarities among the members (i.e., age, developmental level, culture, knowledge, skills, and motivation on the group topic), whether the group is open or closed, the size of the group, its duration, the time of day and frequency with which it occurs, and how long it meets.

Membership

An important element in group structure is the makeup of the membership. Matching clients with the right groups is critical for success of the group as well as the individual who participates in them. As mentioned earlier in the chapter, when selecting individuals for groups, the occupational therapy practitioner must consider the nature of the available groups as well as existing strengths, functional limitations, skill levels, and individual treatment goals of potential members. In addition, the occupational therapy practitioner must consider the program's resources, such as staffing, the availability and location of group rooms, and the type and amount of supplies available for the group.

Not all groups are appropriate for everybody. The client's readiness to participate is one critical ingredient for success. In order to arrive at a decision on a client's readiness and appropriateness for group treatment, the data obtained from formal evaluation and clinical observation are analyzed along with information obtained from the treatment team and unit staff. Readiness is also determined, in part, by how a client understands and deals with his or her illness and whether he or she views the topic of a group as personally relevant. In the acute setting, one can anticipate that these factors will change as the client progresses in treatment; therefore, the type of group and the individual's suitability for groups in general will likely change from one day to the next.

Similarities among members may lead to increased cohesion in the group, but there can also be advantages to creating a diverse membership with respect to chronological or developmental age, life experiences, and/or skill levels. A diverse population increases the opportunity for an assortment of feedback and role models. It increases the variability of social interactions, which is more reflective of the "real world" that exists outside of the group.

At times, membership for those groups that are held on inpatient units or in outpatient programs may be predetermined by program structure, availability of staff, and requirement of third-party payers. For example, on most acute care mental health units with "bundled" treatment costs, the expectation is that all clients will attend occupational therapy groups. If admission on a behavioral unit in a large hospital is open to adults aged 18 or over with any type of mental illness, there will likely be a wide variation in abilities and skills among group members. The occupational therapist may address the variation by selecting a group activity that can be adapted to skill level and/or by creating smaller subgroups of individuals that work together on the task within the larger group. For maximum learning and interaction, these subgroups should be composed of individuals who are compatible in developmental interaction skills and abilities.

Open Versus Closed Groups

Another consideration when selecting an appropriate treatment group is to consider whether the group is open or closed. Groups in which the membership remains stable are termed *closed groups*. Because membership is fixed, the development of trust and cohesiveness is maximized. This encourages members to take risks and experiment with new roles and skills that can lead to behavioral change outside the group setting (Yalom, 1983). Closed groups are usually small, with 15 or fewer members. Each week, new learning builds on what has taken place in prior meetings, which necessitates that members be in the group from its start.

Two variations of the closed group include a time-limited group and the ongoing group in which members fill vacancies as they occur. An example of a time-limited group is cohort of individuals with substance abuse issues who are attending a recovery program on an inpatient unit. These individuals attend a specified number of groups during their 28-day program, starting and finishing treatment together. An example of an ongoing closed group would be an outpatient therapy group for adolescents with eating disorders who attend an after-school program. The size of the group would never be more than a specified number of individuals, and the leader would fill vacancies with individuals with a similar diagnosis as members graduate from high school and therefore "graduate" from the program.

In an *open group*, membership changes from one group to the next, which is termed *revolving membership*. Revolving membership requires that the group dedicate time and effort to acclimate new members at the beginning of each session. Open groups may have no absolute limit on the number of members, and as such, can make it difficult for participants to feel heard and understood and for members to feel a sense of connection to the group.

Open groups are usually found in acute care inpatient treatment programs, as well as partial hospitalization programs and outpatient support groups. Revolving membership provides increased opportunity for members to interact with a greater number of people, which more accurately reflects real life. However, because individuals must adjust to frequent, unpredictable membership changes, the structure of these groups may have a negative impact on group climate. Open groups, therefore, will require more structure and active leadership in order to develop cohesion. Specific information on group leadership will be addressed in the next chapter.

Size, Frequency, and Duration of Group

Other factors that have a significant influence on group climate and cohesiveness are the size, frequency, and duration of the group. The term *frequency* refers to how often the group meets—for example, twice per week or once per day. The term *duration* refers to the length of time that individuals meet—for example, one 60-minute session or six 30-minute sessions held over the period of 6 weeks. The term *size* refers to the number of members allowed to participate in a group.

In terms of size, in order to be effective, small groups must consist of at least three people. Frequently, however, there is no set upper limit on the number of group members in most treatment settings; rather, the number of participants is determined by the size of the room and the amount of seating. However, the ideal number of group members should be viewed as the smallest number needed to competently complete the group's task or achieve the group's purpose (Corey, Corey, Callahan & Russell, 2003). In smaller groups, more social interaction is likely to occur because there is more time (and therefore opportunity) for each member to speak. In addition, speaking with a smaller number of people may be experienced as less anxiety provoking than speaking in a large group.

Research has shown that groups become less productive as they increase in size. Castore (1962) studied the impact of group size on the number of member-to-member interactions in therapy groups. He found that there was a significant decrease in the number of interactions once group size reached nine or more members. This phenomenon has been attributed to the **Ringelmann effect** (Levinger, Ingham, Graves, & Peckham, 1974), and is said to be caused by the reduction of individual effort when people work together in a group. Generally, as the group gets larger and individual contributions become increasingly difficult to identify, group members perceive their input as less meaningful. When individuals feel as though their level of effort cannot be determined because the task is a collective one, social loafing is likely. Likewise, when people feel that they are being evaluated, they tend to exert more effort and their productivity increases.

Large groups foster anonymity, as only the most vocal individuals have the opportunity to speak. When individuals feel anonymous in a large group, they may exhibit less social responsibility. For example, a group member may not offer feedback to another participant who is struggling with a task, or he or she may hesitate to demonstrate the skills that are needed to successfully complete an undertaking, as it is assumed that somebody else will step up and take that responsibility. As a consequence, the individual who is experiencing the problem may be denied the opportunity to receive constructive peer criticism or observe modeling of more appropriate behavior. Thus, the potential for new skill development decreases. Lack of social responsibility may lead to less task involvement from the group as a whole and lower morale among group participants (Baron & Norbert, 2003, p. 7).

A positive aspect to larger groups, however, is that they are more likely to include people with a range of skills and a variety of opinions. Depending on the goals of the group, this can be a huge advantage. A wide range of skills allows for more specialization of labor in activity groups, as well as more opportunities for observation and modeling of social behavior and work skills. Research has shown that modeling is an effective instructional strategy. According to social learning theorist Albert Bandura (1977), "Learning would be exceedingly laborious, not to mention hazardous, if people had to rely solely on the effects of their own actions to inform them what to do. Fortunately, most human behavior is learned observationally through modeling: from observing others one forms an idea of how new behaviors are performed, and on later occasions this coded information serves as a guide for action" (p. 22).

So, what is the ideal size for a group? Research studies have shown that the optimal size of a group depends on several factors, including the purpose of the group, individual client factors (i.e., age and functional level of the participants), the knowledge and experience of the leader, and type of group. In general, groups consisting of four to nine members are considered the ideal when frequent interaction and group cohesiveness are objectives (Johnson & Johnson, 2013). As mentioned earlier, however, the group leader may have limited control over the size of the group due to a predetermined program schedule and location, especially on acute care psychiatric units. In that case, the leader should consider breaking activity groups or teaching groups of over 12 members into smaller subgroups of 3 to 6 members in order to maximize interaction and learning (Corey, Corey, & Corey, 2010).

The duration of the group also has an impact on whether goals are met. As with group size, individual client factors need to be considered. For example, if the group is held in a school setting, the meeting times should correspond to regularly scheduled class periods whenever possible. As a general rule, younger children should be placed into smaller groups with shorter sessions, and members should be kept within two academic grade levels to ensure that members have the skills to successfully participate in the group. With older children and adolescents, it is better to meet more frequently and for a shorter time in order to match their attention span. A 1-hour session is typically used with adults in order to allow adequate time to complete goals. For a group of lower-functioning members who need maximum direction, such as individuals diagnosed with dementia who reside in an assisted living program, the frequency should be lowered to one to two groups per day and the duration shortened to 30- to 45-minute sessions.

The time of day at which the group is held is also important. For example, individuals diagnosed with major depression or people who have been prescribed antipsychotic medicine can be slow to awaken in the morning, making participation in morning groups more difficult for them. Elderly clients may have a need to take a nap mid-afternoon due to fatigue. Any group held immediately after mealtime has the potential to be interrupted by members requiring a restroom break. All of these examples highlight the importance of considering individual client factors.

Whenever possible, the frequency and duration of a scheduled group should remain consistent to promote the development of schedules and routines among members. **Schedules** represent the big picture—the main activities to be completed daily. **Routines** represent the steps done to complete the schedule. Consistency in routines and schedules helps group members feel secure, avoid confusion, and understand leader expectations, all of which support engagement in the group.

Communication Patterns

Communication patterns describe the flow of information within the group. As stated earlier in this chapter, as a group increases in size, the opportunity that each individual has to interact with other members decreases. But size of the group is not the only factor that affects the amount of social interaction within the group. The arrangement of the physical and social environment affects communication patterns as well. By proper arrangement of space and equipment, the occupational therapy assistant can encourage varying levels of group interaction.

Research has proved that groups behave differently depending on seating pattern (Forsythe, 2006). Seating arrangements significantly influence patterns of interaction, communication, and leadership. For example, studies show that individuals tend to speak immediately after the person sitting opposite from them (Steizor, 1950), and leadership is associated with sitting at the end of the table. Some arrangements, like a circle of chairs, promote interaction by increasing the potential for eye contact and verbal communication. Other arrangements, such as chairs organized into a row, discourage interaction. In general, people prefer seating patterns that promote social interaction, but research shows that preferences vary according to the type of task being attempted by the group (Sommer, 1969).

Personal space refers to the distance required between two or more people as they interact in order for a person to feel comfortable. It provides a boundary that limits the amount of physical contact between individuals (Hall, 1966). The preferred distance is influenced by a number of elements, including psychosocial issues related to mental illness, familiarity with the other person, and the type of situation in which people meet. In addition, personal space extends further in front of the person than behind. In general, when people feel that their personal space is being violated, they respond physiologically—heart rate and blood pressure increase and faster breathing. In some cases, this anxiety can trigger a "flight or fight" response in which a participant leaves the group or uses aggressive behavior to create additional space between himself or herself and others. Therefore, it is very important that a leader consider the need for personal space when creating a group. Table 13-2 explains personal boundaries using five classifications, which are (1) remote zone, (2) public zone, (3) social zone, (4) personal zone, and (5) intimate zone.

PART 5: TYPES OF GROUPS

There are many types of treatment groups led by occupational therapy practitioners working in mental health settings, which range on a continuum from very structured activity groups to minimally structured psychotherapy groups. All of the groups on this continuum contain both task and interpersonal elements; however, the goals of the most structured groups focus more on the development and refinement of basic work skills, whereas the goal of psychotherapy groups focus on the use of group process to increase participants' knowledge of themselves and others. Such knowledge can aid an individual in the decision of whether, when, and how to make difficult and important changes in their lives.

Figure 13-1 illustrates the continuum of groups mentioned earlier. A continuum refers to a continuous sequence (visualize a line) in which adjacent elements are not perceptibly different from one another, but the extreme endpoints are very distinct. In other words, in Figure 13-1, each of the groups found on the line will have something in common with the group alongside of it, but will also have distinct differences. The level of self-disclosure required by group members in order to meet their goals increases as one moves across the continuum from left to right—from participation in skill-based (teaching) activity groups toward the (interpersonal) psychodynamic endpoint. As such, nonverbal, acutely ill individuals or individuals with significant cognitive impairment are usually most appropriate for the groups to the left side of the continuum, whereas individuals in outpatient programs, such as day hospitals, are usually appropriate for groups across the continuum.

The skill level of group leaders and the knowledge they must possess of the theoretical foundations underlying the treatment of mental illness also increases as one moves across the continuum from left to right. It should be noted that although information on all of the groups found on the continuum is included in this text, it is not expected that an entry level occupational therapy assistant be prepared to facilitate all of these groups without additional training beyond graduation and supervision from an experienced leader. Typically, the entry-level occupational therapy assistant with group experience from Level II fieldwork placement will be competent to lead activity and task groups. Group leaders should never attempt to use group techniques or modalities for which they are not trained, and occupational therapy practitioners should always be cognizant of practice laws in their states. Therefore, when new techniques are used with any group, the occupational

TABLE 13-2		
PERSONAL SPACE		
ZONE	DISTANCE	ACTIVITIES
Intimate	Touching to 18 inches	Hugging; kissing; slow dancing; comforting
Personal	18 inches to 4 feet	Handshakes; conversation; discussion; car travel
Social	4 feet to 12 feet	Dining; dealing with a counter person in a fast food restaurant; speaking with a receptionist
Public	12 feet or more	Lectures; plays; recitals
Remote	Various locations	Email; telephone calls
Adapted by from Forsyth, D. R. (2006). *Group dynamics* (4th ed.). Belmont, CA: Thomson Wadsworth Publishing.		

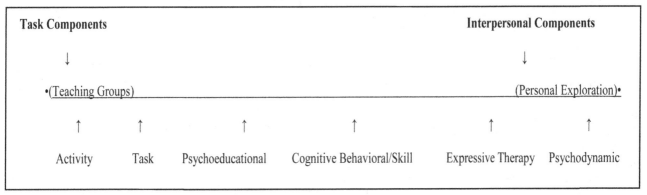

Figure 13-1. Continuum of groups.

CHECKPOINT 13-4. ANALYZE
Go online and explore the occupational therapy practice act in your state as well as another state (your choice). Compare the responsibilities of the occupational therapist and occupational therapy assistant who are using groups as a treatment modality in each state.

therapy assistant should be certain to have appropriate training and supervision from experts who are familiar with the techniques to be employed. Checkpoint 13-4 encourages the student to analyze the occupational therapy practice laws from at least two different states to determine the role of the occupational therapy assistant in conducting therapeutic groups.

Activity Groups

The word *activity*, as commonly defined in the Occupational Therapy Practice Framework (AOTA, 2014), refers to a class of human actions that are goal directed, and includes a broad range of treatment interventions utilized by occupational therapy practitioners. People engage in activities in order to fill their time and give life meaning. The term *activity group* has been described in various ways by different professions; however, all of these definitions

include an action-oriented component that differentiates this group from other therapy groups. Activity groups have been used for rehabilitation purposes by occupational therapists from the earliest days of the profession, and they continue to play an important role in occupational therapy programming for both inpatient and outpatient treatment programs. The content of the group is usually defined by the activity (i.e., cooking group, arts and crafts group, exercise group, relaxation group, work skills group) and is based on the needs and skill levels of the identified group members, as well as general program format and available resources. Activity groups engage participants in focused tasks that are designed to enable change in performance skills, occupations, habits, and routines. They are particularly effective for nonverbal clients, as they typically foster a sense of community and promote social interaction among members. Occupational therapy practitioners frequently use activity groups as an arena in which to observe participants for response to treatment and readiness for discharge.

Task Groups

A **task group** is an assembly of individuals who are brought together to accomplish a specific action or produce a product. Examples of a task group include creating a newsletter or decorating an inpatient treatment unit. According to Fidler (1969):

> Task as it relates to groups is defined as any activity or process directed toward creating or producing an end product or demonstrable service for the group as a whole and/or for persons outside of group ... The intent of the task-oriented group is to provide a shared work experience wherein the relationship between feeling, thinking and behavior is analyzed, and where members explore the impact that their behavior has on others and on task accomplishment. (p. 45)

As individual participants work side by side with other members to complete a clearly defined task, they demonstrate functional capabilities and deficits. Here, the focus of the group is on the interpersonal communication among members rather than task completion. The task group provides the opportunity for members to develop and refine communication skills and experiment with new roles within the group as they deal with issues of control, conflict, and consensus.

Psychoeducational Teaching Groups

Effective **psychoeducational groups** are highly organized and time limited, and integrate principles of teaching and learning with traditional group intervention strategies. The primary purpose of this group is to develop performance, emotion regulation, and cognitive skills of the members by imparting, discussing, and integrating factual information. Content may focus on, among other things, self-improvement and self-awareness; emphasize learning about a specific problem; and/or teach life skills for the purpose of prevention, growth or remediation (Coursey, Curtis, & March, 2000). Psychoeducational groups are structured by the leader and include didactic teaching. In **didactic teaching**, the focus is primarily on the leader who attempts to engage participants in the subject being taught using teaching materials such as diagrams, handouts, photos, and pictures. Psychoeducational groups may include experiential components as well. New information is usually incorporated into the group through planned skill-building activities and/or preplanned curriculum that includes handouts and discussion. These groups offer information that is intended to have direct application to clients' lives. They focus on developing a solid knowledge base upon which sound decisions can be made and effective action taken to remediate or develop skills that may promote wellness, prevent illness, and improve the quality of life (Colum, 2011). When groups consist of members who share a common diagnosis, the content tends to focus on developing knowledge to cope with that specific disorder. In more diverse groups where members have a range of diagnoses and abilities, the educational focus will most likely be on one of the many skills needed to successfully live within the community, such as money management, communication skills, work skills, relaxation, and time management. Members can practice these skills with each other, observe how different people use the same skills, and benefit from the positive reinforcement of a peer group when they use skills effectively.

The leader of a psychoeducational group must always keep in mind that the process of learning and incorporating new skills may be difficult for participants, especially if the previous approach has been used for a long time. Learning new information does not automatically transfer into action; therefore, reviewing one handout on a topic seldom, if ever, results in change since real learning must incorporate knowledge, skills, and motivation. Planning for adequate time in which to practice new skills is essential, and consideration of the context in which the skills will be utilized must also be taken into account when planning the group. Occupational therapy practitioners, with their education in activity analysis, can be extremely effective leaders of psychoeducational groups.

Because client needs vary considerably from one group member to another, the focus of a skill development group should be on a topic that takes into account the unique occupational profile of each participant and includes consideration of client factors, knowledge, skills, and motivation to learn. This information is gathered during the initial occupational therapy assessment. The appropriateness of an individual for a skills development group will depend on the particular needs of the individual along with the skill(s) being taught. Skills development groups may run for a limited number of sessions or consist of a revolving curriculum. The size of the group should be limited, with an ideal range of 8 to 10 participants, as the group should be small enough for members to practice the skills being taught.

With the shorter duration of mental health treatment and the regulations and requirements of managed health care, many professionals utilize the techniques of psychoeducation (Sadock, Sadock, & Ruiz, 2009). To help clients get the most out of psychoeducational sessions, group leaders need to possess basic teaching skills. Teaching components include creating learning goals, group objectives, and participant outcomes; organizing the content to be taught; selecting appropriate teaching modalities; planning for participant involvement in the learning process; and delivering information in a culturally relevant and meaningful way. These techniques are discussed in more detail in Chapter 14.

In addition to understanding the teaching/learning process, the effective leader of psychoeducational groups must meet other criteria. First, although content may be taught using videotapes, PowerPoint slides, handouts, discussions, and/or lecture, the leader should possess content knowledge in the topic area (Galanter, Castaneda, & Franco, 1998) and be prepared to demonstrate the set of skills that the participants are trying to develop. Depending on the skill being taught, certain educational or certification requirements may be required as well. Second, an effective leader should be able to help each group member understand the relevance of the educational topics to his or her life in order to promote motivation, group participation, and learning. Third, leaders need to possess a basic understanding of group dynamics. This includes the ways that groups grow and evolve, as well as knowledge of how people usually relate to one another in a group setting. Finally, and perhaps most importantly, they should be skilled in group facilitation skills and be able to manage the conflict that inevitably arises among members in a group environment. It is crucial that leaders of skill development groups remain sensitive to the struggles of the participants and possess the ability to be positive and patient with individuals who may appear, at times, to be overwhelmed by the task. These topics will also be discussed in Chapter 14.

Occasionally the occupational therapy practitioner may identify a mismatch between the initial analysis of the group members selected to participate in a group and their actual ability to function within it. The importance of appropriately graded psychosocial education in acute illness is supported in the literature (Lieberman & Kopelowicz, 2000; Medaliea, Dorn, & Watras-Gans, 2000). A mismatch will result in frustration for all parties involved—the participant, the leader, and fellow group members. For example, an individual diagnosed with severe anxiety who is too distracted to focus on discussion may begin to demonstrate fidgeting behavior and rocking in his or her chair, distracting the group. Likewise, an individual who is diagnosed with schizophrenia and is unable to deal with the stimulus of a large group of people debating the correct answer to a question may begin to respond to auditory hallucinations and blurt out comments that are not seemingly related to the group topic. Such issues must be addressed during the group and not ignored. Two ways to address mismatches are adapting the task that is creating difficulty for the individual member, or grading the task for the entire group.

Adaptation is a change that facilitates performance. Adaptation may require a change in the task itself or in the environment in which it is accomplished (Early, 2012). Modifications to the task may include, among other things, changing the type of tools (i.e., glue stick versus glue bottle for the individual who has difficulty with fine motor tasks), the type of instructions (i.e., written versus verbal directions for the individual who is suspicious of others and prefers to work alone), and procedures (i.e., designating the color of paint versus allowing the client who has difficulty with decision making to select his or her own colors; alternating short discussion periods with hands-on activities to help distracted individuals remain focused during group). Adaptation of the environment may focus on physical aspects (i.e., decreasing the size of work tables and increasing the contrast between the work surface and project tools to facilitate participation for individuals with low vision who have difficulty scanning the environment and locating their tools; providing hand fidgets for the individual who needs to "work out" his or her anxiety while participating in a group that requires that he or she remain seated), as well as social demands (i.e., allowing individuals to work in teams of two rather than mandating participants with limited social skills and ability to handle verbal conflict to negotiate problem solving in a large group).

Successful adaptation of an activity for an individual requires knowledge of activity analysis and synthesis. "*Activity analysis* is the process of analyzing the activity to distinguish its component parts. *Activity synthesis* is the process of combining component parts of the human and nonhuman environment so as to design an activity suitable for evaluation or intervention relative to performance" (Mosey, 1981, p. 114).

Gradation is the process of gradually advancing the skills required to complete a group activity, step by step (Early, 2012). The occupational therapy practitioner designs a skill-development group that allows clients to begin work at the level at which they are capable, but permits them to progress as skills are developed. Over the course of future sessions, the leader adds content and skill challenges so that clients can improve performance by building on what they have learned. If group members do not have the skills to complete a task and work together effectively, the decisions they make will not be effective. A mismatch may occur when group participants are asked to participate in an activity for which they have not yet learned basic performance skills.

An example is a case in which young adults participating in a clubhouse program were asked to participate in a values clarification group in which they broke into small work groups of three to four individuals to collaborate on a project. During the group, it soon became clear to the occupational therapy assistant that the participants had little knowledge of how to resolve group conflict constructively in order to arrive at a common decision and difficulty with anger management. The focus of the group was subsequently changed to a general discussion on frustration, the physical symptoms that accompany it, and options for dealing with it—both positive and negative. In the next group, participants were taught the difference between passive, assertive, and aggressive communication and the consequences associated with the use of each of those communication styles. They also practiced strategies to "cool down" as frustration escalated to anger. As their knowledge of effective anger management and communication strategies grew, participants were challenged to develop their personal coping skills by participating in role-plays where they had to negotiate compromise with just one other individual. Once the young adults demonstrated growth in basic anger management, decision making, and assertive communication skills, they were able to return to the values clarification group where they were now ready to practice conflict negotiation and learn about the process of compromise within a larger group.

Cognitive Behavior Groups

Cognitive behavior groups focus on the member's thoughts (self-talk) and feelings, and subsequent behavior. People often draw generalizations from their life experiences and apply the generalizations to the current environment, even when doing so is inappropriate or counterproductive. These "cognitive distortions" may serve to maintain habits people would otherwise like to change. For example, a young man who has just enrolled in college and does not know anybody tries to initiate conversation with a woman on the bus, who brushes him off. He feels humiliated and says to himself, "Why do I bother to try to talk with this woman? Nobody in this town will ever talk to me!" He subsequently chooses to refrain from initiating conversation with people on the bus, as well as in the classroom. He becomes even lonelier, which leads to depression. He begins to isolate himself in his room, telling himself he is an outcast.

The purpose of cognitive behavior groups is to change learned behavior (such as isolating from others) by changing maladaptive thinking patterns, beliefs, and/or perceptions. Such groups are frequently used to help individuals develop effective ways to cope with stress and depression. The leader focuses on providing a structured environment within which the members examine their thoughts and beliefs and explore patterns of behavior. Some approaches focus more on behavior, others on core beliefs, and still others on developing problem-solving capabilities. Research has shown that if the focus of group work is on what people are doing, chances are greater that members will be able to make changes to their thinking and feeling (McEvoy & Nathan, 2007). Regardless of the particular focus, however, the group leader conducting cognitive behavior groups must have foundation knowledge of the broader theory of cognitive behavior therapy.

Expressive Groups

Expressive groups include a range of therapeutic activities that allow clients to express feelings and thoughts—conscious or unconscious—that they might have difficulty communicating with spoken words alone. The actual characteristics of an expressive therapy group vary depending on the form of expression clients are asked to use (art,

music, drama, games, dance, free movement, or poetry). These groups generally foster social interaction among group members as they engage either together or independently in a creative activity. Expressive therapy groups often can be "the source of valuable insight into patients' deficits and assets, both of which may go undetected by treatment staff members concerned with more narrowly focused treatment interventions" (Galanter, Castaneda, & Franco, 1998, p. 528).

The effective expressive group leader must have the ability to focus the group's attention on creative activities while remaining mindful of group process issues. These groups require skilled leaders, as the activities can stir up very powerful feelings and memories; they are therefore not appropriate for the novice group leader unless supervised by an experienced practitioner. The leader of an expressive group often will be trained in the particular modality to be used (for example, art or music therapy). He or she must possess the ability to recognize the signs of reactions to trauma and be able to contain clients' emotional responses when needed. It is important to be sensitive to a client's ability and willingness to participate in an expressive activity. To protect participants who may be in a vulnerable emotional state, the leader must be assertive enough to set and maintain boundaries with all group participants. For example, in a movement therapy group, participants need to be aware of each other's personal space and understand that touching may not be allowed.

Psychodynamic Groups

Psychodynamic group therapies can be thought of as a generic name encompassing ways of looking at the dynamics that take place in groups. Psychodynamic groups aim at remediation of in-depth psychological problems, and explore how past influences affect the present. From a psychodynamic point of view, starting in early childhood, developmental issues are a key concern, as are environmental influences. Originally, these dynamics were described by Freud, who placed a heavy emphasis on sexual and aggressive drives and conflicts and attachments between parents and children. The psychodynamic approach recognizes that conflicting forces in the mind, some of which may be outside one's awareness, determine a person's behavior, whether healthy or unhealthy. Attachment to others is one of the contending forces.

Over time, the psychodynamic approach has changed from a lengthy, insight-oriented process to more of a short-term, action-oriented approach. Interpersonal process groups use **psychodynamics**, or knowledge of the way people function psychologically, to promote change and healing. The nature of this group is to create a safe environment in which to experiment with getting and giving feedback and exploring new behaviors and responses in a social context.

The object of interest in the psychodynamic approach is the here-and-now interactions among members. The main purposes of the group are to increase people's knowledge of themselves and others, help them clarify the changes they want to make in their lives, and teach them the tools necessary to make those changes. Of less importance is what happens outside of the group or in the group member's past. As faulty relationship patterns are perceived and identified, group members can begin to change dysfunctional, destructive behavioral patterns and become increasingly able to form mutually satisfying relationships with other people.

The effective leader of a psychodynamic group must always be aware of flux in a wide variety of group dynamics, including the current stage of group development, how leadership is emerging within the group, the strengths each individual is bringing to the group as a whole, and how an individual's resistance to change is interacting with and influencing overall group functioning (Brown, 1998). These factors are discussed in more detail in Chapter 14.

Occupational Therapy Groups

The groups listed in Figure 13-1 can be led by a variety of health professionals. In addition to those groups, there are two other sensory-based groups designed to be used by occupational therapy practitioners with specific populations, which are described next.

The Directive Group

The **directive group** was designed to meet the needs of the most severely and acutely mentally ill who have significant cognitive impairment and are receiving treatment on an inpatient psychiatric unit or in a long-term facility (Ross & Burdick, 1981). The structure of the group consists of five steps:

1. Orientation to the group and introduction of individual group members

2. Motor-based warm-up activity

3. Perceptual motor task

4. Cognitive discussion of the activities

5. Closure

In stage 1, the leader may pass around an object to evoke memories, such as a postcard, or ask participants to share a piece of information, such as their favorite food, in order to promote interaction with others during introductions. In stage 2, which requires movement, the members are asked to participate in stretching exercises, perform range of motion, or perhaps do simple weight-lifting exercises using everyday items. Stage 3 entails member participation in a 10- to 15-minute perceptual–motor activity, such as working on a group collage or puzzle. In stage 4, the occupational therapy practitioner encourages members to sit and

listen to one another as they discuss what has been learned by participation in the group activities and how it may be applied to oneself. An essential outcome of stage 5 is to help members feel calm, alert, and ready to move on to the next activity of the day; therefore, the choice of the closing activity will depend on how the members have responded to the activities performed in previous stages. For example, if they need calming, they may be asked to move heavy furniture to another location, whereas a need for increased alertness may lead to a closure activity where each member addresses one another by name as they shake hands before leaving the room. The major assumption behind this group structure is that the members learn by receiving, processing, and responding to sensory stimulation. The group is kept to a length of just 30 minutes in order to ensure maximum participation of all members. Although the activities may change, the format of the group is kept consistent to facilitate goals of initiation, attention, participation, and interaction. In this type of group, the leader must be very active in order to move the group through all five stages.

Sensory Modulation

Sensory integration is "the neurological process that organizes sensations from one's body and from the environment and makes it possible to use the body effectively in the environment" (Ayres, 1979, p. 9). Research supports the presence of sensory-processing disorders and sensory modulation difficulty among people diagnosed with mental illness (Butler, 2009; Kinnealey & Fuiek, 1999; Olson, 2010). **Sensory processing disorder** is a condition that exists when sensory signals don't get organized into appropriate responses. Sensory processing disorder has been compared to a neurological traffic jam that prevents certain parts of the brain from receiving the information needed to interpret and act upon sensory information correctly, affecting an individual's ability to perform everyday tasks (Ayres, 1979; King, 1974). **Sensory modulation** is a clinical intervention that focuses on the use of environments, equipment, and activities to regulate an individual's sensory experience and optimize physiological and emotional well-being (Ross, 1997).

The use of sensory approaches for treatment has expanded as the mental health treatment paradigm shifted from one focused on illness to one of recovery (New Freedom Mental Health Commission, 2003). Champagne and Stromberg (2004) and Champagne (2008, 2011) have developed sensory-processing groups and sensory modulation programs for mental health inpatient treatment and systems. These groups utilize activities that motivate clients and are targeted to their sensory challenges (Champagne & Stromberg, 2004). Groups using a sensory integrative approach safely and effectively require a leader who possesses (1) knowledge of sensory integration theory to design the activity, (2) training and practice in sensory integration therapy in order to closely monitor and grade the activity in the moment as needed, and (3) the ability to skillfully adapt the group according to the members' responses during the session.

Community-Based Groups

It has been said that the combined efforts of many individuals who passionately support a particular issue or cause is the best method to initiate change at the local, regional, and even national levels (Osborne & Gaebler, 1992). This is certainly the case with community-based mental health advocacy groups (New Freedom Commission on Mental Health, 2003). In a community-based health group for individuals diagnosed with mental illness, the members define the issues to be addressed, work together to make decisions, and develop solutions that are consumer driven. These groups are congruent with the shift from an illness to a recovery-based paradigm, and are primarily the work of the members from the community; however, they may be facilitated by occupational therapy practitioners, depending on the setting. Such groups can be sponsored by particular organizations or populations and occur in psychosocial rehabilitation, clubhouse, and assertive community treatment settings (AOTA, 2014), or they may be conducted in public facilities such as schools or churches. Two types of community groups to which occupational therapy clients may be referred—the support group and the self-help group—are described next.

Support Groups

Support groups meet for the purpose of giving emotional support and information to persons with a common problem. They are based on the beliefs that lifestyle change associated with major life transitions is a long-term goal and that support groups can play a major role in adjusting to those transitions (Kurtz, 1997). Support groups are often facilitated by professionals who are linked to a social agency or larger formal organization, but they may also be peer led. The National Alliance for the Mentally Ill is an example of such an organization. Support groups provide a psychosocial network and offer opportunities for problem sharing, usually for individuals with chronic illness and/or their families. Although a support group will always have a clearly stated purpose, the purpose varies according to its members' motivation and stage of recovery. Many of these groups are open ended, with a changing population of members. As new clients move into a particular stage of recovery, they may join a support group appropriate for that stage until they are ready to move on again. Groups may continue indefinitely, with new members coming in and old members leaving. Members typically talk about their current situation and recent problems that have arisen. They are encouraged to share and discuss common experiences and problem solve how to address challenges, whether those challenges are at the individual, community, or national level.

The leadership style for someone running a support group typically will be active, but less directive than for activity and task groups. The leader's primary role is to facilitate group discussion and help group members share their experiences.

Self-Help Groups

The intent of **self-help groups** is to promote change within an individual. They may be based on a condition (i.e., wounded warrior) or a common disorder (i.e., anxiety disorder). They seldom have professional facilitators. Rather, they are usually organized and managed by the members and are conducted in public buildings such as schools, churches, and community centers. Self-help groups share many of the principles of support groups, such as unconditional acceptance of other group members, open and honest interpersonal interaction, and self-reflection (Jacobs & Goodman, 1989; Silverman, 2002). Alcoholics Anonymous and Toastmasters are examples of two well-known self-help groups.

PART 6: PUTTING IT ALL TOGETHER: THE GROUP PROTOCOL

So far we have defined the term *group*, summarized the benefits of using (and participating) in a group, analyzed the elements used to frame the group, delineated the impact that these factors have on the level of participation among members, and evaluated the structural elements on a continuum of groups, including the level of skill required by the individual who leads them. But how are these components brought together? The answer to that question is the group protocol. The **group protocol** is a way to organize your thoughts about the design of a group and share them with other members of the treatment team. It is a written plan that describes the goals of the group and the methods by which these goals will be achieved. Writing out a group protocol on paper before the group is implemented ensures that it is well thought out and allows your supervisor to share feedback and ask any questions.

Protocols vary in form from one facility to the next, but usually include similar content. They should, at a minimum, include the following:

- Title of the group
- Rationale for its use
- Group goals
- Description of the group format and content

- Selection criteria for participants
- Necessary materials
- Description of the role that the leader takes with the group

This information is needed to ensure that clients who are selected to participate are appropriate for the group and will benefit from it. It allows different facilitators to replicate the group in the future and helps them to explain its relevance to clients, promoting "buy-in" for group participation.

There are preparatory steps that should be conducted and questions that must be answered before designing a new group (Cara & MacRae, 2013; Cole, 2012). Answering these questions will help clarify and focus your thinking, thereby simplifying the group development process. The first step is to conduct a needs assessment of the clients within your practice setting. What knowledge or skills are required by the individuals with whom you work in order for them to achieve their individual treatment goals? Are those skills related to the performance areas of instrumental activities of daily living, activities of daily living, work, education, or social participation? What are the existing motor performance skills, process performance skills, communication, interaction performance skills, and mental functions within the group? Do your clients need to develop performance habits, routines, and roles? What activities do *they* want to accomplish? Are those needs able to be met utilizing existing groups? If not, identify those clients for whom your group would serve that purpose. How could you, as an occupational therapy assistant, use this group to help them achieve those goals?

Consider the general level of group skills demonstrated by this population, as well as other client factors, in particular, cognitive skills. What do the clients already know about this topic? What do they *want* to know? Are there any safety concerns—is this a group for acutely ill individuals or a psychoeducational group for adolescents in a clubhouse program? This will help you determine the general learning goals and suggest the appropriate format, content, member inclusion criteria, and group structure. The answers to these questions will also help to determine the specific outcome measures for the group.

The next step is to identify what resources are required, as well as any constraints of the existing program and setting. What size and type of room is needed (i.e., a small kitchen, a large room with tables, a room with access to the Internet)? Does the budget allow for supplies (i.e., grocery items, kitchen utensils, laptop computers)? Are there enough staff available to help facilitate the group? Are you able to dictate the group size, or is attendance mandatory for all clients currently admitted to the program? Are existing groups open or closed? What is the anticipated length of stay? How often would this group need to meet in order for participants to achieve the goals? What is the frame of reference or model that will be used to design the group? A frame of reference is used as a general guide to help the occupational therapy practitioner determine the following:

- Primary purpose of the group (for example, symptom reduction versus wellness and illness prevention)
- Nature of the activity (i.e., creative, expressive, educational, sensory based, etc.)
- Role of the leader (i.e., teacher directed versus client self-exploration)
- Type of group that is most appropriate for the population (i.e., activity, task, psychoeducational, directive, etc.)

Although ideally, the occupational therapy practitioner would be able to select the frame of reference that best addresses the therapeutic goals and problem areas of potential members, at times the context of the program dictates the model. For example, in a behavioral treatment program in which observable behavior is considered the only appropriate focus for intervention, the exploration of values or emotions would be contradicted.

Title

Once these preliminary questions have been answered, you should be ready to create the written protocol. The first step is to decide on a name for the group. The name should reflect the goals of the group rather than offer a description of the activity used to achieve the goals. For example, if the purpose of the group is to assess work habits or develop basic work skills and the activity for that purpose is craft projects, the group should be entitled "Work Skills" rather than "Arts and Crafts." This enables participants and staff members to understand the rationale for the group and encourages referrals to it.

Rationale

The next step in creating the protocol is to describe the rationale for the existence of the group. Reflect on the answers to the questions formulated in the needs assessment. Summarize the findings and the clinical reasoning used to design the group, making sure to include any evidence found in the literature that supports the need for the group and/or the activity selected to achieve group goals. This section should be brief—no more than a paragraph—but thorough enough to address any concerns regarding this area.

Goals

The next section of the protocol lists the goals. When working with individuals who are participating in occupational therapy groups, two levels of goals co-exist: personal goals (as noted on the individual treatment plans) and group goals. Although the group is working to attain general goals, members will be addressing individual goals as well. For example, a general group goal might be for all members to engage in a 45-minute progressive muscle relaxation exercise in order to develop stress management skills. An individual participant with a high level of social anxiety might simultaneously be working on a goal of remaining in a therapeutic group (such as stress management) for at least 30 minutes.

General goals should describe what all members will achieve by actively participating in the group and the way they will go about doing it. They consist of observable outcomes stated in behavioral terms using action verbs and should be attainable by every participant, given the length and duration of the group. An outcome is "the measured or observed consequence of an action" (Cara & MacRae, 2013, p. 604). Since outcomes serve as one of the standards by which a group is judged, the group protocol should include a list of three to five goals. Fewer than two goals might not offer enough justification to run the group, but more than five may be unrealistic, given that every participant who actively participates should be able to attain them. Variables that affect whether the group goals are met include whether the members see the goals as meaningful; the extent to which goals have clearly defined outcomes; the cohesiveness of the group; the degree of compatibility with individual treatment goals; the skill of the group leader; and the availability of resources to meet goals, including but not limited to, budget, time, and number of staff available to assist the leader in group facilitation.

Group Format

The next section of the written protocol is the group format. The format includes a description of the setting and preparation that must occur prior to the group, the ideal number of participants, the duration and frequency of the group, and the overall time structure. In some protocols, the role of the group leader is specified in this section as well, since the format of the group dictates the actions of the leader. The subjects of time structure and group leadership styles will be covered in more detail in Chapter 14.

Group Content

Group content is the activity that is planned and carried out in a group (Denton, 1987) and what is said in group (Cole, 2012). In order to decide on the content, the occupational therapy practitioner reflects on the combined individual goals of potential members. In reviewing these goals, a theme will usually emerge, which is used to guide the selection of an appropriate activity. Common group themes addressed by occupational therapy practitioners who work on acute care units include anger management and coping skills, time management, work skills and behaviors, stress management, communication, and life skills. Within these themes, the occupational therapy practitioner must then decide on the activity and how the content will be presented.

The content area of the protocol includes details on how the group will run. It begins with the group introduction, which includes the rationale for use of the group activity. This is followed by an explanation of the warm-up exercise, the verbal instructions given to participants about the activity, and questions that will be used to prompt participation during the sharing and processing of the group. In addition, the protocol should include any printed materials that are to be distributed to the members. For groups that run more than one session, the protocol should contain all of the lesson plans.

Selecting a therapeutic activity may initially appear to be a simple task, given that groups are formed with clients who have similar goals and treatment priorities. However, this process involves the use of clinical reasoning; the occupational therapy practitioner must take into consideration the context and the environment in which the group is held, as well as his or her role on the treatment team in that setting. Combining the use of activity analysis and synthesis and the application of the selected frame of reference, the occupational therapy group leader determines a variety of potential activities that could be used to address the general goals of the group intervention process. Ultimately, the selection of the activity should be based on the best *fit* between the activity and the clients after taking into consideration the resources and constraints of the program in which the group will be held. To determine that fit, the occupational therapy practitioner must consider several variables. For example, can the clients do this activity given their current functional level and performance skills? Is the activity compatible with the participants' chronologic ages, sex, and sociocultural backgrounds? How does this activity help clients cultivate or maintain developmentally appropriate occupational roles? Is it providing the "just right" challenge to develop needed skills?

If the topic and activity are not a "fit" with the members, even the best planned group will fall flat and participants will not reach their goals. A common mistake made by the student who is learning how to develop a group is to select an activity based on his or her personal interest rather than careful analysis of the population and then working "backward" to justify its use. This usually results in a poor fit with the preferences and needs of the group, and is evidenced by a student leader who struggles to engage the group in the activity or sustain discussion among group members. In those instances, the group leader works harder than the group itself!

Inclusion Criteria

The inclusion criteria section describes the minimum skills or behaviors needed in order to participate successfully in group. Since group treatment is most effective when clients have comparable functional abilities, assessment of occupational performance should always precede client selection for group membership. Formal assessment and informal observations can be used for that process. As an example, the inclusion criteria might specify that the individual will possess the ability to do the following:

- Attend to group topic for a minimum of 15 minutes without staff prompts
- Refrain from aggressive behavior
- Respect the personal space of others
- Refrain from interrupting the discussion when someone else is speaking

The occupational therapy assistant will often find that thoughtful analysis of the inclusion criteria, combined with minor changes in the format of the group, will usually increase the potential number of appropriate group members within a setting. For example, minor accommodations, such as changing the length of the group (say from 60 minutes to 30 minutes), the size of the group (12 members to 6 members), the physical environment (i.e., increasing the number of tables, thereby ensuring every participant his or her own personal space), and changing the role of the leader from facilitative to directive (i.e., directing a question to a specific group member rather than the entire group) will allow a group to be replicated or expanded to include individuals with lower cognitive abilities.

Required Materials

This section specifies what supplies are required to conduct the group. In some facilities, it is recommended that the cost per group member be calculated. Administrators frequently request this list in order to solicit donations or to inform individuals who are eager to make material donations as to what type of items they might purchase.

Evaluation

This section of the protocol describes how achievement of group goals will be assessed. For example, if the group is focused on disseminating information on a particular topic, a questionnaire may be distributed to participants before and after the group to determine if their level of knowledge has changed. In a skill-based group, participants may be asked to independently demonstrate the skill upon completion of the group. If a published assessment tool exists to measure specific group goals, it may be used as well. It is important for occupational therapy practitioners to evaluate their groups in order to refine existing protocols and improve the efficacy of their treatment. These evaluations should be shared with program administrators to justify the use of occupational therapy groups for treatment and the role of the occupational therapy practitioner as an essential member of the treatment team.

SUMMARY

In 1947, Lewin coined the term *group dynamics* as the way that groups and individuals act and react to changing circumstances. He theorized that when a group is established, it becomes a unified system with qualities that cannot be understood by evaluating members individually. This notion, that a group is composed of more than the sum of its individual members, quickly gained support from sociologists and psychologists, who understood the significance of this emerging field.

Group treatment is a planned process for creating changes in individuals, bringing them together for this purpose. In the practice area of mental health, much of occupational therapy is carried out in activity-based groups, with the goals of developing skills and encouraging social interaction among members. The skills required to design and lead groups involve a combination of artistic and scientific abilities, and the occupational therapy assistant, under the supervision of an occupational therapist, is competent to assist in the design and execution of group interventions. Historically, occupational therapy activity groups were used primarily to treat mental illness; however, over the years the focus of groups has broadened from treatment of the mentally ill population to include client education in the "well population" as a means for illness prevention.

Although there are numerous advantages to the use of group treatment, there are also limitations, given that the group must also meet the needs of every individual client. Common properties are used to characterize the core elements that frame any type of group. These include the goals of the group, group climate, group membership, group composition, and the communication patterns between the group leader and group participants. These elements can be varied, depending on the type and purpose of the group, as well as the needs and functional level of its members.

There are many types of treatment groups led by occupational therapy practitioners working in mental health settings, which range on a continuum from very structured activity groups to minimally structured psychotherapy groups. In addition to those groups, there are several types of sensory-based groups designed to be used by occupational therapy practitioners with specific populations.

The group protocol is a way to organize your thoughts about the design of a group and share them with other members of the treatment team. It is a written plan that describes the goals of the group and the methods by which these goals will be achieved. Writing out a group protocol on paper before the group is implemented ensures that it is well thought out and allows your supervisor to share feedback and ask any questions that he or she may have.

PART 7: APPLICATIONS

The following activities will help you identify key aspects of this chapter, which were highlighted in this text. In particular, these questions highlight the chapter objectives at the start of the chapter. Activities are suggested to be completed individually, in a small group, or as a class to enhance learning.

1. You are an occupational therapy assistant working in the public school setting. Your supervising occupational therapist has asked you to design an educational group for 15 kindergarten students on the topic of good nutrition. Before you design this group, there are important factors to consider. List those factors, and explain the significance of each in regard to your population.

2. Create a title for your group, and write three group goals.

3. Now that you have selected your goals, write a description of your group. Remember, the description must address how your goals will be accomplished. Include the format. How much time is allotted for each step of the group?

4. You have been informed that one of the children in the group has cerebral palsy. She uses a wheelchair for mobility and has limited use of her right arm. What adaptations would you make to ensure that she is able to participate in your group?

5. Using the same topic, you now have to create a group for 10 adults hospitalized on an acute care psychiatric unit for clients with severe and persistent mental illness. Respond to questions 1 to 3.

6. Using the same topic, your target population is an outpatient after-school program for 10 adolescents diagnosed with mood disorders. Respond to questions 1 to 3.

7. You have been informed that the size of the group has been increased to 20 individuals, with the assistance of one aide. What aspects of your group will need to be changed? Be specific.

REFERENCES

Accreditation Council for Occupational Therapy Education. (2013). *Standards and interpretive guide.* Retrieved from www.aota.org/-/media/Corporate/Files/EducationCareers/Accredit/StandardsReview/guide/2006ACOTEStandardsInterpretiveGide8-2012.pdf

Allen, C. K. (1987). Activity: Occupational therapy's treatment method. *American Journal of Occupational Therapy, 41,* p. 563-575.

Allen, C. K. (1999). *Structures of the cognitive performance modes.* Ormond Beach, FL: Allen Conferences, Inc.

American Occupational Therapy Association. (2010). Specialized knowledge and skills in mental health promotion, prevention, and intervention in occupational therapy. *American Journal of Occupational Therapy, 64,* 313-323.

American Occupational Therapy Association. (2014). Occupational therapy practice framework: Domain and process (3rd ed.). *American Journal of Occupational Therapy, 68* (Supplement 1).

Ayres, A. J. (1979). *Sensory integration and the child.* Los Angeles, CA: Western Psychological Services.

Bandura, A. (1977). *Social learning theory.* New York, NY: General Learning Press.

Baron, R., & Norbert, K. (2003). *Group process, group decision, group action.* Buckingham, UK: Open University Press.

Baumeister, R. F., & Leary, M. R. (1995). The need to belong: Desire for interpersonal attachments as a fundamental human motivation. *Psychological Bulletin, 117,* 497-529.

Bell, P. A., Green, T. C., Fisher, J. D., & Baum, A. (2011). *Environmental psychology* (5th ed,). Orlando, FL: Harcourt.

Bickes, M. B., Deloache, S., Dicer, J., & Miller, S. (2001). Effectiveness of experiential and verbal occupational therapy groups in a community mental health setting. *Occupational Therapy in Mental Health , 17*(1), 51-72.

Brown, N.W. (1998). *Psychoeducational groups.* Philadelphia, PA: Accelerated Development, 1998.

Bruce, M., & Borg, B. (2002). *Psychosocial frames of reference.* Thorofare, NJ: Slack.

Bullock, A. & Bannigan, K. (2011). Effectiveness of activity-based work in community mental health: A systematic review. *America Journal of Occupational Therapy, 65,* 257-266.

Butler, P. D. (2009). Early-stage visual processing deficits in schizophrenia. In A. Lajtha (Ed.) & D. C. Javitt, & J. T. Kantrowitz (Eds.), *Handbook of neurochemistry and molecular neurobiology* (pp. 332–352). New York, NY: Springer.

Cara, E. & MacRae, A. (2013). *Psychosocial occupational therapy: An evolving practice.* Clifton Park, NY: Delmar.

Castore, C.F. (1962). Number of verbal interrelationships as a determinant of group size. *Journal of Abnormal and Social Psychology, 64,* 456-458.

Champagne, T. (2008). *Sensory modulation & environment: Essential elements of occupation* (3rd ed.). Southampton, MA: Champagne Conferences & Consultation.

Champagne, T. (2011). *Sensory modulation and the environment: Essential elements of occupation* (3rd ed.; rev.). Sydney, Australia: Pearson Assessments.

Champagne, T., & Stromberg, N. (2004). Sensory approaches in inpatient psychiatric settings: Innovative alternatives to seclusion and restraint. *Journal of Psychosocial Nursing, 42,* 35–44.

Cole, C. (2012). *Group dynamics in occupational therapy*. Thorofare, NJ: SLACK.

Colum, F. (2011). Keeping therapies simple: Psychoeducation in the prevention of relapse in affective disorders. *The British Journal of Psychiatry, 198*, 338-340.

Corey, G., Corey, M., Callahan, P., & Russell, J. (2003). *Group techniques*. Pacific Grove, CA: Brooks/Cole-Thompson Learning.

Corey, M., Corey G., & Corey, C. (2010). *Groups: Process and practice*. Belmont, CA: Brooks/Cole.

Coursey, R., Curtis, L., & Marsh, D. (2000). Competencies for direct service workers who work with adults with severe mental illness: Specific knowledge, attitudes, skills and biography. *Psychiatric Rehabilitation Journal, 23*, 378-392.

Cowls, J., & Hale, S. (2005). It's the activity that counts: What clients value in psychoeducational groups. *Canadian Journal of Occupational Therapy, 16*, 176-182.

Denton, P. (1987). *Psychiatric occupational therapy: A workbook of practical skills*. Chicago, IL: Lippincott, Williams & Wilkens.

Duncombe, L., & Howe, M. C. (1985). Group work in occupational therapy: A survey of practice. *American Journal of Occupational Therapy, 39*, 163-170.

Early, M. B. (2012). *Mental health concepts & techniques*. (4th ed.). Philadelphia, PA: Lippincott, Williams & Wilkins.

Fidler, G. S. (1969). The task oriented group as a context for treatment. *American Journal of Occupational Therapy, 23*, p. 43-48.

Fidler, G. & Fidler J. (1963). *Occupational therapy: A communication process in psychiatry*. New York, NY: MacMillan Group.

Forsyth, D. R. (2006). *Group Dynamics*. (4th ed.). Belmont, CA: Thomson Wadsworth Publishing.

Galanter, M., Castaneda, R., & Franco, H. (1998). Group therapy, self-help groups, and network therapy. In Frances, R. J., & Miller, S. I., (Eds). *Clinical textbook of addictive disorders*. (2nd ed.). New York, NY: The Guilford Press, pp. 521–546.

Gieryn, T. F. (2000). A pace for place in sociology. *Annual Review of Sociology, 39*, 60-70.

Hagedorn, R. (2000). *Tools for practice in occupational therapy: A structural approach to core skills and practices*. Edinburgh, UK: Churchill Livingstone.

Hagedorn, B., & Hirshhorn, M. (2009). When talking won't work: Implementing experiential group activities with addicted clients. *The Journal for Specialists in Group Work , 34*(1), 43-67.

Hall, E. T. (1966). *The hidden dimension*. New York, NY: Doubleday.

Hare, A. P. (1982). *Creativity in small groups*. Thousand Oaks, CA: Sage.

Hildenbrand, W., & Lamb, A. (2013). Occupational therapy in prevention and wellness: Retaining relevance in a new health care world. *American Journal of Occupational Therapy, 67*(3), 266-271.

Howe, M., & Schwartzberg, S. (2001). *A functional approach to group work in occupational therapy*. Baltimore, MD: Lippincott, Williams and Wilkins.

Jacobs, M. K., & Goodman, G. (1989). Psychology and self-help groups: Predictions on a partnership. *American Psychologist, 44*(3), 536-545.

Johnson, D., & Johnson, P. (2013). *Joining together: Group therapy and group skills*. (11th ed.). Saddle River, New Jersey: Pearson.

King, L. J. (1974). A sensory-integrative approach to schizophrenia. *American Journal of Occupational Therapy, 28*, 529–536.

Kinnealey, M., & Fuiek, M. (1999). The relationship between sensory defensiveness, anxiety, depression and perception of pain in adults. *Occupational Therapy International, 6*, 195–206.

Kolb, D. A. (1984). *Experiential learning*. Englewood Cliffs, NJ: Prentice Hall.

Kurtz, F. (1997). *Self-help and support groups: A handbook for practitioners*. Thousand Oaks, CA: Sage Publications.

Levinger, J., Ingham, A. G., Graves, J. & Peckham, P. (1974). The Ringelmann effect: Studies of group size and group performance. *Journal of Experimental Social Psychology, 10*(4), 371-384.

Lewin, K. (1947). Frontiers in group dynamics: Concept, method and reality in social science; social equilibria and social change. *Human Relations, 1*, 41.

Lewin, K. (1951). *Field theory in social science; selected theoretical papers*. New York, NY: Harper & Row.

Lieberman, R., & Kopelowicz, A. (2000). Editorial introduction to overcoming barriers to individualized psychosocial rehabilitation in an acute treatment unit of a state hospital. *Psychiatric Services, 51*(3), 313-317.

Lloyd, C., & Mass, F. (1997). Occupational therapy group work in psychiatric settings. *British Journal of Occupational Therapy, 60*, 415-419.

McEvoy, P., & Nathan, P. (2007). Effectiveness of cognitive behavioral therapy for diagnostically heterogeneous groups: A benchmarking study. *Journal of Consulting and Clinical Psychology, 75*(2), 344-350.

Medaliea, A., Dorn, H., & Watras-Gans, S. (2000). Treating problem-solving deficits on an acute care psychiatric inpatient unit. *Psychiatry Research, 97*, 70-88.

Mosey, A. C. (1970). *Three frames of reference*. Thorofare, NJ: SLACK.

Mosey, A. C. (1973). *Activities therapy*. New York, NY: Raven Press.

Mosey, A. (1981). *Occupational therapy: Configuration of a profession*. New York, NY: Raven Press.

Olson, L. (2010, March). Examining schizophrenia and sensory modulation disorder: A review of the literature. *Sensory Integration Special Interest Section Quarterly, 33*(1), 1–3.

Osborne, D. & Gabeler, T. (1992). *Reinventing government: How the entrepreneurial spirit is transforming the public sector*. New York, New York: Penguin Books.

Penny, N., Mueser, K., & North, C.T. (1995). The Allen Cognitive Level test and social competence in adult psychiatric patients. *American Journal of Occupational Therapy. 49*, 420-427.

Poole, C. (1995). Learning. In C. Trombly (Ed.). *Occupational therapy for physical dysfunction* (3rd ed.). Baltimore, MD: Williams and Wilkins.

Pratt, J. H. (1922). The principle of class treatment and their application to various chronic diseases. *Hospital Social Services, 6*, 401-417.

President's New Freedom Commission on Mental Health. (2003). *Achieving the promise: Transforming mental health care in America*. (DHHS Publication No. SMA-03-3832). Rockville, MD: Author. Retrieved from www.mentalhealthcommission.gov/reports/FinalReport/toc.html.

Ross M., & Burdick D (1981). *Sensory Integration: A training manual for therapists and teachers for regressed, psychiatric and geriatric patient group*. Thorofare, NJ: Slack Incorporated.

Ross, M. (1997). *Integrative group therapy – mobilizing coping abilities with the five-stage group*. Bethesda, MD: American Occupational Therapy Association.

Sadock, B., Sadock, V., & Ruiz, P. (2009). *Kaplan and Sadock's comprehensive textbook of psychiatry* (9th Ed.). Philadelphia, PA: Lippincott, Williams & Wilkins

Schindler, V. P. (1999). Group effectiveness in improving social interaction skills. *Psychiatric Rehabilitation Journal, 22*(4), 1999, 349-354.

Schwartzberg, S., Howe, M., & Barnes, M. A. (2008). *Groups: Applying the functional group model*. Philadelphia, PA: F. A. Davis.

Silverman, P. (2002). *The self-help group sourcebook: Your guide to community and online support groups*. (7th ed.). Denville, NJ: Saint Clare's Health Services.

Sommer, R. (1969). *Personal space*. Englewood Cliffs, NJ: Prentice Hall.

Steizor, B. (1950). The spatial factor in face to face discussion groups. *Journal of Abnormal and Social Psychology, 45*, 552-555.

Townsend, E. (1996). Enabling empowerment: Using simulations versus real occupation. *Canadian Journal of occupational Therapy, 49*, 114-128.

Yalom, I. D. (1983). *Inpatient group psychotherapy*. New York: Basic Books.

14

The Group Leader

Christine A. Manville, EdD, OTR/L

KEY TERMS

- Acting Self
- Active Listening
- Advisory Leadership
- Autocratic Leader
- Bloom's Taxonomy
- Body Language
- Boundary Violations
- Communication Network
- Conflict
- Democratic Leader
- Directive Leader
- Discrimination
- Educational Process
- Facilitative Leader

- Functional Approach
- Group Dynamics
- Group Process
- Instructional Materials
- Instructional Method
- Interpersonal Learning
- Laissez-Faire Leader
- Leader
- Leadership
- Learning
- Learning Goals
- Learning Needs
- Learning Styles
- Mixed Signals

- Norm
- Perceived Self
- Power Struggle
- Prejudice
- Professional Boundaries
- Racism
- Rapport
- Relational Leadership
- Sanction
- Scaffolding
- Socialization
- Stereotype
- Task Leadership
- Teaching

CHAPTER LEARNING OBJECTIVES

After completing this chapter, students will be able to:

1. Define the term leadership and compare six different leadership styles.

2. Discuss how the attitude of the group leader may enhance or detract from the development of rapport between a group leader and the members.

3. Summarize the elements that contribute to self-awareness in the group leader.

Manville, C.A., & Keough, J. L.
Mental Health Practice for the Occupational Therapy Assistant (pp 335-366).
© 2016 Taylor & Francis Group.

4. Demonstrate the use of specific communication techniques, including body language, that enhance the development of rapport between the group leader and members.

5. Identify the components that contribute to group dynamics.

6. Compare and contrast two different styles of group development.

7. Categorize the roles that typically develop within a group.

8. Draw a communication continuum and provide examples of each of the communication styles located on it.

9. Role-play expression of an "I" message.

10. List the elements that must be taken into consideration in effective instructional design, and offer an explanation to support the importance of each element.

CHAPTER OUTLINE

INTRODUCTION

At one time, leadership was thought to be a quality that was possessed naturally by certain individuals. A study by Stogdill in the 1940s, however, found that personal traits made no difference in leadership in most situations. Instead, he reported that leadership is a relationship that exists among individuals within a social context. "The evidence suggests that leadership is a relationship that exists between persons in a social situation, and that persons who are leaders in one situation may not necessarily be leaders in other situations" (Stogdill, 1948, p. 48). In the 1980s, new research emerged that brought the leader-trait view back into prominence (Zaccaro, 2007). Those studies suggested that leadership potential is based on multiple traits that operate in an integrated way.

The term traits was used to refer not only to personality attributes, but also cognitive abilities, motives, values, social and problem-solving skills, and expertise. It was proposed that the expression of leadership traits adjusted in order to conform to the current situation. Therefore, because situations change, the expression of the leader's traits will change as well; however, the research also indicated that some traits remain stable during this accommodation process. More recent definitions of leadership combine elements of both studies (Barge, 2003; Gouran, 2003). According to Johnson and Johnson (2013), "a leader is a person who can influence others to be more effective in working to achieve mutual goals and maintain effective working relationships among members" (p. 162). Leadership, on the other hand, is "the process through which leaders exert their influence" (p. 162). The consequence of good leadership is cooperation among individuals in pursuit of a common goal.

PART 1: THE OCCUPATIONAL THERAPY ASSISTANT AS A GROUP LEADER

The ability to lead groups effectively is a skill that the occupational therapy assistant can use in any work setting. *Leaders* influence their groups in a variety of ways, and clients benefit when groups are led by good leaders (Larson & Christiansen, 1996). For example, in a psychoeducational group, members may try to focus on their past rather than exploring new problem-solving methods unless an assertive leader can redirect them back to the present. Likewise, leaders may miss a "teachable moment" by rigidly following the group protocol rather than dealing with an important issue that has emerged that would be better dealt with in the here and now.

Leadership is a process, and based on the type of group, the leader guides, organizes, directs, coordinates, supports, and motivates the efforts of members to varying degrees at different points in the group. Running an effective group requires that a balance be maintained between adhering to the task and meeting the interpersonal needs of group members. To illustrate this point, consider the leader of an educational group who is focused solely on reviewing a written handout. Consequently, he or she may not take the time to survey the group to determine whether participants understand the information as it is being taught or even whether they are interested in the topic. If written material is not understood and/or members do not see how it applies to their lives, the group will most likely be ineffective.

Leadership Styles

Research has shown that the same group of people will demonstrate significantly different behaviors under individuals with varied leadership styles (Lewin, Lippitt & White, 1939). According to Stogdill (1974), the most effective leader promotes group productivity, cohesiveness, and satisfaction by demonstrating concern for the well-being of the members while at the same time defining group structure. This structure is created by clearly explaining one's role as a leader and clarifying what is expected from the group members. In other words, there are two important dimensions to consider as a leader of an activity group:

1. How the task will be completed

2. The relationship between the leader and the members

Task leadership is focused on the work that will be done within the group to achieve goals. Here the leader creates structure by planning activities, setting goals, defining the group roles and responsibilities of the members, developing operating procedures, monitoring compliance with those procedures, offering feedback, proposing solutions, and stressing productivity to facilitate the achievement of group goals (Yukl, 2005). In contrast, when considering the dimension of *relationship leadership*, the leader focuses on the development of interpersonal relationships within the group and shows concern for members by boosting morale, providing support and encouragement, reducing interpersonal conflict, and establishing rapport among participants.

Some studies have focused on a functional approach to group leadership within an organization. The *functional approach* to leadership refers to the ability of the leader to manage the group in order to complete the task while working together as a team. In 1938, a study known as "Leadership and Group Life" was conducted under the leadership of Kurt Lewin. As a result of this study, three specific styles of functional leadership were identified, along with the impact that each style has on the social climate within the group (Lewin et al., 1939). Those styles of leadership are described next. Although further research has determined that there are additional types of leadership, this early study was very influential within the field. Table 14-1 summarizes the advantages and disadvantages associated with the autocratic, democratic, and laissez-faire leadership styles as defined by Lewin.

The Autocratic Leader

An *autocratic leader* is task oriented and less focused on the individual group members than other types of leaders. In a group with an autocratic leader, there is a clear division between the leader and the participants. This style is also known as *authoritarian*, as the leader has all of the authority and power within the group. The group leader with this leadership style decides what needs to be done without involving other members in the decision making and dictates all the work methods and processes to be used. The autocratic style is beneficial when decisions need to be made quickly or when a leader is working with members who have significant cognitive limitations. By eliminating the need to make decisions, the leader allows the group members the ability to focus all of their energy on completing the assigned task.

TABLE 14-1			
LEWIN'S LEADERSHIP STYLES			
STYLE	CHARACTERISTICS	ADVANTAGES	DISADVANTAGES
Autocratic	The leader exerts maximum authority and control over group members. Members are not encouraged to participate, interact, or offer input into decision making.	Conserves time and energy as roles and responsibilities are assigned to members. Most effective when used in emergencies.	May cause dependency on the leader and limit growth potential in members.
Democratic	The leader encourages group interaction, problem solving, and decision making.	Input from group members is valued by the leader. Spontaneous and honest communication among group members is encouraged. The leader seeks input and tailors the group's work toward common goals. Higher commitment from members, greater productivity, and creative problem solving are associated with this style.	The group may need significant time and effort to accomplish goals; therefore, this style is not appropriate when quick or immediate action is required.
Laissez-Faire	Group members are free to function as they choose.	Effective when members are highly knowledgeable or skilled, task oriented, and motivated. Higher motivation levels are associated with this style.	This style is time consuming and frequently inefficient in regard to accomplishment of group goals.

The Democratic Leader

In order to promote group engagement, the **democratic leader** encourages group members to share their ideas and opinions; however, he or she reserves the right to have the final say on decisions. The increased level of involvement among participants that results from this leadership style can lead to creative solutions to problems, higher productivity within the group, and increased commitment to completion of a task. This leadership style is also known as participatory, as the leader requests the cooperation of other group members. After facilitating conversation among group members, the democratic leader analyzes all of the proposed solutions in order to determine the best possible direction for the group and then communicates the final decision back to the participants. Democratic leadership works best with skilled, knowledgeable group members. It is important that a group under this style of leadership have a schedule that allows them enough time to share ideas, develop a plan, and then vote on the best course of action.

The Laissez-Faire Leader

The **laissez-faire leader** allows group members to make all of the decisions. Although this individual may provide resources and support to the group, he or she does not make suggestions, offer direction, or exert control over the group in any way. This level of autonomy can lead to high levels of satisfaction among group members, but it can also be damaging if participants do not manage their time well, or if they lack the knowledge, skills, or self-motivation to work effectively.

Leadership Styles for the Occupational Therapy Assistant

The concepts of power, influence, and authority affect leadership in a group setting. As a group leader, the decision must be made on how to best distribute responsibility between the leader and group members, the amount of structure to provide (maximum to minimum), and the

		TABLE 14-2	

FACTORS THAT INFLUENCE OCCUPATIONAL THERAPY LEADERSHIP STYLE

FACTORS	DIRECTIVE LEADERSHIP	FACILITATIVE LEADERSHIP	ADVISORY LEADERSHIP
Client factors	Low cognitive level. Psychiatric symptoms create barriers to social interaction.	Medium cognitive level. Members are capable of problem solving and insight.	High cognitive level. Members are highly motivated.
Group focus	Task achievement	Learning oriented	Focused on socialization and problem solving.
Group maturity	Low. Little connection or cohesiveness among members.	Medium. Members are learning relationship skills.	Highly cohesive.
Leadership control and influence	The leader provides the activity and structures the task. Members rely on him or her for support.	Medium control. The leader seeks input from the group in decision making, and encourages members to support one another.	Least influence.–The leader intervenes on an as-needed basis.
Goals	Productivity; basic social skills.	Learning oriented; development of self-awareness and insight.	Socialization; solving problems and developing support systems.
Theoretical base	Sensory motor; cognitive disabilities	Cognitive behavior; psychoeducational; psychodynamic	Developmental; system-oriented approach

role the leader will assume (directive to nondirective). Leadership styles for the occupational therapy assistant that address these factors can best be visualized on a continuum, with directive leadership and advisory leadership as the endpoints and facilitatory leadership in the middle. On this continuum, the directive leader may be compared with the authoritarian leader, the facilitatory leader with the democratic leader, and advisory leadership with the laissez-faire leader; however, there are distinct differences, which are described next.

Those groups with a leader-centered focus are termed directive, with the leader in the center of all communication. On the other end of the continuum, members communicate primarily with one another in groups under a nondirective (advisory) leader. It is important to note that one style of leadership is not necessarily better than the others, and different approaches will be more effective depending on the situation. For example, if a new skill is being taught, the group will probably require more direction, whereas a group that is using expressive therapy will benefit from a nondirective approach. Many factors must be considered in determining which leadership style to use for a given group, including but not limited to, client factors, existing skill levels, group goals, and theoretical approach used to design the group. Table 14-2 summarizes factors associated with directive, facilitative, and advisory leadership.

Directive Leadership

The *directive leader* exerts the most control over the group; therefore, this leadership style is the appropriate choice for clients functioning at a low cognitive level. Psychoeducational groups that focus on educating clients regarding a specific topic or teaching a particular skill frequently utilize directive leadership as well, since the content that must be covered is clearly defined, usually in lesson plans. The directive leader does not function in the same way as the autocratic or authoritarian leaders. Unlike autocratic leadership, which is focused on retaining control, directive leadership is only used by the occupational therapy assistant when clients require direction in order to benefit from the group activity.

For example, the longer it takes an individual with cognitive dysfunction to process information, the more likely that individual will miss important cues that are relevant to successfully completing the group task. As a directive group leader, the occupational therapy assistant will choose the group activity, direct the task process, and carry the responsibility for the majority of communication with the group. It is important that the directive group leader remain aware of the tone of his or her voice so as not to come across as demeaning or patronizing and role-model the use of respect (i.e., using phrases like "thank you" and

TABLE 14-3
STEPS IN AN ACTIVITY ANALYSIS
Step 1: Specify the activity
Step 2: List the steps of the activity
Step 3: Define the objects, properties, social demands, and space associated with performance of the activity
Step 4: Define the body functions required to successfully perform the activity
Step 5: List required body structures
Step 6: Define the required actions and performance skills required in order to successfully perform the activity
Step 7: Analyze for intervention

"please") at all times. The leader should not do the activity for the members, but rather guide them through the process. If the members are unable to complete the task as designed, it should be graded in such a way that the members can be successful in their efforts.

Grading is used to increase or decrease the demands of the activity. As a general rule, members should be given as much responsibility as they can handle within the group. Sometimes, however, careful observation by the leader during the group activity shows that there has been a mismatch between the therapist's expectation and the client's abilities. For example, if the members appear confused or if they shut down during group (i.e., become silent and reclusive), they have most likely been given too little structure, too much independence, and/or the group activity is too difficult. If, on the other hand, they are argumentative with the group leader or are not working to capacity (based on prior assessment), they are probably not being given enough responsibility, the group is too structured, and/or the activity needs to provide greater challenge. Once these mismatches have been identified, grading of the activity is done in small steps so as to allow the clients to develop the necessary skills, but not overwhelm them.

Grading should be accompanied by scaffolding. *Scaffolding* occurs when the occupational therapy practitioner provides assistance and support to the client at those times that the client cannot complete a step on his or her own and then gradually removes that support as the individual learns to perform the activity. Finding the "just right" challenge in an activity group is often difficult for novice leaders. Observation of the functional skills of potential group members prior to their selection for the group, combined with a thorough analysis of the activity, promotes success in this task. Table 14-3 summarizes the steps that should be used in the activity analysis.

Facilitative Leadership

The term *facilitate* is defined as "to make something easier; to help cause something" (Facilitate, n.d.). Under a *facilitative leader*, a group will make its own decisions, with the leader remaining in the background. This leadership style is perhaps the most familiar to students who have worked together in small groups under the guidance of an instructor; it has been compared to a democratic approach. Facilitative leaders use an array of communication techniques to enable group participation, which will be described later in this chapter. The effective facilitative leader successfully encourages communication among members, promotes group problem solving, and models and reinforces social learning. In groups with highly skilled members, group-centered leadership may emerge, in which the facilitative leader permits members to share the leadership responsibilities (Shimanoff & Jenkins, 2003). Facilitative leadership is preferred over other styles when the goals of the group are to develop self-awareness and insight and members possess the ability to problem solve and negotiate conflict.

Advisory Leadership

Advisory leadership is typically used in community-based support and self-help groups. The leader exercises little authority over the group and acts primarily as a resource, but only when absolutely necessary. This can be particularly difficult for leaders who are more accustomed to a facilitative role, as a lack of structure (and therefore control) may increase their anxiety level (Johnson & Johnson, 2009). *Advisory leadership* can only be applied with clients who have the ability to independently organize and conduct the group. Using this type of leadership, the occupational therapy assistant would step in only when members are unable to solve a problem on their own or when support is needed to effectively and appropriately deal with conflict among the members, as this may turn into a safety issue. It is used in groups where the goal is to learn problem-solving, decision-making, cooperation, and/or compromise skills.

Determining the appropriate level of responsibility to give to members is sometimes a problem for new group leaders and is an area in which an experienced supervisor can help. The entry-level occupational therapy practitioner who desires to further develop his or her group leadership

CHECKPOINT 14-1. IDENTIFY

- How do you recollect yourself as a group member?
- Were you a leader or a follower?
- What was your pattern of behavior when functioning within those groups?
- Did you spontaneously offer ideas, or did you wait for others to share their thoughts first?
- What were your strengths in the role of group member?
- How did you deal with conflict?
- How did you feel when faced with conflict?
- Did you spontaneously seek feedback or wait for it to be offered by your peers?
- How did you handle constructive feedback from your peers?

CHECKPOINT 14-2. UNDERSTAND

Consider the questions that you answered in Checkpoint 14-1. Now ask your peers with whom you have worked in groups those same questions.

- How do they view you as a fellow group member?
- How would they describe your typical pattern of behavior when working within groups?
- What do they see as your strengths?
- How did you deal with conflict within the group?
- How did you handle their feedback?
- What skills, in their opinion, do you need to develop?

skills should seek ongoing clinical supervision from an expert group leader and co-lead groups with that individual as often as possible. Co-leading a group offers at least two advantages. First, novice group leaders can observe a more experienced leader in action and gradually assume leadership function as they become more comfortable in that role. Second, inexperienced leaders have an opportunity to validate their perception of group process.

PART 2: THE ROLE OF THE EFFECTIVE GROUP LEADER

Before you lead a group, it is important to consider how you function as a team member. Self-reflection is a powerful learning tool in this process. Look back on all of the group projects that you completed as a student. Answer the questions in Checkpoint 14-1.

Equally important as self-reflection is an understanding of how we come across to others in our communication. Although self-reflection is an important element of the learning process and is used to develop skills, an individual's self-perceptions may not correspond with how he or she is viewed by others. For example, Mary may see her strength as the ability to solve problems within a group. Her peers, however, may view her as bossy. In another example, Mark may see himself as a leader who asks probing questions, whereas fellow group members merely find his questions off-target and annoying. In order to be therapeutic when working with others, the occupational therapy practitioner must have a clear sense of his or her communication abilities and challenges. This requires seeking feedback from the people with whom you have worked. Respond to the questions in Checkpoint 14-2.

The world we live in and how we perceive it is created in large part from our prior experiences. It consists of a set of predictions and expectations that are applied to the current situation, which are based on feedback received from other people during similar events from our past. The *perceived self* includes aspects such as physical and intellectual abilities, emotions, values, and standards that have been developed through our interactions with other people and the successes and failures to which they led. What gradually emerges from these interactions are consistent ways of behaving, which are elicited by certain situations having something in common—what may be termed the *acting self*. Therapeutic use of self requires the awareness of both the perceived and acting self, accompanied by a clear understanding of what needs to be done given the context of the situation and how it can best be accomplished. When considering all of these elements, it becomes clear that the role of an effective group leader requires much more than learning how to write a detailed group protocol.

Attitude

Before you begin to develop your skills for the role of group leader, it is important to consider how your attitude may affect your ability to establish the development of **rapport** when working with individuals experiencing mental illness. Clients like to feel that they are respected and are active participants in their treatment (Horvath, 2000). "Rapport occurs when two or more people feel that they are *in sync* or *on the same wavelength* because they feel similar or relate well to each other" (Stewart, 1998, p. 282). This includes agreement on therapy goals and the methods that are used to achieve them. According to Anderson (1979), five attitudes can be used to build rapport when working with individuals experiencing a mental illness. These attitudes include the following:

- *Friendliness*: Friendliness can be considered a feeling of warmth that reaches out to the other person. Its components include respect and politeness. Friendliness can be conveyed through body language as well as words. It comes from a person who has unconditional positive regard for others.

- *Patience*: In the context of therapy, patience can be thought of as persistent interest in the achievement of the clients' goals, no matter how long it may take the individual to achieve a task. For example, research has shown that individuals diagnosed with chronic schizophrenia do not generalize new information learned in one particular setting to another without extensive practice (Shohamy et al., 2010). Recognize that the speed of learning may not be a choice; avoid labelling the client as "unmotivated" if he or she does not learn at the speed to which you are accustomed.

- *Truthfulness*: The essence of truthfulness is that it is based on reality. However, truthfulness should not be brutal, nor should it be coated in a "white lie." It is demonstrated by earnestness of manner and sincerity of purpose.

- *Calmness*: Calmness is a great asset when working with people who are emotionally upset, as display of emotion can stir up the emotions of others. By demonstrating anger or anxiety, you may unintentionally upset clients who look to you for feelings of stability and safety.

- *Nonjudgemental attitude*: An individual experiencing psychosis may have very different beliefs, standards, and values from your own. Avoid laughing at or criticizing clients for those differences. Students unfamiliar with mental health practice settings and individuals being treated for mental illness may approach the client with fear and anxiety, assuming that they are unpredictable and therefore "dangerous." These misconceptions are usually based on preconceived ideas learned from movies or books. It is important to view clients without such preconceived expectations, viewing them as individuals with unique client factors, skills, and challenges. Remember that a judgemental attitude may be conveyed both verbally and nonverbally through body language. For example, disapproval can be communicated by a look of disdain or a shrug, even if your words are nonjudgemental.

Communication Skills

In addition to demonstrating the characteristics listed earlier, rapport may be enhanced by using specific communication techniques. These techniques are summarized in Table 14-4. It is important to understand that these skills do not exist on an all-or-nothing basis. Rather, they should be considered on a competency continuum from none to fully mastered skills. In other words, they can be learned and refined through practice. Another important point is that these skills overlap with one another; therefore, an effective group leader must develop the ability to multitask in the group. Continually scanning the group, correctly noting verbal and nonverbal communication, and responding appropriately to clients while simultaneously tracking progress toward individual goals are some of the most difficult challenges that a novice group leader faces. It cannot be stressed enough that leading a group should be practiced under the supervision of an experienced co-leader until the occupational therapy assistant has demonstrated competency in these basic skills.

Once rapport has been established, it is important that the group leader build a therapeutic relationship with members of the group. The therapeutic relationship is a helping relationship built upon trust, which fosters collaboration (Hagerty & Patusky, 2003). Carl Rogers, the individual responsible for developing the term *client-centered*, argued that the therapeutic relationship is a critical element in effective therapy. He hypothesized that the relationship is determined by the quality of communication as well as the type of experiences available to the client in treatment (Horvath, 2000). Mosey defined the therapeutic relationship as "a conscious, planned interaction with another individual in order to exchange information, alleviate fears, and assist the individual in gaining increased use of inner resources" (1981, p. 199). Davis (1998) described a therapeutic interaction as incorporating the occupational therapy practitioner's ability to develop trust, listen, and speak. Those three points are discussed next.

Trust is the foundation of close relationships. It involves taking a risk and sharing oneself with another despite the fact that it could result in being judged, embarrassed, or

TABLE 14-4

GROUP COMMUNICATION TECHNIQUES

COMMUNICATION TECHNIQUE	DEFINITION	EXAMPLE
Clarification	To seek to make clear that which is vague. To check that your understanding is accurate.	"I'm not sure I understand what you mean by 'angrier than usual.' What is different now?"
Confrontation	Helping a client become aware of inconsistencies in feelings, attitudes, beliefs, and behaviors.	"You said you have already made up your mind, but you keep asking the group for feedback." "You are talking about something that you stated made you angry, but have a smile on your face..."
Empathize	To express that you understand what other the individual is going through from his or her perspective; to accurately perceive feelings and to communicate understanding.	"It must be very frustrating to know what you need and not be able to get it."
Link	To find a way to relate what one person is saying to the concerns of another person in the group.	"Can anyone else in the group relate to the situation that Ron is in?"
Model	To demonstrate the attitudes and skills desired by members in the group.	The occupational therapy assistant accepts negative feedback in a nondefensive manner and thanks the individual for bringing it up. "I didn't know that my comment came across as sarcastic. I will try to be mindful of differences in humor—thank you for bringing it up."
Paraphrase	Restating another's message using one's own words.	Client: "I can't do it. My mind keeps wandering." Occupational Therapy Assistant: "You're having difficulty concentrating?"
Question	Seeking clarification to ensure you have the whole story and that you understand it thoroughly.	"How are you coping with the stress you are under?" *Note:* Asking, "How does that make you feel?" and "Why do you feel that way?" is overused.
Reflect	State the essence of what a person has communicated.	Client: "I don't want to be here. I'm bored." Occupational therapy assistant: "You sound discouraged about the possibility of getting anything constructive out of this group."
Summarize	Pulling together what has been said. This technique is often used to decide in which direction the group should go next or what has been learned.	"Let's see. So far you have said..."

hurt. People with mental illness are frequently in emotional pain and often fear being misunderstood. Consequently, they may be particularly reluctant to trust others (Deering, 2009). Behaviors that foster trust in a group leader include the verbalization of clear expectations and demonstration of consistency and predictability. Examples include the following:

- Showing the same degree of respect and interest toward every group member every time the group meets

- Maintaining consistent start and stop times for groups

- Holding all group members to the same level of accountability for their behavior

- Establishing and maintaining rules that support safety and respect for one another in the group

Providing a safe environment for members is one of the most important functions of a group leader. Individuals will not participate in a group if they do not feel safe. Promoting and maintaining a safe environment is demonstrated, for example, when the leader establishes the rule that the use of aggressive behavior or language will not be permitted within the group; the consequence for engaging in that behavior will be one verbal warning before the individual is asked to leave the room. It is important that the leader consistently upholds this rule and that any warnings that are articulated in a firm, but nonshaming manner. This type of communication is termed assertive. How to develop assertive communication skills will be presented later in this chapter.

Active listening is the keystone in the process of building a therapeutic relationship. It has been defined as being attentive to what the client is saying, verbally and nonverbally, while allowing him or her to determine the content of what is said, as well as the level of self-disclosure. It requires that the occupational therapy assistant possess the abilities to perceive and correctly interpret verbal messages and nonverbal language given the context in which it is demonstrated. Effective listening demands energy and concentration. The occupational therapy assistant must be able to remain silent while focusing objective, empathetic attention on the speaker. If the listener is thinking about something else or planning what he or she is going to say next, nonverbal cues and subtleties in the conversation may be missed. Active listening requires the ability to stay focused on the moment-to-moment experience. Therefore, it preferably occurs in an area without environmental distractions (i.e., other people, traffic, a loud radio or television) or interruptions.

People send and receive wordless signals every time they interact with others. The nonverbal behaviors that send these signals are termed *body language*. Body language includes things like facial expressions, hand gestures, eye contact, body movement, how a person sits and stands (posture and stance), how fast and how loudly he or she speaks, and how close he or she chooses to position himself or herself to others. Body language is an often-overlooked component of effective social skills and an important consideration in the development of rapport. For example, eye contact is important in maintaining the flow of conversation, as well as gauging the other person's interest in what is being said. Likewise, the way a person moves and positions his or her body sends a plethora of information to the observer. Body language can reveal clues to unspoken intentions or feelings, as well as the attitude or state of mind of a person. The physical proximity selected to another person, for example, may signal feelings of attraction, affection, anxiety, dominance, or even aggression, depending on the culture and the situation. Table 14-5 offers a list of nonverbal behaviors and how they may be interpreted by others. It should be noted that not everyone reacts or behaves in identical ways. Context in which the body language is demonstrated should always be considered in the interpretation.

Sometimes what is being communicated verbally and what is being expressed with body language are two totally different things. When faced with these *mixed signals*, the listener must choose whether to believe the verbal or the nonverbal message (Bugental, Kaswan, & Love, 1970). If an individual is sharing that he or she feels angry but has a smile on his or her face, the listener may minimize or discount the verbalized message altogether. Likewise, if a group member states that he or she feels "fine" but is observed to be crying, the group will most likely not believe the verbalized message. Research has shown that when confronted with mixed messages, the listener tends to believe the body language as opposed to the verbalized message (Mehrabian, 1971). It is important that the group leader be aware of his or her body language at all times in order to prevent giving mixed messages. When nonverbal signals match up with the words being spoken, they promote feelings of trust toward the leader, improve clarity of content, and increase rapport. When they don't match, they may generate confusion among members and promote feelings of anxiety and mistrust toward the leader of the group.

Two behaviors that bear special consideration when discussing body language are the use of gestures and how a person speaks. The meaning of gestures can be very different across cultures and regions, making them open to misinterpretation. Therefore, their use may need to be limited when working with a diverse population. Likewise, *what* is said by a person (the content) may be misinterpreted based on *how* it is said. People "read" voices similar to the way they read body language. The timing and pace of the spoken word, how loudly it is uttered, and the tone and inflection with which words are stated can change how the message is understood. Take, for example, the simple

TABLE 14-5	

BODY LANGUAGE

NONVERBAL BEHAVIOR	INTERPRETATION
Sitting with legs crossed, swinging one foot	Boredom
Sitting with legs crossed, rapidly shaking or swinging one foot	Anxiety
Sitting, legs apart	Open and relaxed
Sitting with tightly locked ankles	Anxiety or apprehension
Sitting with hands clasped behind head	Confidence or superiority
Sitting or standing with arms crossed on chest	Closed off, defensive or anxious
Sitting with hand resting on cheek, eyes on speaker	Evaluating or thinking
Sitting with head/chin resting on hand, eyes downcast	Bored
Walking briskly (upright – head erect)	Confidence
Walking with shoulders hunched, eyes downcast	Depression or dejection
Pacing	Anger or anxiety
Standing with hands on hips	Aggression
Standing with hands clasped behind back	Expectancy, frustration, or aggression
Drumming fingers	Impatience
Steeling fingers	Authoritative
Clenched fists	Anger
Tugging on ear	Indecision
Rubbing hands	Anxiety or anticipation
Playing with hair	Insecurity or attraction
Pushing back hair in a grooming gesture	Anger
Tilted head	Interest
Shoulders pushed back with chin jutting forward	Aggression

phrase "Not you!" which could indicate sarcasm, surprise, anger, and even affection, depending on its presentation.

Self-Awareness

In order to make authentic connections with others, an occupational therapy practitioner must be conscious of personal feelings, motives, and behaviors during the communication process. In occupational therapy literature, the therapeutic sense of self has been defined as "planned use of … personality, insights, perceptions and judgments as part of the therapeutic process (Mosey, 1981, p. 628). Based on her research, Flores (1997) stated that many therapists "do not fully appreciate the impact of their personalities or values" on helping the group to explore changes in behaviors and lifestyle that affect their relationships with others (p. 456). An effective group leader will be skilled at promoting interpersonal learning in the group using the therapeutic sense of self. **Interpersonal learning** is defined as "all of the processes or relationships among individuals that result in change in behavior, knowledge, or attitude on the part of any one or more of the people involved" (Early, 2013, p. 351). The occupational therapy assistant must utilize all of the resources that are available within the group in order to promote the development of interpersonal learning. Resources include "all of the possibilities for different kinds of interactions and learning among group members, each of whom has different knowledge, skills, feelings, and beliefs to share with others" (Early, 2013, p. 352). To elicit these interactions, the occupational therapy assistant can draw upon his or her personal characteristics. Although it is difficult to identify all of the traits of an effective group leader, numerous researchers have created a variety of lists with different characteristics. Some of the most commonly cited characteristics include:

- *Willingness to model*: The group leader can teach by example and demonstrate behavior that is expected from group members. Behavior can be used to support group norms such as respect for diversity, acceptance of others, willingness to participate, and seriousness of group purpose. For example, when a leader admits error appropriately, group members learn that they can make and admit mistakes while retaining positive relationships with others. The leader encourages participants to do the same by role-modeling how to admit errors when they occur. The leaders can also role-model how to offer support to peers, disagree with what is being said, and verbalize anger.

- *Use of humor*: Humor can be used to support the accomplishment of therapeutic goals and is a great asset to the group leader. For example, being able to detect the humor in situations can help members deal with the stress of an unexpected occurrence in a group, such as a fire alarm going off. It can also help to decrease the tension in a new group as members get to know one another. A leader who smiles, makes frequent eye contact, jokes, and uses an animated tone of voice can pass on enthusiasm to group members who may be reluctant to engage in a novel activity and keep the group moving.

- *Maintaining integrity*: Ethical issues will inevitably arise in any group. Ethical issues include topics such as confidentiality, physical and emotional abuse, and expressed threats of self-harm, as well as intent to harm others. Although the latter are more often expressed in interpersonal groups, all leaders should be familiar with their institution's policies and with pertinent laws and regulations regarding these topics. The occupational therapy assistant should also understand the Occupational Therapy Code of Ethics as it relates to these topics. Appendix D covers these topics as well as others.

- *Coping with feedback*: A leader may be criticized for many reasons; for example, the group topic is not perceived to be important, the activity sounds boring, or members are not being treated equally. Regardless of the rationale behind the complaints and whether or not they are justified, it is important that the leader nondefensively explore with the group the feelings behind them. Modeling how to appropriately share feelings provides members with the opportunity to learn to express their emotions in a similar manner. It also sends the message that openness and sharing of feedback are encouraged within the group.

- *Caring*: Caring implies acceptance. It involves valuing, respecting, and showing a sincere interest in group members. Caring offers group members warmth and support. It is demonstrated by being watchful of the client's needs, listening to his or her concerns, and staying alert to the effects of the group process on him or her.

- *Awareness of diversity*: The term *culture* addresses the beliefs, values, and behaviors shared by a group of people. It can refer to groups based on gender, age, socioeconomic status, race, religion, ethnicity, and sexual identity. Culture influences how an individual views the world and affects how he or she is perceived by others. Differences in cultural backgrounds may affect, among other things, the expectations that members have of a leader, how conflict is (or is not) managed, and expectations of gender-specific roles. If a leader believes that cultural traditions might be a factor in a client's participation in group and/or lead to misunderstandings among group members, the leader should always check the accuracy of those perceptions with the client.

- Barriers that exist to interacting effectively with peers within a diverse group membership include stereotypes, prejudice, and racism. A *stereotype* is a label used to describe differences among groups and to predict how others will behave. Stereotypes can become a type of shorthand that unfairly defines others when the person holding the stereotype does not take the time to interact and view each person as an individual (i.e., "He is overweight; therefore, he must be lazy."). *Prejudice* is defined as an unjustified negative attitude toward a person based solely on the person's membership in a group ("She is too pretty to be smart—we shouldn't even interview her for the job."). They are stereotypes taken to extremes. Prejudices are judgments made about others that establish a superiority/inferiority belief system. *Racism* is prejudice directed at people specifically because of their race or ethnic membership. When prejudice is acted upon, it is *discrimination.* The effective group leaders must address these issues immediately if they are exhibited within a group.

- *Presence*: Presence requires being fully attentive to what is happening in the moment. This provides the group leader with the ability to be compassionate and empathetic with others. The characteristic of presence is closely related to openness.

- *Openness*: Openness refers to the use of appropriate and facilitative self-disclosure. The leader reveals only enough of himself or herself to provide members with a sense of who he or she is as a person in order to help them feel comfortable in the group. Appropriate use of openness by the leader encourages the same from group members. The concept of personal and therapeutic boundaries, however, is often difficult for the novice group leader to grasp. Checkpoint 14-3 illustrates the Therapeutic Boundaries Quiz, which the reader can take to examine his or her knowledge of professional boundaries.

CHECKPOINT 14-3. BOUNDARY QUIZ

1. The best way to prevent boundary crossing is to:

   a. Not see a client alone

   b. Treat all people equally

   c. Never compliment a client

   d. All of the above

2. It is okay to hire a client to paint your house as long as he or she has been discharged:

   a. True

   b. False

3. Rules regarding professional boundaries may vary according to the setting, so if you cross one, it is not your fault:

   a. True

   b. False

4. The concept of therapeutic or professional boundaries applies to anyone who has contact with people and to whom a client entrusts his or her welfare:

   a. True

   b. False

5. It is okay to touch a client without permission if you are just trying to make a point or offer support:

   a. True

   b. False

6. Boundary violations occur when there is a blurring between the needs of the occupational therapy assistant with client needs:

   a. True

   b. False

7. If the occupational therapy assistant encounters a client outside of the treatment setting, he or she should:

   a. Initiate conversation by calling the person's name

   b. Bring up the client's treatment goals and ask how he or she is doing with them

   c. Wait to be addressed by the client

   d. Ask him or her if they are still in recovery

8. A potentially destructive relationship may involve:

   a. Self-disclosure

   b. Trading advice

   c. Allowing the client to freely hug you

   d. All of the above

9. Which of the following statements best illustrates a social, and not therapeutic, relationship?

   a. Sharing mutual experiences, feelings, and ideas

   b. No time limit on length of interactions or frequency of interactions

   c. Encouraging the client to choose the discussion topic

   d. All of the above

(continued)

CHECKPOINT 14-3. BOUNDARY QUIZ (CONTINUED)

10. The following is a danger signal for violation of personal boundaries:
 	
   a. Reporting only positive aspects of the individual's performance in team meetings
 	
   b. The client rearranges his or her schedule in order to meet you on your shift
 	
   c. Both a and b
 	
   d. None of the above

TABLE 14-6

DANGER SIGNALS TO BOUNDARY CROSSING

Warning Signal 1:	You receive gifts, cards, letters, and/or telephone calls from the individual. You accept their invitation to be a friend on Facebook.
Warning Signal 2:	You spend a disproportionate amount of time with that individual, even though you are "off duty."
Warning Signal 3:	You feel that you are the only one who understands that individual.
Warning Signal 4:	The client sticks around or stays up to see you on your shift.
Warning Signal 5:	You keep secrets with the client and do not share information with the treatment team.
Warning Signal 6:	You are guarded and defensive when someone questions your interaction or relationship with that individual.
Warning Signal 7:	Your style of dress has changed since working with this individual.
Warning Signal 8:	The client speaks freely and spontaneously with you, but remains silent and defensive with other staff.

Ask yourself the following questions:

- During level 1 fieldwork, did you find yourself talking about your personal problems with clients?
- Did you tell the clients personal things about yourself in order to impress them?

If the answer was yes, professional boundaries probably were violated. Therapeutic or *professional boundaries* are the limits of the relationship that allow for a safe and healthy connection between the occupational therapy assistant and the client. They are the theoretical "line in the sand" that separates the relationship that an occupational therapy practitioner has with the consumer from his or her personal relationships. Boundaries imply professional distance and respect, and are established in order to protect the client from harm. Because the occupational therapy assistant is supporting the client's personal journey through the recovery process, there are numerous opportunities for overt or inadvertent boundary violations. *Boundary violations* are forms of boundary crossing that involve a professional misusing his or her power to exploit a consumer for personal gain. These violations are at a minimum unethical and can be illegal. Boundary violations with clients include, but are not limited to the following:

- Loaning or borrowing money
- Inappropriate sharing of personal information with the individual
- Sexual advances on the part of the occupational therapy practitioner *or* failure to properly respond to a client's sexual advance
- Staff/client dating
- Verbal threats and derogatory comments made toward the client
- Inappropriate physical contact *or* allowing a client to touch you inappropriately

Table 14-6 contains a list of danger signals that should raise a red flag and cause the occupational therapy practitioner to re-examine a relationship with a person in his or her care.

Even with excellent communication skills and preexisting knowledge of effective communication techniques, learning the role of group leader can be difficult for an entry-level practitioner. For the novice leader, a concrete structure for group leadership designed by Cole (2012) may be useful. This is a client-centered, seven-step model.

TABLE 14-7

COLE'S SEVEN STEPS

Step 1: Introduction

The leader conducts group introductions, explains the group's purpose, outlines how the group will run, and sets the tone by conducting a warm-up activity. The warm-up activity should be 5 minutes or less in length and prepare the members for the main activity to come. Since a warm-up activity can calm or promote arousal, the leader should select it based on the observed need of the group during their introductions.

Step 2: Activity

The activity is the vehicle by which the group achieves its goals. The activity should be based on individual client goals, client factors, and health conditions, and take into consideration an analysis of the demands of the activity.

Step 3: Sharing

After the activity is completed, the product is shared. For activities that include group discussion, this step is not necessary.

Step 4: Processing

In this step, the members discuss how they felt about the activity, the leader, and each other.

Step 5: Generalizing

Members describe what they learned from participating in the group.

Step 6: Application

Members are encouraged to articulate how they can use that information or skill in their personal lives outside of the group.

Step 7: Summary

The leader involves the members in a review of the group that highlights each step and reinforces the main points. The leader thanks the group for their participation and reminds them of when they will meet again for the next session.

It is designed to facilitate client participation at each step. Table 14-7 provides a summary of Cole's model.

PART 3: GROUP DYNAMICS

Group dynamics are the forces that influence the relationship among members and the group outcome (Cole, 2012). Many relationships develop within a group, and these relationships shift or change in response to a number of factors. The term group dynamics expresses this constantly evolving quality of groups, which includes group process. *Group process* refers to *how* group members approach a task to get things done. Yalom (1995) stated that group process includes reflection about the interrelationships of members and how this interaction affects the outcomes of the group. Group process gives members the opportunity to develop an awareness of how their behavior affects others. It also helps to identify what must be changed in order to develop meaningful relationships outside of the group. Three important elements that affect group process are norms, roles, and networks of communication among members. An effective group leader will utilize keen observation skills to monitor for ongoing changes in all three elements. Questions to consider include the following:

- How do members treat one another?
- Is their behavior consistent from one group to the next?
- How cohesive is the group?
- Who takes responsibility for what aspects of the group activity?
- Do members talk to each other or only to the leader?
- Who talks the most?
- Who sits where?
- Who has stopped talking?

Understanding and using group process is a skill that is only developed with repeated practice over time. "Because of the subtle yet complex qualities of group process, [occupational therapy] leaders only become skilled at observing and facilitating through experience. For this reason, supervision is necessary for students to become fully aware of these very powerful but often invisible forces within their groups" (Cole, 2008, p. 324).

Norms

The term *norm* refers to the shared expectations among members that outline the parameters of what is desirable and acceptable behavior, as well as discouraged or prohibit certain actions in a particular setting or group. A group's norms are a statement of what that group believes is an appropriate way of thinking, feeling, and acting. They are basically rules of conduct for the group. The use of group norms contributes to the development of cohesion within a group and promotes feelings of safety and trust among members. An atmosphere of trust is essential for group members to feel safe enough to disclose their feelings and problems and risk trying out new skills and behaviors. When a group is cohesive, the members are more engaged in the group and the change-promoting process. Without cohesion, feedback is not accepted, norms may not be respected, and groups do not accomplish their goals.

Norms are set in part by how the group leader models desirable behaviors and deals with unwanted behavior. For example, a norm of talking directly to each other is sanctioned when the leader asks an individual who is discussing the behavior of another member to direct his or her comments instead to the person about whom he or she is speaking. Another example can be seen when the group leader requests that a member refrain from talking about a peer who is absent from the group that day and wait until that individual returns to discuss the issue. Confidentiality, respect for the differences among the group members, taking responsibility for one's own behavior, listening to others, and participation in group are examples of norms commonly found in most groups. It should be noted, however, that each member inherently has a right to choose whether to interact, what to disclose, and what to do in the group (Corey, Corey, & Corey, 2010). Additional norms might include explicitly stated expectations that members will shut off cell phones during group and refrain from the use of aggressive behavior and language at all times. Research has shown that the less members follow group norms, the less effective the group will be. Norms provide direction and motivation, organize social interactions, and make other people's responses predictable and meaningful (Mullen & Copper, 1994).

Norms are usually openly shared at the start of the group. New members may not be aware of norms, which may be taught by the group through a process called *socialization.* In socialization, the new group member learns the knowledge, social skills, language, and values required to conform to the norms of the group. When the person understands these norms, he or she knows what is expected and is able to predict what other group members will do. A group member who does not act in accordance with group norms is subject to sanction by the group. *Sanction* is a consequence for violating group norms. It may involve the following:

- Telling a person that he or she is doing something that is not acceptable to the group
- A threat of punishment
- Temporary dismissal from the group
- Permanent dismissal

In therapeutic groups, the leader has the most responsibility for monitoring and enforcing norms, although group members are able to assume this responsibility as well. It is a good idea to have norms for a group that reflect the social norms of the community. Once learned, they can be generalized to life outside of the group. Group norms need to be attended to throughout the life of the group; when a norm is ignored by group members for a long period, it ceases to be functional.

Roles

A *role* is described as a tendency to behave, contribute, and interrelate with others in a particular way (Belbin, 1981). Johnson and Johnson (2009, p. 24) state, "Roles define the formal structure of the group and differentiate one position from another." If you watch any small group interact for a time, you will see that individuals in the group behave in different ways. Some members are supportive, others are more concerned with getting the task done, and still others cause friction and conflict within the team. Roles specify the types of behaviors expected of individuals who occupy particular positions in a group. A role in a group can be compared to a role in a play. Once an individual is "cast" in a role, the other members will interact with him or her in a particular way. People can fulfil the same role in slightly different ways, but much like actors, group members cannot wander too far off character from the basic role requirements in order to be effective in that position (Forsythe, 2010).

Some roles are more satisfying the others, and most people prefer to occupy roles that are prestigious and important. They also like roles that require specialized skills and talents (Bettencourt & Sheldon, 2001). Roles may be assigned by the leader or they may emerge spontaneously from within the group. Sometimes the assumption of particular roles may result in shared leadership of the group, especially when the members can accomplish the group goals with minimal assistance from the leader using the roles that they have selected. On the opposite end of the continuum, when members are unwilling or unable to assume roles, the leader must provide directive leadership. Facilitative leadership falls between the two, with the leader enabling members to take on some of the group roles while retaining the others for himself or herself. Ultimately, the

	TABLE 14-8	

FUNCTIONAL TASK ROLES IN THE GROUP

ROLE	PURPOSE
Coordinator	Identifies and explains the relationships between ideas. Pulls them together and makes them cohesive.
Elaborator	Takes other people's initial ideas and builds on them with examples, relevant facts, and data. Looks at the consequences of proposed ideas and actions.
Energizer	Concentrates the group's energy on forward movement. Challenges and stimulates the group to take further action.
Evaluator/critic	Evaluates proposals against a predetermined or objective standard. Assesses the reasonableness of a proposal and looks at whether it is fact based and manageable as a solution.
Information giver	Provides factual information to the group. Is seen as an authority on the subject and relates own experience when relevant.
Information seeker	Requests clarification of comments in terms of their factual adequacy. Seeks expert information or facts relevant to the problem. Determines what information is missing and needs to be found before moving forward.
Initiator/contributor	Proposes original ideas or different ways of approaching group problems or goals. Initiates discussions and move groups into new areas of exploration.
Opinion giver	Expresses his or her own opinions and beliefs about the subject being discussed in terms of what the group "should" do.
Opinion seeker	Asks for clarification of the values, attitudes, and opinions of group members. Checks to make sure different perspectives are given.
Orienter	Reviews and clarifies the group's position. Provides a summary of what has been accomplished, notes where the group has veered off course, and suggests how to get back on target.
Procedural technician	Facilitates group discussion by taking care of logistical concerns like where meetings are to take place and what supplies are needed for each meeting.
Recorder	Acts as the secretary or minute-keeper. Records ideas and keeps track of what goes on at each meeting.

Adapted from Benne, K., & Sheats, P. (1948). Functional roles of group members. *Journal of Social Issues, 4*(2), 41-49.

style of the group leader, the goals of the group, and the skills of the members will determine which roles members assume within the group.

Two influential theorists of group behavior were Benne and Sheats (1948), who defined 26 distinct roles that can be played by one or more people within a group. In addition, they delineated three categories in which to place these roles: (1) task roles, (2) personal and social roles, and (3) dysfunctional or individualistic roles. Benne and Sheats stated that the functional roles that are selected by individuals will depend on their experience, as well as which roles are deemed necessary in order for the group to accomplish its goals. Although research continues to be conducted on this topic, their original study remains useful and interesting way of looking at group behavior.

Functional Task Roles

The purpose of task roles is to assist the group in coordinating its efforts to define and solve common problems. These are the roles that relate to getting the work done and address the different parts of a project, from start to finish. Individuals may assume several different roles during the life of a project. They may also share roles with more than one person. Table 14-8 lists each of the functional task roles in a group and the responsibilities associated with them.

Functional Personal and Social Roles

These roles focus on group-building processes. Their purpose is to strengthen, regulate, and maintain the group. The members who assume these roles influence

	TABLE 14-9	
	FUNCTIONAL, PERSONAL, AND SOCIAL ROLES IN THE GROUP	
ROLES	**DESCRIPTION**	
Compromiser	Offers to change his or her position for the good of the group, or meets others halfway.	
Encourager	Affirms, praises, and supports the efforts of fellow group members. Demonstrates warmth toward others and maintains a positive attitude in meetings.	
Follower	Seen as a listener not a contributor. Accepts without comment what is shared and decided by others.	
Gatekeeper/ expediter	Regulates the flow of communication. Makes sure all members have the opportunity to speak. Encourages shy and quiet members to contribute their ideas. Limits participation of those who dominate the conversation.	
Harmonizer	Mediates differences between individuals in order to overcome hostility. Seeks ways to reduce tension in the group. May diffuse a situation by providing further explanation, seeking clarification, or using humor.	
Observer/ commentator	Provides feedback to the group about how it is functioning. Usually speaks when a group wants to set, evaluate, or change its standards and processes.	

Adapted from Benne, K., & Sheats, P. (1948). Functional roles of group members. *Journal of Social Issues, 4*(2), 41-49.

the relationships among members, assisting them to work together through behaviors such as showing concern for the feelings of others, promoting trust, and reducing conflict within the group. Table 14-9 identifies functional, personal, and social roles in a group.

Dysfunctional Individualistic Roles

The individualistic role is concerned exclusively with the satisfaction of individual needs. Although assumption of these roles may "work" for the individual, the behaviors associated with them usually block the group's progress. Even members with the ability to take on productive group roles will occasionally adopt a dysfunctional role. This usually occurs when the leader is too authoritarian or permissive, or if there is a mismatch between the skill level required to complete the task and the skills that actually exist within the group (i.e., the activity is too easy or too challenging). If the individuals who have assumed dysfunctional roles are not redirected, they will inevitably take up the group's time with irrelevant issues. Table 14-10 identifies dysfunctional and individualistic roles in the group. It also lists the roles and the responsibilities associated with each role.

After discussing the various types of roles found within a group and the responsibilities associated with each of them, it becomes clear that the greater the ability of the members to effectively assume a variety of functional roles—in other words, the greater the leadership capacity within the group—the greater the potential for the group to be effective. The challenge for the leader is to enable and support members to take on the risk of assuming functional task roles that they have not tried previously. Although

it is natural for group members to assume certain roles based on their personal preference, experience, and skills, all members benefit from the opportunity to experience the different aspects of themselves required to effectively fulfill a wide variety of different roles. The following are some of the techniques that can be used by the group leader to promote role development and variation among group members (Forsythe, 2010; Howe & Schwartzburg, 2010):

- The leader does not assume all of the roles needed for a group to function in a given situation. Rather, he or she assumes only the roles that members are currently unable to take on because of insufficient group interaction skills.

- The leader delegates the role functions to members that are needed in order for them to develop their group interaction skills to the next level, supports their work in that role, and allows time for error learning. This allowance would include such things as allocating extra time to complete a task or simplifying an activity so that it can be completed using a smaller number of steps.

- The leader begins a group with a discussion about the various membership roles, then provides concrete examples of how a person may act within each of them in order to fulfill these roles.

- A group member is given special attention or praise when he or she takes on a role that he or she has never assumed before in the group.

- The group role-plays how to behave in a specific role (i.e., harmonizer, elaborator, gate keeper, etc.), thereby

	TABLE 14-10

DYSFUNCTIONAL AND INDIVIDUALISTIC ROLES IN THE GROUP

ROLE	RESPONSIBILITIES
Aggressor	Makes personal attacks using belittling and insulting comments, usually in an attempt to decrease another member's status.
Blocker	Opposes every idea or opinion that is put forward, yet refuses to make own suggestions, thereby stalling the group with resistance.
Disruptor play-boy/playgirl	Distracts other people by telling jokes, playing pranks, and discussing unrelated material. Uses group as a time to have fun.
Dominator	Tries to control the conversation. Dictates what people should be doing. Exaggerates his or her knowledge—monopolizes the discussion by claiming to know more about the situation and have better solutions than anybody else.
Help seeker	Actively looks for sympathy by expressing feelings of inadequacy and acting helpless.
Recognition seeker	Uses group meetings to draw personal attention to himself or herself. Brags about past accomplishments or shares irrelevant stories that paint him or her in a positive light.
Self-confessor	Uses the group meetings as an avenue to disclose personal feelings and issues. Relates group actions to his or her personal life (i.e., "This reminds me of a time in my life when...").
Special-interest pleader	Makes suggestions based on what others would think or feel. Avoids revealing his or her personal opinions by using a stereotypical position (i.e., "The boss wouldn't like that idea.").

Adapted from Benne, K., & Sheats, P. (1948). Functional roles of group members. *Journal of Social Issues, 4*(2), 41-49.

allowing members to experiment with roles without the pressure of acting in a real group situation.

- The members view a group as outside observers in order to see how roles are carried out during the group process.
- The leader requests that the group stop what it is doing in order to look at what roles have been assumed in the last 20 to 30 minutes, what has been accomplished by individuals in those roles, what remains to be done, and what roles need to be assumed in order to complete those tasks.

As members begin to realize that the choice of roles within a group is more than "leader" or "follower," the array of functional roles that they can choose to assume in the group process will increase. This variation in roles provides group members with an opportunity to take note of their individual strengths and challenges. Role variation keeps a group dynamic, and the effective group leader will use the skills listed earlier to promote role development and growth of interpersonal skills in every group member.

The Communication Process Within the Group

Effective communication is a prerequisite for group function, since it is through communication that group members interact. In this process members are required to simultaneously receive and interpret information, offer suggestions, and provide feedback. If a group is to function effectively, its members must be able to communicate efficiently. Communication is only successful when both the sender and the receiver understand the same information as a result of the communication.

The pattern of interaction and communication among group members will differ from group to group. **Communication networks** refer to the regular patterns of information exchange among members of a group. The efficiency of these networks determines whether group goals are achieved, and will also affect individual outcomes in regard to member satisfaction and performance within the group. Communication networks become more complicated as a group increases in size.

Communication within the group needs to be arranged so that ideas and information flow freely among group members. This flow (or lack of it) has been found to influence the emergence of group roles, the morale of group members, and the efficiency of problem solving within the group (Leavitt, 1951; Shaw, 1964). The way group members seat themselves in relation to one another affects their communication flow and exerts significant influence on the perception of status among members. For example, a member who perceives himself or herself as having relatively high status may sit at the head of a rectangular table, where he or she is then viewed as a leader by the other members. Likewise, there is a strong tendency for individuals to communicate with members facing them rather than members seated adjacent to them.

Research has shown that the increased opportunity for eye contact among members seated in a circle will enhance frequency of interaction, friendliness, cooperativeness, and liking for the members of the group, whereas sitting in long rows will decrease the likelihood of eye contact and social interaction. Why does seating position influence so many group processes? One explanation, based on the equilibrium model of communication, suggests that personal space, body orientation, and eye contact define the level of intimacy of any interaction and consequently the amount of interaction. If group members feel that a low level of intimacy is appropriate, they may sit far apart, make little eye contact, assume a relatively formal posture, and initiate little, if any, conversation. If, in contrast, members desire to discuss personal topics, they may move closer together, make more eye contact, and adopt more relaxed postures (Patterson, 1991). Relaxed, less formal groups are associated with increased levels of social interaction.

A communication network may be interactive, in which every member communicates with every other member as well as the group leader, or leader mediated, where the group communicates only with or through the group leader. Opportunities for interpersonal learning are greatest with a pattern of interactive communication. In groups that include persons at lower levels of group interaction skill (parallel or project), the members are not expected to interact freely. Instead, the leader will direct the discussion, asking members for their feelings or reactions to what another member has said. At higher levels of groups (egocentric-cooperative and above), the leader should refrain from answering the members' questions, instead redirecting them back to the group or a specific group member in order to create more interaction (Mosey, 1986).

Dealing With Conflict

Interaction can be predominantly verbal, as in interpersonal groups, or physical, as in a task group. The interactional pattern may be highly structured where members wait to be called upon, or informal and spontaneous, where members may talk as they choose. The style of leadership, nature of the group goals, and the type of activity will influence the interactional pattern within the group. When groups are working cooperatively, communication tends to be more frequent, open, complete, accurate, and honest (Deutsch, 1973; Johnson & Johnson, 2009). When group members are competing with one another, communication tends to be lacking or deliberately misleading. Competition within a group can lead to conflict.

When *conflict* occurs in a group, the actions or beliefs of one or more members of the group are viewed as unacceptable and/or are resisted by the other members. Many group and individual factors can create conflict in a group, but the most common sources are competition and power struggles. *Power struggles* occur in groups where members vie for control in leadership, status, and/or position. Some additional examples of potential sources of conflict include being assigned a nonpreferred functional role, dislike of other group members, and dislike of the group task.

Most people, if given the choice, will avoid conflict. However, group conflict can be useful, as it provides the opportunity for a leader to teach problem solving to participants in the group. A group, by its very nature, brings individuals into contact with one another, each with their own interests, preferences, motivations, and viewpoints. Such differences of opinion are generally the base source of conflict. If conflict does not occur within a group, the chances are that different points of view are intentionally being withheld from other members, or participants are bored and uninvolved in the task (Fisher, 1980). A leader can assist a group to deal with conflict by:

- Increasing openness within the group (modelling self-disclosure; use of nonverbal and verbal mirroring to teach clarity of communication; using open-ended questions to elicit additional information; checking out perceptions rather than making assumptions).

- Reinforcing and commenting on positive group action that has been taken up to the point of conflict.

- Identifying hidden agendas among members (operating goals that influence group process even though they are not openly acknowledged) that may be contributing to the conflict.

- Facilitating win/win solutions to conflict (i.e., focus on defeating the problem, not each other; seek facts to resolve dilemmas; view conflict as helpful; avoid self-oriented behavior; focus on others' needs).

- Changing seating arrangements (i.e., a circle is conducive to problem solving; break up subgroupings by having members sit next to someone different; the leader can choose to sit next to an anxious individual to show support or a hostile group member to signal a desire for communication).

- Teaching problem-solving skills:

  ○ Define the problem.

  ○ *Brainstorm*: Write down all possible ideas without judging the merits of each. Then rank them in order of usability.

  ○ *Discussion*: In this stage, each person is asked for his or her perspective.

○ *Proposal/counteroffer:* Repeated until a compromise is reached.

- Teaching and promoting the use of assertive communication. Before a leader can teach group members how to use assertive communication to deal with conflict, he or she must possess a thorough understanding of the concept (knowledge) and the ability to phrase an assertive message (skill). The next section in this chapter offers an overview of passive, aggressive, and assertive communication styles; cites reasons for acting assertively; explains how to articulate an assertive message; and provides examples of assertive messages that can be used to deal with disruptive behaviors in a group.

PART 4: THE ASSERTIVE GROUP LEADER

Research indicates a need to educate students on how to negotiate conflict, handle confrontation, set limits, and deal with aggressive behavior (Davidson, 2011; Haertl, 2008). Students who are unable to effectively cope with these behaviors will not be prepared for common practice challenges, regardless of the setting in which they work. When an individual uses assertion, he or she is expressing thoughts, feelings, and beliefs in a direct, honest, and appropriate manner. The use of assertive communication involves respect for oneself, as well as the other person's needs and rights. It is not a strategy for getting one's way; rather, it is a way for negotiating mutually satisfactory solutions to a variety of problems.

If assertiveness entails finding a win/win solution, what behaviors and outcomes are associated with passive and aggressive communication? To answer that question, first try to envision a continuum of communication, with passive communication at one endpoint and aggressive communication at the other. It is important to emphasize that people do not consistently use just one style of communication in every situation. Rather, they move up and down the continuum depending on the topic, the person with whom they are speaking, and the context of the situation. It is also important to point out that a person can be known as outgoing, yet not be assertive, as assertiveness involves expressing *feelings* and not only involvement in general conversation.

Passive Communication

When an individual chooses to be nonassertive and utilizes passive communication, he or she fails to express feelings or expresses them with little confidence. Consequently, he or she permits others to violate his or her rights. If this person does try to verbalize his or her emotions, they may come across in an apologetic, timid, and self-effacing manner (i.e., "Uh, it kind of bothers me … If you can stop, I would appreciate it … It's not that big of a deal."); therefore, the content of the message is disregarded by others. The unspoken message is that the individual's feelings don't really count and that this person can be taken advantage of. A person is behaving passively when he or she allows others to push him or her around and consistently does what he or she is told, even when he or she disagrees and is aware that it is not in his or her best interest. The advantage of being passive is that the person rarely experiences direct rejection (since he or she has not articulated his or her needs) and avoids conflict. The disadvantage is that the passive person will consistently be taken advantage of (the "doormat" syndrome) and stores up a heavy burden of resentment and anger toward the individuals who treat him or her this way.

Aggressive Communication

On the other end of the spectrum is the aggressive (controlling) individual who does stand up for his or her rights and articulates his or her feelings but does so by:

- Threatening (i.e., "You better stop or you will be sorry!")

- Accusing ("I can't help my temper … You make me so mad!")

- Labeling ("You are such a nag … You are a slob.") and generally stepping on people without regard for their feelings

The usual goal of this communication style is to dominate and win, forcing the other person to lose by humiliating, degrading, and overpowering him or her. The message is that what the aggressive person wants, feels, or thinks is more important than what anyone else wants, feels, or thinks. This controlling individual is "right" and knows "how it should be done."

The advantage of aggressive communication is that other people do not push this individual around, and the aggressive individual feels "important." The disadvantage is that people do not want to be around this person any more than necessary. It is important to pause for a moment to reflect on the fact that people employed as occupational therapy practitioners, as well as other health care professionals, may unintentionally be communicating aggressively in their zeal to "help" others, telling them exactly what needs to be done and precisely how to do it.

The information listed earlier offers just a glimpse into the communication continuum and is intended to assist the reader in understanding the basic differences between communication styles. To supplement this information, Table 14-11 describes body language that accompanies each of those styles.

TABLE 14-11			
NONVERBAL MESSAGES ASSOCIATED WITH PASSIVE, ASSERTIVE, AND AGGRESSIVE COMMUNICATION			
CHARACTERISTICS	**PASSIVE**	**ASSERTIVE**	**AGGRESSIVE**
Eye contact	Usually avoided. Eyes tend to be cast downward.	Frequent but broken by occasional horizontal glances away.	Direct and fixed—"stares you down."
Facial expression	Often anxious or apologetic. The person may blush or exhibit nervous smiling or inappropriate laughter.	Appropriate to the content of the message.	Holds muscle tension in the jaw. Appears angry.
Flow of words	Considerable hesitation—searches for words to please the other person. Sentences may be left incomplete (drifts off). May also be stalling/pausing before getting to the point. Pace will be slow or the words pour out all at once.	Even and conversational, without rushing or hesitating.	May be faster or slower than usual in pace. Occasionally less fluent, as anger level overwhelms the person.
Movement and gestures	Few gestures or quick/unfocused gestures (i.e., fidgeting, picking cuticles). Shrugs shoulders with palms and hands outward.	Movements are relaxed and fluid. Gestures are open. Hands appear relaxed.	Gestures are sharp and rapid (i.e., karate-like movements). May gesture with the index finger pointed. Balled fists.
Physical contact	Minimal touching, if any.	Varies by culture. If it occurs, it is usually gentle, with open palms.	Firm—jabbing the air (or the person) with finger. May become physically assaultive.
Physical distance	Greater than 3 feet.	Varies depending on culture. Usually conversational distance (2 to 3 feet).	Closer than usual, "invading" the other person's space.
Posture	The body is hunched, making it appear smaller. The body is tilted toward the ground or angled away from the other person. Face is tilted down and away. Shoulders may be raised toward ears.	Upright posture with shoulders straight. The body faces the other person directly. Face is not tilted up or down.	The body looks bigger, as shoulders are thrown back. Body is angled downward and toward the other person. The position communicates that this person is "ready to charge" and fight.
Tone of voice	Quiet. May have an upward swing at the end, as though asking a question (communicates uncertainty).	Warm, firm, and modulated. Normal tone of voice.	Yelling; shouting or deadly cold, with little emotion. Tone can also be condescending or sarcastic.

Assertive Communication

Knowing when assertive communication is needed and the reasons that people choose (or not) to use it still does not inform the student how to articulate an assertive message. The key to clear and assertive communication of feelings is the "I message" (Gordon, 1970). An "I message" is a way of communicating feelings without assigning blame for them to another. The individual expressing the statement is taking responsibility for the feeling and "owning" it. Another person is not being accused of causing the problem. Disclosing what one is feeling is the beginning of effective communication, as it invites the other person to do the same. "I" language is particularly useful as a guide for helping people express negative feelings. The following format is used to verbalize an assertive message:

1. The situation is … (speaker objectively describes the person's behavior, not his or her subjective opinion of it).

2. I feel … (speaker describes how he or she is feeling).

3. Because (speaker expresses the self-talk/rationale that contributes to the feeling).

4. I would like … (suggest the compromise, or pose a question to gain more information).

Imagine this scene. You are busy writing a progress note in a chart when your supervisor abruptly steps into the staff room and announces in a loud voice, "I have something important to discuss with you, but I can't talk about it right now. We will meet later." The supervisor's facial expression is angry, he is moving quickly, and he is using sharp, abrupt hand gestures.

A passive response would be to say nothing, then sit and worry for the rest of the day as to whether you have done something wrong. An aggressive response would be to follow the supervisor out of the room while stating loudly, "You can't just come in and announce something like that without an explanation! I insist that you talk with me now!" Neither of these options would provide both of you with what is needed—you want to decrease your anxiety level, and your supervisor has something else that needs to done. An "I message' that would allow for the needs of both individuals to be met would be, "You have something important to discuss with me and don't have time to do it right now (situation). I am concerned (feeling) because your facial expression appears angry to me (self-talk/rationale for the feeling). I realize that you are in a hurry, but can you just let me know if I have done something to upset you?"

This was a real-life situation; the outcome of the "I message" was the following response from my supervisor: "I need to go over your performance evaluation before the end of the week. You didn't do anything wrong—quite the contrary. I am just upset because my car broke down on the way here and I am late for a meeting with a client's family." My anxiety alleviated, I was able to focus on my documentation, and my supervisor got to his meeting. Table 14-12 presents characteristics of dysfunctional communication.

In the group setting, assertive "I messages" may be used to address a variety of issues, including, but not limited to:

- A member who is engaging in a behavior that is impeding the progress of the group

- A group norm that has been violated

- The leader needs clarification on an issue occurring in the group

- There is a member who is nonparticipative and needs encouragement to join in discussion

When the group leader utilizes "I messages" to seek clarification or to confront members who are exhibiting negative behavior in the group, these individuals are provided with the opportunity to understand the impact that their behavior is having on others and decide what, if anything, they want to do about it. When confrontation is done assertively, it improves the chances that it will be heard, as group members will be more likely to remain nondefensive. The effective group leader must remember to always utilize the following guidelines when utilizing assertive communication:

- Be descriptive (objective) rather than judgmental (subjective).

- Be specific (concrete) rather than general.

- Provide feedback at the time the behavior occurs.

The following are some of the situations commonly encountered by the leader in a group. Examples of "I messages" are included that could be used to address each issue.

Monopolizing

Monopolizing occurs when one group member talks nonstop. When the purpose of the group is to share ideas, learn from one another, or make group decisions, a member who fails to let others contribute affects group movement. Sometimes an overtalkative group member may speak for an extended period because the group does not address his or her behavior. In this case, the leader might provide opportunity for feedback by stating, "Mark, you have shared your thoughts with the group on this topic for several minutes—thank you for your participation (situation). I am concerned (emotion), however, because other group members have not shared their thoughts yet, and it needs to be a group decision (self-talk). What are the rest of you thinking?"

Silence

A group member's nonparticipation, silence, or withdrawal is not an obvious problem, but it does influence the other group members. It may occur because the individual is not cognitively competent to handle the demands of the group or because symptoms, such as hallucinations, may be a barrier to participation. An example of an "I message"

	TABLE 14-12	

CHARACTERISTICS OF DYSFUNCTIONAL COMMUNICATION

CHARACTERISTICS	BEHAVIOR
Blame	You blame your problems on other people.
Counterattack	You respond to constructive criticism by criticizing the person who offers it to you.
Defensiveness	You refuse to admit to any wrongdoing.
Demanding	You want better/more, but refuse to ask for what you need in a direct, straightforward way.
Denial	You insist that you feel fine, even when you actually feel sad, angry, or hurt.
Diversion	Instead of expressing your feelings about something happening in the moment, you list past grievances.
Helper role	Instead of permitting other people to share their feelings of hurt, sadness, or anger, you try to solve their problem.
Hopeless	You give up and don't say anything ("There's no point in trying—nothing ever changes").
Martyrdom	You play the role of an innocent victim ("Someday he will realize how hard I work to keep this family together...").
Passive aggression	You pout or withdraw, then expect people to understand the reason behind your behavior.
Put down	You claim that people *"always"* misbehave or *"never"* make an effort to change.

in this situation could be, "Rosie, you have been sitting in group for 10 minutes without joining in discussion, but I have observed you muttering under your breath and looking over your shoulder (situation). I am concerned (emotion) because it is not clear to me to whom you are speaking (self-talk). Do you feel able to participate in the group?" Depending on Rosie's response, she may be excused from group, or the leader may specifically direct questions and comments to Rosie in order to help her focus on group discussion.

Physical Aggression

The leader cannot allow any aggressive behavior among group members. This includes touching group members who do not want to be touched, throwing objects, and hitting or hurting others. Some "I messages" that could be used in these situations include the following: "Joe, you just pounded the table, shouted, and swore as you described the anger you feel toward your doctor for putting you on meds (situation). I am worried (emotion) because the rules of the group prohibit aggressive behavior, but I think you need to share your feelings (self-talk). In order to remain in group, you have to refrain from pounding the table and swearing." The leader would then suggest that Joe take a short break from group in order to calm down. Later, after welcoming

Joe back to the group, the group could be addressed with the following comment: "Joe had difficulty verbalizing anger earlier without swearing and pounding the table (situation). I am curious (emotion) how all of you felt while he demonstrated this behavior; I saw several of you jump in your seats (self-talk). Is there anybody who is willing to share their thoughts or feelings about the situation with Joe?"

Interrupting

Clients who interrupt group may be demonstrating dysfunctional group roles, such as the dominator and aggressor. Such interruptions disrupt the flow of discussion in the group, with frustrating results. An example of an "I message" that could be used in this scenario follows: "Dean, you did not let Mary finish her last three sentences before you shared your thoughts (situation). I am concerned (emotion) because Mary asked you to refrain from that behavior, and you have not complied (self-talk)." Group norms regarding respectful behavior in group would then be reviewed, and the consequences for disregarding the norms made clear.

These are just a few of the many scenarios that a group leader may encounter. Based on the brief overview of group process, the rationale for developing effective interpersonal communication skills as a leader is clear. Humans are not born with these skills; they must be learned (Johnson & Johnson, 2013). In much the same way that individuals go through developmental phases when learning interpersonal skills, the effective group must go through stages of development as well.

PART 5: STAGES OF GROUP DEVELOPMENT

Studies have suggested that the success of the group depends to a large extent on its movement through successive stages of development (Bion, 1961; Gerseck, 2003; Poole, 2005; Yalom, 1995). Models that describe stages of group development are based on the fact that it is the *system itself* that changes during the developmental stages, and not the individual group members. These stages of a group can happen over an extended length of time or in as little as one session.

Tuckman's Five-Stage Theory

Probably the most famous sequential stage theory was formulated by Bruce Tuckman (1965), who reviewed over 50 studies on group development. Although at first glance, these descriptions appeared to vary widely, upon further exploration, Tuckman found a significant amount of agreement among theorists. Using the data from his study, he hypothesized five successive stages of group development (Tuckman, 1965): forming, storming, norming, performing, and adjourning. It was suggested that the path of development does not always occur in a straight line, and stages may overlap. In addition, regression to a previous stage can occur if a group is experiencing an abnormal level of stress.

Forming

In this stage, the group has to confront issues of getting to know one another and learning about the task they need to perform. It is a period of uncertainty, as members try to determine their place in the group. While they learn the procedures, norms, and rules of the group, members are usually on their "best behavior" and try to determine whether they will be accepted or excluded by their peers based upon their similarities and differences. Consequently, they may be hesitant to express their points of view. Once they become accustomed to the group and their anxiety level decreases, however, participants usually begin sharing personal information and decide whom they will trust and like. In this stage the leader outlines the structure of the group, assists members to establish a trusting atmosphere, and role-models appropriate participation in the group.

Storming

In the second stage of group development, conflict emerges. For example, there may be disagreement regarding group leadership or the process that will be used to complete the task. Group members may discover that they just don't get along with one another. Conflict may erupt over group goals. Competition may develop between individual group members for authority and preferred roles. While in the forming stage, members may have accepted the leader's guidance with few questions, but now, as the group matures and enters the storming stage, conflict between the leader and group members may disrupt the group's functioning. Expressed conflict may result in a response of "flight" or "fight"; those members who are unable to tolerate anxiety may leave the group, whereas their peers openly challenge the leader's policies and decisions. Coalitions and subgroups may form in response to the bickering. Once stable patterns of communication and authority develop, however, conflict usually subsides, but until then, members struggle with "risk taking and compliance, control, and confrontation" (Cara & MacRae, 2013, p. 680). Participants may be concerned about feeling safe and being accepted. The role of the leader in this stage is to help members recognize personal resistance and the issues behind the interpersonal conflicts. Group members should be encouraged to give their input, with the leader explaining that differences in opinion are to be expected. Conflict is described as part of a healthy group process and is not considered failure.

Norming

By this stage, the group has designed and implemented norms and procedures to carry out activities, and it is getting down to work. Cohesion among members has grown. As a result, members communicate openly with one another, offering and accepting constructive feedback. The problems that led to earlier conflicts have been resolved. The group shares leadership functions, and there is a willingness to take risks. The leader functions as a role model who balances support and confrontation, interprets the meaning of behavior demonstrated within the group, links the work of the individual member to life outside of the group, and encourages members to take on new group roles and practice new skills.

Performing

In this stage, the group spends the majority of time working effectively on the task at hand. Group members become proficient in working together to achieve the group's goals and are more flexible in working with one another. Not all groups get to this stage, for even cohesive groups are not necessarily productive.

Adjourning

In this phase, the members address their feelings about the group ending. They discuss what has been accomplished, offer feedback to others, complete any unfinished business left in the group, and generalize what has been learned from working in the group to their everyday life.

Group Life Cycle Approach

With the onset of managed health care and shorter treatment duration, therapeutic groups may not have sufficient time to move through all five of Tuckman's stages. These factors, in addition to the move toward a public health model, have led to another way in which to address group development: the phase-specific approach (Smith, 2001). Every group has a beginning, middle, and end, and these phases occur at different times for different types of groups. Whatever the type or length of a group, the group leader is responsible for attending to certain key elements in each of the phases of the group's development, which are better viewed on a continuum rather than distinct phases. The phases found on the group life cycle continuum are initiation, exploration and clarification, conflict, resolution, and dissolution. Each is described next.

Initiation

Initiation consists of group introductions, statement of purpose, and efforts on the part of participants to become acquainted with one another, usually in a warm-up activity. The members establish basic norms for group behavior, such as how often, when, and where the group will meet. The length of time required for this stage depends on the size of the group; the complexity of the problem; and the personal, social, and organizational differences among members. If the group members have had previous experience with one another, this stage may be quite short.

Exploration and Clarification

The second stage, exploration and clarification, is a testing stage in which members define the problem (if there is one), clarify the task, discover who the leaders are, and distribute group roles that specify how the members will relate to one another. Norms and expectations are defined further by this role distribution. The group decides, for example, who will introduce new ideas in what way and how decisions will be made.

Conflict

Conflict may occur in a group because of differences of opinion about how best to solve the problem or address the task, differences between ascribed and earned leadership, and differences of opinion about procedure. Conflict may require a return to exploration and clarification as group members seek new understandings of each other and the problem.

Resolution

Resolution is the "performing" stage of the group life cycle. The group is ready to engage in the task process.

Dissolution

Dissolution, the final stage in the life cycle, brings the group to a close. The group may lose its reason for being in a number of ways. With a problem-solving group, there has been resolution of the problem, and in a task group, completion of the task eliminates the need for the group. A support group may dissolve when it no longer meets the needs of individual members. Other groups may have term limits and dissolve after a certain period.

PART 6: EDUCATIONAL STRATEGIES TO PROMOTE LEARNING

In Chapter 13, it was suggested that the novice occupational therapy assistant group leader is usually responsible for conducting activity, task, and psychoeducational groups under the supervision of the occupational therapist. In those groups, teaching activities are used to help clients develop new skills, remediate problems, and promote wellness. **Teaching** is defined as a deliberate intervention that involves sharing information and experiences to meet learner outcomes in cognitive, affective, and psychomotor domains (Carpenter & Bell, 2002). When teaching, it is critical that the occupational therapy assistant facilitate whatever method of learning is most effective for the **learner**—the individual who is being taught the skills. Teaching is a component in the **education process**, which is defined as a systematic, sequential, logical, scientifically based, planned course of action consisting of two major operations: teaching and learning (Carpenter & Bell, 2002). The outcome of the education is **learning**. Learning is indicated by a change in behavior (knowledge, attitudes, or skills) that can be observed or measured.

The education process fosters growth in both the teacher and learner. Effective education has been associated with increased client satisfaction, improvement in the quality of care being given to clients, decreased client anxiety, and increased compliance in the learning process. It can empower clients to live the lives that they desire (Bastable, Gramet, Jacobs, & Sopczyk, 2011). Learning to assume the role of the educator (teacher) is of critical importance to health care providers.

To be a competent educator, the occupational therapy assistant must be able to identify the information that is required to learn a skill and evaluate the client's readiness, ability, and motivation to learn that content. He or she then helps the client understand the value of knowing that information. In other words, the provision of information alone does not ensure that learning will occur. Research has demonstrated that adults are much more likely to learn through active exploration than they are through passively listening to lecture and reading from handouts. Consequently, it is the responsibility of the group leader to design learning experiences that actively engage participants in the learning process; this is called *instructional design*. In order to do this, the occupational therapy assistant, under the supervision of an occupational therapist, must perform the following steps:

- Assess the learner's problems and deficits

- Provide only needed information (so as not to overwhelm the individual) and present it in appropriate ways.

- Take time to check on the progress being made in the learning process

- Provide appropriate feedback

- Reinforce learning in the acquisition of knowledge, skills, and attitudes

- Evaluate outcomes/learner abilities

What factors affect the teaching and learning process? Research has shown that there are three basic elements that contribute to effective teaching and learning, whether it occurs on a one-on-one level with a client, or in a group setting. They include (1) the characteristics of the learner; (2) the content that needs to be taught; and (3) the methods, media, and materials that are used to teach it. These elements are discussed in more detail next.

The Learner

Assessment of a learner's needs, readiness to learn, and learning styles is the most important step in instructional design, but is also the most likely to be neglected. It is not unusual that clients with the same condition who receive services at one facility or program are taught the same information with the same instructional materials in the same manner (Haggard, 1989). The outcome is that the information is neither individualized nor based on adequate educational assessment of learning needs.

Learning needs are defined as the gaps in knowledge that exist between a desired level of performance and the actual level of performance (Healthcare Education Association, 1985). These gaps exist because of a lack in knowledge, skill, or attitude (motivation) within the client. It is important to note that differences frequently exist between the client's perception of needs and the needs identified by the occupational therapy practitioner. Such a mismatch in readiness to learn results in frustration on the part of both the learner and the educator—the learner feels that the group is a waste of time, whereas the educator may view the learner as unmotivated. For example, if the adolescent residents of a group home are being taught about

retirement and pension plans but currently have no job or source of income, the information that is being discussed is difficult for them to "apply" to real life, and consequently is soon forgotten.

In addition to emotional readiness to learn, the educator must consider, among other things, the complexity of the task being taught, the environment in which it will be taught (stimulation level), the health status of the learner (how much energy does he or she have to devote to the task), the anxiety level (which affects ability to concentrate), the available support in the community to perform that task once it is learned, and the level of risk-taking behavior typically demonstrated by that individual (affects the willingness of the individual to implement new skills). In addition, the learner's cultural background, present fund of knowledge, cognitive ability, reading ability, literacy level, and learning styles must all be ascertained (Bastable et al., 2011).

Learning styles refer to the way in which the learner most effectively perceives, processes, stores, and recalls what he or she is attempting to learn (James & Gardner, 1995). Every individual processes information in his or her own way, even though he or she may share some learning patterns, preferences, and approaches with others. The three primary learning styles are (1) visual, (2) auditory, and (3) tactile/kinesthetic. Checkpoint 14-4 offers the reader a comparison of these styles.

Given the same content, most learners can take in the information with equal success, but how they master that content is determined by their individual learning style, as well as how that information is presented by the educator. Six teaching principles have emerged from research about learning styles (Friedman & Alley, 1984). These principles are important for the educator to consider when approaching the task of instructional design for educational groups:

1. Both the style by which the educator prefers to teach and the style by which the learner prefers to learn should be identified.

2. Educators need to guard against relying on the teaching methods and tools that match their preferred learning style.

3. Educators are most helpful when they assist the learner to identify and learn according to his or her own style preferences.

4. Learners should initially have the opportunity to learn through their preferred style.

5. Later, learners should be encouraged to diversify their style preferences.

6. Educators should develop learning activities that reinforce all three styles.

Once the characteristics of the learner have been determined and the occupational therapy assistant has identified

CHECKPOINT 14-4. ANALYSIS OF LEARNING STYLES			
Activity	*Visual*	*Auditory*	*Kinesthetic and Tactile*
Spell	Do you try to picture or see the word?	Do you sound out the word?	Do you write the word down to explore if it "feels right"?
Talk	Do you favor words such as "see," "picture," and "imagine"?	Do you use words such as "hear," "listen, and "say"?	Do you gesture and use expressive movements? Do you use words such as "feel" and "touch"?
Concentrate	Does untidiness distract you?	Does noise distract you?	Does activity distract you?
Meet people again	Do you forget the name but remember the face or the location where you met?	Do you forget the face but remember the name and the topic of the conversation?	Do you remember what you did together?
Contact people	Do you prefer direct, face-to-face meetings?	Do you prefer the telephone?	Do you prefer to talk while participating in an activity together?
Read	Do you enjoy viewing descriptive writing, and pausing to "picture" the scene?	Do you enjoy dialog and conversation written into the story?	Do you prefer action stories?
Learn something new	Do you like to see demonstrations, diagrams, slides, and posters?	Do you prefer verbal instructions?	Do you prefer to jump right in and try it?
Put something together	Do you look at the directions and prefer pictures?	Do you enjoy having somebody "talk you through it"?	Do you ignore directions and figure it out as you go along?
Adapted from Rose, C. (1985). *Accelerated learning.* Bucks, UK: Accelerated Learning Systems Ltd.			

the gap in the client's knowledge and skills that must be addressed in order for him or her to achieve treatment goals, the educator can identify the specific content that will be taught.

Content

The content addresses what the learner is expected to accomplish or know. In order to decide on the content to be covered in a group, the occupational therapy assistant educator must examine individual client needs and treatment goals. This information is then used to formulate learning goals and objectives for the group. **Learning goals** are the final outcome of what is achieved at the end of the teaching–learning process, and are usually achieved in weeks or months. A **learning objective**, on the other hand, is short term and achievable at the end of one group session. It provides direction for the design of the group protocol. Trying to run a group without predetermined learning objectives is like driving to an unknown destination without a road map—you may waste lots of time and effort without getting to where you want to go. Learning objectives keep the educator's thinking on target and learner centered, and provide a sound basis for the selection of teaching methods and materials. They are written in the same way that treatment

goals are written, using the ABCD method (Heinich, Molenda, Russell, & Smaldino (2001):

A—audience/learner (who)

B—behavior (what is demonstrated)

C— condition (under what circumstances the behavior will be observed)

D—degree (how much, how well, to what extent)

Using the ABCD approach, here is an example of a learning objective: "Following participation in a 60-minute group on assertiveness (condition), the group member (learner) will be able to list (performance) at least two differences between passive, assertive, and aggressive communication styles (criterion)." It should be noted that all learning objectives should be achievable by every participant if the proper inclusion criteria are used when selecting group members.

Many educators use **Bloom's taxonomy** as a framework for determining and clarifying learning objectives. Bloom's taxonomy is a mechanism for the classification and categorization of different levels of learning. It was created in 1956 under the leadership of educational psychologist Dr. Benjamin Bloom in order to promote higher forms of thinking in education. It is a multitiered model of classifying thinking according to six cognitive levels of complexity. The taxonomy is hierarchical in that each level is subsumed

TABLE 14-13		
BLOOM'S TAXONOMY		
CATEGORY	**KEY VERBS**	**EXAMPLES**
Remembering: Recall previous learned information.	defines, describes, identifies, knows, labels, lists, matches, names, outlines, recalls, recognizes, reproduces, selects, states	The occupational therapy assistant student lists the parts of a treatment plan.
Understanding: Comprehending the meaning, translation, and interpretation of instructions and problems. State a problem in one's own words.	comprehends, converts, defends, distinguishes, estimates, explains, extends, generalizes, gives an example, infers, interprets, paraphrases, predicts, rewrites, summarizes	The occupational therapy assistant student summarizes the differences between each part of the treatment plan.
Applying: Uses a concept in a new situation; applies what was learned in the classroom into novel situations.	applies, changes, computes, constructs, demonstrates, discovers, manipulates, modifies, operates, predicts, prepares, produces, relates, shows, solves, uses	The occupational therapy assistant student modifies an existing treatment plan to incorporate the client factors and contextual factors listed in a case study.
Analyzing: Separates material or concepts into component parts so that its organizational structure may be understood. Distinguishes between facts and inferences.	analyzes, breaks down, compares, contrasts, diagrams, deconstructs, differentiates, discriminates, distinguishes, identifies, illustrates, infers, outlines, relates, selects	The occupational therapy assistant student differentiates between the use of the biomechanical, Person-Environment-Occupation, and Model of Human Occupation frames of reference as applied to the same case study.
Evaluating: Make judgments about the value of ideas or materials.	appraises, compares, concludes, contrasts, criticizes, critiques, defends, describes, discriminates, evaluates, explains, interprets, justifies, relates, summarizes	The occupational therapy assistant student evaluates the frames of reference listed above in order to suggest the best match for a client in a case study.
Creating: Builds a structure or pattern from diverse elements. Puts parts together to form a whole, with emphasis on creating a new meaning or structure.	categorizes, combines, compiles, composes, creates, devises, designs, explains, generates, modifies, organizes, plans, rearranges, reconstructs, relates, reorganizes, revises, rewrites, summarizes, tells	The occupational therapy assistant student creates a treatment plan for an individual in a case study based on a frame of reference specified by the instructor.

by the higher levels. In the 1990s the original model was altered slightly. Table 14-13 lists the six categories of learning according to the revised Bloom's taxonomy.

Once the educator knows the students and has a clear idea of what they need to get out of the lesson, he or she is ready to select the instructional strategy, which is the overall plan for a teaching–learning experience. It involves the use of one or more instructional methods.

Instructional Methods and Materials

An ***instructional method*** is the way in which information is taught. There is no one perfect method to teach all learners in all settings. Decisions about which methods to choose are based upon a number of factors, including the instructional setting, the learning objectives, characteristics of the learner, the educator's expertise, and cost

	TABLE 14-14	
	COMPARISON OF INSTRUCTIONAL METHODS	
METHOD	**ADVANTAGES**	**DISADVANTAGES**
Demonstration by instructor	Client gets to preview the skill and see how it is used. May increase motivation to learn it.	The learner is passive. If the members are not visual learners, the skill may not be learned.
Group discussion	Cost effective. Stimulates sharing of ideas and emotions; promotes development of social skills and interaction.	Shy members can hide behind vocal peers. Difficult for some individuals to anchor discussion topics to their personal lives and see how it applies to them.
Lecture	Cost effective; can be used with large groups.	Not individualized. Learner is passive.
One-on-one instruction	Can be tailored to individual client factors and treatment goals. Easier for individuals with limited social skills.	Labor intensive. Isolates client from peer learning.
Role modeling	Helps members learn new roles.	Requires trust and rapport with the educator leader. The learner is passive.
Role playing	Develops understanding of the perspectives of others. The learner is active.	Too threatening for some individuals when done in a group setting if strong emotions are evoked.
Simulation	Practice is done in a "safe" setting. Learner is very active.	Learning may not generalize to "real life." May require purchase of expensive equipment.

effectiveness. Some examples of methods include discussion, lecture, and role playing. Table 14-14 lists a variety of instructional methods, along with the advantages and disadvantages to using each of them.

Instructional materials or tools are the objects, such as books, videos, PowerPoint slides, and handouts, that are used to transmit information and that supplement the task of teaching. They help the student master the material that he or she is required to learn. They include written materials (i.e., handouts, books, brochures, posters, and instruction sheets), demonstration materials (visual hands-on nonprint material such as models or actual equipment, like an iron and ironing board), and audiovisual materials (i.e., PowerPoint, overhead transparencies, compact discs, video and television, radio, and computer learning resources). The decision as to which instructional materials are most appropriate should always be based on the size of the group and characteristics of the members, the predetermined learning objectives, and the availability of resources. For example, although printed materials may be the most popular tool for client education, effective use requires a determination of readability of the selected materials and literacy levels of the group members. The occupational therapy assistant educator must always remember that instructional materials are only used to *support* learning and complement teaching, not substitute for it.

SUMMARY

In this chapter, the concept of leadership was defined and a variety of leadership styles were discussed. An overview was provided of the knowledge, skills, and attitude that are required by the occupational therapy assistant functioning in the role of an effective group leader, along with suggestions on how these elements can be developed. The components of group dynamics were outlined, and two variations of group process were described. Three styles of communication—passive, assertive, and aggressive—were discussed, and the reader was given instructions on how to compose an "I message." Finally, educational strategies were presented as a way to improve the teaching and learning process inherent in all treatment, whether it is provided on a one-on-one basis or in the group setting.

PART 7: APPLICATIONS

These activities should be directed by the instructor while working with the entire class.

1. Elect five students to go to the front of the classroom. These students are charged with the task of teaching the story of the Three Little Pigs to the rest of the class. They have 10 minutes to plan their lesson. After observing the planning process, students should answer the following questions:

   a. What role(s) did each individual assume in the group?

   b. What style of leadership was used? Be prepared to justify your selection.

   c. List the steps in Tuckman's group process. Describe how these stages evolved in the planning group that you observed. What occurred in each step? Be specific.

   d. What method(s) and material(s) were selected to teach the story? To which learning style would they appeal the most? Why?

   Students share their responses in a large classroom discussion. An alternative would be to break the observers into small groups in order to answer the same questions.

2. *Stop and Play*: Each student is given a note card and instructed to write down a detailed example of a recent conflict in which they chose to be passive or aggressive, but in hindsight wished they had been assertive. The instructor collects the cards and asks for two student volunteers to come to the front of the class, pick a card, and role-play the scenario, with one student assuming an assertive role and using an "I message." An alternative would be for the instructor to read the cards and request each student to write an "I message" for every scenario selected.

3. *Draw the Line*: Students take the Therapeutic Boundaries Quiz listed in Spotlight 14-1 and discuss their responses in small groups.

4. *Watch and Listen*: A volunteer comes to the front of the class and speaks for 2 to 3 minutes on the subject of his or her choice (i.e., the best day of my life; who I would like to be and why; my favorite heroes, etc.). The rest of the class notes body language while using active listening. Students are asked to practice effective communication by referring to Table 14-4 and using each of the techniques listed in order to respond to the speaker.

REFERENCES

Anderson, L. (1979). How to develop rapport with a patient. (Class handout). School of Occupational Therapy, Madison, WI: University of Wisconsin.

Barge, J. K. (2003). *Leadership as organizing*. In R. Hirokawa, R. Cathart, & L. Samovar (Eds.). *Small group communication: Theory and practice. An anthology.* (8th ed.). Los Angeles, CA: Roxbury.

Bastable, S. B., Gramet, P., Jacobs, K., & Sopczyk, D. L. (2011). *Health professional as educator: Principles of teaching and learning.* Sudbury, MA: Jones and Bartlett Learning.

Belbin, M. (1981). *Management teams: Why they succeed or fail.* Oxford: Heinemann Professional.

Benne, K., & Sheats, P. (1948). Functional roles of group members. *Journal of Social Issues, 4*(2), p. 41-49.

Bettencourt, B. A., & Sheldon, K. (2001). Social roles as mechanism for psychological need satisfaction within social groups. *Journal of Personality and Social Psychology, 81,* 1131-1143.

Bion, W. (1961). *Experiences in groups and other papers.* New York, NY: Basic Books.

Bugental, D. E., Kaswan, J. W., & Love, L. R. (1970). Perception of contradictory meanings conveyed by verbal and nonverbal channels. *Journal of Personality and Social Psychology, 16,* 647-655.

Cara, E. & MacRae, A. (2013). *Psychosocial occupational therapy: An evolving practice.* Clifton Park, NY: Delmar.

Carpenter, J. A. & Bell, S. K. (2002). What do nurses know about teaching patients? *Journal of Nursing Development, 18*(3), 157-161.

Cole, M. B. (2008). Client-centered groups. In J. Creek, & L. Lougher, (Eds.). *Occupational therapy and mental health.* (4th ed.). Philadelphia, PA: Elsevier.

Cole, M. C. (2012). *Group dynamics in occupational therapy.* Thorofare, NJ: SLACK.

Corey, M., Corey G., & Corey, C. (2010). *Groups: Process and practice.* Belmont, CA: Brooks/Cole.

Davidson, D. (2011). Therapeutic use of self in academic education: A mixed methods study. *Occupational Therapy in Mental Health, 27*(1), 87-102.

Davis, C. M. (1998). *Patient practitioner interaction: An experiential manual for developing the art of health care.* Thorofare, NJ: SLACK.

Deering, C. (2009). Therapeutic relationships and caring. In W. Mohr (Ed.), *Psychiatric mental health nursing.* (7th ed.). Philadelphia, PA: Lippincott, Williams & Wilkins.

Deutsch, M. (1949). A theory of cooperation and competition. *Human Relations, 2,* 129-152.

Deutsch, M. (1973). *The resolution of conflict.* New Haven, CT: Yale University Press.

Early, M. B. (2012). *Mental health concepts & techniques.* (4th ed.). Philadelphia, PA: Lippincott, Williams, & Wilkins.

Facilitate. (n.d.) In *Meriam-Webster's Online Dictionary.* Retrieved from www.meriam-webster.com/dictionary/facilitate.

Fisher, B. A. (1980) *Small group decision making* (2nd ed.). New York, NY: McGraw Hill.

Flores, P. J. (1997). *Group psychotherapy: An integration of twelve-step and psychodynamic theory.* (2nd ed.) New York, NY: The Haworth Press.

Forsythe, D. (2010). *Group dynamics.* Belmont, CA: Cengage Learning.

Friedman, P., & Alley, R. (1984). Learning/teaching styles: Applying the principles. *Theory into Practice, 23*(1), p. 77-81.

Gerseck, C. J. (2003). Time and transition in work teams. In R. Hirokawa, R. Cathart, & L. Samovar (Eds.). *Small group communication: Theory and practice. An anthology.* (8th ed.). Los Angeles, CA: Roxbury Publishing.

Gordon, T. (1970). *Parent effectiveness training.* New York, NY: Peter Wyden.

Gouran, D. (2003). Leadership as the art of counteractive influence in decision making and problem-solving groups. In R. Hirokawa, R. Cathart, & L. Samovar (Eds). *Small group communication: Theory and practice. An anthology.* (8th ed.). Los Angeles, CA: Roxbury.

Haertl, K. (2008). From the roots of psychosocial practice – therapeutic use of self in the classroom: Practical applications for occupational therapy faculty. *Occupational Therapy in Mental Health,* 24(2), 121-134.

Hagerty, B. M., & Patusky, K. L. (2003). Reconceptualizing the nurse-patient relationship. *Journal of Nursing Scholarship,* 35(2), 145-150.

Haggard, M. (1989). Students' metacognitive response to ambiguous literacy tasks. *Reading Research and Instruction, 31*(1), 1-11.

Healthcare Education Association. (1985). *Managing hospital education.* Laguna Niguel, CA: Author.

Heinich, J. D., Molenda, M., Russell, J., & Smaldino, S. (2001). *Instructional methods and techniques for learning* (7th ed.). Upper Saddle River, NJ: Prentice Hall.

Horvath, A. O. (2000). The therapeutic relationship: From transference to alliance. *Psychology in Practice,* 56(2), p. 163-173.

Howe, M., & Schwartzberg, S. (2010). *A functional approach to group work in occupational therapy.* Baltimore, MD: Lippincott Williams and Wilkins.

James, W. B., & Gardner, D. L. (1995). Learning styles. *New Directions for Adult and Continuing Education, 67*(1), 19-32.

Johnson, D. W., & Johnson, F. (2009) *Joining together. Group theory and group skills* (11th ed.). Boston, MA: Pearson.

Johnson, D., & Johnson, P. (2013). *Joining together: Group therapy and group skills.* (11th ed.). Saddle River, NJ: Pearson.

Larson, J. R., & Christensen, C. (1993). Groups as problem-solving units: Toward a new meaning of social cognition. *British Journal of Social Psychology, 32*(1), 5-30.

Leavitt, H. J. (1951). Some effects of certain communication patterns on group performance. *Journal of Abnormal and Social Psychology, 46,* 38-50.

Lewin, K., Lippitt, R. & White, R. (1939). Patterns of aggressive behavior in experimentally created "social climates." *Journal of Experimental Psychology, 34,* 271-299.

Mehrabian, A. (1971). *Silent messages,* Wadsworth, CA: Belmont.

Mosey, A. (1981). *Occupational therapy: Configuration of a profession.* New York, NY: Raven.

Mosey, A. (1986). *Psychosocial components of occupational therapy.* New York, NY: Raven.

Mullen, B., & Copper, C. (1994). The relationship between group cohesiveness and performance: An integration. *Psychological Bulletin, 115,* 210-227.

Patterson, M. L., (1991). A functional approach to nonverbal exchange. In R. S. Feldman & B. Rime (Eds.), *Fundamentals of nonverbal behavior* (pp. 458-495). New York, NY: Cambridge University.=Poole, M. S. (2005). A multiple sequence of group decision development. In R. Hirokawa, R. Cathart, & L. Samovar (Eds.). *Small group communication: Theory and practice. An anthology.* (8th ed.). Los Angeles, CA: Roxbury Publishing.

Rose, C. (1985). *Accelerated learning.* Bucks, UK: Accelerated Learning Systems Ltd.

Shaw, M. (1964). Communication networks. In L. Berkowitz (Ed.), *Advances in experimental psychology* (pp. 111-147). New York, NY: Academic Press.

Shimanoff, S. B., & Jenkins, M. M. (2003). Leadership and gender: Challenging assumptions and recognizing resources. In R. S. Cathcart & L. A. Samovars (Eds.), *Small group communication: Theory and practice* (6th ed., pp. 101-133). New York: Oxford Press.

Shohamy, D., Mihalakos, P., Chin, R., Thomas, B., Wagner, A. D., & Tamminga, C. (2010). Leaning and generalization in schizophrenia: Effects of disease and antipsychotic drug treatment. *Biological Psychiatry, 67*(10), 926-932.

Smith, G. (2001) Group development: A review of the literature and a commentary on future research directions. *Group Facilitation, 3,* 14–45.

Stewart, D. (1998). *Gower handbook of management skills.* Surrey, UK: Gower Publishing.

Stogdill, R. (1948). Personal factors associated with leadership: A review of the literature. *Journal of Psychology, 25,* 35-71.

Stogdill, R. (1974). *Handbook of leadership.* New York, NY: Free Press.

Tuckman, Bruce W. (1965). Developmental sequence in small groups. *Psychological Bulletin, 63,* 384-399.

Yalom, I. (1995). *The theory and practice of psychotherapy.* (4th ed.). New York, NY: Basic Books.

Yukl, G. (2005). *Leadership in organizations.* (6th ed.). Englewood Cliffs, NJ: Prentice-Hall.

Zaccaro, S. J. (2007). Trait-based perspectives of leadership. *American Psychologist, 62*(1), 6-16.

Glossary

Action systems: Brain networks with a neurobiological and human evolutionary purpose.

Active listening: Being attentive to what the client is saying, verbally and nonverbally, while allowing the client to determine the content of what is said as well as the level of self-disclosure.

Activity analysis: The process of analyzing the activity to distinguish its component parts.

Activity group: Action-oriented component that differentiates this group from other therapy groups. The content of the group is usually defined by the activity (i.e., cooking group; arts and crafts group; exercise group; relaxation group; work skills group) and is based on the needs and skill levels of the identified group members, as well as general program format and available resources.

Activity limitations: Level of dysfunction associated with the level of function at the individual or whole-person level.

Activity synthesis: The process of combining component parts of the human and nonhuman environment so as to design an activity suitable for evaluation or intervention relative to performance.

Adaptability: The ability to change behavior in accordance with the occupational demands required by many different roles and activities.

Adaptation: A change that facilitates performance.

Adaptive capacity: Allows for cognitive system flexibility so that stressors can be endured more calmly and recovered from more quickly.

Adaptive response: An appropriate action in which the individual responds successfully to some environmental demand.

Adaptive Response Model: Model to help practitioners recognize naturalistic learning in clients while learning to apply it in their own practice.

Advisory leadership: Typically used in community-based support and self-help groups. The leader exercises little authority over the group and acts primarily as a resource, but only when absolutely necessary.

Advocating: One of the six therapeutic modes, advocating describes when therapists stand up for a client's rights and ensure resources are accessible.

Affordable Care Act (ACA): Passed in 2009, provided changes to the Medicare Improvements for the Patients and Providers Act of 2008. The Affordable Care Act offers the possibility of insurance benefits through an expansion of Medicaid.

Arts and crafts movement: Movement that started out of concern for the ills of industrialization and mass production.

Manville, C.A., & Keough, J. L.
Mental Health Practice for the Occupational Therapy Assistant (pp 367-375).
© 2016 Taylor & Francis Group.

Assertive community treatment (ACT): A service-delivery model that provides comprehensive, locally based treatment to people with serious and persistent mental illnesses.

Asylums: Asylums for the insane, in the Kirkbride tradition, were designed to be "retreats" or places where a patient could escape the pressure of daily life. The pleasant environment and treatment, participation in occupations, and manual labor were designed to cure and return the person to his or her previous home and community.

Attachment: Emerges from a combination of variables and is often presented as being on a continuum. Variables that influence a caregiver's capacity to develop and maintain attunement with their child include one's temperament, mental and physical health factors, developmental abilities and delays, one's own sensory-processing patterns, and cultural and economic influences.

Autocratic leader: Task oriented and less focused on the individual group members than other types of leaders.

Behavioral approach: Emphasizes a person's cognitive dimension. It offers various action-oriented methods to help the person take definite steps to change his or her behaviors.

Behavioral health care: Community-based services available to the mentally ill as well as for the treatment for addiction disorders as a way to help individuals function at optimum levels.

Biopsychosocial model: (a) A model of practice that incorporates the medical model of care delivery and a social model of disability such as found in the International Classification of Functioning. (b) Focuses on the biological components of disease and disability. At the same time it incorporates social and psychological dimensions of health and illness. An example is the medical model. (c) The occupational therapy model as proposed by Anne C Mosey that would later become the Person-Environment-Occupational (PEO) model.

Bloom's taxonomy: Framework for determining and clarifying learning objectives. Hierarchy of learning that identifies three domains of learning, which include the cognitive, affective, and psychomotor domains.

Body functions: Physiological functions of body systems within the International Classification of Functioning.

Body structures: Anatomic parts of the body within the International Classification of Functioning.

Boundary violations: Form of boundary crossing that involves a professional misusing his or her power to exploit a consumer for personal gain.

Brain reward center: Neurological system of the brain that causes stimulation and a sense of well-being.

Caring and empathy: The second theme of the Contemporary Era has been characterized by an emphasis on the qualities of *caring* and *empathy* within the therapeutic relationship. This can be summarized as an emphasis on the emotional exchange between the client and therapist.

Cognitive behavior therapy (CBT): A psychotherapeutic approach that addresses dysfunctional emotions, maladaptive behaviors, and cognitive processes and contents.

Cognitive therapy: Aaron T. Beck developed this approach, which has a number of basic similarities to RET. Beck did his work independently of Ellis, but their approaches have the same goal of assisting clients in recognizing and discarding self-defeating cognitions.

Centering: Activities that promote self-motivation by producing a feeling of personal reward and positive anticipation.

Client-centered: Approach to service that incorporates respect for and partnership with clients as active participants in the therapy process.

Client factors: Domain in the Occupational Therapy Practice Framework. It describes factors within a person that affect the ability to participate or perform in occupations. It includes values, beliefs, spirituality, body functions, and body structures.

Clinical reasoning: Involves thinking about the client–therapist relationship as a component of the occupational therapy process. It includes making sense of assessment findings and developing a treatment plan.

Closed group: Groups in which the membership remains stable.

Co-occupation: When two or more individuals are involved in an occupation together.

Cognitive behavior group: Focus on the member's thoughts (self-talk) and feelings, and subsequent behavior.

Cognitive Disability Theory (CDT): A function-based theory that was organized by Claudia Kay Allen, OTR/L. Instead of solely identifying impairments and disability, the CDT theory identifies what the client may be able to do with his or her remaining skills and abilities.

Collaborating: One of the six therapeutic modes, collaborating emphasizes a partnership with the client to ensure that the client plays an active role in the therapeutic process.

Communication network: Regular patterns of information exchange among members of a group.

Communication patterns: The flow of information within the group.

Community Mental Health Act (CMHA): Facilitated the move from institutions to the community. This act mandated that adults with mental illness be treated in the least restricted environment, mainly in the person's community.

Complexity science: The study of dynamic "systems that change with time" such as human beings.

Conflict: The actions or beliefs of one or more members of the group are viewed as unacceptable and/or are resisted by the other members.

Contemporary Era: The profession of occupational therapy realigned itself back to the centrality of occupation during the latter part of the 20th century. This era was labeled as the Contemporary Era or the "Return to Occupation."

Core knowledge and skills: Shared knowledge and skills of mental health practitioners gained in general education preparation, courses in psychology, and occupational therapy coursework and assignments.

Core mental health professional (CMHP): Professionals who are recognized at the federal level as mental health professionals by meeting requirements in the United States Code of Federal Regulations. Includes psychologists, psychiatrists, clinical social workers, licensed marriage and family therapists, and psychiatric nurses.

Dialectical behavior therapy (DBT): A form of psychotherapy that was originally developed by Marsha M. Linehan, a psychology researcher at the University of Washington.

Deinstitutionalization: The provision of care to meet an individual's needs within the community rather than in an institution.

Democratic leader: Encourages group members to share their ideas and opinions, which helps to promote group engagement.

Developmental frame of reference: Activities are used to facilitate human growth and development by enabling one to explore the environment, establish relationships, acquire knowledge, and adapt successfully to one's world.

Developmental learning: The natural process of learning from patterns of experience that involve ongoing adaptive responses.

Developmental stages: Categorized by developmental milestones that are typically expected to emerge within each given age range. Information related to developmental milestones are often categorized by physical, cognitive (thinking skills), communication, social, and emotional skills.

Developmental theory: Erickson built on Freud's ideas and extended his theory by stressing the psychosocial aspects of development beyond early childhood. Erickson's theory of development holds that psychosexual growth and psychosocial growth take place together.

Diagnostic and Statistical Manual (DSM): Document created by the American Psychological Association to aid in the definition and description of mental health illnesses.

Didactic teaching: The focus is primarily on the leader who attempts to engage participants in the subject being taught using teaching materials such as diagrams, handouts, photos, and pictures.

Directive group: Designed to meet the needs of the most severely and acutely mentally ill who have significant cognitive impairment and are receiving treatment on an inpatient psychiatric unit or in a long-term facility. The structure of the group consists of five steps: orientation to the group and introduction of individual group members, motor-based warm-up activity, perceptual motor task, cognitive discussion of the activities, and closure.

Directive leader: The person who exerts the most control over the group. This leadership style is the appropriate choice for clients functioning at a low cognitive level.

Discrimination: When prejudice is acted upon.

Dynamic Systems Theory (DST): Systems that change over time and are characterized by complexity, randomness, and nonlinearity. The focus of the dynamic system in occupational therapy is the emerging pattern(s) of human engagement in occupation(s).

Early Occupation Era: The earliest era, referred to as the Occupational Era, reflects the values that were held by the founders of occupational therapy.

Early occupations: Occupations that provide a diversion from the pain and troubles of life, occupations that restore mental and physical function, vocational education to return one to gainful employment—either related to past employment or proposed future employment. Also includes "bedside occupational therapy" that gives a start in a kind of avocation, "side-line," or hobby.

Emotion-focused coping cues: Used by occupational therapy assistants to activate the emotional self-regulation action system required for client self-motivation. Positive emotion-focused coping cues may be part of the environment, occupation, or therapeutic exchange.

Emotion-focused coping resources: Underlying emotional self-regulation strategies that can be used to support healthy coping behavior. Rather than activities, these are patterns of thought that support and promote coping, self-motivation, attention, adaptive action, and learning.

Emotional resiliency: Key component of healthy mental and cognitive aging. It includes the emotional capacity to adapt to change, even to a stressful loss.

Empathizing: One of the six therapeutic modes, empathizing is when the therapist seeks to understand the client's thoughts, feelings, and behaviors.

Encouraging: One of the six therapeutic modes, encouraging describes when the therapist takes on the role of a cheerleader or motivator to instill hope and confidence in a client.

Environment/context: Domain in the Occupational Therapy Practice Framework. It includes interrelated factors within and surrounding a person that can affect engagement in occupations. Examples include cultural, personal, physical, social, temporal, and virtual aspects.

Environmental fit: Occupational patterns tend to be shaped through attraction to pleasant feelings such as flow and avoidance of negative emotions associated with unpleasant stress.

Era of Inner Mechanism: In the mid-20th century, a client's underlying impairment became the focus of occupational therapy treatment.

Evaluation process: Process of obtaining and interpreting data necessary for intervention.

Explicit memories: Holistic memories that can be remembered as a unified experience. These are memories of an event, its time of day, where it happened, objects, and people who were present.

Expressive group: Includes a range of therapeutic activities that allow clients to express feelings and thoughts—conscious or unconscious—that they might have difficulty communicating with spoken words alone.

Facilitative leader: A group will make its own decisions, with the leader remaining in the background.

Fight-flight-freeze: Challenging patterns of reactive stress. Hard-wired reactions to negative environmental cues.

Flow: A state associated with meaningful and purposeful activity characterized by complete absorption in the activity and diminished awareness of the external environment, a sense of oneness with the activity, total immersion in the present moment and a lost sense of time, lost fear or anxiety (everyday worries fade as people become increasingly engrossed in the activity), and immense feelings of personal satisfaction (the activity is rewarding in itself).

Functional approach: The ability of the leader to manage the group in order to complete the task while working together as a team.

Generative group engagements: This approach is believed to promote feelings of security and safety within group activities. The feelings of security and safety seem to support the client's capacity to use his or her exploratory action system for developmental learning and sociability.

Gestalt therapy: Frederick Perls developed Gestalt therapy, a form of existential therapy. It is based on the premise that people must find their own way in life and accept personal responsibility if they hope to achieve maturity.

Grounding: Activities promote self-motivation by facilitating the relaxation response and a sense of calm anticipation.

Group: A collection of people who have a shared purpose for being together.

Group climate: The emotional environment within the group.

Group cohesion: The sense of solidarity the members feel toward one another and the group.

Group content: Describes the activities and topics incorporated into a group session.

Group duration: The length of time that individuals meet; for example, one 60-minute session, or six 30-minute sessions held over the period of 6 weeks.

Group dynamics: The forces that influence the relationship among members and the group outcome.

Group frequency: How often the group meets; for example, twice per week or once per day.

Group gradation: Process of gradually advancing the skills required to complete a group activity, step by step.

Group interaction skill: The ability to be a productive member of a variety of primary groups. Through acquisition of the various group interaction subskills, the individual learns to take appropriate group membership roles, engage in decision making, communicate effectively, recognize group norms and interact in accordance with these norms, contribute to goal attainment, work toward group cohesiveness, and assist in resoling group conflict.

Group process: How group members approach a task to get things done.

Group protocol: A way to organize your thoughts about the design of a group and share them with other members of the treatment team.

Group size: The number of members allowed to participate in a group.

Group treatment: A planned process for creating changes in individuals and bringing them together for this purpose.

Identity cues: Implicit memory environment that matches a client's core life identity. These have been embedded in the therapeutic environment of a memory care space with a primary emotion-focused coping purpose.

Impairments: Level of dysfunction associated with the level of function at the body function or body structure level.

Implicit memories: Step-by-step procedures in the brain that can often be performed without conscious thought. A second form of implicit memory is the association between a feeling or emotion and a life experience.

Institutionalization: Perceived as an acceptable method of protecting society from individuals with mental illness, as well as providing a safe, supportive, and caring environment for the person. Significantly, society as a whole deemed it necessary to accept responsibility for the care and needs of individuals.

Instructing: One of the six therapeutic modes, instructing is when the therapist takes on the role of teaching through clear explanations of the plan, sequence, and events of therapy.

Instructional method: The way in which information is taught.

Intensive individualized services: One of the three major tiers of service in the multi-tiered system of support, intensive individualized services (tier 3) focus services individually for those diagnosed with mental illness.

Intentional Relationship Model (IRM): Model developed in an attempt to clarify and provide more detailed guidance on how to develop and utilize therapeutic use of self in occupational therapy. It explains therapeutic use of self and its relationship with occupational engagement.

Interactive reasoning: When therapists do much of their clinical reasoning during therapy sessions while they are interacting with the client. It is an internal process during which the occupational therapy practitioner selects the most appropriate mode for interacting with a client at a particular time.

Interdisciplinary team: Composed of nursing aides, nurses, social workers, recreational staff, music therapists, psychologists, occupational therapists, physical therapists, dietitians, speech therapists, family members, physicians, and psychiatrists.

International Classification of Functioning (ICF): A document created by the World Health Organization to provide a common language to describe health and health-related states.

Interpersonal characteristics: Individual characteristics of each person that include communication style, capacity for trust, need for control, capacity to assert needs, response to change and challenge, affect, predisposition to giving feedback, capacity to receive feedback, response to human diversity, orientation toward relating, preference for touch, and capacity for reciprocity.

Interpersonal dynamics: A dynamic defines the distinctive pattern, emotional tone, and interpersonal events that comprise the interaction between individuals. They can be positive or negative.

Interpersonal learning: All of the processes or relationships among individuals that result in change in behavior, knowledge, or attitude on the part of any one or more of the people involved.

Intensive outpatient program (IOP): Similar to partial hospital programs. Patients in these programs, however, do not meet the criteria of being at risk for immediate hospitalization if the services were not provided.

Laissez-faire leader: Allows group members to make all of the decisions.

Leader: A person who can influence others to be more effective in working to achieve mutual goals and maintain effective working relationships among members.

Leadership: The process through which leaders exert their influence.

Learning styles: The way in which the learner most effectively perceives, processes, stores, and recalls what he or she is attempting to learn.

Lifespan development approach: Approach that includes the understanding that development occurs across the lifespan. Development is also affected by societal, cultural, psychological, and other environmental variables that occur over the life course.

Medicaid: Program funded jointly by the federal government and the states, but is administered at the state level. It was established to provide health care services to low-income children deprived of parental support, their caretaker relatives, the elderly, the blind, and individuals with disabilities.

Mindfulness: The awareness that emerges through paying attention on purpose, in the present moment, and nonjudgmentally to the unfolding of experience moment by moment.

Model: A body of theory that explains some aspect of human behavior addressed by occupational therapy practitioners.

Motivational interviewing (MI): A semi-directive, client-centered counseling style for eliciting behavior change by helping clients to explore and resolve ambivalence.

Medical model: Medicine's view of mankind as mechanistic—the view of man as a machine—and reductionistic—the view of man as body parts. The goal of treating the parts to return the system to its previous level of ability.

Medicare: Title 18 of the Social Security Act was enacted in 1965 and administered by the federal government. Medicare initially was created as a health insurance plan for the elderly.

Mental health: It is not merely the absence of mental illness, but the presence of something positive. The continuum of mental health as described by Keyes can be viewed as ranging from mental illness and/or "languishing in life" at one end to "moderately mentally healthy" and "complete mental health and flourishing" at the other end.

Mental health literacy: Focuses on providing all children and youth with a working knowledge of how to develop and maintain positive mental health. It also provides children and youth a method to recognize, manage, and seek intervention for mental illness.

Mental illness: The terms *mental illness* and *mental disorders* are commonly used to refer to diagnosable psychiatric conditions that significantly interfere with a person's functioning, such as schizophrenia, bipolar disorder, and dementia.

Mindful state of consciousness: Good self-awareness and the positive sense of being in control of one's own Person-Environment-Occupational (PEO) fitness decisions.

Mixed signals: At times, what is being communicated verbally and what is being expressed with body language are two totally different things.

Model of Human Occupation (MOHO): Occupation-based model that views how people participate in life occupations and achieve positive adaptations.

Modeling: The therapeutic process of demonstrating the occupational pattern before asking the client to demonstrate it independently.

Moral treatment: Providing one with laborious or interesting occupation and treating one with kindness and firmness to treat mental illness.

Multisensory environment: Provides a therapeutic environment that is filled with emotion-focused coping cues for clients who do not have the capacity to self-regulate their emotions.

Multi-tiered system of support: A three-tiered model focusing on mental health promotion, prevention, and intervention, which can be used to guide occupational therapy services for children and youth in multiple types of settings.

Narrative approaches: Focuses on how the client conceptualizes and summarizes key events in his or her life. Narrative approaches seek to organize and make sense of information.

Neuroplasticity: The ability to create new neuronal connections in the brain.

Neuroadaptation: May be thought of as a brain–mind–body system. It is involved in the adaptive response required for coping with stress, setting and achieving goals, and ongoing developmental learning.

New Freedom Commission: President George W. Bush created the New Freedom Commission in 2002 to better understand the problems in the current mental health service delivery system that prevent people from getting the excellent health care they need.

Norm: Shared expectations among members that outline the parameters of what is desirable and acceptable behavior.

Occupation: Domain of the Occupational Therapy Practice Framework that includes a host of activities that can be grouped under activities of daily living, rest/sleep, education, work, play, leisure, and social participation.

Occupational analysis: See *activity analysis.*

Occupational identity: One's sense of who he or she is and wants to become.

Occupational pattern adaptation: Developmental learning that occurs during Person-Environment-Occupational (PEO) exchanges.

Occupational performance fit: The result of the interaction of the person, environment, and occupation at a given time.

Occupational performance patterns: The habits, roles and rituals used in the process of engaging in occupations or activities.

Occupational performance skills: Observable elements of actions that have an implicit functional purpose; skills that are considered a classification of actions, encompassing multiple capacities.

Occupational profile: Summary of the information provided and obtained during the occupational therapy evaluation. It helps to summarize the client's background information, needs, values, priorities, desire, outcomes, occupational history, patterns of daily living, strengths, and interests.

Occupational Therapy Practice Framework (OTPF): Document created by the American Occupational Therapy Association that describes the general domains and processes of occupational therapy and expresses the occupation-based, client-centered, and evidence-based nature of occupational therapy.

Occupational therapy process: Way in which occupational therapy practitioners operationalize their expertise to provide services to clients.

Open group: Membership changes from one group to the next.

Occupational Performance History Interview (OPHI): An instrument designed to gather an accurate and clinically useful history of an individual's work, play, and self-care performance for adolescents and adults.

Palliative: An adaptive response within the context of dementia care and treatment.

Participation in structured recreation and leisure activities: Occupation-based practice when promoting mental health in children. Structured leisure activities are associated with many qualities present in paid work. They include regular participation schedules, rule-guided interaction, direction by one or more adult leaders, an emphasis on skill development that increases in complexity and challenge, performance that requires sustained active attention, and the provision of feedback.

Participation restrictions: Level of dysfunction associated with the level of functioning at the societal level.

Peer learning: Learning from those one perceives as equals rather than those one perceives as authorities.

Perceived self: Includes aspects such as physical and intellectual abilities, emotions, values, and standards that have been developed through our interactions with other people.

Performance modes: Key performance levels of ability which distinguishes how a client will be able to function in meaningful occupational tasks in the Cognitive Disability Model.

Person-centered therapy: Based on the belief that humans can develop in a positive and constructive manner if a climate of respect and trust is established.

Person-Environment-Occupation (PEO) model: Provides an explanation for the complex dynamic relationship between the person, environment, and occupation. It provides a systematic approach to identify and address occupational performance.

Personal space: The distance required between two or more people as they interact in order for a person to feel comfortable.

Partial hospital program (PHP): Partial hospital programs provide services to individuals who, without these services, would most likely require an inpatient level of care.

Play therapy: Combines the comforting support of empathic therapeutic exchanges with the clinical skill of facilitating the neuroadaptive response.

Positive approach: A way to approach and interact with clients with dementia that signal they are safe, secure, and respected.

Positive behavioral interventions and supports (PBIS): Provides a framework for preventing problem behaviors by proactively altering a situation before problems escalate. Concurrently teaching appropriate alternatives also aids in preventing problem behaviors.

Power struggle: Group members vie for control in leadership, status, and/or position in a group.

Praxis: Action planning for a client-centered treatment session.

Prejudice: An unjustified negative attitude toward a person based solely on the person's membership in a group.

Prevention: Efforts focused both on reducing the incidence and seriousness of problem behaviors and mental health disorders.

Professional boundaries: The limits of the relationship that allow for a safe and healthy connection between the occupational therapy assistant and the client.

Priming: The therapeutic process of physically assisting the occupational pattern once or twice before asking for the client to demonstrate it independently.

Problem-focused coping cues: Used by occupational therapy assistants to trigger context-specific neuroadaptive responses. Positive problem-focused coping cues support a client's capacity to take intentional adaptive actions designed to change life problems.

Problem-focused coping resources: The environmental resources that support healthy coping behavior. These are commonly the social, cultural, and economic resources a person has that support coping rather than activities, emotional, or cognitive states.

Problem solving: One of the six therapeutic modes, problem solving describes when the therapist acts as a facilitator.

Promotion: Efforts emphasize competence enhancement, which includes building on strengths and resources. Mental health promotion includes creating supportive school, home, and community environments.

Psychoanalytic theory: The Freudian view of human nature is deterministic. According to Freud, the behavior of people is determined by irrational forces, unconscious motivations, biological and instinctual drives, and certain psychosexual events during the first 6 years of life.

Psychobiology model: The holistic view of man included a mind–body union; a term coined by Dr. Adolph Meyer.

Psychodynamic group: A generic name encompassing ways of looking at the dynamics that take place in groups. Psychodynamic groups aim at remediation of in-depth psychological problems and explore how past influences affect the present.

Psychoeducational group: Highly organized, time limited, and integrates principles of teaching and learning with traditional group intervention strategies. The primary purpose of this group is to develop performance, emotional regulation, and cognitive skills of the members by imparting, discussing, and integrating factual information.

Psychosocial rehab: Training in life skills. This training includes the areas of social skills, independent living, prevocational skills, stress management, and assertion.

Qualified mental health professional (QMHP): Often used by states to identify licensed mental health professionals. Includes psychologists, psychiatrists, clinical social workers, licensed marriage and family therapists, and psychiatric nurse practitioners. Criteria and requirements vary from state to state.

Racism: Prejudice directed at people specifically because of their race or ethnic membership.

Rapport: Occurs when two or more people feel that they are in sync or on the same wavelength because they feel similar or relate well to each other.

Reality testing: The ability to tell the difference between reality and fantasy and to share the same general ideas about reality as everyone else.

Recovery model/movement: A civil rights movement that emphasizes a person-centered and empowering manner of health care.

Relaxation response: State of emotional integration; the "triangle of well-being" associated with a higher capacity for empathetic relationships, brain energy flow, and coherent thought processes.

Resilience: The adaptive capacity that supports healthy adjustments to the inevitable internal and external system stressors common during the aging years.

Rational-emotive Therapy (RET): Developed by Albert Ellis. Its basic hypothesis is that our emotions stem mainly from our beliefs, evaluations, interpretations, and reactions to life situations.

Revolving membership: Membership changes from one group to the next.

Role: A set of expectations about the ways in which people are supposed to behave in different situations.

Routines: Represent the steps done to complete the schedule.

Sanction: A consequence for violating group norms.

Scaffolding: When the occupational therapy practitioner provides assistance and support to the client only at those times that the client cannot complete a step on his or her own. The occupational therapy practitioner then gradually removes that support as the individual learns to perform the activity.

Schedules: Represent the big picture—the main activities to be completed daily.

Self-actualization: Advanced state of social and emotional wellness that can be achieved during the late lifespan.

Self-help group: Promotes change within an individual.

Self-organized learning system: Consists of a positive and encouraging therapist, self-motivating therapeutic activities, a well-designed environment, an active exploratory learning approach, and cues to trigger the adaptive response cycle.

Self-organization: Rewarding and relaxing feelings act as behavioral attractors that shape a person's personality and occupational patterns through the approach-and-avoidance system.

Self-regulation: Capacity to self-regulate is developed by relational capacities that are influenced from genetic predispositions and experiences over time.

Sensory integration: The neurological process that organizes sensations from one's body and from the environment and makes it possible to use the body effectively in the environment.

Sensory integration frame of reference: Jean Ayres developed sensory integration. In her efforts to formulate explanations about sensory integrative dysfunction, Ayres described children's gross motor play activities in terms of sensory integrative properties and the organizing effects of movement in human functioning. Movement requires the integration of all sense, and generates important tactile, proprioceptive, kinesthetic, and vestibular sensations.

Sensory integration group: Use of sensory integration theory to closely monitor and grade the activity in the moment as needed and adapt the group according to the members' responses during the session.

Sensory modulation: A clinical intervention that focuses on the use of environments, equipment, and activities to regulate an individual's sensory experience and optimize physiological and emotional well-being.

Sensory processing: Well-regulated sensory systems can contribute to important outcomes in social-emotional, physical, communication, self-care, cognitive, and adaptive skill development.

Service competency: A clinician's attainment of skills or abilities that may be utilized or expected at a particular setting.

Social and emotional learning (SEL): Refers to the process of helping children recognize and manage emotions, think about their feelings and how one should act, regulate behavior based on thoughtful decision making, and acquire important social skills for developing healthy relationships in life.

Social model: Looks at social relationships, environmental barriers, and social stressors to promote social relationships and social advocacy.

Socialization: New group member learns the knowledge, social skills, language, and values required to conform to the norms of the group.

Specialized knowledge and skills: Profession-specific specialized knowledge and skills that occupational therapy assistants gain during educational preparation.

Spirituality: The aspect of humanity that refers to the way individuals seek and express meaning and purpose.

Stereotype: A label used to describe differences among groups and to predict how others will behave.

Supervision: Interaction and collaboration that occurs between the occupational therapist and occupational therapy assistant that facilitates health care services to meet the needs of the client. Supervision is the responsibility of both the occupational therapist and the occupational therapy assistant.

Support group: Meeting for the purpose of giving emotional support and information to persons with a common problem.

Supported/transitional center: They are designed to assist an individual in transitioning to a more independent living situation. They also help an individual remain stable in his or her current residential setting.

Systems theory: The interdisciplinary study of systems in science and society.

Targeted services: One of the three major tiers of service in the multi-tiered system of support, targeted services (tier 2) focus services on individuals at risk of those diagnosed with mental illness.

Task group: An assembly of individuals who are brought together to accomplish a specific action or produce a product.

Task leadership: Focuses on the work that will be done within the group to achieve goals.

Temperament: All people are born with their own unique combination of temperament traits that can include biological regularity, adaptability, approach/withdrawal, intensity of emotional response, distractibility, quality of mood, and persistence/attention.

Theory: A contemplative and rational type of abstract or generalized thinking, or the result of such thinking.

Theory of retrogenesis: A reverse developmental theory whereby the progression of dementia corresponds to the developmental sequence of the brain earlier in life.

Therapeutic adaptation: An adaptive response facilitated by a practitioner in treatment to promote the natural process of developmental learning.

Therapeutic cues: Motivation, ability, and a personally relevant cue must be present for developmental learning to occur.

Therapeutic modes: A style of relating to a client. The Intentional Relationship Model identifies six therapeutic modes.

Therapeutic rapport: Description of the interaction between the therapist and client.

Therapeutic use of self: A term that is used to describe how an occupational therapy practitioner uses personal understanding about relationships, emotions, and experiences in an intentional way in order to communicate with the client.

Trauma-informed care: A model of care that requires all practitioners working with clients with mental health concerns be aware of the high prevalence of trauma incidence among mental health service users, the pervasive influence of trauma (particularly when trauma occurs in early childhood), and the provision of services that address the impact of trauma.

Universal services: One of the three major tiers of service in the multi-tiered system of support, universal services (tier 1) focus services on the whole population for those diagnosed with mental illness.

Wellness Recovery Action Plan (WRAP): A self-management and recovery system.

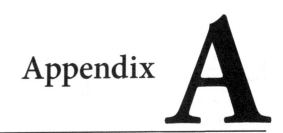

Appendix A

Website Resources

TABLE A-1		
WEBSITE RESOURCES IN THE EARLY LIFESPAN		
WEBSITE NAME	**WEBSITE**	**DESCRIPTION**
Administration for Children and Families	www.acf.hhs.gov	Foster health and well-being by providing federal leaderships, partnerships, and resources for the compassionate and effective delivery of human services.
American Academy of Pediatrics	www.aap.org/en-us/Pages/Default.aspx	Attain optimal physical, mental and social health, and well-being for all infants, children, adolescents, and young adults.
American Occupational Therapy Association (AOTA)	www.aota.org	Advances the quality and availability and use and support of occupational therapy services.
Anti-Bullying	www.stopbullying.gov	Provides information from government agencies on bullying, cyberbullying, and how to respond to and prevent bullying.
Anti-Defamation League	www.adl.org/education/curriculum_connections/winter_2005	Fight anti-Semitism and all forms of bigotry, defend democratic ideals, and protect civil rights for all.
Association for Behavioral and Cognitive Therapies	www.abct.org/home/	Multidisciplinary organization committed to the integration and application of behavioral, cognitive, and other evidenced-based principles to understand and improve human functioning.
Association for Treatment and Training in the Attachment of Children	www.attach.org	Recognizes and promotes healthy attachment and its critical importance to human development.

(continued)

Manville, C.A., & Keough, J. L.
Mental Health Practice for the Occupational Therapy Assistant (pp 377-383).
© 2016 Taylor & Francis Group.

TABLE A-1 (CONTINUED)		
WEBSITE RESOURCES IN THE EARLY LIFESPAN		
WEBSITE NAME	**WEBSITE**	**DESCRIPTION**
Bazelon Center for Mental Health Law	www.bazelon.org	The Bazelon Center for Mental Health Law works on a broad array of children's mental health issues.
Brain Gym	www.braingym.org	Optimize learning through movement-based programs to optimize the joy of living.
BrainWorks	www.sensationalbrain.com	Online tools for creating sensory diets.
Carnegie Library of Pittsburgh	www.carnegielibrary.org/ research/parentseducators/ parents/bibliotherapy/	Words that heal: using children's literature to prevent bullying
Centers for Disease Control and Prevention (CDC)	www.cdc.gov	Fights disease and supports communities and citizens to do the same. Conducts science, provides health information, and attempts to protect the United States from health safety and security threats.
Centers for School Mental Health Technical Assistance Centers	www.smhp.psych.ucla.edu UCLA www.csmha.umaryland.edu (University of Maryland at Baltimore	In 1995, two national training and technical assistance centers focused on mental health in schools were established with partial support from the U.S. Department of Health and Human Services (USDHHS) and the Center for Mental Health Services. The websites include information and resources on school-based mental health programs.
Child Welfare League of America (CWLA)	www.cwla.org	Coalition of private and public agencies who provide services to vulnerable children and families.
Coalition for Evidence-Based Policy	http://toptierevidence.org	Nonprofit, nonpartisan organization to increase government effectiveness through the use of rigorous evidence about what works.
Collaborative for Academic, Social, and Emotional Learning	www.casel.org	Helps make social and emotional learning (SEL) an integral part of education for preschool through high school.
Dialectical Behavioral Therapy Behavioral Tech, LLC	http://behavioraltech.org/ resources/whatisdbt.cfm	Trains professionals and treatment teams to provide compassionate, evidence-based treatments and evaluate the use of these treatments in service settings.
Eyes on Bullying Toolkit	www.eyesonbullying.org/ pdfs/toolkit.pdf	What Can You Do? (free downloadable)
Greenspan Floortime Approach	www.stanleygreenspan.com	Approach that incorporates time with a child in his or her context to excite his or her inherent drive to connect and challenge him or her to be creative, curious, and spontaneous. Approach created by Dr. Stanley Greenspan.

(continued)

	TABLE A-1 (CONTINUED)	

WEBSITE RESOURCES IN THE EARLY LIFESPAN

WEBSITE NAME	WEBSITE	DESCRIPTION
Healthy Children	www.healthychildren.org/english/ages-stages/teen/Pages/default.aspx	Committed to the attainment of optimal physical, mental, and social health and well-being for all infants, children, adolescents, and young adults.
How Does Your Engine Run?	www.alertprogram.com	Therapy Works, Inc. provides services and education related to the Alert Program with children with disabilities and impairments. The goal is to enhance children's lives.
Minnesota Children's Mental Health Association	www.macmh.org	The mission is to promote positive mental health for all infants, children, adolescents, and their families through education and resources.
Multisystemic Therapy	www.mstinstitute.org	Encourages the use and quality use of multisystemic therapy (MST). Monitors the implementation of MST through quality assurance standards.
National Center for Child Traumatic Stress	www.nctsn.org	Improve access to care, treatment, and services for traumatized children and adolescents.
National Center for Learning Disabilities (NCLD)	www.ncld.org	Improve the lives of all people with learning difficulties by empowering parents and youth, transforming schools, and providing advocacy.
National Child Traumatic Stress Network	www.nctsn.org	Raise public awareness, advance interventions and services, establish systems of care, and foster community collaboration.
National Early Childhood Technical Assistance Center	www.nectac.org	Funded by the Office of Special Education Programs to improve state early intervention and early childhood special education.
National Institute of Mental Health (NIMH)	www.nimh.nih.gov/health/publications/children-and-adolescents-listing.shtml	Transfer the understanding and treatment of medical illness through research, prevention, recovery, and care.
OSEP Technical Assistance Center on PBIS	www.pbis.org	Bully Prevention Manual: Elementary School Level; Bully Prevention Manual: Middle School Level -Authors: Stiller, B., Ross, S., Horner, R. (free downloadable manuals)
Office of Special Education and Rehabilitative Services (OSERS), US Department of Education	http://www2.ed.gov	"To provide leadership to achieve full integration and participation in society of people with disabilities by ensuring equal opportunity and access to, and excellence in, education, employment, and community living."
PACER National Center for Bully Prevention	www.pacer.org/bullying/	Free resources, information sheets, bookmarks, etc.
Peer Advocacy Guide	www.pacer.org/bullying/resources/activities/toolkits/pdf/PeerAdvocacyGuide.pdf	How to address bullying of students with disabilities by engaging, educating, and empowering their peers with advocacy skills.

(continued)

TABLE A-1 (CONTINUED)

WEBSITE RESOURCES IN THE EARLY LIFESPAN

WEBSITE NAME	WEBSITE	DESCRIPTION
Positive Behavioral Interventions and Supports (PBIS)	www.pbis.org	OSEP Center on positive behavioral interventions and supports. Effective school-wide interventions.
Promising Practices	www.promisingpractices.net	Group of individuals and organizations dedicated to providing quality evidence-based interventions about improving lives of children, families, and communities.
Rehabilitation Services Administration (RSA), US Department of Education	https://www.rsa.ed.gov	Provides grant program funds to vocational rehabilitation programs to provide counseling, medical and psychological services, job training, and other individualized services.
SchoolMentalHealth.Org.	www.schoolmentalhealth.org	This site offers school mental health resources for clinicians, educators, administrators, parents/caregivers, families, and students. The resources included in the site emphasize practical information and skills based on current research, including prominent evidence-based practices, as well as lessons learned from local, state, and national initiatives.
Sensory Modulation Program	www.ot-innovaitons.com	Promotes embodied, comprehensive, and person-centered practices by providing a resource for collaboration, support, and education.
Sensory Processing Disorder Foundation	www.spdfoundation.net	Sensory Processing Disorder (SDF) Foundation: World leader in research, education, and advocacy for sensory-processing disorders.
Sensory Stories	www.sensorystories.com	Stories to teach children to engage in social activities in the home, school, and community.
Social and Emotional Learning and Bullying Prevention	http://casel.org/wp-content/uploads/SEL-and-Bullying-Prevention-2009.pdf	Collaborative for Academic, Social, and Emotional Learning (CASEL) focuses on student academic, social, and emotional ability growth (free downloadable).
Social Profile	www.social-profile.com/references.html	Assessment to identify a group's social level.
Social Stories™	www.thegraycenter.org/social-stories	Assist all individuals in the shared challenge of building and maintaining effective social connections.
Steps to Respect	www.cfchildren.org/steps-to-respect.aspx	Focuses on bully prevention and friendship development; developed by Committee for Children

(continued)

TABLE A-1 (CONTINUED)		

WEBSITE RESOURCES IN THE EARLY LIFESPAN

WEBSITE NAME	WEBSITE	DESCRIPTION
SticKids	www.stickids.com	Software and activity-based kits of friendly therapeutic strategies for use in school, home, and the community.
Tony Attwood	www.tonyattwood.com	Understanding and teaching friendship skills; friendship checklists.
Trauma-Focused Cognitive Behavior Therapy	http://tfcbt.musc.edu	Web-based learning of trauma-focused cognitive behavioral therapy.
Yoga Kids	www.yogakids.com	Yoga for children around the world that addresses the needs and capabilities of children.

TABLE A-2		

WEBSITE RESOURCES IN THE MIDDLE AND LATE LIFESPAN

WEBSITE NAME	WEBSITE	DESCRIPTION
A Place For Mom	www.aplaceformom.com	A comprehensive senior living resource for people that provides information, resources, and services by connecting families to senior care.
Administration on Aging	www.aoa.gov	Services the Older Americans Act; home and community-based care, elder rights, and health, prevention, and wellness information. Provides funding for 27 resource centers on topics of aging.
Alzheimer's Association	www.alz.org	Group with goal to eliminate Alzheimer's disease
American Association of Retired Persons (AARP)	www.aarp.org	Provides information for seniors as well as advocates for seniors.
American Occupational Therapy Association (AOTA)	www.aota.org	Advances the quality, availability, use, and support of occupational therapy through standard setting, advocacy, education, and research on behalf of its members and the public.
American Psychological Association (APA)	www.apa.org	Advance the creation, communication, and application of psychological knowledge to benefit society and improve people's lives.
Assistant Secretary for Planning and Evaluation, USDHHS	www.aspe.hhs.gov	"National plant to address Alzheimer's Disease" along with other interesting research.
Centers for Disease Control and Prevention (CDC)	www.cdc.gov/ncbddd/childdevelopment/index.html	To protect Americans from health, safety, and security threats and support communities and citizens to do the same.
Centers for Medicare and Medicaid Services (CMS)	www.cms.gov/	"As an effective steward of public funds, CMS is committed to strengthening and modernizing the nation's health care system to provide access to high quality care and improved health at lower costs."

(continued)

TABLE A-2 (CONTINUED)		
WEBSITE RESOURCES IN THE MIDDLE AND LATE LIFESPAN		
Commission on Accreditation of Rehabilitation Facilities (CARF)	www.carf.org	"To promote the quality, value, and optimal outcome of services through a consultative accreditation process and continuous improvement services center on enhancing the lives of person's served."
The Gerontological Society of America	www.geron.org	Promote multidisciplinary research, disseminate gerontological knowledge, and promote, support, and advocate for aging education.
Health People 2020	www.healthypeople.gov	Healthy people initiative managed by the Office of Disease Prevention and Health Promotion (ODPHP) of the USDHHS.
International Council on Active Aging	www.icaa.cc	Connect individuals who share the goal of changing society's perception on aging, improve quality of life within the seven dimensions of wellness.
International Mental Health Research Organization (IMHRO)	www.imhro.org	"To alleviate human suffering from mental illness by funding scientific research into causes, prevention, and new treatments."
Internet Mental Health	www.mentalhealth.com	Free encyclopedia of mental health information created by Dr. Phillip Long.
National Alliance on Mental Illness (NAMI)	www.nami.org	NAMI is a grassroots organization consisting of individuals with mental illness, family members, and friends with the mission: "To advocate for effective prevention, diagnosis, treatment, support, research, and recovery that improves the quality of life of persons of all ages who are affected by mental illnesses."
National Center on Elder Abuse: Administration on Aging	www.ncea.aoa.gov/	"Up-to-date information regarding research, training, best practices, news and resources on elder abuse, neglect and exploitation."
National Council for Behavioral Health (NCHB)	www.thenationalcouncil.org	"Advance our members' ability to deliver integrated healthcare" through advocating and consulting, coordinating the Mental Health First Aid program, operating the SAMHSA-HRSA Center for integrated Health Solutions, and offering the National Council for Behavioral Health Conference.
National Institute of Mental Health (NIMH)	www.nimh.nih.gov	The mission of NIMH is to diminish the burden of mental illness through research.
The Joint Commission	www.jointcommission.org	"To continuously improve health care for the public, in collaboration with other stakeholders, by evaluating health care organizations and inspiring them to excel in providing safe and effective care of the highest quality and value."
Substance Abuse and Mental Health Services Agency (SAMHSA)	www.samhsa.gov	Leads the public health efforts to advance the behavioral health of the nation. Reduce the impact of substance abuse and mental illness.
Surgeon General Reports	www.surgeongeneral.com	In 1999, Surgeon General David Satcher issued A Comprehensive Report on mental health.

(continued)

TABLE A-2 (CONTINUED)		
WEBSITE RESOURCES IN THE MIDDLE AND LATE LIFESPAN		
U.S. National Library of Medicine	www.nim.nih.gov	Searchable databases and free full text articles, as well as other services.
World Health Organization (WHO)	www.who.org	Coordinating authority for health in the United Nations systems.

Appendix B

Psychotropic Medications

J. Michael McGuire, PharmD, BCPP and Cathy H. Ficzere, PharmD, BCPS

CHAPTER OUTLINE

Introduction
Antipsychotic Agents
Antidepressant Agents
Drugs for the Treatment of Bipolar Disorder: Mood Stabilizers
Drugs for the Treatment of Anxiety
Sedative-Hypnotics
Cognitive Enhancers
Drugs for the Treatment of Attention Deficit Hyperactivity Disorder
Drugs for the Treatment of Substance Use Disorders

INTRODUCTION

Psychotropic medications include a variety of categories of medications. Since the 1990s, there has been an increase in the number of available psychotropic medications, the prevalence of mental disorder diagnoses, and the frequency of psychotropic medication prescriptions (Glied & Frank, 2009). Almost all psychotropic medications increase or decrease the effect of chemicals called neurotransmitters. These chemicals are located in the central nervous system (CNS), and include serotonin, norepinephrine, dopamine, acetylcholine and gamma-aminobutyric acid (GABA). Deficiency or excess of one or a combination of neurotransmitters is thought to cause depression, anxiety, schizophrenia, bipolar disorder, and other mental illnesses (Stahl, 2008). These neurotransmitters cause changes in symptoms by acting on a receptor which is a site of action specific for a particular neurotransmitter, i.e., serotonin affects serotonin receptors.

As with all medications, clinicians must weigh the risks of psychotropic therapy with the potential benefits. Patient response to psychotropic medications is highly variable and not all patients will benefit from the same drug or combination of drugs. Additionally, psychotropic medications are associated with serious side effects, many of which can negatively impact a patient's daily functioning. This appendix will briefly review the most commonly prescribed psychotropic medications, discuss the most common reasons each category is prescribed, and address common adverse events. The following is not intended to be an exhaustive review of the clinical use of these agents.

Manville, C.A., & Keough, J. L.
Mental Health Practice for the Occupational Therapy Assistant (pp 385-407).
© 2016 Taylor & Francis Group.

TABLE B-1		
ANTIPSYCHOTIC MEDICATIONS		
	GENERIC NAME	BRAND NAME
First-Generation (Typical)	Chlorpromazine	Thorazine
	Fluphenazine	Prolixin
	Haloperidol	Haldol
	Loxapine	Loxitane
	Perphenazine	Trilafon
	Thioridazine	Mellaril
	Thiothixene	Navane
	Trifluoperazine	Stelazine
Second-Generation (Atypical)	Aripiprazole	Abilify
	Asenapine	Saphris
	Brexpiprazole	Rexulti
	Cariprazine	Vraylar
	Clozapine	Clozaril, FazaClo
	Iloperidone	Fanapt
	Lurasidone	Latuda
	Olanzapine	Zyprexa
	Paliperidone	Invega
	Risperidone	Risperdal
	Quetiapine	Seroquel
	Ziprasidone	Geodon

ANTIPSYCHOTIC AGENTS

Historically, antipsychotic agents have been used primarily in the treatment of patients with schizophrenia; however, over the last decade there has been an increase in the use of antipsychotics for other psychiatric illnesses, including bipolar disorder, depression, and autism spectrum disorders. Antipsychotics are currently divided into first-generation (typical antipsychotics) and second-generation agents (atypical antipsychotics) (Tandon, 2011). Due to adverse effects, use of first-generation antipsychotics is commonly limited to acute management of psychiatric disorders and for patients who fail to respond to second-generation antipsychotics. Two to four weeks of therapy is typically required for full antipsychotic effect (Lehman et al., 2004; Tandon, 2011). Table B-1 lists the antipsychotic medications available in the United States. Table B-2 provides a summary of these additional indications.

Use of both generations of antipsychotics may result in unintended side effects including sedation, dry mouth, blurred vision, constipation, dizziness, heart rhythm disturbance (arrhythmia) and orthostatic hypotension (sudden decrease in blood pressure upon standing). Although the second-generation antipsychotics may also be associated with these adverse effects, the incidence and severity are generally not as great as with the first-generation agents (Crismon, Argo, & Buckley, 2011). The second-generation antipsychotics may result in improved tolerability, especially less extrapyramidal symptoms (EPS), which are discussed later (Stahl, 2008). The Food and Drug Administration (FDA) requires that all antipsychotics carry a major warning, i.e., black-box warning, against use of these agents in elderly patients with dementia-related psychosis due to an increased risk of death (U.S. Food and Drug Administration, 2008). Table B-3 describes the antipsychotics and the relative incidence of adverse effects.

EPS may be caused by both generations of antipsychotics, but the incidence is substantially higher with the first-generation agents. These adverse effects may be divided into early and late-onset EPS. Early-onset EPS develops within hours to days or weeks and includes acute dystonic reactions, akathisia, and pseudoparkinsonism. Acute dystonic

TABLE B-2

SECOND-GENERATION ANTIPSYCHOTICS: FDA-APPROVED INDICATIONS

ANTIPSYCHOTIC	SCHIZOPHRENIA, ADULT	SCHIZOPHRENIA, ADOLESCENTS (13 TO 17 YEARS)	BIPOLAR MANIA, ADULT	BIPOLAR DISORDER, PEDIATRICS (10 TO 17 YEARS)
Aripiprazole (Abilify)	X	X	X	X
Asenapine (Saphris)	X		X	X
Brexpiprazole (Rexulti)	X			
Cariprazine (Vraylar)	X		X	
Clozapine (Clozaril)	X treatment resistant			
Iloperidone (Fanapt)	X			
Lurasidone (Latuda)	X			
Olanzapine (Zyprexa)	X	X	X	X (13 to 17 years)
Paliperidone (Invega)	X			X (12 to 17 years)
Quetiapine (Seroquel)	X	X	X	X
Quetiapine XR (Seroquel XR)	X	X	X	X
Risperidone (Risperdal)	X	X	X	X
Ziprasidone (Geodon)	X		X	

(continued)

TABLE B-2 (CONTINUED)				
SECOND-GENERATION ANTIPSYCHOTICS: FDA-APPROVED INDICATIONS				
ANTIPSYCHOTIC	BIPOLAR DEPRESSION	BIPOLAR DISORDER, MAINTENANCE ADULT	MAJOR DEPRESSIVE DISORDER, (ADJUNCT TO ANTIDEPRESSANT)	IRRITABILITY IN AUTISTIC DISORDER
Aripiprazole (Abilify)		X (alone or adjunct to mood stabilizer)	X	X (6 to 17 years)
Asenapine (Saphris)				
Brexpiprazole (Rexulti)			X	
Cariprazine (Vraylar)				
Clozapine (Clozaril)				
Iloperidone (Fanapt)				
Lurasidone (Latuda)	X alone or adjunct to mood stabilizer			
Olanzapine (Zyprexa)	X combined with fluoxetine	X	X combined with fluoxetine	
Paliperidone (Invega)				
Quetiapine (Seroquel)	X	X adjunct to mood stabilizer		
Quetiapine XR (Seroquel XR)	X	X adjunct to mood stabilizer	X	
Risperidone (Risperdal)				X (5 to 16 years)
Ziprasidone (Geodon)		X adjunct to mood stabilizer		

Compiled from Abilify [package insert]. Tokyo, Japan: Otsuka Pharmaceuticals Co, Ltd.; February, 2012.; Clozaril [package insert]. East Hanover, NJ: Novartis Pharmaceuticals Corporation; March 2013.; Fanapt [package insert]. East Hanover, NJ: Novartis Pharmaceuticals Corporation; January, 2013.; Geodon [package insert]. New York, NY: Pfizer Inc.; October, 2012.; Invega [package insert]. Titusville, NJ: Jansen Pharmaceuticals, Inc.; June, 2011.; Latuda [package insert]. Marlborough, MA: Sunovion Pharmaceuticals, Inc.; July, 2013.; Rexulti [package insert]. Tokyo, Japan: Otsuka Pharmaceuticals Co. Ltd.; July, 2015.; Risperdal [package insert]. Titusville, NJ: Janssen Pharmaceuticals, Inc.; August, 2012.; Saphris [package insert]. Whitehouse Station, NJ: Merck & Co, Inc.; March, 2013.; Seroquel [package insert]. Marlborough, MA: Sunovion Pharmaceuticals, Inc.; July, 2013.; Seroquel XR [package insert]. Wilmington, DE: AstraZeneca; July, 2013.; Vraylar [package insert]. Parsippany, NJ: Actavis; September, 2015.; Zyprexa [package insert]. Indianapolis, IN: Lilly USA, LLC; July, 2011.

TABLE B-3

ANTIPSYCHOTICS: RELATIVE INCIDENCE OF ADVERSE EFFECTS

ANTIPSYCHOTIC	SEDATION/ SOMNOLENCE	WEIGHT GAIN/ METABOLIC ADVERSE EFFECTS	ORTHOSTATIC HYPOTENSION/ DIZZINESS	PROLACTIN ELEVATION	EXTRAPYRAMIDAL SYMPTOMS
First Generation Antipsychotics					
Chlorpromazine (Thorazine)	++++	++	++++	+++	+++
Haloperidol (Haldol)	+	+	+	++++	++++
Perphenazine (Trilafon)	++	+	+	++++	+++
Second Generation Antipsychotics					
Aripiprazole (Abilify)	+	+	+	-	+
Asenapine (Saphris)	++	+	+	+	++
Brexpiprazole (Rexulti)	+	+	+		+
Cariprazine (Vraylar)	+	++	+		++++
Clozapine (Clorazil)	++++	++++	++++	+	+
Iloperidone (Fanapt)	+	++	+++	++	+
Lurasidone (Latuda)	++	+	++	+	++
Olanzapine (Zyprexa)	+++	++++	++	+	++
Paliperidone (Invega)	++	+	+	++++	++
Quetiapine (Seroquel)	+++	+++	++	+	+
Risperidone (Risperdal)	++	++	++	++++	++
Ziprasidone (Geodon)	+	+	+	+	++

Key: + = 1% to 10%; ++ = 11% to 20%; +++ = 21% to 30%; ++++ = 31% or greater
*Please note, these above are estimates based on prescribing information and many adverse events such as extrapyramidal symptoms and sedation/somnolance and weight gain are experienced more frequently in children and adolescents. Rates also vary by disease state (i.e., for quetiapine, somnolence/sedation is more common in patients with depression vs patients with schizophrenia).

Compiled from Abilify [package insert]. Tokyo, Japan: Otsuka Pharmaceuticals Co, Ltd.; February, 2012.; Chlorpromazine. (2012). Drugs.com. Retrieved from www.drugs.com/chlorpromazine.html.; Clozaril [package insert]. East Hanover, NJ: Novartis Pharmaceuticals Corporation; March 2013.; Fanapt [package insert]. East Hanover, NJ: Novartis Pharmaceuticals Corporation; January, 2013.; Geodon [package insert]. New York, NY: Pfizer Inc.; October, 2012.; Haloperidol [package insert]. Schaumberg, IL: Sagent Pharmaceuticals, Inc.; August, 2011.; Invega [package insert]. Titusville, NJ: Jansen Pharmaceuticals, Inc.; June, 2011.; Latuda [package insert]. Marlborough, MA: Sunovion Pharmaceuticals, Inc.; July, 2013.; Perphenazine. (2012). Drugs.com. Retrieved from www.drugs.com/pro/perphenazine.html; Rexulti [package insert]. Tokyo, Japan: Otsuka Pharmaceuticals Co. Ltd.; July, 2015.; Risperdal [package insert]. Titusville, NJ: Janssen Pharmaceuticals, Inc.; August, 2012.; Saphris [package insert]. Whitehouse Station, NJ: Merck & Co, Inc.; March, 2013.; Seroquel [package insert]. Marlborough, MA: Sunovion Pharmaceuticals, Inc.; July, 2013.; Vraylar [package insert]. Parsipanny, NJ: Actavis; September, 2015.; Zyprexa [package insert]. Indianapolis, IN: Lilly USA, LLC; July, 2011..

TABLE B-4		
LONG-ACTING INJECTABLE ANTIPSYCHOTICS		
DRUG	BRAND NAME	DOSING FREQUENCY
Aripiprazole	Abilify Maintena	Every 4 weeks
	Aristada	Every 4 to 6 weeks
Fluphenazine	Prolixin Decanoate	Every 2 to 3 weeks
Haloperidol	Haldol Decanoate	Every 4 weeks
Olanzapine	Zyprexa Relprevv	Every 2 or 4 weeks
Paliperidone	Invega Sustenna	Every 4 weeks
	Invega Trinza	Every 3 months
Risperidone	Risperdal Consta	Every 2 weeks

Compiled from Abilify Maintena [package insert]. Tokyo, Japan: Otsuka Pharmaceutical Co., Ltd.; February, 2013.; Aristada [package insert]. Waltham, MA: Alkermes, Inc.; October, 2015.; Fluphenazine decanoate [package insert]. Bedford, OH: BenVenue Laboratories, Inc., Bedford Laboratories; December, 2010.; Haloperidol decanoate [package insert]. Toronto, ON: Apotex, Inc.; December, 2004.; Invega Sustenna [package insert]. Titusville, NJ: Janssen Pharmaceuticals, Inc.; August, 2012.; Invega Trinza [package insert]. Titusville, NJ: Jansen Pharmaceuticals, Inc.; May, 2015.; Risperdal Consta [package insert]. Titusville, NJ: Janssen Pharmaceuticals, Inc.; June, 2012.; Zyprexa Relprevv [package insert]. Indianapolis, IN: Lilly USA, LLC; July, 2011.

reactions are characterized by continuous muscular contractions typically in the neck, jaw, back, extremities, eyes, throat, and tongue. Acute dystonias may develop quickly, are painful, and are considered a medical emergency. Antipsychotic-induced parkinsonism or pseudoparkinsonism presents similarly to Parkinson's disease with rigidity, bradykinesia (slow movement), and tremor. Additional symptoms may include shuffling gait and stooped posture. Patients with akathisia describe an inner sense of motor restlessness plus observed restlessness. Patients may be pacing or rocking. Akathisia is often accompanied by dysphoria, or emotional discomfort (Pierre, 2005).

Late-onset EPS includes tardive dyskinesia (TD) and develops after prolonged treatment with antipsychotics. TD is characterized by involuntary movements of the tongue, jaw, trunk, or extremities. The movements may be described as choreiform or rapid, jerky, nonrepetitive; athetoid, or slow, sinuous, continual; and rhythmic, or senseless, repetitive (APA, 2013). It may develop after months or years of therapy and can be irreversible (Sachdev, 2000). In general, second-generation antipsychotics are associated with reduced rates of both early and late-onset EPS effects (Leucht et al., 2009). The difference in incidence of EPS among the second-generation agents varies. Despite the reduced rates of EPS with the second-generation compared to first-generation antipsychotics, patients may still experience EPS with these agents (Rummel-Kluge et al., 2012).

The second-generation antipsychotics are associated with metabolic adverse events including weight gain, increased blood sugar, increased cholesterol, and type 2 diabetes mellitus. Therefore, monitoring of weight, blood glucose, and cholesterol is necessary (Consensus Development Conference on Antipsychotic Drugs and Obesity and Diabetes, 2004; Newcomer & Haupt, 2006). Children and adolescent patients may be particularly vulnerable to the metabolic adverse effects associated with the second-generation antipsychotics (Corell et al., 2009). As with adult patients, routine monitoring of body weight, blood sugar, and cholesterol is required children and adolescents receiving second-generation antipsychotics (Pringsheim, Panangiotopoulos, Davidson, & Ho, 2001; Walkup, 2009).

Patients with schizophrenia are at risk for nonadherence such as stopping medication use or lack of follow-up with office visits (Gilmer et al., 2004; Valenstein, Ganoczy, McCarthy, Kim, Lee, & Blow, 2006). Nonadherence to antipsychotic medications increases the risk of relapse, hospitalization, and health care costs (Gilmer et al., 2004). In order to overcome this obstacle, several of the first-generation and second-generation antipsychotics are available in long-acting injectable formulations. Table B-4 describes long-acting injectable antipsychotics.

These formulations are administered via intramuscular injection every 2 to 4 weeks depending on the agent. Just as these formulations provide a prolonged therapeutic response, the duration of any adverse effects will be prolonged as well. Additionally, patients may neglect to report use of long-acting antipsychotic formulations since these are not taken on a daily basis.

Clozapine

Clozapine is unique among the second-generation antipsychotics in that it is effective in patients with schizophrenia who have failed treatment with previous antipsychotics

TABLE B-5
FIRST-GENERATION ANTIPSYCHOTICS SUMMARY: COMMON ADVERSE EFFECTS

- Breast milk production
- Constipation
- Decreased urination
- Dizziness
- Dry mouth
- Extrapyramidal symptoms (movement difficulties)
  - More likely with first generation than second generation antipsychotics
  - Patients may unable to fasten their clothes or walk with a normal gait
- Photosensitivity (sunburn-like reaction after limited exposure to sunlight)
- Sedation
  - Occurs early in treatment and may decrease over time
  - May contribute to cognitive, perceptual, and motor dysfunction
  - Patients should be warned about the risk of using hazardous machinery or driving while sedated

(Kane, Honigfield, Singer, & Meltzer, 1988). It is FDA approved for patients with schizophrenia who have failed treatment with other antipsychotic agents as well as for patients with suicidal behavior in schizophrenia and schizoaffective disorder (Clozaril, 2013). Clozapine is associated with a rare and serious side effect called agranulocytosis, or severely decreased white blood cell count. This necessitates continuous lab monitoring for the duration of treatment—weekly for the first 6 months, biweekly for next 6 months, then monthly for the remainder of treatment. Common adverse effects of clozapine include significant sedation and anticholinergic effects (constipation, increased heat rate), sialorrhea (excessive salivation), urinary incontinence, and orthostatic hypotension and dizziness (Clozaril, 2013).

Table B-5 lists common adverse effects of first-generation antipsychotic medications. Table B-6 lists common adverse effects of second-generation antipsychotic medications.

ANTIDEPRESSANTS

According to the American Psychiatric Association (APA) treatment guidelines for major depressive disorder (MDD), antidepressants are recommended as initial treatment of choice in patients with mild to moderate MDD, and definitely should be provided for those with severe MDD unless electroconvulsive therapy is planned (Gelenberg et al., 2010). Although the effectiveness of antidepressant medications is generally comparable, these agents differ regarding their side effects which are often the main determinant of initial agent selection. Although the exact mechanism of action for treating depression is unknown, all currently available antidepressants increase the concentration of one or more of the following neurotransmitters: serotonin, norepinephrine, or dopamine (Stahl, 2008). Antidepressants are typically categorized based on their mechanism of action or chemical structure. The categories of antidepressants include monoamine oxidase inhibitors (MAOIs), tricyclic antidepressants (TCAs), selective-serotonin reuptake inhibitors (SSRIs), serotonin-norepinephrine reuptake inhibitors (SNRIs), and norepinephrine dopamine reuptake inhibitor (NDRIs). Table B-7 lists antidepressant medications available in the United States.

Initial response to an antidepressant may be seen in 2 weeks, but full effect should not be expected until the patient has completed at least 4 to 8 weeks of therapy. Antidepressant therapy is generally continued for about 1 year after a full response is achieved after a single episode of depression. For patients with a history of depressive episodes, long-term antidepressant therapy may be advised. In patients who do not respond to antidepressants alone, a second antidepressant or a nonantidepressant medication may be added. Nonantidepressant medications which may be added to antidepressant therapy include thyroid hormone, buspirone (BuSpar), lithium carbonate (Lithobid, Eskalith), second-generation antipsychotics, stimulants, and anticonvulsants (Gelenberg et al., 2010).

In addition to treatment of MDD, antidepressants may be used to treat depression associated with bipolar disorder;

TABLE B-6
SECOND-GENERATION ANTIPSYCHOTICS SUMMARY: COMMON ADVERSE EFFECTS

- Breast milk production
- Constipation
- Decreased urination
- Dizziness
- Dry mouth
- Metabolic adverse effects: increased blood glucose, increased cholesterol, weight gain
- Extrapyramidal symptoms (movement difficulties)
  - Less likely with second-generation than first-generation antipsychotics
  - Patients may unable to fasten their clothes or walk with a normal gait
- Sedation
  - Occurs early in treatment and may decrease over time
  - May contribute to cognitive, perceptual, and motor dysfunction
  - Patients should be warned about the risk of using hazardous machinery or driving while sedated

however, their use is controversial (Amit & Weizman, 2012; Sachs et al., 2007). Antidepressants are commonly prescribed for patients with anxiety disorders such as panic disorder, generalized anxiety disorder, and social anxiety disorder as well as for obsessive-compulsive disorder and post-traumatic stress disorder. Certain antidepressants may also be used for other conditions including insomnia (tricyclic antidepressants, trazodone), chronic pain (certain tricyclic antidepressants, duloxetine), prevention of migraine headaches (tricyclic antidepressants), and premenstrual dysphoric disorder (selective-serotonin reuptake inhibitors). Table B-8 identifies SSRI and SNRI antidepressants and additional FDA-Approved indications.

The FDA requires that all antidepressants carry a major warning, (i.e., a black-box warning), for the risk of increased suicidality. Suicidality is defined as suicidal thinking and behaviors. The risk of suicidality must be weighed against the clinical need for the medication. Regardless of age, patients should be monitored for clinical worsening, suicidality or unusual changes in behavior (U.S. Food and Drug Administration, 2010). Antidepressants may also cause dry mouth, blurred vision, constipation, orthostatic hypotension, dizziness, sedation, and weight gain.

Monoamine Oxidase Inhibitors

The MAOIs are effective antidepressants; however, use has been limited to patients with treatment-resistant depression due to significant dietary restrictions and numerous drug-drug interactions. Common side effects associated with MAOIs include insomnia or sedation, orthostatic hypotension, dizziness, nausea, weight gain, edema, muscle pain, myoclonus (involuntary jerking of muscles), paresthesia (abnormal tingling sensation), and sexual dysfunction (VanDenberg, 2012).

MAOIs prevent breakdown of tyramine in the gastrointestinal tract (Stahl, 2008). Consumption of dietary tyramine while receiving an MAOI can lead to a rapid increase in blood pressure (hypertensive crisis), which may be fatal (Golwyn & Sevlie, 1993; Stahl, 2008). Patients receiving an MAOI must follow a low-tyramine diet for the duration of treatment and for 2 weeks after cessation of the agent. Tyramine is found in moderate to high concentrations in some foods and drinks including aged meats and cheeses, pickled herring, fava beans, yeast extracts, sauerkraut, tap beers, and others. Dietary restrictions are not necessary for one MAOI, transdermal selegiline, when given at a lower dose (6 mg/24 h); dietary restrictions are necessary at higher doses (9 to 12 mg/24 h) (Schulman, Walker, MacKenzie, & Knowles, 1989).

In addition to dietary restrictions, use of many medications in combination with an MAOI must be avoided due to the numerous serious drug–drug interactions. The combined use of an MAOI with other antidepressants, some over-the-counter cough/cold preparations, stimulants, selected opiate pain relievers, and some other medications may lead to serotonin syndrome or hypertensive crisis, which may be fatal (Flockhart, 2012).

TABLE B-7		
ANTIDEPRESSANTS		
	GENERIC NAME	*BRAND NAME*
Monoamine Oxidase Inhibitors (MAOIs)	Isocarboxazid	Marplan
	Phenelzine	Nardil
	Selegiline transdermal	EMSAM
	Tranylcypromine	Parnate
Tricyclic Antidepressants (TCAs)	Amitriptyline	Elavil
	Clomipramine	Anafranil
	Desipramine	Norpramin
	Doxepin	Sinequan, Silenor
	Imipramine	Tofranil
	Nortriptyline	Pamelor
	Protriptyline	Vivactil
	Trimipramine	Surmontil
Selective Serotonin Reuptake Inhibitors (SSRIs)	Citalopram	Celexa
	Escitalopram	Lexapro
	Fluoxetine	Prozac
	Fluvoxamine	Luvox, Luvox CR
	Paroxetine	Paxil, Pexeva
	Sertraline	Zoloft
Serotonin-Norepinephrine Reuptake Inhibitors (SNRIs)	Desvenlafaxine	Pristiq
	Duloxetine	Cymbalta
	Levomilnacipran	Fetzima
	Venlafaxine	Effexor, Effexor XR
Norepinephrine-Dopamine Reuptake Inhibitors (NDRIs)	Bupropion	Wellbutrin, Aplenzin, Forfivo XL
Other	Mirtazapine	Remeron
	Nefazodone	Serzone
	Trazodone	Desyrel
	Vilazodone	Viibryd
	Vortioxetine	Brintellix

Tricyclic Antidepressants

The TCAs are so named because their chemical structure contains three rings. The TCAs increase the concentrations of serotonin and norepinephrine (Stahl, 2008). Use of TCAs in depression is limited by their side effect profile and toxicity on overdose; however, these agents continue to be frequently prescribed (Bartholow, 2011). Continued prescribing of these agents is likely due to their beneficial use for other uses including pain, migraine headache prevention, sleep and others. Common side effects with the TCAs include sedation, weight gain, dry mouth, blurred vision, urinary retention, constipation, orthostatic hypotension, and dizziness (Teter, Kando, & Wells, 2011). Overdoses with TCAs are serious and may be fatal due to cardiovascular toxicity, which includes heart rhythm disturbances (arrhythmias), and substantially reduced blood pressure (hypotension) (Thanacoody & Thomas, 2005).

Table B-8

SSRI and SNRI Antidepressants: Additional FDA-Approved Indications

Antidepressant	Generalized Anxiety Disorder	Panic Disorder	Social Anxiety Disorder	Post-Traumatic Stress Disorder	Obsessive-Compulsive Disorder
SSRI Antidepressants					
Citalopram (Celexa)	–	–	–	–	–
Escitalopram (Lexapro)	X	–	–	–	–
Fluoxetine (Prozac)	–	X	–	–	X
Fluvoxamine (Luvox, Luvox CR)	–	–	–	–	X
Paroxetine (Paxil)	X	X	X	X	X
Sertraline (Zoloft)	–	X	X	X	X
SNRI Antidepressants					
Desvenlafaine (Pristiq)	–	–	–	–	–
Duloxetine (Cymbalta)	X	–	–	–	–
Levomilnacipran (Fetzima)	–	–	–	–	–
Venlafaxine (Effexor, Effexor XR)	X	X	–	–	–

Compiled from Celexa [package insert]. St. Louis, MO: Forest Pharmaceuticals, Inc.; December 2012.; Cymbalta [package insert]. Indianapolis, IN: Eli Lilly and Company; November, 2012.; Effexor XR [package insert]. Philadelphia, PA: Pfizer, Inc.; December, 2012.; .Fetzima [package insert]. St. Louis, MO: Forest Pharmaceuticals, Inc.; July, 2013.; Lexapro [package insert]. St. Louis, MO: Forest Pharmaceuticals, Inc.; December, 2012.; Luxor CR [package insert]. Palo Alto, CA: Jazz Pharmaceuticals, LLC; October, 2012.; Paxil [package insert]. Research Triangle Park, NC: GlaxoSmithKline; January, 2013.; Pristiq [package insert]. Philadelphia, PA: Pfizer, Inc.; February, 2013.; Prozac [package insert]. Indianapolis, IN: Lilly USA, LLC; January, 2013.; Zoloft [package insert]. New York, NY: Pfizer, Inc.; June, 2013.

Selective-Serotonin Reuptake Inhibitors

The SSRIs increase the concentration of serotonin in the brain (Stahl, 2008). Among all classes of antidepressants, the SSRIs are considered by many to be the first choice for treatment of patients with MDD as well as many anxiety disorders. SSRIs have become widely prescribed because they are much better tolerated and have less severe adverse effects on overdose compared to the MAOIs and TCAs (Mann, 2005). The most common side effects associated with the SSRIs include gastrointestinal upset (nausea, vomiting, constipation/diarrhea), central nervous system activation (anxiety, insomnia), possible sedation, and sexual dysfunction (Mann, 2005; Teter et al., 2011).

Serotonin-Norepinephrine Reuptake Inhibitors

The SNRIs increase the concentrations of serotonin and norepinephrine in the brain. The SNRIs may be used as a first-choice antidepressant; however, many primary care physicians prefer SSRIs as first-line treatment (Gelenberg et al., 2010; Thase, 2008). Common adverse events of the

SNRIs include insomnia, agitation, possible sedation, elevated blood pressure, gastrointestinal upset (nausea, vomiting), and sexual dysfunction (Mann, 2005).

Other Antidepressants

Bupropion (Wellbutrin) is thought to increase the concentrations of norepinephrine and dopamine in the brain (Stahl, 2008). Bupropion is also used for smoking cessation under the brand name Zyban (Zyban, 2011). Bupropion is associated with less sedation and less sexual dysfunction than other antidepressant medications; however, this agent is associated with an increased risk of seizures, especially at higher doses (Moreira, 2011). Common adverse effects include but are not limited to the following: nausea/vomiting, tremor, insomnia, and dry mouth (Teter et al., 2011).

Mirtazapine (Remeron) increases concentrations of both serotonin and norepinephrine, but it is not considered an SNRI. The most common side effects of mirtazapine include sedation, increased appetite, and weight gain (Croom, Perry, & Plosker, 2009). As with bupropion, mirtazapine is associated with less sexual dysfunction than other antidepressant medications (Croom et al., 2009; Clayton & Montejo, 2006). Trazodone (Desyrel), nefazodone (Serzone), vilazodone (Viibryd), and vortioxetine (Brintellix) share a similar effect of increasing serotonin for the treatment of depression, but they are not considered SSRIs. Neither trazodone nor nefazodone are frequently utilized as antidepressants. Relatively low doses of trazodone are frequently prescribed at bedtime for sleep (Mendelson, 2005). Nefazodone is not frequently used in the treatment of depression due to a risk of fatal hepatotoxicity (Gelenberg et al., 2010). Vilazodone and vortioxetine are newly approved antidepressants. Table B-9 provides a summary of the most common adverse effects of antidepressant medications.

DRUGS FOR THE TREATMENT OF BIPOLAR DISORDER: MOOD STABILIZERS

Although there is no accepted definition of a "mood stabilizer" according to the FDA (Stahl, 2008), the term is commonly used to refer to medications for the treatment of patients with bipolar disorder. Bipolar disorder is characterized by fluctuations in mood from extreme elevation in mood (manic episode) to depression (depressive episode) (APA, 2013). The classic mood stabilizers include lithium, valproate (divalproex, [Depakote], valproic acid [Depakene]), carbamazepine (Tegretol, Carbatrol, Equetro), and lamotrigine (Lamictal). The second-generation antipsychotics discussed previously are considered by many to be mood stabilizers. Table B-10 lists drugs used in the treatment of bipolar disorder. The combination of classic mood stabilizers and second-generation antipsychotics is commonly seen in the treatment of patients with bipolar disorder.

Lithium

Lithium is a first choice for treatment for bipolar disorder and is effective for the treatment of manic and depressive episodes. It is also effective at preventing relapse (Grunze et al., 2013; Licht, 2012). Therapy with lithium requires periodic laboratory monitoring of the level of lithium in the body as well as kidney function and thyroid function. Side effects of lithium include cognitive impairment (difficulty thinking or processing information), acne, tremor, decreased thyroid function, weight gain, nausea, vomiting, diarrhea, and increased urination (Grandjean & Aubry, 2009; Moreira, 2011). Lithium levels that are only slightly elevated above goal may be associated with toxicity; substantially increased levels may be fatal. Elevated lithium levels and toxicity may be caused by drug–drug interactions or dehydration. Signs of toxicity include worsening tremor, confusion, drowsiness, severe gastrointestinal upset, dizziness, increased urination, and increased thirst (Grunze et al., 2013; Ng et al., 2009). Lithium toxicity is a medical emergency.

Anticonvulsants

Valproate (valproic acid, divalproex) is a first choice for treatment of bipolar disorder and is effective for the treatment of acute mania. It is frequently used for maintenance therapy of bipolar disorder (Crismon, Argo, Bendele, & Suppes, 2007; Grunze et al., 2013). Valproate is also used for the treatment of various seizure disorders and prevention of migraine headaches (Depakote, 2013). Valproate is available as either valproic acid (Depakene) or divalproex (Depakote, Depakote ER). Divalproex is formulated to have less gastrointestinal side effects than valproic acid. As with lithium, valproate levels may be monitored (Crismon et al., 2007). Common adverse events of valproate include hair loss (alopecia), muscle incoordination (ataxia), difficulty thinking or processing information (cognitive impairment),

TABLE B-9

ANTIDEPRESSANTS SUMMARY: COMMON ADVERSE EFFECTS

MONOAMINE OXIDASE INHIBITORS (MAOIs)

- Dizziness, orthostatic hypotension
- Edema
- Low tyramine diet required
- Numerous drug-drug interactions
- Sexual dysfunction
- Weight gain

TRICYCLIC ANTIDEPRESSANTS (TCAs)

- Dizziness
- Dry mouth, decreased urination, constipation
- Sedation
- Use caution in elderly patients

SELECTIVE-SEROTONIN REUPTAKE INHIBITORS (SSRIs)

- Central nervous system activation (anxiety, insomnia)
- Gastrointestinal upset (nausea, vomiting, constipation/diarrhea)
- Sedation, possibly
- Sexual dysfunction

SEROTONIN-NOREPINEPHRINE REUPTAKE INHIBITORS (SNRIs)

- Agitation
- Elevated blood pressure
- Gastrointestinal upset (nausea, vomiting)
- Insomnia or sedation
- Sexual dysfunction

BUPROPION

- Insomnia
- Risk of seizures

MIRTAZAPINE

- Increased appetite, weight gain
- Sedation

VILAZODONE

- Diarrhea
- Insomnia
- Nausea/vomiting

VORTIOXETINE

- Nausea/vomiting
- Constipation

TABLE B-10

DRUGS FOR TREATMENT OF BIPOLAR DISORDER

	GENERIC NAME	BRAND NAME
Lithium	*Lithium Carbonate*	*Eskalith, Lithobid*
Anticonvulsants	Carbamazepine	Tegretol, Carbatrol, Equetro
	Lamotrigine	Lamictal
	Oxcarbazepine	Trileptal
	Valproic acid or Divalproex	Depakene
		Depakote, Depakote ER
Antidepressants*	Ex. SSRIs, SNRIs, Bupropion (See Table B-8)	
Second-Generation Antipsychotics	Ex. Olanzapine, Risperidone, Quetiapine (See Table B-1 and B-2)	

* Use of antidepressants in patients with bipolar disorder is controversial.

dizziness, gastrointestinal upset, rash, sleepiness (somnolence), tremor, and weight gain (Crismon et al., 2007).

Carbamazepine (Tegretol, Carbatrol, Equetro), like valproate, is an anticonvulsant (medication for seizure disorder) and is considered a second-choice for treatment of patients with bipolar disorder (Crimson et al., 2007; Grunze et al., 2013; Yatham et al., 2009). The usefulness of carbamazepine is limited by reduced tolerability and numerous drug–drug interactions (Grunze et al., 2013). It is effective for the treatment of acute mania and may be used for maintenance therapy as well, although it is not recommended as a first-line treatment (Crimson et al., 2007; Grunze et al., 2013; Yatham et al., 2007). Common side effects of carbamazepine include muscle incoordination (ataxia), double-vision (diplopia), dizziness, joint pain (dysarthria), gastrointestinal upset, abnormal eye movement (nystagmus), and sedation (Crimson et al., 2007). Oxcarbazepine (Trileptal) is chemically similar to carbamazepine and may be used for the treatment of bipolar disorder. Adverse effects are similar to those seen with carbamazepine (Drayton, 2011).

Lamotrigine (Lamictal), also an anticonvulsant, is effective for the treatment of depression in patients with bipolar disorder and is FDA-approved for the prevention of relapse in patients with bipolar disorder (Crimson et al., 2007; Lamictal, 2012). Common side effects of lamotrigine include muscle incoordination (ataxia), dizziness, headache, nausea, rash, and sleepiness (somnolence) (Crimson et al., 2007). Lamotrigine-induced rash can be serious and potentially fatal. The rash is associated with rapid dose escalation; therefore, the dose must be increased slowly (Rogers & Cavozos, 2011). Table B-11 provides a summary of mood stabilizers.

DRUGS FOR THE TREATMENT OF ANXIETY

A number of different medications are used for treatment of anxiety and anxiety disorders, which include benzodiazepines, antidepressants, buspirone (BuSpar), and hydroxyzine (Vistaril). Anxiety disorders include generalized anxiety disorder, panic disorder, and social anxiety disorder. Although no longer considered anxiety disorders in DSM-5, obsessive-compulsive disorder (OCD), post-traumatic stress disorder (PTSD) symptoms may be managed with anti-anxiety medications (The DSM-5 Task Force, 2013). Table B-12 identifies the currently available anti-anxiety medications.

Treatment guidelines recommend antidepressants as a first-choice therapy for the anxiety disorders and OCD and PTSD (Bandelow, Zohar, Hollander, Kasper, & Moller, 2008; Davidson et al., 2010; Stein et al., 2010). The therapeutic benefit of antidepressants and buspirone in the treatment of anxiety may take several weeks. Therapy should generally be continued for one year once patient's symptoms have improved. In contrast, therapeutic benefit with benzodiazepines may occur quickly; however, long-term treatment with benzodiazepines is generally not recommended due to the potential for abuse and dependency (Dell'osso & Lader, 2013).

Benzodiazepines are used to relieve anxiety and promote muscle relaxation. They are also used for sedation and anticonvulsant effects (Stahl, 2008). Benzodiazepines may be used for a variety of indications: anxiety disorders, insomnia, alcohol withdrawal, agitation, sleep and anxiety in patients with other mental illnesses (Dell'osso & Lader, 2013). Due to their habit-forming and abuse potential, all benzodiazepines are controlled substances and subject to prescribing limitations enforced by the Drug Enforcement Agency of the United States. Adverse effects associated with initial therapy include sedation, drowsiness, impairment of learning, psychomotor slowing (delayed motor response time), and anterograde amnesia (difficulty with acquiring new information/memories). These effects may continue with long-term therapy. Benzodiazepines may affect driving performance and increase the risk of involvement in a traffic accident (Melton & Kirkwood, 2011). Use of benzodiazepines in elderly patients is not recommended because they increase the risk of falls and fractures (Fick, Cooper, Wade, Waller, Maclean, & Beers, 2003). Since physical dependence may occur with long-term use, abruptly stopping benzodiazepine therapy may cause significant withdrawal symptoms including seizures which can be life-threatening (Dell'osso & Lader, 2013). Due to their sedative effects, benzodiazepines should not be co-administered with alcohol or other medications that depress the CNS (Melton & Kirkwood, 2011).

Buspirone (BuSpar) affects serotonin receptors and is approved by the FDA for the treatment of generalized anxiety disorder. Buspirone is generally well tolerated, with dizziness, nausea and headache being the most commonly reported adverse events (Melton & Kirkwood, 2011). Buspirone is also commonly combined with antidepressants in the treatment of both depression and anxiety disorders (Shelton, 2007). Hydroxyzine (Vistaril) is an antihistamine that may be used in the treatment of anxiety. Common adverse effects include drowsiness and dry mouth (McEvoy, 2012). Other medications that may be used for the treatment of anxiety in patients who do not adequately respond to initial treatment include TCAs, MAOIs, second-generation antipsychotics, and anticonvulsants such as pregabalin (Lyrica) and gabapentin (Neurontin). Table B-13 provides a summary of the common adverse effects of drugs used to treat anxiety disorder.

TABLE B-11

MOOD STABILIZERS SUMMARY: COMMON ADVERSE EFFECTS

ANTICONVULSANTS		Lithium
Carbamazepine	*Oxcarbazepine*	• Cognitive dysfunction
• Ataxia (muscle incoordination)	• Ataxia	• Diarrhea
• Diplopia (double-vision)	• Diplopia (double-vision)	• Increased urination
• Dizziness	• Dizziness	• Nausea/vomiting
• Dysarthria (joint pain)	• Headache	• Tremor
• Gastrointestinal upset/nausea	• Itching	
• Nystagmus (abnormal eye movement)	• Nausea	*Second-Generation Antipsychotics* (see Table B-3 and B-6)
• Sedation or somnolence (sleepiness)	• Rash	
	• Sedation or somnolence (sleepiness)	
	• Tremor	
Lamotrigine	*Valproate*	
• Ataxia	• Ataxia	
• Dizziness	• Cognitive impairment	
• Gastrointestinal upset/nausea	• Dizziness	
• Headache	• Gastrointestinal upset/nausea	
• Rash	• Sedation or somnolence (sleepiness)	
• Sedation or somnolence (sleepiness)	• Tremor	
	• Weight gain	

TABLE B-12

DRUGS FOR ANXIETY DISORDER

	GENERIC NAME	BRAND NAME
Benzodiazepines	Alprazolam	Niravam, Xanax
	Chlordiazepoxide	Librium
	Clonazepam	Klonopin
	Clorazepate	Tranxene
	Diazepam	Valium
	Lorazepam	Ativan
	Midazolam	Versed
	Oxazepam	Serax
	Temazepam	Restoril
Other	Buspirone	BuSpar
	Hydroxyzine	Atarax, Vistaril

TABLE B-13
DRUGS FOR ANXIETY DISORDER SUMMARY: COMMON ADVERSE EFFECTS

Benzodiazepines	*Buspirone*
• Delayed motor response time	• Dizziness
• Drowsiness, sedation	• Headache
• Falls and fractures	• Nausea
• Impaired driving performance	*Hydroxyzine*
• Impairment of learning, anterograde amnesia (difficulty with acquiring new information/memories)	• Drowsiness
	• Dry mouth

TABLE B-14
SEDATIVE-HYPNOTICS

	GENERIC NAME	*BRAND NAME*
Benzodiazepines	Ex. Clonazepam, Lorazepam, Oxazepam, etc. (See Table B-12)	
Non-Benzodiazepine GABA Agonists	Eszopiclone	Lunesta
	Zaleplon	Sonata
	Zolpidem	Ambien, Intermezzo
Melatonin Receptor Agonist	Ramelteon	Rozerem

SEDATIVE-HYPNOTICS

Sleep disorders are a common problem encountered in both a primary care and specialty care setting and often accompany other psychiatric and nonpsychiatric medical conditions (APA, 2013). Sedative-hypnotics are intended to assist in the treatment of sleep disorders. Sedative-hypnotics should generally be administered when the patient is ready to go to bed due to their relatively quick onset and potentially prolonged duration of action. A number of different sedating medications may be used including benzodiazepines, non-benzodiazepine GABA agonists, ramelteon (Rozerem), certain antidepressants, some low-dose second-generation antipsychotics, antihistamines, and some herbal remedies. Table B-14 identifies the available sedative-hypnotic medications.

Side effects of all sedative-hypnotics may include drowsiness, sedation, excessive daytime sleepiness (i.e., hangover), cognitive impairment, decreased motor coordination, amnesia, and dependence (Buscemi et al., 2007; Guideline Development Group, 2009). Because these agents may be associated with daytime drowsiness, patients may experience impaired work performance (Melton & Kirkwood, 2011). Elderly patients are at an increased risk of falls (Fick et al., 2003). Certain sedative-hypnotics have been associated with complex behaviors such as sleepwalking, sleep driving, sleep eating, or sleep telephone calling, (i.e., zolpidem; Ambien, 2013). Sedative-hypnotics should not be co-administered with alcohol or other medications that depress the CNS (Melton & Kirkwood). Table B-15 provides a summary of the common adverse effects of the sedative-hypnotics.

Melatonin is a neurotransmitter that is naturally produced and released in the brain in the evening. Melatonin is available without a prescription (i.e., over the counter) and is an effective hypnotic. Ramelteon (Rozerem) is a prescription medication that affects melatonin receptors in the brain to improve sleep onset (Stahl, 2008). Unlike many of the hypnotics, both melatonin and ramelteon are not controlled substances. Antihistamines such as diphenhydramine or doxylamine may be used to promote sleep and are found in over the counter sleep aids (e.g., Unisom) (Drug Facts & Comparisons, 2013).

COGNITIVE ENHANCERS

Cognitive enhancers are primarily used in the treatment of Alzheimer's disease, which is the most common type of dementia. Currently, there is no cure for dementia;

TABLE B-15

SEDATIVE-HYPNOTICS SUMMARY: COMMON ADVERSE EFFECTS

Benzodiazepines (see Table B-13)	*Ramelteon*

Benzodiazepines
(see Table B-13)

Non-Benzodiazepine GABA Agonists
- Amnesia
- Cognitive impairment
- Decreased mental alertness
- Decreased motor coordination
- Dependence
- Drowsiness/sedation
- Excessive daytime sleepiness (i.e., hangover)
- Impaired driving performance

Ramelteon
- Dizziness
- Headache
- Somnolence (sleepiness)

Trazodone
- Dizziness
- Orthostatic hypotension
- Sedation

Antihistamines
- Blurred vision
- Constipation
- Dry mouth
- Sedation
- Urinary retention

TABLE B-16

COGNITIVE ENHANCERS

	GENERIC NAME	BRAND NAME
Acetylcholinesterase Inhibitors	Donepezil	Aricept
	Rivastigmine	Exelon
	Galantamine	Razadyne
	Tacrine	Cognex
NMDA Receptor Antagonist	Memantine	Namenda

medications are used to delay progression of the illness and to improve symptoms (Qaseem et al., 2008). Small improvement in cognition and activities of daily living may be seen. Response to therapy occurs slowly and should be evaluated after a period of approximately 6 months (Farlow & Cummings, 2007). Currently, only five agents are FDA-approved for the treatment of Alzheimer's disease, and they are divided into two categories: acetylcholinesterase inhibitors (AChI) and an NMDA receptor antagonist. Table B-16 identifies the available cognitive enhancers.

There is no convincing evidence that any one of these agents is more effective than another. As a result, treatment selection is often based on prescriber comfort, patient tolerance, and cost (Qaseem et al., 2008). Table B-17 provides a summary of the adverse effects of cognitive enhancers.

DRUGS FOR THE TREATMENT OF ATTENTION DEFICIT HYPERACTIVITY DISORDER

Stimulant medications increase the concentration of dopamine and norepinephrine in the brain and are the first choice treatment for attention deficit hyperactivity disorder (ADHD) (Subcommittee on ADHD, 2011). Due to their abuse potential, all of the stimulant medications are regulated as schedule II controlled substances and, as such, are subject to prescribing limitations. Stimulant medications have a rapid onset of effect, which may be seen shortly after dose administration (Dopheide & Pliszka,

TABLE B-17

COGNITIVE ENHANCERS SUMMARY: COMMON ADVERSE EFFECTS

ACETYLCHOLINESTERASE INHIBITORS (ACHEI)	*MEMANTINE*
• Anorexia	• Confusion
• Diarrhea	• Constipation
• Dizziness	• Dizziness
• Nausea/vomiting	• Hallucinations
	• Headache

TABLE B-18

ATTENTION DEFICIT HYPERACTIVITY DISORDER (ADHD) MEDICATIONS

	GENERIC NAME	*BRAND NAME*
Stimulants*	Methylphenidate	Ritalin, Methylin, Ritalin LA+, Ritalin SR†, Metadate CD+, Metadate ER+, Daytrana+, Aptensio XR+ Quillivant XR+, Concerta+
	Dexmethylphenidate	Focalin, Focalin XR+
	Mixed amphetamine salts	Adderall, Adderall XR+
	Dextroamphetamine	Dexedrine, Dexedrine Spansule+, Procentra Solution, Zenzedi
	Lisdexamphetamine	Vyvanse
Nonstimulants	Atomoxetine	Straterra
	Guanfacine, extended release	Intuniv
	Clonidine, extended release	Kapvay
Certain Antidepressants (listed agents only)	Bupropion, Imipramine, Norptriptyline	

* All stimulants listed are C-II controlled substances.

† Extended-release formulation.

2011). Nonstimulant medications are used adjunctively with stimulant medications and may be preferred in individuals with substance abuse history because these agents are not controlled substances and are not subject to abuse or diversion. They are, however, generally not as effective for the treatment of ADHD as the stimulants (Pliszka, 2007). Table B-18 identifies the available medications for ADHD.

There are many formulations of stimulants available including immediate and extended-release preparations. Immediate-release formulations must be taken two to three times daily, whereas extended or sustained-release preparations have a longer duration of effect and may be dosed once or twice daily. The extended/sustained-release preparations are more convenient for the patient and family and are associated with greater adherence to therapy. In general, all of the stimulant medications have been shown to be equally effective. Treatment selection is based upon prescriber comfort, patient or family preference, and cost (Pliszka, 2007). The most common adverse effects related to stimulants are decreased appetite, weight loss, and insomnia. Stimulant medications may be associated with increased blood pressure and pulse and have been associated with sudden cardiac death in patients with heart problems or heart defects. Children should be screened for cardiac risk factors prior to receiving a stimulant medication. Because stimulant medications have abuse potential, clinicians should monitor for evidence of misuse or diversion (Dopheide & Pliszka, 2011; Pliszka, 2007). To minimize the effect of stimulants on appetite and sleep, they should

TABLE B-19
DRUGS FOR ATTENTION DEFICIT HYPERACTIVITY DISORDER SUMMARY: COMMON ADVERSE EFFECTS

Stimulants	*Atomoxetine*
• Decreased appetite	• Decreased appetite
• Dizziness	• Fatigue
• Insomnia	• Increased blood pressure
• Mood lability	• Increased pulse rate
• Poor growth	• Insomnia
Guanfacine and Clonidine	• Nausea
• Constipation	• Sedation
• Dizziness	
• Hypotension	
• Sedation	

not be administered late in the day, (i.e., close to dinner or bedtime; Dopheide & Pliszka, 2011).

The nonstimulant agents guanfacine (Intuniv) and clonidine (Kapvay) were initially marketed as blood pressure treatments; however, both have been reformulated into extended release formulations for treatment of ADHD (Intuniv, 2013; Kapvay, 2013). These agents may also be useful for the treatment of comorbid aggression or insomnia in ADHD (Pliszka, 2007). The most common adverse effects for these agents are sedation, hypotension, dizziness, and constipation (Dopheide & Pliszka, 2011).

Atomoxetine (Strattera) is FDA-approved for the treatment of ADHD in adults and children (Stahl, 2008). The most common adverse events for atomoxetine include nausea, anorexia, increased blood pressure, increased pulse rate, insomnia, fatigue, and sedation. Similar to antidepressant medications, atomoxetine carries a warning regarding increased suicidality; however, it is not FDA-approved for the treatment of depression (Dopheide & Pliszka, 2011; Strattera, 2012). Unlike stimulant medications, 2 to 4 weeks of treatment with atomoxetine may be required before therapeutic effect is seen (Dopheide & Pliszka). Table B-19 summarizes the common adverse effects of drugs for ADHD.

DRUGS FOR THE TREATMENT OF SUBSTANCE USE DISORDERS

Currently, there are several medications that are FDA-approved for the treatment of substance use disorders.

Naltrexone (ReVia, Vivitrol), acamprosate (Campral), and disulfiram (Antabuse) are used for alcohol dependence. Methadone (Dolophine), buprenorphine (Subutex), and buprenorphine/naloxone (Suboxone, Zubsolv) are used for opiate dependence. Table B-20 identifies available drugs for treatment of substance use disorders and other medications commonly prescribed in mental health.

Alcohol Use Disorder

Benzodiazepines such as diazepam (Valium), chlordiazepoxide (Librium), and lorazepam (Ativan) are used to manage acute alcohol withdrawal, which may be fatal if not appropriately managed (Doering & Moorman, 2011). Once a patient has been safely and successfully detoxed from alcohol, maintenance treatment may be initiated with naltrexone (ReVia/Vivitrol), acamprosate (Campral) or disulfiram (Antabuse) (Center for Substance Abuse Treatment, 2009; Doering & Moorman, 2011). Naltrexone is FDA-approved for the management of alcohol dependence (Vivitrol, 2010). It is available in an oral formulation under the trade name ReVia or as a monthly intramuscular injection under the trade name Vivitrol. Naltrexone blocks opioid receptors in the body and has been shown to reduce the craving for alcohol and its rewarding effects (Center for Substance Abuse Treatment, 2009). The most common side effect of naltrexone is nausea. Acamprosate (Campral) is FDA-approved for maintenance of abstinence from alcohol in patients who are abstinent. Common side effects of acamprosate include diarrhea and somnolence (Doering & Moorman, 2011).

TABLE B-20		
DRUGS FOR SUBSTANCE USE DISORDER AND OTHER MEDICATIONS COMMONLY PRESCRIBED IN MENTAL HEALTH		
	GENERIC NAME	*BRAND NAME*
Opioid and alcohol use disorder medications	Buprenorphine	Suboxone
	Buprenorphine plus Naltrexone	Subutex, Buprenex
	Disulfiram	Antabuse
	Methadone	Dolophine, Methadone
	Naltrexone	ReVia, Vivitrol
Anticholinergic—for management of EPS caused by antipsychotic drugs	Benztropine	Cogentin
	Trihexyphenadyl	Artane
Anticonvulsant	Gabapentin	Neurontin, Gralise
	Topiramate	Topamax
Antihistamine	Cyproheptadine	Periactin
	Hydroxyzine	Vistaril, Atarax
Other	Amantadine	Symmetrel

Disulfiram (Antabuse) is FDA-approved for the treatment of alcoholism. If alcohol is consumed while a patient is taking disulfiram, the patient experiences a reaction of flushing, sweating, nausea, and increased heart rate. This reaction may be fatal. Patients should not consume any alcohol (including alcoholic beverages, cough/cold preparations with alcohol, mouthwashes, etc.) while receiving disulfiram and for 14 days after discontinuation. Common side effects of disulfiram include drowsiness, metallic taste, dermatitis, and headache (Center for Substance Abuse Treatment, 2009).

Opioid Use Disorder

Opioid addiction is defined as physical dependence upon and a subjective need and craving for opioid drugs such as prescription pain medicines (i.e., hydrocodone, oxycodone) and heroin. Opioid dependence is most successfully managed with a combination of pharmacological and behavioral interventions (Center for Substance Abuse Treatment, 2005a). Buprenorphine (Subutex), buprenorphine/naloxone (Suboxone) and methadone (Dolophine) are all controlled substances which can be utilized for the management of acute opiate withdrawal and dependence (Doering & Moorman, 2011).

Buprenorphine is a schedule III controlled substance (C-III) which partially stimulates opioid receptors in the body, thereby reducing opioid craving and withdrawal. Buprenorphine may be initiated on an inpatient basis for patients who are experiencing acute withdrawal or in an outpatient setting when patients present with withdrawal symptoms such as nausea, diarrhea, sweating, yawning, and drug craving. The most common side effects of buprenorphine include nausea, vomiting, and constipation (Center for Substance Abuse Treatment, 2004).

Methadone (Dolophine, Methadose) is a controlled substance that may be used for the treatment of chronic pain or opiate dependence. When used for the treatment of opioid dependence, methadone is only available through specially licensed physician practices or health care facilities. Methadone fully stimulates opioid receptors in the body, which, like buprenorphine, can decrease opioid craving and withdrawal. There are strict prescribing limits on the use of methadone for the treatment of opioid dependence. The most common side effects of methadone include sedation, dizziness, nausea, vomiting, and constipation (Center for Substance Abuse Treatment, 2005b). Table B-21 provides a summary of the common adverse effects of drugs used to treat substance abuse disorder.

TABLE B-21
DRUGS FOR SUBSTANCE USE DISORDER SUMMARY: COMMON SIDE EFFECTS

ALCOHOL USE DISORDER	OPIOID USE DISORDER
Naltrexone	*Buprenorphine*
• Nausea	• Constipation
Acamprosate	• Nausea
• Diarrhea	• Vomiting
• Somnolence (sleepiness)	*Methadone*
Disulfiram	• Constipation
• Dermatitis	• Dizziness
• Drowsiness	• Nausea
• Headache	• Vomiting
• Metallic or garlic-like taste	• Sedation

REFERENCES

Abilify [package insert]. Tokyo, Japan: Otsuka Pharmaceuticals Co., Ltd.; February, 2012.

Abilify Maintena [package insert]. Tokyo, Japan: Otsuka Pharmaceutical Co., Ltd.; February, 2013.

Ambien [package insert]. Bridgewater, NJ: Sanofi-Aventis U.S. LLC; 2013.

American Psychiatric Association. (2013). *Diagnostic and statistical manual of mental disorders*, 5th ed. Arlington, VA: American Psychiatric Publishing.

Amit, B. H., & Weizman, A. (2012). Antidepressant treatment for acute bipolar depression: An update. *Depression Research and Treatment.* Article ID 684725, 10 pages. doi:10.1155/2012/684725.

Aristada [package insert]. Waltham, MA: Alkermes, Inc.; October, 2015.

Bandelow, B., Zohar, J., Hollander, E., Kasper, S., & Möller, H. J. (2008). WFSBP Task Force on Treatment Guidelines for Anxiety Obsessive-Compulsive and Post-Traumatic Stress Disorders. World Federation of Societies of Biological Psychiatry (WFSBP) guidelines for the pharmacological treatment of anxiety, obsessive-compulsive and post-traumatic stress disorders: first revision. *World Journal of Biological Psychiatry, 9*(4), 248-312.

Bartholow, M. (2011). Top 200 drugs of 2011. *Pharmacy Times.* Retrieved from www.pharmacytimes.com/publications/issue/2012/July2012/Top-200-Drugs-of 2011.

Buscemi, N., Vandermeer, B., Friesen, C., Bialy, L., Tubman, M., Ospina, M.,...Witmans, M. (2007). The efficacy and safety of drug treatments for chronic insomnia in adults: A meta-analysis of RCTs. *Journal of General Internal Medicine, 22*(9), 1335-1350.

Celexa [package insert]. St. Louis, MO: Forest Pharmaceuticals, Inc.; December 2012

Center for Substance Abuse Treatment. (2004). *Clinical Guidelines for the Use of Buprenorphine in the Treatment of Opioid Addiction.* Treatment Improvement Protocol (TIP) Series 40. DHHS Publication No. (SMA) 04-3939. Rockville, MD: Substance Abuse and Mental Health Services Administration.

Center for Substance Abuse Treatment. (2005a). *Quick Guide for Clinicians: Based on TIP 43: Medication-Assisted Treatment for Opioid Addiction in Opioid Treatment Programs.* Rockville, MD: Substance Abuse and Mental Health Services Administration.

Center for Substance Abuse Treatment. (2005b). *Medication-Assisted Treatment for Opioid Addiction in Opioid Treatment Programs.* Treatment Improvement Protocol (TIP) Series 43. HHS. Publication No. (SMA) 12-4214. Rockville, MD: Substance Abuse and Mental Health Services Administration.

Center for Substance Abuse Treatment. (2009). *Incorporating Alcohol Pharmacotherapies into Medical Practice.* Treatment Improvement Protocol (TIP) Series 49. HHS Publication No. (SMA) 09-4380. Rockville, MD: Substance Abuse and Mental Health Services Administration.

Clayton A. H., & Montejo A. L. (2006). Major depressive disorder, antidepressants, and sexual dysfunction. *Journal of Clinical Psychiatry. 67*(Suppl 6), 33-37.

Chlorpromazine. (2012). Drugs.com. Retrieved from www.drugs.com/chlorpromazine.html.

Clozaril [package insert]. East Hanover, NJ: Novartis Pharmaceuticals Corporation; March 2013.

Coe, H. V., & Hong, I. S. (2012). Safety of low doses of quetiapine when used for insomnia. *The Annals of Pharmacotherapy, 46,* 718-22.

Consensus Development Conference on Antipsychotic Drugs and Obesity and Diabetes (2004). *Diabetes Care, 27*(2), 596-601.

Correll, C. U., Manu, P., Olshanskiy, V., Napolitano, B., Kane, J. M., & Malhotra, A.K. (2009). Cardiometabolic risk of second-generation antipsychotic medications during first-time use in children and adolescents. *Journal of the American Medical Association, 302*(16), 1765-1773.

Crismon, M. L., Argo, T. R., & Bendele, S. D., & Suppes, T. (2007). *Texas Medication Algorithm Project Procedural Manual: Bipolar Disorder Algorithms.* Austin, TX: The Texas Department of State Health Services.

Crismon, M. L., Argo, T. R., & Buckley, P. F. (2011). Schizophrenia. In J. T. DiPiro, R. L. Talbert, G. C. Yee, G.R. Matzke, B. G. Wells, & L. M. Posey (Eds.), *Pharmacotherapy: A Pathophysiologic Approach* (8th ed, pp. 1147-1172). New York, NY: McGraw Hill.

Croom K. F., Perry C. M., & Plosker G. L. (2000). Mirtazipine: a review of its use in major depression and other psychiatric disorders. *CNS Drugs.* 23(5), 427-452.

Cymbalta [package insert]. Indianapolis, IN: Eli Lilly and Company; November, 2012.

Davidson, J. R., Zhang, W., Connor, K. M., Ji, J., Jobson, K., Lecrubier, Y.,...Versiani, M. (2010). A psychopharmacological treatment algorithm for generalised anxiety disorder (GAD). *Journal of Psychopharmacology, 24,* 3-26. . doi:10.1177/0269881108096505.

Dell'osso, B., & Lader, M. (2013). Do benzodiazepines still deserve a major role in the treatment of psychiatric disorders? A critical reappraisal. *European Psychiatry, 28,* 7-20.

Depakote [package insert]. North Chicago, IL: AbbVie Inc.; May 2013.

The DSM-5 Task Force. *Diagnostic and Statistical Manual of Mental Disorders,* (5th ed.). Arlington, VA: American Psychiatric Association.

Doering, P. L., & Moorman, R. (2011). Substance-related disorders: alcohol, nicotine, and caffeine. In J. T. DiPiro, R. L. Talbert, G. C. Yee, G.R. Matzke, B. G. Wells, and L. M. Posey (Eds.), *Pharmacotherapy: A Pathophysiologic Approach,* (8th ed., pp. 1131-1146). New York, NY: McGraw Hill.

Dopheide, J. A., & Pliszka, S. R. (2011). Childhood disorders, In J. T. DiPiro, R. L. Talbert, G. C. Yee, G.R. Matzke, B. G. Wells, and L. M. Posey (Eds). *Pharmacotherapy: A Pathophysiologic Approach,* (8th ed., pp. 1087-1099). New York, NY: McGraw Hill.

Drayton, S. J. (2011). Bipolar disorder, In J.T. DiPiro, R. L. Talbert, G. C. Yee, G.R. Matzke, B. G. Wells, and L. M. Posey (Eds). *Pharmacotherapy: A Pathophysiologic Approach,* (8th ed., pp. 1191-1208). New York, NY: McGraw Hill.

Drug Facts and Comparisons. Facts & Comparisons (2013) [database online]. St. Louis, MO: Wolters Kluwer Health, Inc. Accessed July 22, 2013.

Effexor XR [package insert]. Philadelphia, PA: Pfizer, Inc.; December, 2012.

EMSAM [package insert]. Morgantown, WV: Somerset Pharmaceuticals Inc.; November 2012.

Fanapt [package insert]. East Hanover, NJ: Novartis Pharmaceuticals Corporation; January, 2013.

Farlow, M. R., & Cummings, J. L. (2007). Effective pharmacologic management of Alzheimer's disease. *American Journal of Medicine, 120,* 388-397.

Fetzima [package insert]. St. Louis, MO: Forest Pharmaceuticals, Inc.; July, 2013.

Fick, D. M., Cooper, J. W., Wade, W. E., Waller, J. L., Maclean, R., & Beers, M. H. (2003). Updating the Beers Criteria for potentially inappropriate medication use in older adults: results of a US consensus panel of experts. *Archives of Internal Medicine, 163,* 2716-2724.

Flockhart, D. A. (2012). Dietary restrictions and drug interactions with monoamine oxidase inhibitors: an update. *Journal of Clinical Psychiatry, 73*(Suppl 1), 17-24.

Fluphenazine decanoate [package insert]. Bedford, OH: BenVenue Laboratories, Inc., Bedford Laboratories; December, 2010.

Geodon [package insert]. New York, NY: Pfizer Inc.; October, 2012.

Gelenberg, A. J., Freeman, M. P., Markowitz, J. C., Rosenbaum, J. F., Thase, M. E., Trivedi, M. H., & Van Rhoads, R. S. (2010). Practice Guideline for the Treatment of Patients with Major Depressive Disorder, 3rd Ed. Arlington, VA: American Psychiatric Association.

Gilmer, T. P., Dolder, C. R., Lacro, J. P., Folsom, D. P., Lindamer, L., Garcia, P., & Jeste, D. V. (2004). Adherence to treatment with antipsychotic medication and health care costs among Medicaid beneficiaries with schizophrenia. *American Journal of Psychiatry, 161,* 692-699.

Glied, S. A., & Frank, R. G. (2009). Better but not best: recent trends in the well-being of the mentally ill. *Health Affairs, 28*(3), 637-648.

Golwyn, D. H., & Sevlie, C. P. (1993). Monoamine oxidase inhibitor hypertensive crisis headache and orthostatic hypotension. *Journal of Clinical Psychopharmacology, 13*(1), 77-78.

Grandjean, E. M., & Aubry, J. M. (2009). Lithium: updated human knowledge using an evidence-based approach. *CNS Drugs, 23*(5), 397-418.

Grunze, H., Vieta, E., Goodwin, G. M., Bowden, C., Licht, R. W., Möller, H. J.,...WFSBP Task Force on Treatment Guidelines for Bipolar Disorder. (2013). The World Federation of Societies of Biological Psychiatry (WFSBP) guidelines for the biological treatment of bipolar disorders: update 2012 on the long-term treatment of bipolar disorder. *World Journal of Biological Psychiatry, 14,* 154-219.

Guideline Development Group for the Management of Patients with Insomnia in Primary Care. (2009). *Clinical Practice Guidelines for the Management of Patients with Insomnia in Primary Care.* Clinical Practice Guidelines in the NHS: UETS No. 2007/5-1. Community of Madrid: National Health System Quality Plan, Ministry of Health and Social Policy, Health Technology Assessment Unit. Laín Entrago Agency.

Haloperidol [package insert]. Schaumberg, IL: Sagent Pharmaceuticals, Inc.; August, 2011.

Haloperidol decanoate [package insert]. Toronto, ON: Apotex, Inc.; December, 2004.

Intuniv [package insert]. Wayne, PA: Shire US Inc.; February 2013.

Invega [package insert]. Titusville, NJ: Jansen Pharmaceuticals, Inc.; June, 2011.

Invega Sustenna [package insert]. Titusville, NJ: Janssen Pharmaceuticals, Inc.; August, 2012.

Invega Trinza [package insert]. Titusville, NJ: Janssen Pharmaceuticals, Inc.; May, 2015.

Kane, J., Honigfield, G., Singer, J., & Meltzer, H. (1988). Clozapine for the treatment-resistant schizophrenic. *Archives of General Psychiatry, 45,* 789-796.

Kapvay (package insert). Florham Park, NJ: Shionogi Inc.; February 2013.

Lamictal [package insert]. Research Triangle Park, NC: GlaxoSmithKline; 2012.

Latuda [package insert]. Marlborough, MA: Sunovion Pharmaceuticals, Inc.; July, 2013.

Lehman, A. F., Lieberman, J. A., Dixon, L. B., McGlashan, T. H.,Miller, A. L., Perkins, D.O.,...Steering Committee on Practice Guidelines. (2004). Practice guideline for the treatment of patients with schizophrenia, 2nd ed. *American Journal of Psychiatry, 161*(2 Suppl), 1-56.

Leucht, S., Corves, C., Arbter, D., Engel, R. R., Li, C., & Davis, J. M. (2009). Second-generation versus first-generation antipsychotic drugs for schizophrenia: A meta-analysis. *Lancet, 373,* 31-41.

Lexapro [package insert]. St. Louis, MO: Forest Pharmaceuticals, Inc.; December, 2012.

Licht, R. W. (2012). Lithium: Still a major option in the management of bipolar disorder. *CNS Neuroscience & Therapeutics, 18,* 219-226.

Luxor CR [package insert]. Palo Alto, CA: Jazz Pharmaceuticals, LLC; October, 2012.

Mann, J. J. (2005). The medical management of depression. *New England Journal of Medicine 353*(17), 1819-1834.

McEvoy, G. K., (Ed.). (2012). *AHFS Drug Information 2012.* Bethesda, MD: American Society of Health-System Pharmacists.

Melton, S. T., & Kirkwood, C. K. (2011). Anxiety disorders I: generalized anxiety, panic, and social anxiety disorders. In J. T. DiPiro, R. L. Talbert, G. C. Yee, G.R. Matzke, B. G. Wells, and L. M. Posey (Eds.). *Pharmacotherapy: A Pathophysiologic Approach* (8th ed., pp. 1209-1227). New York, NY: McGraw Hill.

Mendelson, W. B. (2005). A review of the evidence for the efficacy and safety of trazodone in insomnia. *Journal of Clinical Psychiatry*, 66(4), 469-76.

Moreira, R. (2011). The efficacy and tolerability of bupropion in the treatment of major depressive disorder. *Clinical Drug Investigation*, 31(Suppl 1), 5-17.

Newcomer, J. W., & Haupt, D. W. (2006). The metabolic effects of antipsychotic medications. *Canadian Journal of Psychiatry* 51(8), 480-491.

Ng, F., Mammen, O. K., Wilting, I., Sachs, G. S., Ferrier, I. N., Cassidy, F.,...International Society for Bipolar Disorders. (2009). The International Society for Bipolar Disorders (ISBD) consensus guidelines for the safety monitoring of bipolar disorder treatments. *Bipolar Disorders*, 11, 559-595.

Paxil [package insert]. Research Triangle Park, NC: GlaxoSmithKline; January, 2013.

Perphenazine. (2012). Drugs.com. Retrieved from www.drugs.com/pro/perphenazine.html.

Pierre, J. M. (2005). Extrapyramidal symptoms with atypical antipsychotics: incidence, prevention and management. *Drug Safety*, 28(3), 191-208.

Pliszka, S. (2007). AACAP Work Group on Quality Issues. Practice parameter for the assessment and treatment of children and adolescents with attention-deficit/hyperactivity disorder. *Journal of the American Academy of Child and Adolescent Psychiatry*, 46(7), 894-921.

Pringsheim, T., Panangiotopoulos, C., Davidson, J., & Ho, J. (2011). Evidence-based recommendations for monitoring safety of second-generation antipsychotics in children and youth. *Paediatrics and Child Health*, 16(9), 581-589.

Pristiq [package insert]. Philadelphia, PA: Pfizer, Inc.; February, 2013.

Prozac [package insert]. Indianapolis, IN: Lilly USA, LLC; January, 2013.

Qaseem, A., Snow, V., Cross, T., Forceia, M. A., Hopkins, R., Shekelle, P.,...Owens, D. K. (2008). Current pharmacologic treatment of dementia: A clinical practice guideline from the American College of Physicians and the American Academy of Family Physicians. *Annals of Internal Medicine* 148, 370-378.

Rexulti [package insert]. Tokyo, Japan; Otsuka Pharmaceuticals Co. Ltd.; July, 2015.

Risperdal [package insert]. Titusville, NJ: Janssen Pharmaceutricals, Inc.; August, 2012.

Risperdal Consta [package insert]. Titusville, NJ: Janssen Pharmaceuticals, Inc.; June, 2012.

Rogers, S. J., & Cavazos, J. E. (2011). Epilepsy, In: J. T. DiPiro, R. L. Talbert, G. C. Yee, G.R. Matzke, B. G. Wells, and L. M. Posey (Eds.). *Pharmacotherapy: A Pathophysiologic Approach* (8th ed., pp. 979-1005). New York, NY: McGraw Hill.

Rummel-Kluge, C., Komossa, K., Schwarz, S., Hunger, H., Schmid, F., Kissling, W.,...Leucht, S. (2012). Second-generation antipsychotic drugs and extrapyramidal side effects: A systematic review and meta-analysis of head-to-head comparisons. *Schizophrenic Bulletin*, 38(1), 167-177.

Sachdev, P. S. (2000). The current status of tardive dyskinesia. *The Australian and New Zealand Journal of Psychiatry*, 34(3), 355-369.

Sachs, G. S., Nierenberg, A. A., Calabrese, J. R., Marangell, L. B., Wisniewski, S. R., Gyulai, L.,...Thase, M. E. (2007). Effectiveness of adjunctive antidepressant treatment for bipolar depression. *New England Journal of Medicine*, 356(17), 1711-1722.

Saphris [package insert]. Whitehouse Station, NJ: Merck & Co, Inc.; March, 2013.

Seroquel [package insert]. Marlborough, MA: Sunovion Pharmaceuticals, Inc.; July, 2013.

Seroquel XR [package insert]. Wilmington, DE: AstraZeneca; July, 2013.

Schulman, K. I., Walker, S. E., MacKenzie, S., & Knowles, S. (1989). Dietary restriction, tyramine and the use of monoamine oxidase inhibitors. *Journal of Clinical Psychopharmacology*, 9(6), 397-402.

Shelton, R. C. (2007). Augmentation strategies to increase antidepressant efficacy. *Journal of Clinical Psychiatry*, 68(Suppl 10), 18-22.

Stahl, S. M. (2008). *Stahl's Essential Psychopharmacology*, 3rd ed. Cambridge, UK: Cambridge University Press.

Stein, M. B., Goin, M. K., Pollack, M. H., Roy-Byrne, P., Sareen, J., Simon, N. M., & Campbell-Sills, L. (2010). *Practice guideline for the treatment of patients with panic disorder*. Arlington, VA: American Psychiatric Association.

Strattera [package insert]. Indianapolis, IN: Lilly USA, LLC; August 2012.

Subcommittee on Attention-Deficit/Hyperactivity Disorder, Steering Committee on Quality Improvement and Management. (2011). ADHD: clinical practice guideline for the diagnosis, evaluation, and treatment of attention-deficit/hyperactivity disorder in children and adolescents. *Pediatrics*, 128(5), 1007-1022.

Tandon, R. (2011). Antipsychotics in the treatment of schizophrenia: An overview. *Journal of Clinical Psychiatry*, 72(suppl 1), 4-8.

Teter, C. J., Kando, J. C., & Wells, B. G. (2011). Major depressive disorder, In J. T. DiPiro, R. L. Talbert, G. C. Yee, G.R. Matzke, B. G. Wells, and L. M. Posey (Eds.). *Pharmacotherapy: A Pathophysiologic Approach* (8th ed., pp. 1173-1190). New York, NY: McGraw Hill.

Thanacoody, H. K., & Thomas, S. H. (2005). Tricyclic antidepressant poisoning: cardiovascular toxicity. *Toxicological Reviews*, 24(3), 205-214.

Thase, M. E. (2008). Are SNRIs more effective than SSRIs? A review of the current state of the controversy. *Psychopharmacology Bulletin*, 41(2), 58-85.

U.S. Food and Drug Administration. (2008). FDA requests boxed warnings on older class of antipsychotic drugs. U.S. Food and Drug Administration, U.S. Department of Health and Human Services. Retrieved from www.fda.gov/NewsEvents/Newsroom/PressAnnouncements/2008/ucm116912.htm.

U.S. Food and Drug Administration. (2010). Antidepressant use in Children and Adolescents. U.S. Food and Drug Administration, U.S. Department of Health & Human Services. Retrieved from www.fda.gov/Drugs/DrugSafety/InformationbyDrugClass/UCM096273. Updated August 12, 2010.

Valenstein, M., Ganoczy, D., McCarthy, J. F., Kim, H. M., Lee, T. A., & Blow, F. C. (2006). Antipsychotic adherence over time among patients receiving treatment for schizophrenia: A retrospective review. *Journal of Clinical Psychiatry*, 67(10), 1542-1550.

VanDenBerg, C. M. (2012). The transdermal delivery system of monoamine oxidase inhibitors. *Journal of Clinical Psychiatry*, 73(Suppl 1), 25-30.

Vivitrol [package insert]. Waltham, MA: Alkermes, Inc.; October 2010.

Vraylar [package insert]. Parsipanny, NJ: Actavis; September, 2015.

Walkup, J., & The Work Group on Quality Issues (2009). Practice parameter on the use of psychotropic medication in children and adolescents. *Journal of the American Academy of Child and Adolescent Psychiatry, 48*(9), 961-973.

Yatham, L. N., Kennedy, S. H., Schaffer, A., Parikh, S. V., Beaulieu, S., O'Donovan, C.,...Kapczinski, F. (2009). Canadian Network for Mood and Anxiety Treatments (CANMAT) and International Society for Bipolar Disorders (ISBD) collaborative update of CANMAT guidelines for the management of patients with bipolar disorder. *Bipolar Disorders, 11*, 225–255.

Zoloft [package insert]. New York, NY: Pfizer, Inc.; June, 2013.

Zyban [package insert]. Indianapolis, IN: Lilly USA, LLC; June 2011.

Zyprexa [package insert]. Indianapolis, IN: Lilly USA, LLC; July, 2011.

Zyprexa Relprevv [package insert]. Indianapolis, IN: Lilly USA, LLC; July, 2011.

Appendix C

Ethical and Legal Issues in Mental Health

Yvette Hachtel, JD, MEd, OTR/L and Lea C. Brandt, OTD, MA, OTR/L

CHAPTER OUTLINE

Introduction
Autonomy/Informed Consent
Competency/Incompetence
Involuntary Commitment
The Emergency Doctrine
Confidentiality
Use of Physical Restraints and Seclusion
Summary
References

INTRODUCTION

As an occupational therapy assistant student or practitioner working in mental health, you will face situations that raise ethical and/or legal issues. The Occupational Therapy Code of Ethics (2015) (referred to as the "Code of Ethics," [AOTA], 2015) provides principles that guide safe and competent professional practice with clients across all diagnostic categories and treatment settings. Certain principles, however, have particular relevance to mental health practice. Although the Code of Ethics (AOTA, 2015) states that occupational therapy practitioners should adhere to relevant laws, regulations, and policies, the information discussed in this appendix is in no way intended to provide legal advice.

AUTONOMY/INFORMED CONSENT

The Code of Ethics (AOTA, 2015) deal with issues related to autonomy, which is an individual's right to self-determination. To honor this right, occupational therapy practitioners must ensure that the client is actively involved in the decision-making process. The Patient Care Partnership, which replaced the American Hospital Association's (AHA) Patients' Bill of Rights, explicitly states that individuals seeking treatment, or their legal representative, must give their informed consent (permission; AHA, 2003). The Code of Ethics (AOTA, 2015) also state that occupational therapy personnel shall obtain consent before administering any occupational therapy service. The exact requirements that must be met for informed consent vary state to state;

Manville, C.A., & Keough, J. L.
Mental Health Practice for the Occupational Therapy Assistant (pp 409-412).

however, in general in order for a patient to give consent he or she must be mentally competent and have been told what is likely to occur in treatment. Patients must be told, and demonstrate an understanding of, the risks and benefits of the proposed treatment, as well as those of alternative treatments, including any possible side effects. The patient must also enter into treatment in a freely voluntary manner, without coercion, duress, or deceit. The Patient Care Partnership (AHA, 2003) and the Code of Ethics (AOTA, 2015) also acknowledge the client's right to refuse treatment. Any clinical consequences of refusing treatment must also be disclosed to the patient. Patients must be made aware that they may refuse or discontinue treatment and that their refusal will not interfere with their receipt of any other desired care.

Competence/Incompetence

In order for a patient to give consent to treatment, it must first be determined that the person is competent. Incompetence is technically left for courts to determine. In reality, however, it is often the physician who determines a patient's decision-making capacity and who decides when to seek substituted consent. It is important to realize that determinations of a person's capacity to give informed consent should not be based on a diagnostic category. In general the presumption should be that the vast majority of people are capable of making their own decisions. Unless there is a reason to question a patient's decision-making ability, the person should be presumed to be competent. Requirements for determining someone's capacity to make decisions vary between states, but generally someone must be able to communicate his or her wishes (express a choice) and those wishes must be consistent over time. The person must also be able to understand relevant information on which to base the choice. The third element is that patients need to be able to understand the consequences of their choices in light of their personal values and the effect their decisions will have on them. Finally, they must have the ability to weigh their options to arrive at a decision (Applebaum, 2007).

When clients are not able to consent to treatment—either because they have been found to lack decision-making capacity, are deemed incompetent, or because the client is a minor—the occupational therapy practitioner must obtain the client's consent to treat from a legitimate representative (or substitute) decision maker. These alternative decision makers are often referred to as surrogates, proxies, or guardians. In the absence of a legally appointed surrogate (durable power of attorney for health care or guardian), family members are often called upon to make clinical decisions. Many states have laws that indicate the order in which family members should be utilized.

There are generally two types of incompetent patients: those who were never competent and those who were once competent but are no longer. Some examples of patients who were never competent include newborns, minors, and individuals who have been severely mentally impaired since birth. When "never competent" individuals become patients, a patient representative needs to be involved in the plan of care. Often this person is the parent. In the case of a mature child and/or an adult who has marginal capacity, it is best practice to involve both the patient and the representative in the shared decision-making process. In some states, when the child is nearing the age of majority (generally considered 18), he or she may be able to consent to elective abortions, treatment for substance abuse, and/or the treatment of sexually transmitted diseases without the knowledge of a parent or guardian. In cases where the individual was previously competent but is not now (due to organic brain damage or adult psychoses), the patient representative must attempt to make decisions based on what they believe the patient would have wanted were he or she still competent. Examples include: A young child is brought to the emergency department of a community hospital by his parents because he has threatened to harm his sibling. In order for the medical staff to treat the child, they will first need to receive informed consent from the child's parents. Another patient, Ms. X, is a resident in a skilled nursing facility and has recently been diagnosed with dementia. Due to her confusion Ms. X believes that aliens are trying to kill her by poisoning her food, and she has stopped eating. She is taken to a hospital for evaluation and treatment. Because Ms. X has dementia, her representative will need to give consent before she can be evaluated. Gillick (2012) points out that the patient's surrogate needs to have a full and realistic understanding of dementia, including how patients respond to medical interventions, before he or she can be expected to make sound decisions for the patient.

Although the legal determination of patient competence is a question for the courts, as an occupational therapy assistant you can offer important input into the patient's capacity in making health care-related decisions based on your observations and interactions with clients. When you suspect that a client may lack the ability to make informed decisions, you are encouraged to raise the issue with the occupational therapist, your supervisor, the client's physician, facility administrators, and/or the facility's legal counsel. Practitioners should also be alert to possible situations where clients are being unfairly discriminated against and being presumed incapable of decision making, when they are in fact capable. Even in situations involving minors, or others who have been determined to be incompetent, this does not relieve the practitioner of the responsibility of explaining to the patient, as fully as the patient can understand, what is going to happen and why (Golub, 2011).

INVOLUNTARY COMMITMENT

There are, however, times when a patient may not have the right to refuse treatment. There are also incidences when it may not be necessary to obtain a patient's informed consent before initiating treatment. As previously discussed, in addition to assuring that the client is competent, the client must have been able to enter into the agreement voluntarily without coercion, duress, or deceit. What happens though when a client is committed to a mental health facility involuntarily?

The Code of Ethics (AOTA, 2015), in part, states that occupational therapy practitioners should comply with relevant laws, regulations, policies, procedures, standards, and guidelines. Involuntary commitment is a legal process through which an individual with symptoms of severe mental illness is court ordered into treatment in a hospital (inpatient) or in the community (outpatient). Involuntary commitment is governed by state law and procedures vary from state to state. In *O'Connor v. Donaldson* (1975) the U.S. Supreme Court ruled that involuntary hospitalization and/or treatment violated an individual's civil rights. They found that the grounds for involuntary commitment must be higher than merely having a mental disorder and being in need of treatment. This ruling forced individual states to change their laws so that an individual must be exhibiting behavior that is a danger to himself or herself or others in order to be held, and the hold must be only for the purpose of evaluation by mental health professionals. In addition, a court order must be received for more than very short-term treatment or hospitalization (typically no longer than 96 hours). The courts then determine whether further civil commitment is appropriate or necessary. In general, once the person is under involuntary commitment, treatment may be instituted without further requirements. Some treatments, such as electroconvulsive therapy, however, often require further procedures to comply with the law before they may be administered involuntarily. In the New Jersey case *Rennie v. Klein (1978)*, the court found that even an involuntarily committed patient has a qualified/conditional right to refuse psychotropic medication if he or she has not been found incompetent and is not in the midst of an emergency situation. For example, Mr. W is home on leave from a tour of duty in Afghanistan where he has been involved in a lot of combat. The day after he gets home his wife goes into the bedroom to gently wake him up for a special homecoming breakfast she has prepared for him. Mr. W. is startled and bolts out of bed screaming and begins trying to strangle his wife. His wife manages to break away and runs to the neighbor's house where she calls for an ambulance. Mr. W. is rushed to the emergency room where he is admitted to the psychiatric unit for observation and treatment of what they suspect is posttraumatic stress disorder. Once there Mr. W. begins throwing things and screaming, "Get me out of here, you can't keep me here." Due to exhibiting behaviors that posed a potential for harm to his wife, Mr. W. may be involuntarily committed without his consent. In cases where the patient is unable to effectively exercise his or her autonomous choice secondary to psychosis or potential harm to others, the ethical principle of beneficence would prevail. Beneficence requires practitioners to promote good, prevent harm to others, and protect persons in danger (Beauchamp & Childress, 2009).

THE EMERGENCY DOCTRINE

Berg, Applebaum, Lidz, and Parker (2001) describe a related exception to the requirement of obtaining patient informed consent referred to as the "emergency doctrine." This principle presumes that clients would consent to reasonable, life-saving medical intervention when they are unable to express their wishes in a life-threatening emergency. For example, Mr. Y is a 75-year-old male with no psychiatric history. After 50 years of marriage his wife died unexpectedly. Prior to her death, Mrs. Y had taken responsibility for making sure her husband took his medicines as prescribed. Mr. Y has been appropriately upset by his wife's death and has fallen out of his regular routines. His daughter has been coming by daily and today she finds her father on the floor unconscious with an empty bottle of pills next to him. When he is rushed to the emergency department of the local hospital he is immediately admitted and treated for an apparent overdose. In this situation informed consent is not needed. The emergency doctrine applies because he is unconscious and unless it is clearly evident that Mr. Y would refuse treatment, it is presumed that he would want to live.

CONFIDENTIALITY

The Code of Ethics (AOTA, 2015) also deal with confidentiality. All occupational therapy practitioners must comply with Health Insurance Portability and Accountability Act regulations and keep all patient information confidential with very few exceptions. State and federal laws mandate that under certain limited circumstances, health professionals are required to reveal confidential patient information. These include, but are not limited to, release of information concerning infectious and sexually transmitted diseases to governmental agencies, or release of information to law enforcement agencies.

The legal case *Tarasoff v. Regents of the University of California* (1976) is known for requiring disclosure of otherwise confidential information when a patient has communicated his or her intent to harm or kill a specific person. This case relates to threats that represent a real and imminent harm and should be exercised prudently as to not unduly violate confidentiality. Occupational therapy practitioners should involve the authorities if they believe their patient presents a real and imminent threat to others. In addition, occupational therapy practitioners may be required to breach confidentiality if they suspect their patient is being abused by others.

USE OF PHYSICAL RESTRAINTS AND SECLUSION

The Code of Ethics (AOTA, 2015) also deal with nonmaleficence and require that occupational therapy practitioners not engage in any activity that could cause harm to a patient, even if the harm was not done maliciously or intentionally. This principle would have particular relevance to restraint use.

In 1987 the Omnibus Budget Reconciliation Act (OBRA) included legislation addressing quality of care issues in nursing homes (Health Care Financing Administration [HCFA], 1989). Much of the change in long-term care service delivery can be directly linked to the implementation of the Nursing Home Reform Act in 1990, an amendment within OBRA. OBRA clearly states that residents have a right to be free of physical restraints imposed for purposes of discipline or convenience which are not required to treat a specific medical symptom (Center for Medicare and Medicaid Services). A physical or mechanical restraint is defined as any device attached or adjacent to one's body that restricts freedom of movement or normal access to one's body (HCFA, 1992). By definition, a wide variety of materials could be classified as restraints, including vests, belts, wrist/ankle straps, sheets, bed rails, or geriatric chairs with fixed tray tables. Any time an able-bodied individual is not able to easily release the device and voluntarily regain freedom of movement the definition of physical restraint has been met.

The Joint Commission and the HCFA require that seclusion and restraint be used only as a last resort, as an emergency response to a crisis situation that presents imminent risk of harm to the patient, staff, or others. Compliance with the mandates requires that facilities consider and document all less restrictive alternatives that have been attempted before employing the physical restraint. Restricting a person's mobility has been shown to result in a wide range of negative physical and psychological consequences for the person being restrained, including stress; fear; humiliation; agitation; combativeness; anger; immobility; deconditioning; incontinence; skin breakdown; increased infections, contractions, and/or edema; decreased circulation and/or appetite; nerve injuries; strangulation; and asphyxiation, among others. (Engberg, Castle, & McCaffrey, 2008).

SUMMARY

Working in mental health may pose unique challenges for the occupational therapy practitioner. It is important to remember that in all instances it is the legal and ethical duty of the practitioner to put the well-being of the client above all else. Mental health professionals have an obligation to facilitate client self-determination, including the client's autonomous right to obtain valued and clinically beneficial treatments in environments free from discrimination. By adhering to the ethical and legal principles outlined in this appendix, occupational therapy practitioners can remain client centered while promoting the safety and dignity of all involved.

REFERENCES

American Hospital Association. (2003). The patient care partnership. Retrieved from www.aha.org/advocacy-issues/communicatingpts/pt-care-partnership.html.

American Occupational Therapy Association. (2015). Occupational therapy code of ethics (2015). *American Journal of Occupational Therapy, 69*(Suppl. 3), 6913410030p1-6913410030p8.. doi: 10.5014/ajot.2015.696S03.

Appelbaum, P. S. (2007). Assessment of patient's competence to consent to treatment. *New England Journal of Medicine, 357*:1834-40.

Beauchamp, T. L., & Childress, J. F. (2009). *Principles of biomedical ethics* (6th ed.). New York: Oxford University Press.

Berg, J. W., Applebaum, P. S., Lidz, C. W., and Parker, L. (2001). *Informed consent: legal theory and clinical practice* (2nd ed.), New York: Oxford University Press.

Center for Medicare and Medicaid Standards, Tag number F203/Regulation number 483.13(a), Retrieved from https://www.cms.gov/Regulations-and-Guidance/Guidance/Manuals/downloads/som107ap_pp_guidelines_ltcf.pdf.

Engberg, J., Castle, N. G., and McCaffrey, D. (2008). Physical restraint initiation in nursing homes and subsequent resident health. *The Gerontologist 48*(4), 442-452.

Gillick, M. G. (2012). Doing the right thing: A geriatrician's perspective on medical care for the person with advanced dementia. *Journal of Law, Medicine & Ethics*, 2012 Spring; 40 (1), 51-56.

Golub, M. (2011). Informed consent. In Bucky, S., Callan, J., Stricker, G. (Ed). *Ethical and legal issues for mental health professionals: A comprehensive handbook of principles and standards* (pp. 101-115). New York: Routledge.

Health Care Financing Administration. (1992). State operations manual. Department of Health and Human Services, Transmittal No. 250, 76-78.

Health Care Financing Administration. (1989). State operations manual. Department of Health and Human Services, Transmittal No. 232.

O'Connor v. Donaldson, 422 U.S. 563 (1975).

Rennie v. Klein, 462 F. Supp. 1131, 1145 (D. N. J. 1978).

Tarasoff v. Regents of University of California, 17 Cal 3d425 (1976).

Financial Disclosures

Dr. Lori T. Andersen has no financial or proprietary interest in the materials presented herein.

Dr. Susan S. Bazyk has no financial or proprietary interest in the materials presented herein.

Dr. Lea C. Brandt has no financial or proprietary interest in the materials presented herein.

Dr. Tina Champagne has no financial or proprietary interest in the materials presented herein.

Lee Ann Fallet has no financial or proprietary interest in the materials presented herein.

Dr. Cathy H. Ficzere has no financial or proprietary interest in the materials presented herein.

Dr. Yvette Hachtel has no financial or proprietary interest in the materials presented herein.

Jeremy L. Keough has no financial or proprietary interest in the materials presented herein.

Dr. Christine A. Manville has no financial or proprietary interest in the materials presented herein.

Dr. J. Michael McGuire is a previous employee and current stockholder of Bristol-Myers and Squibb, has been on the speakers bureau for Sunovion Pharmaceuticals and Forest Pharmaceuticals, and has been a consultant for Otsuka America Pharmaceuticals Inc.

Dr. Janice Ryan has no financial or proprietary interest in the materials presented herein.

Dr. Renee R. Taylor has no financial or proprietary interest in the materials presented herein.

Su Ren Wong has no financial or proprietary interest in the materials presented herein.

Index